Alzheimer's Disease: Basic Mechanisms, Diagnosis and Therapeutic Strategies

This publication was made possible through the support of
Parke-Davis, Division of Warner-Lambert Company

Alzheimer's Disease: Basic Mechanisms, Diagnosis and Therapeutic Strategies

Edited by

Khalid Iqbal
New York State Institute for Basic Research, New York, USA

Donald R. C. McLachlan
Centre for Research on Neurodegenerative Diseases,
University of Toronto, Canada

Bengt Winblad
Department of Geriatric Medicine, Karolinska Institute, Stockholm, Sweden

Henry M. Wisniewski
New York State Institute for Basic Research, New York, USA

A Wiley-Interscience Publication

JOHN WILEY & SONS

Chichester · New York · Brisbane · Toronto · Singapore

Other Wiley Editorial Offices

John Wiley & Sons, Inc., 605 Third Avenue,
New York, NY 10158-0012, USA

Jacaranda Wiley Ltd, G.P.O. Box 859, Brisbane,
Queensland 4001, Australia

John Wiley & Sons (Canada) Ltd, 22 Worcester Road,
Rexdale, Ontario M9W 1LI, Canada

John Wiley & Sons (SEA) Pte Ltd, 37 Jalan Pemimpin 05-04,
Block B, Union Industrial Building, Singapore 2057

Library of Congress Cataloging-in-Publication Data:
Alzheimer's disease : basic mechanisms, diagnosis, and therapeutic
   strategies / edited by K. Iqbal ... [et al.].
       p.   cm.
   Contains selected papers from the Second International Conference
on Alzheimer's Disease & Related Disorders held in Toronto, Canada,
from July 15-20, 1990.
   Includes bibliographical references and index.
   ISBN 0 471 92927 1
   1. Alzheimer's disease—Congresses.   I. Iqbal, Khalid.
II. International Conference on Alzheimer's Disease and Related
Disorders (2nd : 1990 : Toronto, Ont.)
   [DNLM: 1. Alzheimer's Disease—congresses. WM 220 A78205 1990]
RC523.A396   1991
616.8'31—dc20
DNLM/DLC
for Library of Congress   90-13135
                                                                         CIP

British Library Cataloguing in Publication Data:
Alzheimer's disease.
   1. Alzheimer's disease
   I. Iqbal, K. (Khalid)
   616.831

   ISBN 0 471 92927 1

Typeset by Dobbie Typesetting Limited, Tavistock, Devon
Printed in Great Britain by Courier International, Tiptree

Contents

VI RISK FACTORS AND EPIDEMIOLOGY

VII ENVIRONMENTAL FACTORS

VIII GENETIC MECHANISMS

Preface

Alzheimer's disease is one of the most devastating diseases of the human brain that affects so many lives all over the world. With improvements in modern medicine, human longevity continues to be extended and so too does the problem of this age-associated dementia.

At present, neither the etiology nor the pathogenesis of Alzheimer's disease is understood. It is most exciting that since the first conference held in Las Vegas in September 1988, considerable progress has been made towards understanding the basic mechanisms of the disease and toward developing diagnostic and therapeutic strategies. This volume provides a comprehensive coverage of these and other recent advances in the areas of clinical course, neuroimaging, brain energy metabolism, structural and molecular neuropathology, mechanisms of the neuronal degeneration operative in the disease, role of brain amyloidosis, risk factors and epidemiology, environmental factors, genetic mechanisms, biomarkers, animal models and therapeutic strategies. Chapters are also devoted to Alzheimer's disease in the developmentally disabled.

This book contains articles that are at the cutting edge of Alzheimer's disease research selected from papers presented at the Second International Conference on Alzheimer's Disease and Related Disorders. We believe that this single comprehensive source of latest information on Alzheimer's disease and related disorders contributed by some of the most productive scientists in the field will not only be a major reference book for the Alzheimer's disease researchers but also will be equally useful to the clinicians who provide primary care to the unfortunate victims of Alzheimer's disease.

Khalid Iqbal
Donald R. C. McLachlan
Bengt Winblad
Henry M. Wisniewski

Acknowledgments

This book contains articles invited from Alzheimer's disease researchers whose papers were selected from more than 400 presented at the Second International Conference on Alzheimer's Disease and Related Disorders held in Toronto, Canada, from 15–20 July 1990. The abstracts of all the papers presented at the conference were published in *Neurobiology of Aging*, volume 11, issue 3, with the kind help of its editor, Dr Paul Coleman. The scientific program of the conference was organized with the help of an international scientific advisory committee consisting of Drs K. T. Beyreuther (FRG), H. Braak (FRG), A. Brun (Sweden), P. Davies (USA), K. Davis (USA), G. G. Glenner (USA), I. Grundke-Iqbal (USA), L. L. Heston (USA), T. Ishii (Japan), K. A. Jellinger (Austria), A. Klug (UK), D. Price (USA), S. B. Prusiner (USA), B. Reisberg (USA), D. M. A. Mann (UK), G. M. Martin (USA), S. S. Matsuyama (USA), and D. F. Swaab (Holland).

The Conference Secretariat was managed meticulously by Dr Al Snider, with the assistance of Ms Concetta Veneziano, Ms Peggy Clark, and Ms Natalie Perrone of the Institute for Basic Research, Staten Island, New York. Ms Ella Fox of the University of Toronto and Ms Roberta Corey and other volunteers of the Alzheimer Society for Metropolitan Toronto provided invaluable assistance at the conference. Financial support for the conference was generously provided by the National Institute on Aging, United States; New York State Institute for Basic Research; the Ontario Ministry of Health, Health and Welfare, Canada; Alzheimer Society of Canada; Alzheimer's Association (USA); the American Health Assistance Foundation and the French Foundation for Alzheimer Research of the United States, and the following corporate sponsors: Alcan Aluminum Ltd, Aluminum Association, Rhône-Poulenc, Parke-Davis/Warner Lambert, Glaxo Canada, ICI Pharmaceuticals Group, Astra Pharmaceuticals, Azko Organon International, Miles, Inc., Athena Neurosciences, Novopharm Ltd, Bristol-Meyers Squibb Co., Ciba-Geigy Canada, Smith Kline & French Canada, Cortex Pharmaceuticals, Sterling Drug Ltd, Takeda Chemical Industries, The Upjohn Co. and UCB-Brussels.

The editors would like to thank the conference participants, secretariat, and sponsors, the members of the Scientific Advisory Committee and all others who helped with the conference. Special thanks and appreciation of the editors are also due to the chapter contributors, to Parke-Davis/Warner Lambert for their support of this publication, and to Ms Concetta Veneziano for her editorial assistance.

Prevalence and Neurobiology of Alzheimer's Disease: Some Highlights

Cerebral aging is a medical, sociological and economic problem of enormous dimensions in modern society. In the United States alone, nearly 25 million people are 65 years of age or older; this age group has increased from 2.5% of the nation's population in 1850 to more than 10% of the population today. Furthermore, the population of elderly is increasing at 2.5 times the rate of the general population. Among Americans who are 65 years of age and older, 11% have mild to moderate dementia and about 4.4% are severely demented (1). About 55% of the cases of senile dementia are of the Alzheimer type. Another approximate 20% of the population that is demented suffers from a combination of Alzheimer's disease and cerebrovascular dementia. Alzheimer's disease generally occurs at ages greater than 65 years, but in a small number of cases, it strikes people even in their forties and fifties. It is the fourth leading cause of death in adults in the United States after heart disease, cancer, and stroke, claiming more than 100 000 lives a year. If scientific research does not produce discoveries to prevent or cure Alzheimer's disease, the number of individuals affected can be expected to double by the year 2000 and to quintuple by 2040 as the 'baby boomers' reach senescence (US Office of Technology Assessment).

To date, neither the etiology nor the pathogenesis of Alzheimer's disease is understood. Alzheimer's disease is a progressive dementia, the clinical symptoms of which include profound memory loss, decline in ability to perform routine tasks, impairment of judgment, disorientation, personality change, difficulty in learning, and loss of language skills. In the advanced stage of the disease, the victims cannot walk or talk and become totally incapable of caring for themselves (2).

There is no unique pattern of clinical symptoms associated with Alzheimer's disease, and there is no diagnostic test available short of a brain biopsy. The diagnosis of Alzheimer's disease is generally made clinically, with variable degree of uncertainty, by excluding other causes of dementia. The confirmation of the diagnosis is generally made at autopsy by pathological findings, which include atrophy of the brain; some loss of neurons; decrease in the arborizations of the dendritic tree; presence of neurofibrillary tangles, neuritic (senile) plaques, granulovacuolar changes, and amyloid deposits; and accumulation of lipofuscin (3). Large numbers of the tangles and the plaques, which are the two most characteristic lesions of Alzheimer's disease,

Alzheimer's Disease: Basic Mechanisms, Diagnosis and Therapeutic Strategies
Edited by K. Iqbal, D. R. C. McLachlan, B. Winblad and H. M. Wisniewski
© 1991 John Wiley & Sons Ltd

appear to correlate with the degree of dementia (4,5). Both of these types of lesions are also present in normal old people, but in only very small number.

The nature of the primary insult that causes Alzheimer's disease is not yet understood. Old age appears to be the single largest risk factor for Alzheimer's disease. It is likely that this disease has polyetiology that includes genetic makeup, environmental toxins, and chronic infections, all of which might precipitate the disease in old individuals. The major areas of research toward understanding the primary cause of neuronal death in this disease are the identification of the faulty genes, protein abnormalities associated with the formation of the histopathological lesions, and infectious agent or agents of the type seen in transmissible dementias and environmental toxins.

There are families in which 10 or more members, representing four or five generations, have developed Alzheimer's disease. It appears that the disease is transmitted in an autosomal dominant fashion. Furthermore, in nearly all individuals with Down's syndrome, a chromosome-21 disorder, Alzheimer's disease develops in the fourth decade of life. Genetic linkage has been demonstrated between Alzheimer's disease and two anonymous DNA markers D21S1/D21S11 and D21S16 on chromosome 21 in 30 pedigrees with early onset (i.e. at younger than 65 years of age) of the disease (6). However, two other groups (7,8) employing a mixture of early and late onset families, and only late onset families, respectively, have been unable to confirm the linkage to the same chromosome-21 markers. These studies indicate that familial Alzheimer's disease may be genetically heterogeneous. Furthermore, studies of identical twins by Heston (9) in which one twin is affected with Alzheimer's disease and the other is unaffected have suggested that the genetic makeup alone might not be the only factor responsible for the onset of the disease.

To date, neither any abnormal protein nor an abnormal processing of a normally occurring protein unique to Alzheimer's disease has been discovered. Most of the studies in this area have focused on the protein composition of the neurofibrillary tangles and neuritic (senile) plaques. The Alzheimer neurofibrillary tangles are made up mostly of paired helical filaments (PHF) (10). They are sometimes admixed with 15-nm straight filaments. These tangles of the Alzheimer type have also been observed in other disorders such as Guam Parkinsonism dementia complex, postencephalitic Parkinson's disease, dementia pugilistica, and Down's syndrome (11,12). However, PHF of the Alzheimer type has never been reported in any nonhuman species either during aging or as a result of induced disorders. In Alzheimer's disease brains, accumulation of PHF is also seen in the neurites in the neuropil as neuropil threads (13) and in the dystrophic neurites of the neuritic (senile) plaques. The biochemistry of PHF is not yet completely understood. The polypeptide composition of PHF on SDS-polyacrylamide gel electrophoresis has revealed the presence of 45–62 kDa polypeptides as a major component, variable amounts of high-molecular-weight-protein aggregates, and some small-molecular-weight-protein fragments (14–16). The 45–62 kDa PHF polypeptides have been identified as microtubule-associated polypeptide tau by their coelectrophoresis and immunochemical crossreactivity (17,18). Both fragments of tau as well as ubiquitin have been sequenced from preparations of isolated PHF (19,20). Molecular cloning of tau has revealed the presence of a fetal and an adult form of the polypeptides, both of which have been found to be present in PHF (21). Tau in Alzheimer's disease, especially in PHF, has been shown to be abnormally phosphorylated (18,22), and an in-vitro microtubule assembly defect associated with this abnormal phosphorylation of tau in Alzheimer's brain has been shown, too (23). Immunochemical studies have also indicated that some of the tau in PHF might be ubiquitinated (24). The abnormal phosphorylation of tau has been shown to precede the formation of the neurofibrillary tangles, suggesting a protein phosphorylation/dephosphorylation system abnormality as one of the early events in Alzheimer cytoskeletal pathology (25). The high-molecular-weight-protein aggregates seen on gel electrophoresis of isolated PHF are both tau- and ubiquitin-positive. However, the biochemical composition of this PHF polypeptide fraction remains to be established.

Unlike the tangles, the neuritic (senile) plaques are seen in few conditions other than Alzheimer's disease. The three major components of the plaques are (a) wisps or a compact core of amyloid fibers which are surrounded both by (b) dystrophic and degenerating neurites and (c) some reactive cells, the microglia, and astroglial processes. The major protein component of the amyloid fibers, which also accumulates in the walls of the brain vessels (congophilic angiopathy) in Alzheimer's disease, is a 40–42 amino acid protein fragment, called β peptide or A4 peptide (26,27). The β peptide is a fragment of a much larger precursor protein, the β amyloid precursor protein (βAPP), which is 695–770 amino acids long, depending on the size of the inserts (28–33). From its cDNA-derived sequence, the βAPP has been predicted to be a membrane receptor (28). The gene for βAPP, the large form of which contains the Kunitz protease inhibitor insert, has been localized to chromosome 21 in proximity to the putative familial Alzheimer's disease gene but has been shown not to be the latter (34). Neither the mechanism for the processing of the βAPP that gives rise to β peptide nor the biological activity of the βAPP is presently understood. This is a major area of research in the Alzheimer's disease field.

Unlike the plaques in individuals with Alzheimer's disease or Down's syndrome, in aged humans, and in primates—all of which contain amyloid of β peptide—the plaque amyloid of transmissible neurodegenerative diseases, Creutzfeldt-Jakob disease, Gerstmann-Sträussler-Scheinker syndrome, kuru, and their experimental analogues is made from the prion protein (e.g. 35). However, a recent study (36) reported the transmission of a Creutzfeldt-Jakob disease-like histopathology in guinea pigs infected with the buffy coat of the blood from patients with Alzheimer's disease. Confirmation of these findings from other laboratories remains to be reported.

Trace metals are among the environmental factors suspected to contribute to Alzheimer's disease. Injection of aluminum salts into rabbits and cats (but not mice, rats, or monkeys) produces neurofibrillary tangles (37). However, the aluminium-induced CNS changes differ from Alzheimer's disease in topography, ultrastructure, and biochemistry of the filaments (10,38). High concentrations of aluminium in Alzheimer neurofibrillary tangles and of aluminium silicates in neuritic (senile) plaques have been observed (39,40). Heterochromatization and the possible role of aluminium in this process in Alzheimer's disease have been reported (37). Because of the abundance and the ubiquitous nature of aluminium in the environment, understanding of the possible role of aluminium in Alzheimer's disease has been particularly elusive.

Isolation and solubilization of PHF (14); discovery of abnormally phosphorylated tau as a major component of PHF (17-18,22) and the presence of ubiquitin in PHF (20,41); isolation and amino acid sequencing of β amyloid peptide (26); isolation of the β amyloid precursor protein (28-30); and the attempts to link the Alzheimer's disease gene to chromosome 21 have not only opened new, promising areas of research but also tremendously increased the interest of neuroscientists in the field of Alzheimer's disease. Major progress toward understanding the basic mechanisms of Alzheimer's disease is imminent.

Acknowledgments

My heartfelt thanks to Dr Inge Grundke-Iqbal for critical reading of the manuscript, to Ms Maureen Marlow Stoddard for editorial suggestions, and to Ms Concetta Veneziano and Ms Kathy Case for secretarial assistance.

This work was supported in part by the New York State Office of Mental Retardation and Developmental Disabilities, NIH grants AG05892, AG04220, and NS18105, and a grant from the Alzheimer's Disease Research Program of the American Health Assistance Foundation (Rockville, MD).

REFERENCES

1. Katzman R. Arch Neurol 1976; 33: 217.
2. McKhan G, Drachman D, Folstein M, Katzman R, Price D, Stadlan EM. Neurology 1989; 34: 939-44.
3. Khachaturian ZS. Arch Neurol 1985; 42: 1097-1105.
4. Tomlinson BE, Blessed G, Roth M. J Neurol Sci 1970; 11: 205-42.
5. Alafuzoff I, Iqbal K, Friden H, Adolfsson R, Winblad B. Acta Neuropathol (Berl) 1987; 74: 209-25.
6. St George-Hyslop PH, Tanzi RE, Polinsky RJ, Haines JL, Nee L, Watkins PC, Myers RH, Feldman RG, Pollen D, Drachman D, Gordon J, Bruin A, Fauci JF, Slamon D, Frommelt P, Amaducci L, Gorlin S, Placentim S, Stewart GD, Hoblis WJ, Conneally PM, Gusella JF. Science 1987; 253: 885-90.
7. Schellenberg GD, Bird TD, Wijsman EM, Moore DK, Boehnk ML, Bryant EM, Lampe TH, Nochlin D, Sumi SM, Deeb SS, Beyreuther K, Martin GM. Science 1988; 241: 1507-9.
8. Roses AD, Pericak-Vance MA, Yamaoka LH, Haynes CS, Speer MC, Gaskell PC, Wun-Yen H, Clark CM, Heyman AL, Trofatter JA, Earl NL, Gilbert JR, Lee JE, Alberts MJ, Dawson DV, Bartlett RJ, Siddique T, Vance JM, Conneally PM. In Iqbal K, Wisniewski HM, Winblad B (eds) Alzheimer's disease and related disorders. New York: Alan R. Liss, 1989: 201-15.
9. Heston LL. Clinical genetics of Alzheimer's disease. Alz Dis Assoc Disord 1988; 2: 272.
10. Wisniewski HM, Merz PA, Iqbal K. J Neuropathol Exper Neurol 1984; 43: 643-56.
11. Iqbal K, Wisniewski HM, Grundke-Iqbal I, Terry RD. In Nandy K, Sherwin L (eds) The aging brain and senile dementia. New York: Plenum, 1977: 209-27.
12. Wisniewski K, Jervis GA, Moretz RC, Wisniewski HM. Ann Neurol 1979; 5: 288-94.
13. Braak H, Braak E, Grundke-Iqbal I, Iqbal K. Neurosci Lett 1986; 65: 351-5.
14. Iqbal K, Zaidi T, Thompson CH, Merz PA, Wisniewski HM. Acta Neuropathol (Berl) 1984; 62: 167-77.

15. Grundke-Iqbal I, Iqbal K, Tung Y-C, Wisniewski HM. Acta Neuropathol (Berl) 1984; 62: 259-67.
16. Grundke-Iqbal I, Wang GP, Iqbal K, Tung Y-C, Wisniewski HM. Acta Neuropathol (Berl) 1985; 68: 279-83.
17. Grundke-Iqbal I, Iqbal K, Quinlan M, Tung Y-C, Zaidi MS, Wisniewski HM. J Biol Chem 1986; 261: 6084-9.
18. Grundke-Iqbal I, Iqbal K, Tung Y-C, Quinlan M, Wisniewski HM, Binder LI. Proc Natl Acad Sci USA 1986; 83: 4913-17.
19. Goedert M, Wischik CM, Crowther RA, Walker JE, Klug A. Proc Natl Acad Sci USA 1988; 85: 4051-5.
20. Mori H, Kondo J, Ihara Y. Science 1987; 235: 1641-4.
21. Goedert M, Spillantini MG, Potier MC, Ulrich J, Crowther RA. EMBO J 1989; 8: 393-9.
22. Iqbal K, Grundke-Iqbal I, Smith AJ, George L, Tung Y-C. Proc Natl Acad Sci USA 1989; 86: 5646-50.
23. Iqbal K, Grundke-Iqbal I, Zaidi T, Merz PA, Wen GY, Shaikh SS, Wisniewski HM, Alafuzoff I, Winblad B. Lancet 1986; ii: 421-6.
24. Grundke-Iqbal I, Vorbrodt AW, Iqbal K, Tung YC, Wang GP, Wisniewski HM. J Mol Brain Res 1988; 4: 43-52.
25. Bancher C, Brunner C, Lassmann H, Budka H, Jellinger K, Wiche G, Seitelberger F, Grundke-Iqbal I, Iqbal K, Wisniewski HM. Brain Res 1989; 477: 90-9.
26. Glenner GC, Wong DW. Biochem Biophys Res Comm 1984; 120: 885-90.
27. Masters CL, Simms G, Weinman NA, Multhaup G, McDonald BL, Beyreuther K. Proc Natl Acad Sci USA 1985; 82: 4245-9.
28. Kang J, Lemaire H-G, Unterbeck A, Salbaum JM, Masters CL, Grzeschik K-H, Multhaup G, Beyreuther K, Muller-Hill B. Nature 1987; 325: 733-6.
29. Robakis NK, Ramakrishna N, Wolfe G, Wisniewski HM. Proc Natl Acad Sci USA 1987; 84: 4190-4.
30. Goldgaber D, Lerman MI, McBride OW, Saffiotti U, Gajdusek DC. Science 1987; 235: 877-80.
31. Ponte P, Gonzalez-DeWhitt P, Schilling J, Miller J, Hsu D, Greenberg B, Davis K, Wallace W, Lieberburg I, Fuller F, Cordell B. Nature 1988; 331: 525-7.
32. Tanzi RE, McClatchey AI, Lamperti ED, Villa-Komaroff L, Gusella JF, Neve RL. Nature 1988; 331: 528-30.
33. Kitaguchi N, Takahashi Y, Tokushima Y, Shiojiri S, Ito H. Nature 1988; 331: 530-2.
34. Tanzi RE, Gusella JF, Watkins PC, Bruns GAP, St George-Hyslop P, Van Keuren ML, Patterson D, Pagan S, Kurnit DM, Neve RL. Science 1987; 235: 880-4.
35. Prusiner SB. N Engl J Med 1987; 317: 1571-81.
36. Manuelidis EE, DeFigueiredo JM, Kim JH, Fritch WW, Manuelidis L. Proc Natl Acad Sci USA 1988; 85: 4898-901.
37. Crapper-McLachlan DR. Neurobiol Aging 1986; 7: 525-32.
38. Wisniewski HM, Sturman JA, Shek JW. Neurobiol Aging 1982; 3: 11-22.
39. Perl DP, Brody AR. Science 1980; 208: 297-9.
40. Candy JM, Klinowski J, Perry RH, Perry EK, Fairbrain A, Oakley AE, Carpenter TA, Attack JA. Lancet 1986; i: 354-7.
41. Perry G, Friedman R, Shaw G, Chau V. Proc Natl Acad Sci USA 1987; 84: 3033-6.

Address for correspondence:

Dr Khalid Iqbal,
New York State Institute for Basic Research in Developmental Disabilities,
1050 Forest Hill Road, Staten Island, NY 10314, USA
Tel. (718) 494-5259
Fax. (718) 494-5269

Part I

CLINICAL COURSE

1 Leuko-Araiosis and Cognitive Impairment in Alzheimer's Disease

FERNANDO DIAZ, VLADIMIR HACHINSKI, HAROLD MERSKEY, DONALD LEE, MARY BONIFERRO, CINDY WONG AND HANNAH FOX

White matter rarefaction on brain imaging or leuko-araiosis (1) occurs more frequently in Alzheimer's disease than in normal aging (2–4). However, an association between leuko-araiosis and the degree of cognitive impairment in subjects with Alzheimer's disease remains unsettled.

Variables such as age, stroke (5,6), severity of dementia (3,7,8), and, perhaps, duration of the illness are related to both cognitive decline and leuko-araiosis and can, therefore, confound the association. This study explored the relationship between leuko-araiosis and cognitive impairment in Alzheimer's disease, taking into consideration the confounding effect of these variables.

SUBJECTS AND METHODS

The subjects were selected from the University of Western Ontario dementia study, a longitudinal research project described elsewhere (9). All the patients clinically diagnosed as having primary degenerative dementia of the Alzheimer type were reviewed. The clinical diagnosis was established by a research fellow in neurology and reviewed by one of the authors (V.C.H.) on the basis of a systematic comprehensive evaluation as described elsewhere (9,10). Exclusion criteria included a history of stroke, cerebral infarcts on CT, and a primary neuropathological diagnosis other than Alzheimer's disease post-mortem.

All the subjects were reviewed who had undergone a computerized tomography (CT) scan of the head and psychometric testing, completed within a six-month period of each other. The present series therefore included patients who were previously reported (3,7). All the CT scans, however, were read anew by one neuroradiologist (D.H.L.), who interpreted all the CT scans blindly and assessed the presence of leuko-araiosis and infarcts on the basis of specific criteria (11). Cognitive impairment was graded by the Extended Scale for Dementia (ESD) (12). The ESD score derives from 23 weighted sub-scores totalling a maximum of 250 points; the lower the score the more profound the cognitive impairment. One psychometrist completed all the ESD measurements.

Alzheimer's Disease: Basic Mechanisms, Diagnosis and Therapeutic Strategies
Edited by K. Iqbal, D. R. C. McLachlan, B. Winblad and H. M. Wisniewski
© 1991 John Wiley & Sons Ltd

Other variables under study included age, sex, highest level of education attained, duration of the dementia (as elicited from the next of kin), EEG grade of abnormality (13), blood pressure, and hypertension. Hypertension was defined as the presence of one or more of the following: (a) a systolic blood pressure greater than 160 mmHg, (b) diastolic blood pressure greater than 90 mmHg, (c) a previous medical diagnosis of hypertension, and (d) previous or current treatment for hypertension. A univariate analysis, using chi-square for dichotomous or categorical variables and Pearson correlation coefficients and two-tailed t-tests for continuous variables, was performed in order to assess the relationships among the study variables and confounding among the study variables. Analysis of variance was used to explore the association between leuko-araiosis and ESD scores while controlling for confounding and interactive effects. All analyses were done using SPSSX software.

RESULTS

The mean age of the 95 patients was 70.8 ± 9.1 years, the male to female ratio 0.94, the mean duration of the dementia was 3.2 ± 1.5 years, and the mean ESD score was 138 ± 78.2. Forty-two per cent of the patients showed leuko-araiosis on CT scan of the brain.

Patients with leuko-araiosis had significantly lower ESD scores than patients without leuko-araiosis: 106.4 ± 77.0 and 160.3 ± 71.7 respectively ($P < 0.001$), and were significantly older: 75.3 ± 6.1 vs 67.6 ± 9.6 years ($P < 0.0001$). In addition, leuko-araiosis was four times as common in females as in males: 65% vs 17% ($P < 0.0001$).

When controlled for the potentially confounding effects of age, sex and duration of illness, deterioration of the ESD score was dependent on the presence of leuko-araiosis ($P < 0.003$).

DISCUSSION

This study reports an increase in the recognition of leuko-araiosis in patients of whom many were previously studied. The change appears to be due to improved recognition of leuko-araiosis in the light of experience. That the change is real appears highly likely in view of its correspondence with other figures in the literature. The clear association with the independent measures provided by the Extended Scale for Dementia strongly suggests this view.

Results from this study showed that after adjusting for the confounding effect of age, sex, and duration of the illness, the association between leuko-araiosis and cognitive impairment persists.

REFERENCES

1. Hachinski VC, Potter P, Merskey, H. Arch Neurol 1987; 44: 21-3.
2. George AE, de Leon MJ, Gentes CT et al. Am J Neuroradiol 1986; 7: 567-70.
3. Steingart A, Hachinski VC, Lau C et al. Arch Neurol 1987; 44: 36-9.
4. Brun A, Englund E. Ann Neurol 1986; 19: 253-62.
5. Hachinski VC, Lassen NA, Marshall J. Lancet 1974; ii: 207-10.

6. Inzitari D, Diaz JF, Fox A et al. Arch Neurol 1987; 44: 42-7.
7. Steingart A, Hachinski VC, Lau C et al. Arch Neurol 1987; 44: 32-5.
8. Erkinjuntti T, Sulkava R, Palo J, Lenna K. Arch Geront Geriatr 1989; 8: 95-104.
9. Merskey H, Blume WT, Colhoun EG et al. Neuropsychopharmacol Biol Psychiat 1985; 9: 509-14.
10. Wade JPH, Mirsen TR, Hachinski VC et al. Arch Neurol 1987; 44: 24-9.
11. Lee D, Fox A, Vinuela F et al. Arch Neurol 1987; 44: 30-1.
12. Hersch EL. J Am Geriatr Soc 1979; 26: 348-54.
13. Rae-Grant A, Blume W, Lau C et al. Arch Neurol 1987; 44: 50-4.

Address for correspondence:

Dr Vladimir Hachinski,
Department of Clinical Neurological Sciences,
University Hospital,
PO Box 5339, 339 Windermere Road,
London, Ontario N6A 5A5,
Canada

2 Multidisciplinary Validation of Two Dementia Categories

NARAYAN P. VERMA, MARY J. YUSKO,
BETTY J. BERANEK-McCLUNG AND LEON A. WILLIAMS

Dementia comprises diseases of varied etiology. It may occur in over 60 disorders (1). Attempts at classification of dementias are important as they are likely to contribute to understanding the causes of, and developing new therapies for these disorders (2). Albert et al (3) advanced the concept of subcortical dementia (SCD) in relation to that occurring with progressive supranuclear palsy (PSP). Its main feature is a defect of retrieval from stored memory ('tip of the tongue' phenomenon), slowness of mental processing, forgetfulness and impaired ability to manipulate acquired knowledge (4). This is in contrast to cortical dementia (CD), which is characterized by a defect of the stored memory itself, and is traditionally associated with 'dominant' and 'nondominant' hemispheric syndromes: aphasia, amnesia, apraxia, agnosia and acalculia (4).

The concept of SCD has been extended to Huntington's disease (5), Wilson's disease, Parkinson's disease, lacunar state (4), traumatic injuries and multiple sclerosis (6) amongst others. The CD is believed to account for most cases of Alzheimer's disease and Pick's disease (4).

This classification is controversial and has proponents (4,7) and detractors (8). Major reviews (2,6) have outlined the problems with this classification. Firstly, the nomenclature implies an anatomical distinction almost intuitively, although the authors (3,4) insist it is a clinical classification. Secondly, pathologic data indicate prevalence of cortical lesions in SCD and subcortical lesions in CD. For example, lesions of subcortical nucleus basalis of Meynert may well account for cortical cholinergic deficit in Alzheimer's disease (9), cortical lesions similar to Alzheimer's disease are also seen in Parkinson's disease (10) and cortical atrophy may be seen in Huntington's disease as well. Also, an often-quoted neuropsychological study (8) failed to reveal a distinction based on mini-mental state examination. An overlap has been noted in some other neuropsychologic studies as well. For example, constructional apraxia and language deficits, expected in CD, have also been reported in Parkinson's and Huntington's diseases (11). Even nondemented patients with Parkinson's disease show significant visuospatial deficits (12). In addition, the status of bradyphrenia as a cognitive deficit separate from primary motor disturbance is questionable (13–15).

Alzheimer's Disease: Basic Mechanisms, Diagnosis and Therapeutic Strategies
Edited by K. Iqbal, D. R. C. McLachlan, B. Winblad and H. M. Wisniewski
© 1991 John Wiley & Sons Ltd

However, the proponents of this classification argue that the nucleus basalis of Meynert abnormalities in Alzheimer's disease may be nonspecific as they are seen in a number of seemingly unrelated conditions, e.g. Pick's disease (16), Guam disease (17), Parkinson's disease (18) and traumatic brain injuries (19). Also, metabolic studies reveal profound cortical hypometabolism in Alzheimer's disease and subcortical hypometabolism in Huntington's disease (20–22). Electrophysiologic data (23,24) also show distinctive findings. Finally, the lack of distinction in the major negative neuropsychological study (8) may be due to the relative insensitivity of the mini-mental state test as a tool to elicit distinction by virtue of its weightedness towards verbal responses (25) and the rather global nature of the test. The use of specific measures has elicited distinctive information in some studies. Activation of semantic memory is disturbed in Alzheimer's disease but not in Huntington's disease (26). Motor skills learning is, however, more intact in Alzheimer's than in Huntington's disease (27,28). Egocentric spatial perception is more impaired in Huntington's disease and allocentric more so in Alzheimer's disease (29).

The controversy has led reviewers (2,6) to suggest conducting prospective and multidisciplinary studies. Our initial study (30) matched 15 patients with putative CD and 15 with putative SCD for age, sex and severity as measured by the brief cognitive rating scale. Relatively normal EEG on an objective rating scale were found in 14 patients with SCD and only 3 with CD ($P < 0.01$, chi-squared test). Subsequently, our studies with late-event related cognitive brain potentials (24) revealed alterations of early cognitive potentials (N1 and P2) and relative intactness of later potentials (N2 and P3) to be relatively specific of dementias with motoric manifestations (Dem M+, putative SCD), whereas the abnormalities of the late cognitive potential (P3, also called P300) with relative intactness of early potentials N1 and P2 have previously (23,24,31) been reported to be more characteristic of dementias without motoric manifestations (Dem M−, putative CD). This suggests a differential effect of these two classes of dementias on cognitive brain potentials.

A preliminary analysis of our neuropsychological data has been published recently (32). A complete analsis of 92 subjects is given here and results are in line with our preliminary observations. They support the classification at least in mildly to moderately demented subjects.

We have selected presence or absence of motoric disturbance in dementia patients as a novel external criterion reflecting putative subcortical and cortical pathology. This was done because SCD has always been described in patients with motoric abnormalities such as rigidity (e.g. Parkinson's disease and PSP), involuntary movements (e.g. Huntington's disease) or gait disturbance (e.g. normal pressure hydrocephalus). The criteria for dementia with motoric abnormalities (Dem M+) were as follows:

- Mattis Dementia Rating Scale score 133 or less with decline in two or more subtests (33), or WAIS-R full-scale IQ > 15 points less than the predicted premorbid IQ (13).
- Significant motoric disturbance as shown by at least two of the following: (a) Abnormal Involuntary Movement Scale (AIMS) score of 4 or more; (b) clinically significant ratings on the bradykinesia, postural instability, tremor and gait items

of the modified Columbia Unified Parkinson's Scale (CUPS) (34); and (c) Halstead (35) finger-tapping speed less than 35 taps/10 s on the dominant hand.

● Motoric manifestations unrelated to the neuroleptic therapy and having an onset at least six months prior to cognitive decline.

The criteria for dementia without motoric abnormalities (Dem M −) were the same as above; the motoric abnormalities had to be insignificant on the measures stated above, however.

The nondemented patient control group had patients having features the same as the Dem M + group but Mattis scores > 133 or those diagnosed as pseudodementia.

Normal volunteers included subjects recruited from the hospital volunteer service and through newspaper advertisement. They all had Mattis scores > 133. Although no formal motor scales were administered to them, they did not have any motor abnormalities.

Exclusion criteria were severe dementia, evidence of cerebral ischemia (positive history for stroke and/or Hachinski (36) ischemia rating score ⩾ 7), positive serological tests for syphilis, history of significant head trauma, alcoholism, seizures, multiple sclerosis and premorbid psychiatric disorders.

Informed consent was obtained from all subjects and/or their close relatives or legal guardians. The characteristics of the four study groups are listed in Table 1.

All four study groups were matched for age within 3½ years, for education within 1½ grades and for predicted premorbid IQ (37) within 7½ points. Normal and nondemented patient controls were matched for dementia severity within 1 point and the two groups of demented subjects were matched for dementia severity within

Table 1. Group characteristics

	Normal controls n=21 (17M, 4F)		Patient controls n=20 (all M)		Dementia M− n=22 (21M, 1F)		Dementia M+ n=29 (28M, 1F)	
	Mean	SD	Mean	SD	Mean	SD	Mean	SD
Age	60.9	9.7	59.9	10.5	63.6	8.8	64.3	9.5
Education	13.7	3.1	12.6	2.8	11.9	3.2	11.4	3.2
PPIQ	108.5	10.8	106.2	10.1	102.0	12.1	100.6	12.6
Hachinski	NA		1.8	1.5	1.9	1.7	2.6	1.9
Hamilton	2.6	1.7	6.7	5.7	6.6	4.7	8.4	7.2
Mattis Scale								
Total	140.6	3.2	139.3	3.5	117.3	19.5*	114.0	17.0*
Att/conc.	36.3	0.9	36.3	1.0	34.2	2.5*	33.5	4.0*
Ini/pres.	36.6	0.7	35.9	1.5	28.4	7.2*	26.4	7.6*
Construc.	6.0	0.2	5.9	0.5	5.0	1.8	3.8	2.5*
Concept	37.3	2.4	37.7	1.9	31.3	6.8*	31.3	6.8*
Memory	24.4	1.1	23.7	1.3	18.0	6.1*	18.6	5.6*
CUPS	NA		6.2	3.5	1.1	1.4	9.1	4.8†
AIMS	NA		6.7	5.4	0.4	1.0	12.3	9.3†
FT-Dom.	48.5	7.8	41.4	15.4	48.5	5.5	27.3	11.2†
FT-Nondom.	44.5	7.7	40.0	13.0	44.7	5.3	27.5	12.7†

*Significantly different from normal and patient controls at $P < 0.01$.
†Significantly different from dementia M− group at $P < 0.01$.

3 points on the Mattis scale. Nondemented patient controls, Dem M+ subjects and Dem M− subjects were also matched for ischemia scores and depression scores. The Dem M+ group had higher scores on motor impairment rating scales as compared to the Dem M− group, expectedly so. The nondemented patient control group was less impaired than the Dem M+ group on motor scales mainly due to the inclusion of pseudodementia subjects in that group.

The neuropsychological test battery (Table 2) included the following:

Table 2. Neuropsychological data

	Normal controls		Patient controls		Dementia M−		Dementia M+	
	Mean	SD	Mean	SD	Mean	SD	Mean	SD
Mental speed								
Stroop								
name + read	176.0	28.9	142.5	23.5	122.1	38.4	91.7	32.5*
S-T memory								
Free recall								
5 minutes	2.4	1.6	2.6	1.4	1.6	1.4	1.9	1.7
20 minutes	3.4	0.8	3.2	1.1	2.0	1.6	2.0	1.4
w/cues	3.6	0.7	3.5	0.9	2.4	1.4	2.5	1.3
w/multiple ch.	4.0	0.2	3.8	0.9	3.3	0.9	3.0	1.3
Sternberg								
av RT	0.6	0.2	0.7	0.3	0.9	0.4	1.1	0.3*
errors	0.3	0.7	0.4	0.8	0.4	0.7	1.9	2.3*
Wechsler memory								
raw scores	65.2	10.0	58.3	10.9	44.5	10.4	40.6	9.6
stories	10.4	3.3	8.6	4.7	5.9	2.9	5.8	2.3
design	9.2	3.0	8.0	3.5	4.4	3.5	2.7	3.2
Cognitive flexib.								
Stroop								
interference	37.7	7.8	29.7	6.7	19.8	9.9	16.5	9.6
Language								
Western aphasia								
cortical Q	NA		94.7	3.4	82.5	16.4	85.5	10.3
aphasia Q	NA		96.3	2.5	88.1	15.4	91.4	7.8
Boston naming								
w/o cues	55.4	5.0	55.4	4.9	43.0	14.5	41.9	12.5
w/sem. cues	56.0	4.7	55.9	4.6	43.7	14.6	43.4†	11.9
w/phon. cues	57.6	3.4	56.9	4.0	47.3	15.0	46.1	11.9
w/both cues	58.1	3.1	57.4	3.7	48.0	15.3	47.7	11.5
Intelligence								
WAIS-R								
f.s. IQ	115.3	12.6	106.2	15.2	91.8	11.9	84.0	11.3
verb. IQ	115.6	13.9	107.6	15.0	93.6	12.6	87.5	10.9
perf. IQ	111.7	12.6	103.8	13.8	89.4	14.8	80.6	12.1
Parietal lobe								
Stick const.								
memory	10.9	2.3	9.2	3.1	7.8	3.5	4.5	3.1
copy	13.9	0.3	13.3	2.0	12.0	3.7	10.7	3.6
Line orient.	24.3	4.6	25.7	3.3	18.2	7.6	15.1	7.5
Praxis	37.6	3.0	38.3	2.0	34.6	4.0	32.0	6.1
R/L discri.	15.0	2.0	15.3	1.4	14.4	2.5	13.0	3.2

*Only dementia M+ group significantly impaired as compared with normal and patient controls at $P < 0.01$.
†Only dementia M+ group benefits from semantic cues at $P < 0.01$.

Tests for mental speed The Stroop color naming and reading test (38) was used to measure this. The reasons for choosing this test are outlined elsewhere (30). The mental speed in Dem M+ group was maximally slowed and significantly so as compared to controls at $P < 0.01$ (post-hoc Newman-Keuls' multiple range test) (39). The mental speed in Dem M− group, although slowed, was not significantly so as compared with controls.

The average reaction time as measured by Sternberg's rapid memory scanning paradigm (40)—details given elsewhere (24)—was also significantly longer in Dem M+ group as compared with controls at $P < 0.01$ (post-hoc Newman-Keuls' multiple range test) but not so, for Dem M− group. The number of errors made were also maximal in Dem M+ group. That this was a function of bradyphrenia and not motor abnormalities was shown by the presence of significant differences between Dem M+ group and non-demented patient controls even after excluding pseudodementia subjects from the latter and a lack of correlation of Stroop and Sternberg results with motor measures either on Pearson product moment correlation or multiple regression analyses within each group or across the groups.

Tests for short-term memory Simple free recall using a list of four low-frequency words — 'sofa', 'brown', 'cherry' and 'wrench' — was expectedly impaired in the two dementia groups at 5 and 20 min, both with cuing and without. However, there were no differences between the two dementia groups. The Wechsler memory test expectedly revealed lower scores for the two dementia groups as compared with controls but no differences between the two dementia groups.

Intelligence Although lower overall IQ scores were found on WAIS-R in the Dem M+ group as compared with the Dem M− group, the differences were not statistically significant.

Cognitive flexibility This was measured using the Stroop interference test. Both dementia groups were significantly impaired as compared with controls, but did not differ from each other.

Language Cortical and aphasia quotients on Western aphasia battery (41) were lower in Dem M− group as compared to Dem M+ group but the differences were not significant. Scores on Boston naming were expectedly lower in demented subjects but similar in the two dementia groups. Semantic cues, however, significantly benefited group M+ alone.

Parietal lobe functions Stick construction, line orientation, praxis and right–left discrimination were equally impaired in the two dementia groups.

Thus, the dementia M+ and M− groups differed in mental speed and helpfulness of semantic cues for naming. These findings are consistent with the traditional belief that putative subcortical dementia is characterized by bradyphrenia and retrieval defect in memory. This may be related to reduced self-initiation or lowered cortical activation in SCD and word-finding may be facilitated when their semantic network is externally cued. Support for this explanation comes from positron emission tomographic studies showing subcortical hypometabolism in SCD (20-22). On the other hand, some other traditional concepts about this classification, e.g. that apraxia, aphasia, amnesia and agnosia are more frequent and severe in putative CD (4), are not borne out by this study.

There are several possible reasons for our results being different from the most-quoted negative study (8): (a) our data were prospectively collected; (b) the Mattis scale has a much smaller verbal component as compared to mini-mental state examination, preventing mismatch of groups on a variable on which they may naturally differ; (c) the inability of Mayeaux et al to find significant differences may reflect the confounding of the dependent and criterion measures, i.e. the groups were compared on subtests of the global measure they were matched on; and (d) the mini-mental state examination subtests may not be a valid measure of crucial neurobehavioral dimensions differentiating the two groups.

We have retested 7 patients with Dem M− and 8 patients with Dem M+ after a period varying from 7 to 35 months. These two retest groups had equivalent testing intervals (19.7±10.0 and 18.1±9.1 months) and were otherwise matched for age, education and PPIQ. The Mattis scores for both groups fell by an average of 3 points. The scores on Stroop naming and reading fell by an average of 25 points for Dem M− and 17 points for Dem M+. Small follow-up numbers preclude proper statistical treatment but do suggest a faster deterioration of mental speed in group M− as compared with M+ in advanced cases of dementia rendering the former a meaningful differentiating feature only in early stages of dementia. On retest, reaction time measurements by Sternberg's paradigm were precluded in most cases with Dem M− due to their inability to cooperate with this test procedure. A meaningful quantitative comparison with Dem M+ group is therefore not possible. The semantic cues no longer significantly improved naming in Dem M+ group.

This study demonstrates the presence of differences between putative cortical and subcortical dementia and suggests that the differences may disappear as the severity of dementia increases.

REFERENCES

1. Katzman R. N Eng J Med 1986; 314: 964-71.
2. Whitehouse PJ. Ann Neurol 1986; 19: 1-6.
3. Albert ML, Feldman RG, Willis AL. J Neurol Neurosurg Psychiat 1974; 37: 121-30.
4. Cummings JL, Benson F. Arch Neurol 1984; 41: 874-9.
5. McHugh PR, Folstein MF. In Benson DF, Blumer, D (eds) Psychiatric aspects of neurologic disease, vol. 2. New York: Grune & Stratton, 1975: 93-121.
6. Huber SJ, Paulson GW. Am J Psychiat 1985; 142: 1312-17.
7. Goodin DS, Aminoff MJ. Brain 1986; 109: 1103-13.
8. Mayeux R, Stern Y, Rosen J, Benson DF. Ann Neurol 1983; 14: 278-83.
9. Whitehouse PJ, Price DI, Struble RG, Clark AW, Coyle JT, Delon MR. Science 1982; 215: 1237-9.
10. Hakim AM, Mathieson G. Neurology 1979; 29: 1209-14.
11. Scott S, Caird FI, Williams BO. J Neurol Neurosurg Psychiat 1984; 47: 840-3.

12. Boller F. In Grant I, Adams K (eds) Neuropsychological assessment of neuropsychiatric disorders. Oxford, New York: 1986: 375-83.
13. Wilson RS, Kaszniak AW, Klawans HL, Garron DC. Cortex 1980; 16: 67-72.
14. Rafal RD, Posner MI, Walker JA, Friederich FJ. Brain 1984; 107: 1083-94.
15. Rogers D, Lees AJ, Smith E, Trimble M, Stern GM. Brain 1987; 110: 761-76.
16. Uhl GR, Hilt DC, Hedreen JC, Whitehouse PJ, Price DL. Neurology 1983; 33: 1470-3.
17. Nakano I, Hiroan A. Ann Neurol 1983; 13: 87-96.
18. Salazar AM, Gaufam JG. Neurology 1983; 42 (suppl. 2): 104-5.
19. Whitehouse PJ, Hendreen JC, White CL et al. Ann Neurol 1986; 19: 1-6.
20. Benson DF, Kuhl DE, Hawkins RA, Phelps ME, Cummings JL, Tsai SY. Arch Neurol 1983; 40: 711-14.
21. Frackowiak RSJ, Pozzilli C, Legg NJ, Du Boulay GH, Marshall J, Lenzi GL, Jones T. Brain 1981; 104: 753-78.
22. Kuhl DE, Phelps ME, Markhans CH, Metter EJ, Riege WH, Winter J. Ann Neurol 1982; 12: 425-34.
23. Goodin DS, Aminoff MJ. Ann Neurol 1987; 21: 90-4.
24. Verma NP, Nichols CD, Greiffenstein MF, Singh RP, Hurst-Gordon D. Brain Topography 1989; 1: 183-91.
25. Freedman M. Ann Neurol 1984; 15: 506-8.
26. Shimamura AP, Salmon DP, Squire LR, Butters N. Behav Neurosci 1987; 101: 347-51.
27. Martone M, Butters N, Payne M, Becker JT, Sax DS. Arch Neurol 1984; 41: 965-70.
28. Butters N, Wolfe J, Martone M, Granholme E, Cermak LS. Neuropsychologia 1985; 23: 723-43.
29. Brouwers P, Cox C, Martin A. Arch Neurol 1984; 41: 1073-6.
30. Verma NP, Greiffenstein MF, Verma N, King SD, Caldwell DL. Clin Electroenceph 1987; 18: 26-33.
31. Patterson JV, Michelewski HJ, Starr A. Electroenceph Clin Neurophysiol 1988; 71: 450-60.
32. Greiffenstein MF, Verma NP, Nichols CD, DelaCruz CR. Neuropsychiat Neuropsychol Behavioral Neurol 1989; 1: 21-30.
33. Mattis S. In Bellad L, Karash TB (eds) Geriatric psychiatry. New York: Grune & Stratton, 1976.
34. Duvoisin RC. In Monamines noyaux gri centrax et syndrome de Parkinson. Paris: Masson, 1971: 313-25.
35. Halstead WC. In Brain and intelligence. Chicago: University Press, 1947.
36. Hachinski VC, Iliff LD, Zilhka E, Boulay GH, McAllister VL, Marshall J, Russell RW, Symon L. Arch Neurol 1975; 32: 632.
37. Wilson RS, Rosenbaum G, Brown G, Rourke D, Whitman RD, Grisell J. J Consult and Clin Psychol 1978; 46: 1554-5.
38. Stroop JR. J Exp Psychol 1984; 18: 643-62.
39. Bruning JL, Klintz BL. In Computational handbook of statistics. London: Scott Foresman, 1987: 122-4.
40. Sternberg S. American Scientist 1969; 57: 421-57.
41. Kertesz A. In Aphasia and associated disorders. New York: Grune & Stratton, 1979: 35-54.
42. Benton AL, Varney NR, Hamdhey K. Arch Neurol 1978; 35: 364-7.

Address for correspondence:

Narayan P. Verma, MD, FACP,
Associate Professor of Neurology, 6E UHC,
Wayne State University School of Medicine, 4201 St Antoine,
Detroit, MI 48201, USA

3 Heterogeneity of 'Probable Alzheimer's Disease'

K. BLENNOW, A. WALLIN AND C. G. GOTTFRIES

Alzheimer's disease (AD) is characterized by progressive dementia with, in typical cases, memory deficits and parietal-lobe symptoms (1–3). The traditional neuropathological findings, i.e. the Alzheimer encephalopathy, consist of senile plaques and neurofibrillary tangles (4). Originally, the term Alzheimer's disease was reserved for dementia in patients with onset of symptoms before the age of 65 years, while the term senile dementia was used when the onset was at the age of 65 years or after. Today, largely on the basis of similar neuropathological characteristics, presenile AD and senile dementia are usually regarded as only one disease entity.

As both the parietal symptoms (5–7) and the Alzheimer encephalopathy (6–8) are more severe in early-onset AD (EAD) than in late-onset AD (LAD), some authors have, however, questioned the scientific basis for combining the disorders (7–9). The encephalopathy originally described by Alzheimer in 1907 is located in grey matter regions of the brain (4). In the 1980s, however, after the introduction of high-resolution computerized tomography (CT), white-matter lesions, leuko-araiosis (LA), have also been found to be relatively frequent in patients with AD (10–13).

The aim of the study was to further examine the homogeneity of 'probable AD', taking into account the clinical symptomatology, and the relation between the symptomatology and vascular factors, such as concomitant vascular diseases, blood-brain barrier function and leuko-araiosis.

MATERIALS AND METHODS

Forty-one AD patients were included, 17 men and 24 women, mean age ($\pm$SD) 71.2 ± 9.1 years. Nineteen patients, 8 men and 11 women, mean age ($\pm$SD) 63.1 ± 4.5 years, had EAD and 22 patients, 9 men and 13 women, mean age ($\pm$SD) 78.3 ± 5.2 years, had LAD. All patients underwent a thorough examination to exclude other primary (e.g. fronto-temporal dementia) and secondary (e.g. depression) causes for dementia (14). The AD group consisted of all consecutive patients fulfilling the NINCDS-ADRDA criteria for 'probable AD' (15) admitted to the diagnostic unit at our department over a three-year period, except that mildly demented patients were not included in the present study on the grounds that brain regional symptoms have not yet developed in mild dementia (1,3,14).

Alzheimer's Disease: Basic Mechanisms, Diagnosis and Therapeutic Strategies
Edited by K. Iqbal, D. R. C. McLachlan, B. Winblad and H. M. Wisniewski
© 1991 John Wiley & Sons Ltd

In the AD group, vascular factors (mild arterial hypertension, mild non-insulin dependent diabetes mellitus, and mild ischemic heart disease) were recorded. Parietal and confusional symptoms were recorded (for a more detailed description, see 14,15). Parietal symptoms included sensory aphasia, visual agnosia, visuospatial dysfunction and apraxia (3). Symptoms of confusion were defined as clouded consciousness with key symptoms of difficulties in sustaining and shifting attention and incoherent thinking and speech, often accompanied by perceptual and psychomotor disturbances (16). An etiological factor triggering the confusion (e.g. side-reactions of drugs, acute infections) was sought in all patients. The presence of dementia in periods without confusion was always established.

For analysis of the blood–brain barrier (BBB) function in healthy elderly individuals, a control material was drawn, consisting of 50 individuals, 28 men and 22 women, mean age ($\pm$SD) 71.5$\pm$10.8 years, without psychiatric or neurological disease. Lumbar punctures were performed under standard conditions (17), and the albumin ratio — CSF-albumin in mg/l/serum-albumin in g/l — was used as a measure of BBB function (18,19). In 26 of the AD patients, the CT scans were available for evaluation of LA. The CT scans were reviewed by a radiologist without knowledge of the clinical data. LA was defined as periventricular decreased attenuation, mainly around the frontal and occipital horns of the lateral ventricles (10–13,20).

Statistical analysis

The Wilcoxon 2-sample test was used for quantitative parameters, and the chi-square test for qualitative parameters.

The study was approved by the Ethics Committee, University of Göteborg.

RESULTS

Twenty-three patients had predominant parietal symptoms, while 18 patients had a symptomatology without parietal predominance (Table 1). Predominant parietal symptoms were found in 18/19 (95%) of EAD patients and 5/22 (23%) of LAD patients, $P<0.0001$. Symptoms of confusion were present in 22 patients. The confusional symptoms were mild in most cases and were present intermittently in periods of 1–4 weeks during the entire history of dementia. No specific triggering factor could be found. Confusional symptoms were less frequent in patients with predominant parietal symptoms (5/23, 22%) than in patients without such symptoms (17/18, 94%), $P<0.0001$ (Table 1).

Patients with predominant parietal symptoms were significantly younger ($P<0.0001$) and had earlier onset of the disease ($P<0.0001$) than patients without parietal predominance (Table 1). The duration of the disease did not differ between these groups (data not shown). In the group without parietal predominance, vascular factors were more common ($P<0.05$) than in the group with predominant parietal symptoms (Table 1). The albumin ratio did not differ significantly between AD patients with predominant parietal symptoms ($n=23$, albumin ratio$\pm$SD 6.8$\pm$2.4) and controls ($n=50$, albumin ratio$\pm$SD 5.7$\pm$2.1), while the albumin ratio in patients

Table 1. Comparison of clinical data, leuko-araiosis and blood-brain barrier function between Alzheimer patients with and without predominant parietal symptoms

	Predominant parietal symptoms ($n=23$-15)	No predominant parietal symptoms ($n=18$-11)	
Age (years)	66.0 ± 7.2	77.9 ± 6.5	$P<0.0001$
Age at onset (years)	60.3 ± 8.6	72.4 ± 7.2	$P<0.0001$
Duration (years)	5.7 ± 2.5	5.5 ± 2.8	NS
Confusion			
absent	18 (78%)	1 (6%)	$P<0.0001$
present	5 (22%)	17 (94%)	
Vascular factors			
absent	19 (83%)	8 (44%)	$P<0.05$
present	4 (17%)	10 (56%)	
Leuko-araiosis on CT			
absent	10 (67%)	1 (9%)	$P<0.005$
present	5 (33%)	10 (91%)	
Blood-brain barrier function	119% (NS)	147% ($P<0.0001$)	

Values are expressed as mean ($\pm$SD) or number (percentage) of patients. Blood-brain barrier function is expressed as percentage albumin ratio compared with controls (for exact values see text). NS, not significant.

without parietal predominance ($n=18$, albumin ratio $\pm$SD 8.4 ± 3.7) was significantly ($P<0.0001$) higher than in controls.

LA was less frequent in AD patients with predominant parietal symptoms (5/15, 33%) than in AD patients without such symptoms (10/11, 91%), $P<0.005$ (Table 1). AD patients with LA ($n=15$) had significantly ($P<0.005$) higher albumin ratio (7.7 ± 3.0) than controls ($n=50$, albumin ratio 5.7 ± 2.1), while the albumin ratio of AD patients without LA ($n=11$, albumin ratio 6.7 ± 2.3) did not differ significantly from controls.

DISCUSSION

By definition (21), memory deficits were present in all AD patients. Predominant parietal symptoms, however, were mainly found in younger (EAD) patients, while in older (LAD) patients, parietal symptoms were mild or absent (Table 1), the symptomatology being dominated by general cognitive symptoms. These findings are in agreement with other studies (5,6). Symptoms of confusion were more common in the older group of AD patients without predominant parietal symptoms (Table 1). Although structural brain disease has been stressed as a major predisposing factor to confusion (22), confusion in AD patients is often regarded as a complication (21). Since, in the present study, no triggering factors (organic or psychological) for confusion could be found, the confusional symptoms may be considered of more primary nature than a complication. Memory deficits and predominant parietal symptoms are regarded as characteristic of AD (1-3). Thus, the group of older AD patients without predominant parietal symptoms, but with general cognitive and mild confusional symptoms, had atypical (less focal) symptomatology. The finding that five LAD patients had predominant parietal symptoms similar to those in the EAD patients suggests, however, that the symptomatology that is typical of AD may also be found in a minority of LAD patients, and that clinical symptomatology may be a more appropriate factor than chronological age for distinguishing different AD groups.

LA is associated with aging, i.e. it is more frequent at higher ages (10,20,23). Thus, LA may be expected to occur more frequently in older than in younger AD patients, as was also found in the present study (Table 1). Other studies, too, have reported higher frequency of LA in LAD than in EAD (10-13). In the present study, a relation was found between LA and clinical symptomatology: LA was more frequent in the group of older AD patients without predominant parietal symptoms, but with general cognitive symptoms and high frequency of confusional symptoms. General cognitive symptoms and memory deficits are regarded as characteristic of subcortical dementias (2). The fact that LA is located in white matter around the lateral ventricles, i.e. subcortically, may explain the less focal and more generalized symptomatology found in the group of AD patients with LA. Features of subcortical dementia, together with absence of parietal symptoms, were also found in demented patients with LA in another study (24).

A vascular pathogenesis has been suggested for LA (10,25) and also the term 'selective incomplete white matter infarction' (SIWI) (26), because LA is neuropathologically and neurochemically similar to the transitional zone of incomplete white matter infarction between a complete infarct and normal white matter (25,26). This proposed vascular pathogenesis of LA is supported by the finding in this study of higher frequency of vascular factors, i.e. concomitant vascular diseases, in AD patients with LA than in those without LA (Table 1). Such a relationship between vascular factors and LA in patients with AD has also been found in other clinical studies (10,12,13,27).

The pathogenetic basis of LA in patients with AD has been suggested to be a small vessel disease, fibrohyaline nonamyloid arteriolosclerosis in the small penetrating vessels supplying the white matter (10,25,26). Since the BBB is situated in the small vessels of the brain (28), BBB dysfunction may be expected in patients with small vessel disease. In this study, the group of AD patients with LA was found to have impaired BBB function (Table 1). Small vessel disease may be a plausible explanation for this BBB dysfunction, since in the AD patients in this study no other factors, e.g. cerebral infarction/haemorrhage, infectious/autoimmune disease, neoplasms (29), were present that could account for the BBB dysfunction.

The pathogenesis and clinical relevance of LA in AD patients are insufficiently known. If LA in AD patients were caused by the same factor as is the Alzheimer encephalopathy, LA would be as frequent in young as in old AD patients. In this study, however, as in some other studies (10-13), LA was found to be more frequent in older than in younger AD patients. The opposite is true for the grey matter Alzheimer encephalopathy, i.e. this is less severe in older than in younger AD patients (6-8). Thus, grey matter Alzheimer encephalopathy and LA in AD patients do not appear to have a closely linked pathogenesis. In agreement with this suggestion, neuropathologically, LA in AD patients has been suggested to occur independently of grey matter Alzheimer encephalopathy (25,26). If LA in AD patients were an age-related change without clinical relevance, AD patients with and without LA would have similar symptomatologies. In this study, however, AD patients with LA were found to have a less focal (less parietal) symptomatology than AD patients without LA, suggesting that LA in AD patients has clinical significance.

In summary, the results of the present study suggest heterogeneity of 'probable AD', i.e. that, on the basis of clinical symptomatology, two subgroups of patients can be delimited. One subgroup is characterized by memory deficits and marked parietal symptoms but almost no confusional symptoms; the other by memory deficits, general cognitive symptoms, mild confusional symptoms, but no or mild parietal symptoms. The higher age at onset and high frequency of LA in the latter subgroup suggest that age-related changes and/or LA may account for the less focal symptomatology of this subgroup.

Acknowledgments

This study was supported by grants from the Astra Pharmaceuticals Ltd Junior Travel Fellowship; Bohuslandstingets FOU grupp; Kerstin och Bo Pfannenstills Stiftelse för Bekämpande av Själsliga och Nervösa Sjukdomar, Lund, Sweden; Fidia Research Laboratories, Abano Terme, Italy; Faculty of Medicine, University of Göteborg, Sweden; Svenska Läkaresällskapet, Stockholm, Sweden; Swedish Medical Research Council (03X-627 and 21X-05002-14C); Stiftelsen Gamla Tjänarinnor, Stockholm, Sweden; Stiftelsen Handlanden Hjalmar Svenssons Forskningsfond, Göteborg, Sweden and Svenska Sällskapet för Medicinsk Forskning, Stockholm, Sweden.

We would also like to thank Dr Christer Uhlemann, Dept of Radiology, Mölndal's Hospital, Sweden, for invaluable help.

REFERENCES

1. Sjögren T, Sjögren H, Lindgren Å. Acta Psych Neurol Scand 1952 (suppl. 82): 66-115.
2. Cummings JL, Benson DF. Dementia: a clinical approach. Boston: Butterworth, 1983.
3. Lishman WA. Organic psychiatry, the psychological consequences of cerebral disorder. 2nd ed. Oxford: Blackwell, 1987.
4. Tomlinson BE, Corsellis JAN. In Hume Adams J, Corsellis JAN, Duchen LW (eds) Greenfield's neuropathology. London: Edward Arnold, 1984: 951-1025.
5. Lauter H. Psychiatr Clin 1970; 3: 169-89.
6. Constantinidis J. In Katzman R, Terry RD, Bick KL (eds) Alzheimer's disease: senile dementia and related disorders (Aging, vol. 7). New York: Raven Press, 1978: 15-25.
7. Roth M. Br Med Bull 1986; 42: 42-50.
8. Sourander P, Sjögren H. In Wolstenholme GEW, O'Connors M (eds) Alzheimer's disease. Ciba Foundation Symposium. London: Churchill, 1970: 11-36.
9. Gottfries CG. Compr Gerontol 1988; 2: 47-62.
10. George AE, de Leon M, Gentes C et al. Am J Neuroradiol 1986; 7: 561-6.
11. Erkinjuntti T, Ketonen L, Sulkava R et al. Acta Neurol Scand 1987; 75: 262-70.
12. Steingart A, Hachinski VC, Lau C et al. Arch Neurol 1987; 44: 36-9.
13. Wallin A, Blennow K, Uhlemann C et al. Acta Neurol Scand 1989; 80: 518-23.
14. Blennow K, Wallin A, Gottfries CG. Int J Geriatr Psychiatry 1990; in press.
15. McKhann G, Drachman D, Folstein M et al. Neurology 1984; 34: 939-44.
16. Blennow K, Wallin A, Gottfries CG. Aging, in press.
17. Blennow K, Wallin A, Fredman P et al. Acta Neurol Scand 1990; 81: 323-6.

18. Laurell CB. Scand J Clin Lab Invest 1972; 29 (suppl. 124): 21–37.
19. Link H, Tibbling G. Scand J Clin Lab Invest 1977; 37: 391–6.
20. Steingart A, Hachinski VC, Lau C et al. Arch Neurol 1987; 44: 32–5.
21. American Psychiatric Association. Diagnostic and statistical manual of mental disorders. 3rd ed. Washington, DC: APA, 1987.
22. Koponen H. Delirium in the elderly. Dissertation, University of Kuopio, Finland, 1989.
23. Zatz L, Jernigan T, Ahumada A. J Comp Ass Tomogr 1982; 6: 19–23.
24. Gupta SR, Naheedy MH, Young JC et al. Arch Neurol 1988; 45: 637–41.
25. Englund E, Brun A, Alling C. Brain 1988; 111: 1425–39.
26. Brun A, Englund E. Ann Neurol 1986; 19: 253–62.
27. Inzitari D, Diaz F, Fox A et al. Arch Neurol 1987; 44: 42–7.
28. Milhorat T, Hammock K. In Wood JH (ed.) Neurobiology of cerebrospinal fluid. New York, London: Plenum, 1983: 1–23.
29. Rapoport S. Blood–brain barrier in physiology and medicine. New York: Raven Press, 1976: 129–52.

Address for correspondence:

Dr K. Blennow,
Department of Psychiatry and Neurochemistry,
University of Göteborg, S-422 03 Hisings Backa, Sweden

4 Psychopathology and Frontal Lobe Involvement in Organic Dementia

ARNE BRUN AND LARS GUSTAFSON

We have classified organic dementias according to main brain region preferentially involved and thereby also according to the dominating symptomatology, resulting in a close coordination between pathologic and clinical characteristics. The group of organic dementias with a frontal predominance would from a traditional point of view primarily be associated with Pick's disease, although the importance of other degenerative frontotemporal dementias of non-Alzheimer type has been pointed out (1-3). The aim of the present study was to elucidate which disorders of a primary degenerative, vascular or possible other type may commonly cause organic dementia with a mainly frontal symptomatology.

MATERIAL AND METHODS

Out of the 100 last cases in a long-term prospective clinical study those cases were selected that had a frontal symptomatology and a frontal reduction of regional cerebral blood flow (rCBF), measured by the 133-xenon technique. This material was supplemented with a group of 16 cases of frontal lobe degeneration of non-Alzheimer type (FLD) published earlier (1,2). The clinical picture was dominated by personality changes and emotional and language disturbances indicating frontal or frontotemporal cortical involvement, and usually these features appeared as an early manifestation of the dementing process. At autopsy the brains were processed with whole brain coronal semiserial sectioning in 5-μm thick sections for microscopical analysis. Using a large battery of histotechnical methods the changes found were recorded as to type, severity and topographic distribution.

RESULTS

Group 1 contains four female cases aged 83, 77, 81 and 69 years at death (Table 1). The mean duration of the disease was 9.5 years (range 4–17 years). These cases had a severe Alzheimer's disease with brain weights between 960 g and 1050 g. The Alzheimer encephalopathy was pronounced in the limbic and temporoparieto-occipital (TPO) areas but even more so in the frontal lobes with accentuated widening

Alzheimer's Disease: Basic Mechanisms, Diagnosis and Therapeutic Strategies
Edited by K. Iqbal, D. R. C. McLachlan, B. Winblad and H. M. Wisniewski
© 1991 John Wiley & Sons Ltd

Table 1. Patients with brain disease with frontal predominance

Case	Sex	Age at onset	Age at death	Duration (yr)	Diagnosis
1	F	76	83	7	DAT
2	F	67	77	10	DAT
3	F	64	81	17	DAT
4	F	65	69	4	DAT
5	F	52	74	22	SIWI
6	F	55	58	3	SIWI
7	M	76	83	7	SIWI
8	M	59	80	21	PSVE
9	M	60	67	7	PSVE
10	F	70	76	6	PSVE
11-26	M/F 7/9	56.3±7.7 (45-70)	64.3±8.1 (51-77)	8.1±3.4 (3-17)	FLD

DAT, dementia of Alzheimer type; SIWI, selective incomplete white matter infarction (8);
PSVE, progressive subcortical vascular encephalopathy (Binswanger's disease); FLD, frontal
lobe dementia of non-Alzheimer type (1,2).

Table 2. Clinical findings in primary degenerative and vascular dementia with frontal predominance

	FLD ($n=16$)	DAT ($n=4$)	SIWI ($n=3$)	PSVE ($n=3$)
Age at death (yr)	64±8	77.5±6.2	72±12.7	74±6.7
Duration (yr)	8±1.3 (3−17)	9.5±5.6 (4−17)	10.7±10 (3−22)	11±8.4 (6−21)
Early				
personality changes	16	3	2	3
loss of insight	12	3	1	1
disinhibition	8	3	3	1
Euphoria	6	2	1	2
Restlessness	11	1	1	2
Emotional lability	13	2	2	3
Stereotype speech	11	1	1	0
Echolalia	4	0	0	1
Mutism	12	2	0	0
Oral/dietary changes	5	0	1	0
Psychotic episodes	6	1	2	1
Hallucinosis	1	1	2	0
Grand mal	2	1	0	2
Increased muscular tension	4	3	1	1
Early normal EEG	9	0	1	1
Mean blood pressure (mmHg)	103±9.7	93±2.5	96±12	121±12.5

Abbreviations as in Table 1

of sulci and the ventricular system. In only one case were there mild cerebrovascular
lesions in the border zone (case 2). The clinical picture (Table 2) was that of a
progressive dementia which in two cases (cases 1 and 4) had a rather rapid course
during the first two years. Early dysmnesia dominated in three cases; all developed

dysphasia, dyspraxia and dysgnosia, and in three cases there were also extrapyramidal signs such as increase of muscular tension. In addition three cases showed early personality changes such as emotional lability and inadequate laughing (two cases), euphoria (two cases) and loss of insight (three cases). These symptoms indicated a frontal lobe involvement in good agreement with rCBF findings of an accentuated flow pathology in frontal or frontotemporal regions in addition to the temporoparietal flow reduction typical of dementia of Alzheimer type (DAT). The patients had few vascular risk factors and the mean blood pressure was fairly low (93±2.5 mmHg).

The three cases in group 2 (two females and one male), at death aged 83, 74 and 58 years respectively (Table 1), showed bilateral incomplete infarctions selectively in the white matter (SIWI) of the frontal lobes and in two cases also in the parietal lobes. Here there was a partial loss of axons, myelin and oligodendroglial cells with a mild reactive astrogliosis and few macrophages. Apart from an atheromatosis of basal and meningeal arteries of slight to moderate severity, there was a pronounced fibrohyaline narrowing arteriolosclerosis in the white matter areas showing the selective incomplete infarcts. There were no complete cavitating lesions and no or only minimal cerebrovascular lesions in grey matter. The anterior portion of the callosal body was thinned. The frontal lobes showed only a slight atrophy in one case, none in the other two cases. There were no degenerative changes of Alzheimer's type save for what is normal for age and no other pathological brain changes, except in one case a moderately severe degeneration of substantia nigra and a mild loss of Purkinje cells.

The age of onset of clinical symptoms (Table 2) varied from 52 to 76 years and the duration from 3 to 22 years. The onset was insidious and the course was slow in two cases and rapidly deteriorating in one (case 6). Personality changes with disinhibition and emotional lability with spells of anxiety and aggressiveness were frequent. Thus the symptomatology was mainly psychiatric and the neurological symptoms were less obvious. However, dizziness and unsteady gait was observed in two cases and a unilateral Babinski sign was found in the third case. The mean blood pressure was only 96±12 mmHg. RCBF was pathological with frontal abnormalities but with marked changes between repeated measurements. Case 5 showed for many years a marked general hyperemia, returning to normal and even subnormal levels only late in the course.

Group 3, two male and one female cases at death aged 80, 76 and 67 years respectively (Table 1), had Binswanger's disease with intracerebral hypertensive angiopathy and lacunar infarcts in basal ganglia, white matter, cerebellum and pons, and in one case a few somewhat larger infarcts. The lacunes in the white matter were surrounded by large incomplete infarcts where the tissue density was reduced as in group 1 (SIWI). The cortex was spared save for a few minimal infarcts. The subcortical lacunes and their perifocal lesions were most prominent in the frontal lobes in two cases and involved all lobes in the third. The ventricular system was generally enlarged, most pronounced frontally in the two cases with frontal white matter predominance of lesions. There were no Alzheimer changes in one case, slight and physiological for age in one case and mild in the third case.

The age of onset of symptoms (Table 2) varied from 59 to 70 years and the duration from 6 to 21 years. The clinical picture was dominated by emotional lability with periods of euphoria, apathy or depression. Disinhibition and loss of insight were uncommon in the progressive subcortical vascular encephalopathy (PSVE) patients. Two cases had a history of hypertension, and the mean blood pressure was 121 ± 12.5 mmHg at the time of diagnostic examination. Grand mal was reported in two cases.

Group 4, 16 cases aged 55–75 years (Table 1), had a frontal lobe degeneration of non-Alzheimer type reported earlier (1,2). It went with mild to not grossly noticeable frontal or frontotemporal atrophy but without circumscribed or 'knife blade' atrophy. Microscopically, mainly the convexities of the frontal lobes and in some cases also the anterior temporal pole showed a cortical degenerative change marked by a loss of neurons, mild gliosis and microcavitation, involving mainly the three superficial laminae. The amygdala and hippocampus revealed only slight changes in 13 cases and slightly more pronounced alterations in 3 cases. There were no Pick cells or ballooned cells and no plaques or tangles, but moderate diffuse deposits of amyloid without predilection for any region. The nucleus basalis of Meynert was normal and the striate body showed no to slight changes in 13 cases and moderately severe changes in 3 cases.

The typical clinical picture (Table 2) in FLD was that of a slowly progressive dementia with early loss of insight, restlessness, disinhibition, changes of oral/dietary behaviour, stereotypy of speech and behaviour and a progressive loss of expressive speech. A majority of cases became mutistic with reduced minimal activity but relatively spared receptive speech function. RCBF was consistently reduced frontally. Differential diagnosis against Pick's disease was extremely difficult on clinical grounds only, while clinical differentiation from DAT could be based on the clinical symptomatology, especially in the early phases. The confusing mixture of emotional, conative and organic symptoms in FLD also raises the question of differentiation from functional pyschotic states.

DISCUSSION

Whole brain coronal semiserial sectioning proved to be essential for the appreciation of quantity and distribution of the histopathological changes.

The distribution and accentuation of pathological changes correlated well with symptomatology and regional blood flow reductions.

Alzheimer's disease shows according to our experience a basic pattern (4–6) with a postcentral temporoparietal predominance of lesions and less severe involvement of the frontal lobes. This goes also for senile dementia of Alzheimer type (SDAT), although here the frontal involvement is more pronounced than in the presenile cases. All four cases included here were of the SDAT type. Against the background of our experience of more than 200 cases of this type the cases now under consideration showed clearly more frontal involvement than is usually the case even in SDAT. This is also in accord with the clinical impression of a more prominent frontal symptomatolo$_{\mathrm{gy}}$ and more pronounced frontal cerebral blood flow reduction than is usually the case in senile Alzheimer's disease (7). In these cases there was no other pathology and thus no cerebrovascular lesions including selective incomplete white matter infarction. Alzheimer's disease may thus in a limited proportion of cases impress as a mainly frontal lobe disease, an impression that can be explained on the basis of neuropathological data.

A frontal trait may also be added to Alzheimer's disease by selective incomplete white matter infarction (SIWI) which tends to strike most prominently in the frontal white matter in about a third of Alzheimer cases (8). This may add to the frontal symptomatology in a certain proportion of Alzheimer cases.

Besides these two confounding factors in a dementia material the frontal lobe white matter may show SIWI as the only lesion, as evidenced by the three cases in group 2. In the latter situation the symptomatology is vague and the diagnosis difficult, but it may be aided by magnetic resonance imaging (MR), CT or rCBF studies.

In Binswanger's disease the main lesions are widespread incomplete white matter infarctions in the frontal lobes. These surround small complete infarctions in the shape of lacunes which are thus quantitatively much less important. This frontal predominance is known from the literature (16). It results in a symptomatology with some similarities to frontal progressive degenerative brain disease. The Alzheimer encephalopathy in one of our cases was mild, particularly in the frontal lobes, and is not believed to have contributed in any important way to the frontal lobe symptomatology.

The frontal lobe degeneration of non-Alzheimer type reported earlier (1,2) showed a neuropathological and clinical picture that has been verified also in later unpublished cases. It emerges as a relatively common degenerative disease. It is far more common than Pick's disease, with which it has in common the main distribution of the lesions but with important differences relating to intensity and specific microscopical details such as Pick cells and ballooned cells. The cortical changes in FLD are rather more like those seen in amyotrophic lateral sclerosis (ALS) with frontal dementia (3,9,10). Our FLD cases, however, have no or occasionally minimal spinal or muscular pathology. Not included in this material but found in previous studies of FLD is Pick's disease in 2.5%.

Other diseases may have a frontal main point and also a frontal symptomatology. Thus cases of Creutzfeldt–Jakob disease and bilateral thalamic infarction may show a frontal symptomatology (1,11,12). The latter condition may be classified as projected frontal dementia, thus lacking frontal cortical or white matter changes. Other diseases of a similar nature are progressive subcortical gliosis (13), progressive supranuclear palsy (PSP) and some rare familial forms of dementia (14,15).

Thus the frontal lobe symptomatology, which is most easily recognized in Pick's disease and FLD, may also strongly colour the clinical picture of other dementing diseases with frontal predominance. The frontotemporal cortical degeneration in Pick's disease and FLD causes symptoms which stand out against the background of better preserved postcentral cortical functions. This symptom profile contrasts with the cognitive deterioration in DAT caused by the consistently dominant involvement of TPO cortex and posterior cingulate gyrus. Frontal lobe traits are less common in DAT, especially in the presenile group, possibly due to the relative sparing of precentral and anterior cingulate cortex. However, in a small but important group of DAT cases the frontal lobe involvement and symptoms partly overshadow the more typical DAT symptomatology. Then disinhibition, euphoria, and lack of insight may strongly influence the possibilities of the relatives caring for the patients.

The three SIWI cases displayed a productive psychiatric symptomatology and rather unspecific neurological features in combination with the frontal symptomatology. An organic etiology was suspected in all three cases, but the specific type of brain damage could not be settled until the postmortem investigation. A white matter involvement was however indicated by rCBF findings in case 5 and by CT and MR in case 6.

The clinical course in PSVE was of a more vascular type with stepwise deterioration and fluctuations with an ischemic score above 8 points in two cases. The frontal symptomatology was not so severe, especially concerning disinhibition and loss of insight.

Thus in spite of similarities in terms of frontal lobe symptomatology it might be possible to differentiate the four types of dementia with frontal predominance on the basis of additional clinical findings.

In conclusion, dementias of a frontal type account for a considerable percentage of the dementing disorders. They are to a large extent caused by degenerative diseases of the frontal lobes, but also by cerebrovascular frontal disease and by more remote but frontally projecting disorders.

Acknowledgment

The Alzheimer Association (USA) is acknowledged for a Senior International Travel Fellowship to participate in the Second International Conference on Alzheimer's Disease and Related Disorders.

REFERENCES

1. Brun A. Frontal lobe degeneration of non Alzheimer type: I. Neuropathology. Arch Geront Geriatr 1987; 6: 193–208.
2. Gustafson L. Frontal lobe degeneration of non Alzheimer type: II Clinical picture and differential diagnosis. Arch Geront Geriatr 1987; 6: 209–23.
3. Neary D, Snowden JS, Northen B, Goulding P. Dementia of frontal-lobe type. J Neurol Neurosurg Physchiat 1988; 51: 353–61.
4. Brun A. An overview of light and electron microscopical changes. In Riesberg B. (ed.) Alzheimer's disease: the standard reference. New York: Macmillan, 1983; 37–47.
5. Brun A, Gustafson L. Limbic lobe involvement in presenile dementia. Arch Psych Nervenkr 1978; 226: 79–93.
6. Brun A, Gustafson L, Risberg J, Hagberg B, Johansson A, Thulin AK, Englund E. Clinico-pathological correlates in dementia: a neuropathological, neuropsychiatric, neurophysiological and psychometric study. In Bergener M, Finkel SI (eds) Clinical and scientific psychogeriatrics. Vol. 2 The interface of psychiatry and neurology. New York: Springer, 1990: 1–28.
7. Risberg J, Gustafson L. Regional cerebral blood flow in psychiatric disorders. In Knezewic S et al. (eds) Handbook of regional cerebral blood flow. London: Lawrence Erlbaum, 1988: 219–40.

8. Brun A, Englund E. A white matter disorder in dementia of Alzheimer type: a patho-anatomical study. Ann Neurol 1986; 19: 253-62.
9. Morita K, Kaiya H, Ikeda T, Namba M. Presenile dementia combined with amyotrophy: a review of 34 Japanese cases. Arch Geront Geriatr 1987; 6: 263-77.
10. Neary D, Snowden JS, Mann DMA, Northen B, Goulding PJ, Macdermotte N. Frontal lobe dementia and motoneuron disease. J Neurol Neurosurg Psychiat 1990; 53: 23-32.
11. Schulman NS. Bilateral symmetrical degeneration of the thalamus. J Neuropath Exp Neurol 1957; 4: 446-70.
12. Stern K. Severe dementia associated with bilateral symmetric degeneration of the thalamus. Brain 1939; 62: 157-71.
13. Verity MA, Weschler AF. Progressive subcortical gliosis of Neumann: a clinico-pathologic study of 2 cases with a review. Arch Geront Geriatr 1987; 6: 245-62.
14. Kim RC, Collins GH, Parisi JE, Wright AW, Chu YB. Familial dementia of adult onset with pathological finding of a non specific nature. Brain 1981; 104: 61-78.
15. Massé G, Mikol J, Brion S. Atypical presenile dementia. Report of an anatomico-clinical case and review of the literature. J Neurol Sci 1981; 52: 245-67.
16. Ishii N, Nishihara Y, Imamura T. Why do frontal lobe symptoms predominate in vascular dementia with lacunes? Neurology 1986; 36: 340-5.

Address for correspondence:

Dr Arne Brun,
Department of Pathology,
University Hospital,
S-221 85 Lund,
Sweden

5 Myoclonus in Alzheimer's Disease

C. CLARK, A. HEYMAN, N. EARL, C. UTLEY AND C. HAYNES

The role of myoclonus as a marker for a subgroup of patients with Alzheimer's disease (AD) was determined in a cross-sectional and prospective longitudinal study of two separate patient populations.

In the cross-sectional study, 22 patients with myoclonus were matched by age and duration of dementia with an equal number of patients without myoclonus. No differences were observed between the two groups in the Mini-Mental State score, grade of deep tendon reflex, presence of extrapyramidal signs, or history of dementia in a first-degree relative.

In the longitudinal study 93 patients with early onset AD (symptoms before age 65 years) were followed prospectively for as long as eight years. Myoclonic jerks of the limbs or trunk were observed in 5 patients at entry and in 6 others during the period of follow-up observation. All 5 patients with myoclonus at entry were less than 59 years of age and survived for six years or longer. Although none of the 93 patients had major motor seizures at entry, 16 (including 8 with myoclonus) developed recurrent generalized convulsions during the later stages of the illness. The cumulative rates of myoclonus in this cohort were 5.4% and 18.4% respectively five and ten years after onset of the dementia, as compared with 1.2% and 18.2% respectively for generalized seizures in the same time period.

INTRODUCTION

The importance of myoclonus as a clinical characteristic of patients with rapidly progressive AD is controversial. Several papers reported the presence of myoclonus to be associated with rapid clinical deterioration and an average survival rate of less than two years (1,2). Myoclonus and major motor seizures may both appear during the natural course of AD, but the frequency with which they occur together and their relationship to the duration or severity of the dementing process remains uncertain.

In their retrospective study, Hauser and co-workers (1) reported that, during the course of dementia, 8 of 81 autopsy-confirmed cases of AD had generalized seizures and 8 others had myoclonus. Each of the 81 patients had been institutionalized in the late stages of dementia and information on the occurrence of seizure activity was based on a review of the medical records a number of years after the patient's death. Myoclonus was reported to be a late manifestation of AD and was associated

Alzheimer's Disease: Basic Mechanisms, Diagnosis and Therapeutic Strategies
Edited by K. Iqbal, D. R. C. McLachlan, B. Winblad and H. M. Wisniewski
© 1991 John Wiley & Sons Ltd

with a mean survival of less than one year. On the other hand, the study by Mayeux and co-workers (2) reported a 10% prevalence of myoclonus in the early stages of AD. They noted that the patients with myoclonus had a significantly earlier onset of dementia (mean 57.1 years) than those without myoclonus (mean 65.9 years). Kaye and Friedland also observed that myoclonus was associated with an earlier age of onset of dementia and that the illness was usually more severe in such cases (3).

This paper reports two studies of myoclonus in AD. The first is a cross-sectional study designed to determine if the clinical picture of patients with myoclonus differs significantly from those without myoclonus. The second study is a prospective longitudinal evaluation of cases with early onset AD (before age 66) designed to determine the frequency of myoclonus and major motor seizures in this cohort.

METHODS

The population of the cross-sectional study consisted of 285 patients with definite or probable AD based on NINCDS-ADRDA criteria (4) who were admitted between May 1986 and August 1989 to the Memory Disorders Clinic of the Bryan Alzheimer's Disease Research Center at Duke University.

Twenty-two of these 285 patients had the classical picture of myoclonus with isolated, uncontrolled muscle jerks of the arms, legs, or trunk. Each of these 22 patients was matched by age (within three years), and duration of symptoms (within two years) with a patient from the same study population who did not have myoclonus. Comparisons were made between the two groups as to differences in gender, specific clinical signs (i.e. gait disorders, deep tendon reflex abnormalities, and the presence of extrapyramidal changes in muscle tone such as cogwheeling or generalized rigidity), and a history of a first-degree blood relative with dementia.

The statistical evaluation was based on the analysis of the singly matched pairs. Continuous outcomes for matched pairs were compared using the Wilcox signed rank test. Other variables were considered as either absent or present. An exact P-value was determined using McNemar's method (5) which considers whether there is a lack of symmetry in the distribution of the two types of discordant pairs.

The patients in the longitudinal study consisted of 32 men and 61 women who had participated in clinical, genetic and epidemiologic studies of AD at Duke University Medical Center (6-8). Each patient had a standard battery of clinical, psychometric and laboratory studies. The clinical diagnoses of these patients (many of whom entered the study before 1980) were found in retrospect to meet the 1984 NINCDS-ADRDA consensus criteria for probable AD. The mean age at entry of the 93 patients was 62.2 years. Based on the Clinical Dementia Rating Scale described by Hughes et al. (9) 36 patients had mild dementia, 42 had moderate and 15 had severe dementia.

None of the 93 patients were lost during a follow-up period of two to eight years. Cumulative rates for the occurrence of seizure activity during the course of the dementing process were obtained using the method of Kaplan and Meier (10). During follow-up observation, 32 patients died, of whom 21 had pathological examination of the brain. Neuropathological evidence of AD was found in all 21 patients.

RESULTS

In the cross-sectional study the 22 patients with myoclonus had an earlier mean age of onset of dementia (59.3 years, range 57–72) when compared to that in the total group of 285 patients (66.7 years, range 40–86). No correlation was observed between gender and the presence of myoclonus.

Table 1 compares the age of the cases at entry to the study, the ages at onset of dementia, the duration of the illness, and the scores for the Disability Rating Scale (DRS) and the Mini-Mental-State examination. There was no difference between the two groups with respect to their cognitive impairment or functional disability as measured by the scores on either of the two rating measures.

Likewise there was no difference observed between the two groups as to the presence of unsteady gait, hyperactive deep tendon reflexes, presence of extrapyramidal signs or history of a first-degree relative with dementia (Table 2).

In the longitudinal study, 5 patients were observed to have myoclonus on entry to the study and 6 others later during the course of the observation period. The cumulative rate of myoclonus was 5.4% five years after the onset of dementia and increased to 18.4% by the tenth year (Figure 1). Each of the 5 patients with myoclonus on entry had symptoms of dementia prior to age 59. The presence of

Table 1. Comparison of patients with myoclonus to matched patients without myoclonus

		Myoclonus	No myoclonus
Mean age at onset of symptoms		59.3	59.9
	Range	(46–72)	(48–73)
Mean age at time of study		63.8	64.3
	Range	(49–79)	(52–78)
Duration of symptoms at entry		4.6 years	4.4 years
	Range	(1–10)	(1–8)
Disability rating score*		24	29
	Range	(5–45)	(5–37)
Mini-Mental State score**		9	14
	Range	(0–24)	(2–26)

*Scale 0 (no disability) to 55 (maximum disability).
**Scale 0 (no correct answers) to 30 (all answers correct).

Table 2. Outcomes for attribute in matched pairs: AD with myoclonus vs AD without myoclonus

Attribute	Concordant pairs		Discordant pairs		P-value
	+/+	−/−	+/−	−/+	
Abnormal gait	0	13	7	1	0.0703
Hyperactive tendon reflexes	0	15	3	3	1.0000
Extrapyramidal signs	2	10	6	3	0.5078
Family history of dementia	2	11	3	5	0.7266

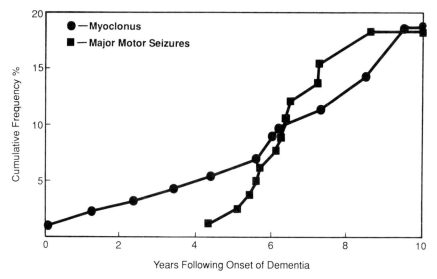

Figure 1. Rates of occurrence according to duration of dementia

myoclonus did not indicate a more severe prognosis, since all 5 patients survived for six years or longer. Three of the patients with myoclonus at entry died and autopsy confirmed the diagnosis of AD.

Although none of the 93 patients had major motor seizures at entry, 16 of them (including 8 patients with myoclonus) developed generalized convulsions during the late stages of the illness. The cumulative rates of major motor seizures were 1.2% and 15.6% respectively five and ten years after the first symptoms of AD (Figure 1). The development of major motor seizures in two patients was associated with a concurrent illness (i.e. hepatitis or pneumonia).

Each of the 5 patients who had myoclonus on entry into the study had an abnormal electroencephalogram with slow background electrical activity which was often associated with intermittent theta or delta waves in both frontal areas. In 2 of these 5 cases epileptiform activity was present. Two showed paroxysmal movements of the limbs and facial musculature on photic stimulation.

DISCUSSION

Myoclonus has long been recognized to develop in a small proportion of AD patients but its importance as a marker of heterogeneity of the illness and its implication for prognosis has never been fully determined. The pathological changes responsible for the appearance of myoclonus in AD remains unclear. In this study the presence of myoclonus did not appear to be associated with a more rapid downhill course of the illness.

The results of our cross-sectional study indicate that, although AD patients with myoclonus tend to have more gait problems and to be slightly more impaired from a functional standpoint, they do not differ significantly from those without myoclonus when matched for age, gender, or duration of dementia. Myoclonus appears to be associated with AD patients who had an earlier onset of dementia.

Our longitudinal study demonstrates that many patients who develop myoclonus will later develop major motor seizures. It seems clear that myoclonic jerks may occur in either the early or late stages of AD, but major motor convulsions usually are associated with the late stages of the illness.

The presence of myoclonus in a patient with dementia often raises the possibility of Creutzfeldt-Jakob disease. The EEG may not be helpful in that a diagnostically characteristic pattern may never, or only transiently, be seen in Creutzfeldt-Jakob disease (11). On the other hand, the EEG associated with myoclonus in AD may have a periodic pattern mimicking that seen in Creutzfeldt-Jakob (12,13).

The severity of myoclonus in AD varies from generalized or asymmetrical twitching of individual muscles to movements of entire muscle groups. Because of the overlap in the clinical manifestations of myoclonus between Creutzfeldt-Jakob and AD, biopsy of brain tissue may be necessary to obtain a completely accurate diagnosis, particularly in patients with a rapid, progressive illness.

The data provided by our longitudinal study indicates that in patients with early onset dementia the presence of myoclonus is not associated with a more rapidly progressive course of the illness. Both groups had a mean survival of 11 years after onset of dementia. Five patients are still alive six years after the onset of myoclonus. In general, myoclonus did not interfere with the patient's routine care.

The myoclonic jerking in our patients was multifocal. Thus, it is not surprising that in the longitudinal study 72% (8 of 11) developed generalized tonic-clonic seizures during the follow-up period. The pathophysiologic relationship between these two is not clear, but it seems reasonable to assume that they represent a continuum. There was no significant difference in the mean age of onset of dementia between the group with myoclonus (56.1 years) and those with major motor seizures (59.3 years).

The generalized tonic-clonic seizures occurred later in the illness and usually were a sign of poor prognosis. The average survival rate after the first major motor seizure was 2.5 years while the average survival rate following the onset of myoclonus was 5.2 years.

In summary, our studies show that the presence of myoclonus does not necessarily indicate a poor prognosis. Secondly, myoclonus can occur in the early stages of Alzheimer's disease, and in some cases may be seen within the first two years of symptoms. The cumulative rate of myoclonus after ten years was 18.4% in this group of 96 patients whose symptoms began at a mean age of 59. The third observation is that major motor seizures frequently develop in patients with myoclonus, but usually appear in the later stages of the disease.

These observations serve to highlight the heterogeneous nature of Alzheimer's disease and the difficulty of using a single clinical feature to define a particular subgroup or predict the course of the illness.

REFERENCES

1. Hauser WA, Morris ML, Heston LL, Anderson VE. Seizures and myoclonus in patients with Alzheimer's disease. Neurology 1986; 36: 1226-30.
2. Mayeux R, Stern Y, Spanton S. Heterogeneity in dementia of the Alzheimer type: evidence of subgroups. Neurology 1985; 35: 453-61.
3. Kaye JA, Moore AM, Friedland RF, Rapoport SI. Distinctive features of patients with dementia of the Alzheimer type and myoclonus. Ann Neurol 1988; 24: 132.
4. McKhann G, Drachman D, Folstein M, et al. Clinical diagnosis of Alzheimer's disease: Report of the NINCDS-ADRDA work group. Neurology 1984; 34: 939-44.
5. McNemar Q. Note on the sampling error of the differences between correlated proportions or percentages. In Fleiss J (ed) Statistical methods for rates and proportions, 2nd ed. New York: John Wiley & Sons, 1981: 114.
6. Heyman A, Wilkinson WE, Hurwitz BJ, Helms MJ, Haynes CS, Utler CM, Gwyther LP. Early-onset Alzheimer's disease: Clinical predictors of institutionalization and death. Neurology 1987; 37: 980-84.
7. Heyman A, Wilkinson WE, Hurwitz BJ, et al. Alzheimer's disease: genetic aspects and associated clinical disorders. Ann Neurol 1983; 14: 507-15.
8. Heyman A, Wilkinson WE, Staffard JA, et al. Alzheimer's disease: a study of epidemiologic aspects. Ann Neurol 1984; 15: 335-41.
9. Hughes CP, Berg L, Danziger WL, et al. A new clinical scale for staging of dementia. Br J Psychiatry 1982; 140: 566-72.
10. Peto R, Pike MC, Armitage P, et al. Design and analysis of randomized clinical trials requiring prolonged observation of each patient. II. Analysis and examples. Br J Cancer 1977; 35: 1-39.
11. Chiofalo N, Fuentes A, Galvez S. Serial EEG findings in 27 cases of Creutzfeldt-Jacob disease. Arch Neurol 1980; 37: 143-5.
12. Ehle A, Johnson P. Rapidly evolving EEG changes in a case of Alzheimer's disease. Ann Neurol 1977; 1: 593-5.
13. Watson CP. Clinical similarity of Alzheimer and Creutzfeldt-Jacob disease. Ann Neurol 1979; 6: 368-9.

Address for correspondence

Chris Clark,
Director, Memory Disorders Service,
Department of Neurology,
The Graduate Hospital,
Philadelphia, PA 19146, USA

Part II

NEUROIMAGING/BRAIN ENERGY METABOLISM

6 Positron Emission Tomography and Alzheimer's Disease

STANLEY I. RAPOPORT, BARRY HORWITZ, CHERYL L. GRADY, JAMES V. HAXBY, CHARLES DECARLI AND MARK B. SCHAPIRO

Measurements of brain functional activity during life, when correlated with the topography of postmortem neuropathology, indicate that Alzheimer's disease (AD) is a neurodegenerative disease which preferentially involves association neocortices and connected regions, and that it is a phylogenic disease. Thus, in AD patients, regional cerebral metabolic rates for glucose, $rCMR_{glc}$, as measured with positron emission tomography (PET), are more disturbed in association than in primary sensory or motor neocortical areas, and neuropathology is more severe in the association neocortices. Association cortical metabolism is asymmetric in mildly and moderately demented patients. The initial direction of asymmetry, which is maintained in a given patient as the disease progresses, predicts whether the patient will develop worse language deficits (lower initial left-sided metabolism) or worse visuospatial deficits (lower initial right-sided metabolism). Thus, PET can be used for the early diagnosis of AD and for characterizing its underlying asymmetric pathology. Despite displaying reduced resting glucose metabolism, visual association areas demonstrate equivalent (as percentage baseline) blood flow responses in mildly to moderately demented AD patients and in healthy controls who are performing a face-matching task. Thus, viability and integrity of these association areas are retained into the intermediate stage of disease.

INTRODUCTION

In the last decade, it has become possible to examine cerebral functional activity in awake men and women by means of positron emission tomography (PET) (1). With the appropriate positron emitting glucose analogue, ^{18}F-2-fluoro-2-deoxy-D-glucose (^{18}FDG), we can determine regional cerebral metabolic rates for glucose, $rCMR_{glc}$, within regions of the human brain as small as 6 mm in diameter, on the cortical surface as well as subcortically. As glucose is the major substrate for brain oxidative metabolism, its rate of consumption is a direct measure of brain functional activity.

Alzheimer's Disease: Basic Mechanisms, Diagnosis and Therapeutic Strategies
Edited by K. Iqbal, D. R. C. McLachlan, B. Winblad and H. M. Wisniewski
©1991 John Wiley & Sons Ltd

In this chapter, we review results of studies using PET and ^{18}FDG by members of the Laboratory of Neurosciences, National Institute on Aging, on patients with Alzheimer's disease (AD), and we relate these results to the topographic distribution of neuropathology in the postmortem AD brain. We conclude that AD is a degenerative disorder selective for brain regions which constitute an association 'system', and that it can be classified as a phylogenic disease.

BRAIN METABOLISM AND COGNITION IN ALZHEIMER'S DISEASE

To measure rCMR$_{glc}$ in an awake subject, ^{18}FDG is injected intravenously, and plasma radioactivity and glucose concentration are determined periodically until, after about 45 min, regional brain radioactivity is determined with PET in horizontal cross-sections of the brain. ^{18}FDG is phosphorylated within the brain, but is not further metabolized nor rapidly dephosphorylated, due to a low activity of brain phosphatase. Its rate of accumulation is used to calculate rCMR$_{glc}$ and to construct metabolic images of the brain (1).

PET was performed when subjects were at rest, with eyes covered and ears plugged with cotton. A medium-resolution PET scanner (ECAT II, Life Sciences, Oak Ridge, TN), with a resolution of 17 mm, was employed initially in our studies, followed — when it became available — by a high resolution scanner (PC 1024-7B, Scanditronix, Uppsala, Sweden), with an in-plane resolution of 6 mm and an axial resolution of 10 mm, and with an empirical attenuation correction.

The regional CMR$_{glc}$ was studied in relation to severity of dementia in AD patients, and in age-matched healthy controls. The AD patients were screened for illnesses other than AD which might contribute to cerebral dysfunction. AD (possible or probable) was diagnosed according to NINCDS-ADRDA criteria for choosing patients for research purposes (2). Severity of dementia was assessed with the Folstein mini-mental state examination (3): mild score 21–30; moderate score 11–20; severe score 0–10.

Subjects also were administered an extensive neuropsychological test battery (4). As a group, mildly demented AD patients had significantly reduced scores in tests of memory (Wechsler memory scale: delayed story recall and delayed figure production) as compared with age-matched healthy controls, but not in tests of language (syntax comprehension, Boston naming) or of visuospatial ability (extended range drawing, Benton facial recognition). Moderately demented patients, however, demonstrated decrements in these language and visuospatial test scores, frequently more so in one score than in the other (syntax/drawing discrepancy, see below).

Differences between mean resting rCMR$_{glc}$ values in AD patients and in healthy controls were statistically significant for severely demented patients but not for moderately or mildly demented patients, due in part to the large 25% standard deviation of the absolute rCMR$_{glc}$ values (5). In the severely demented patients, as illustrated by Figure 1 (see colour plate), association but not primary sensory or motor neocortices had the greatest reductions in rCMR$_{glc}$. However, when the standard deviation of the data was reduced to about 5% of the mean by calculating ratios of association to primary rCMR$_{glc}$ values, the parietal and lateral temporal

Table 1. Relative metabolic rates in Alzheimer's disease

Metabolic ratio*	Controls $n=30$	Mild AD $n=12$	Mod AD $n=15$	Severe AD $n=8$
Parietal/sensorimotor	0.93±0.05	0.83±0.09†	0.85±0.09†	0.72±0.08†
Frontal/sensorimotor	0.97±0.07	0.94±0.06	0.92±0.11	0.87±0.18†
Lat. temporal/occipital	0.85±0.08	0.76±0.11†	0.77±0.11†	0.66±0.09†

*Ratio of rCMR$_{glc}$ values.
†Mean±SD differs from control by Bonferroni t test (P<0.05).
ECAT II data from Haxby et al (4).

cortices were shown to be metabolically abnormal even in the mildly and moderately demented AD patients (Table 1) (4).

METABOLIC AND COGNITIVE ASYMMETRIES IN ALZHEIMER'S DISEASE

To localize small changes in neocortical metabolism in individual AD patients, Haxby et al (6) defined a metabolic asymmetry index (%) for homologous right and left brain regions,

$$\text{Asymmetry index} = \frac{\text{rCMR}_{glc}, \text{ right} - \text{rCMR}_{glc}, \text{ left}}{(\text{rCMR}_{glc}, \text{ right} + \text{rCMR}_{glc}, \text{ left})/2} \times 100 \qquad (1)$$

Metabolic asymmetry indices were calculated for mildly and moderately demented AD patients and for healthy controls, from rCMR$_{glc}$ data obtained with the ECAT II tomograph. Significantly greater variances of asymmetry were demonstrated, as compared with controls, in frontal, parietal, and temporal association regions, but not in primary sensorimotor or occipital (visual) cortices (Figure 2) (6), indicating that AD involves the association neocortices, while sparing comparatively primary sensory and motor regions. When the AD patients were divided according to dementia severity, both the mildly and moderately demented patients were shown to have significantly increased variance of asymmetry in the association neocortices, as compared with controls (Table 2) (4).

Metabolic asymmetries, once evident in the association cortices of mildly demented patients, maintained their direction and increased in magnitude as the disease progressed. This is illustrated in Figure 3 for 11 AD patients who first were studied when mildly impaired, and then were evaluated repeatedly for 25 to 47 months (7,8). These results suggest that AD starts in one or the other hemisphere in an individual patient (initial focus), and that there is an underlying asymmetric pathology. In this regard, Arendt et al (9) reported asymmetrical distributions of senile (neuritic) plaques in the neocortex, and of correlated cell loss in the nucleus basalis of Meynert, in postmortem AD brains.

Studies of patients with focal brain damage suggest that syntax comprehension, mental arithmetic and immediate verbal memory are related to functions of regions in the left parietal and temporal lobes, whereas visuospatial construction is related

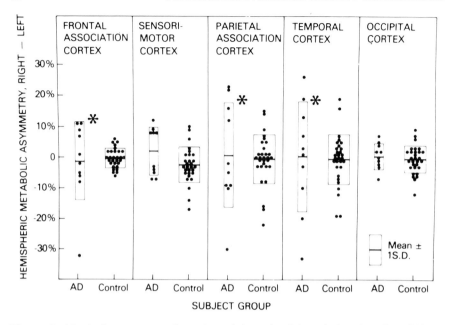

Figure 2. Metabolic asymmetry (eqn. 1, text) in each of 5 cortical regions in mildly to moderately demented AD patients and controls. Values are right minus left $rCMR_{glc}$ values, divided by the mean, per cent.* Coefficient of variation differs from control value. ECAT II data from Haxby et al (6)

Table 2. Metabolic asymmetry indices in Alzheimer's disease patients

Glucose utilization asymmetry index	Controls $n = 29$	Mild AD $n = 10$	Moderate AD $n = 12$
Frontal association cortex	0.00 ± 0.03	-0.01 ± 0.08***	-0.02 ± 0.12***
Parietal association cortex	0.00 ± 0.06	0.00 ± 0.12*	0.02 ± 0.14***
Lateral temporal cortex	-0.01 ± 0.08	-0.05 ± 0.18**	-0.04 ± 0.19***

Mean $\pm$ SD is given. Variance is greater than in controls: *$P < 0.05$; **$P < 0.01$; ***$P < 0.001$. Asymmetry index defined by eqn. 1 (text). ECAT II data from Haxby et al (4).

to right parietal lobe function (4,6,10). To see whether the metabolic asymmetries in AD corresponded to appropriate neocortically mediated cognitive deficits, Haxby et al (4) used the syntax comprehension test to test left hemispheric function, and the extended range drawing test to examine right hemispheric function. AD patients were ranked separately on the test scores; the difference between the ranks was calculated as a 'syntax/drawing discrepancy'.

As illustrated by Table 3, the metabolic asymmetry index was correlated significantly and appropriately with the syntax/drawing discrepancy in moderately demented patients, but not in mildly demented patients or controls. These observations are consistent with evidence that mean language and mean visuospatial test scores are reduced significantly in moderately demented but not in mildly

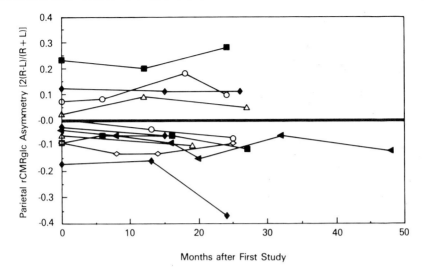

Figure 3. Stability of right–left metabolic asymmetry in parietal association cortices of 11 initially mildly demented patients. From Grady et al (7,8)

Table 3. Correlations between right–left metabolic asymmetries and drawing/syntax comprehension discrepancy

Cortical region	Controls $n=30$	Mild AD $n=12$	Moderate AD $n=15$
Frontal association	−0.30	−0.01	0.71*
Parietal association	−0.11	−0.20	0.73*
Lateral temporal	−0.08	0.01	0.49

*$P<0.05$. From Haxby et al (4).

demented AD patients (see above) (4). Correlations between metabolic asymmetry and cognitive discrepancy were significant and in the expected direction for the frontal and parietal association neocortices, but not for the lateral temporal, sensory or motor regions. Thus, a lower left-sided rCMR$_{glc}$ corresponded to a worse syntax score, and a lower right-sided rCMR$_{glc}$ corresponded to a worse drawing test score.

These cross-sectional results are supported by results of repeated cognitive testing of the 11 AD patients who demonstrated stable metabolic asymmetries for periods of 25 to 47 months (see Figure 3) (7,8). Whereas the mildly demented AD patients on initial evaluation did not display a significant correlation between metabolic asymmetry and discrepancy on syntax/drawing test scores, statistically significant correlations in the appropriate directions (e.g. right-sided hypometabolism and worse visuospatial score, left-sided hypometabolism and worse language score) were evident on follow-up (8,11).

The above data are the first demonstration, in individual AD patients studied repeatedly over extended periods of time, (a) that the direction of metabolic asymmetry is constant in a given AD patient for up to 50 months, (b) that the magnitude of metabolic asymmetry increases with time, and (c) that the heterogeneous metabolic asymmetries that appear early in the disease precede and accurately predict the heterogeneous deficits in neocortically mediated cognitive functions that later appear and establish the individual dementia profile.

PET ACTIVATION STUDIES IN ALZHEIMER'S DISEASE

Grady et al (12) recently determined to what extent association brain regions, whose resting $rCMR_{glc}$ values are reduced, can be activated when an AD patient performs a given cognitive task. They examined regional cerebral blood flow (rCBF) with PET in subjects performing a face-matching task, and found remarkably few differences in the activation pattern between mildly to moderately demented AD patients and controls. Regional CBF was measured with the positron-emitting $H_2^{15}0$, using the Scanditronix PC 1024-7B PET scanner (see above). In each subject, rCBF during a control task was subtracted from rCBF during the face-matching task, and flow differences which exceeded 30% (+2 standard deviations) of the baseline were identified.

As illustrated in Figure 4, 30% or greater activation of normalized rCBF during face matching occurred bilaterally in occipital and occipitotemporal regions — more medial primary visual cortices (not shown) also were activated — in both control and AD subjects. The areas activated are homologous to visual association areas for object recognition in the rhesus monkey (13,14). Thus, although resting metabolism is reduced in visual association areas in mildly to moderately demented AD patients, these areas remain viable and can respond to the same proportional extent in AD patients as in controls during face matching. Their coherent activation demonstrates that the cortical association network which subserves face recognition remains intact in mildly to moderately demented AD patients.

DISCUSSION

PET demonstrates selectively reduced resting glucose utilization in association as compared with primary sensory and motor neocortical regions in living AD patients, and early and maintained asymmetrical metabolic abnormalities, predictive of later-appearing syntax/drawing cognitive discrepancies, in the association neocortices.

On postmortem, numerous studies have demonstrated that neuropathology — cortical atrophy, gliosis, senile (neuritic) plaques, and neurofibrillary tangles — also is more selective for association than primary sensory and motor neocortical areas of the AD brain (15-19). This selectivity is especially evident with regard to neurofibrillary tangles with paired helical filaments (17,18). Indeed, DeCarli et al (20) and Rapoport et al (21) recently showed that cortical association regions which had the most severe reductions in $rCMR_{glc}$ during life in 5 individual AD patients had the highest densities of neurofibrillary tangles, whereas primary and sensory regions with the least metabolic changes had the lowest tangle densities ($P<0.01$). A statistically significant correlation between $rCMR_{glc}$ and neuritic plaque density was not found ($P>0.05$).

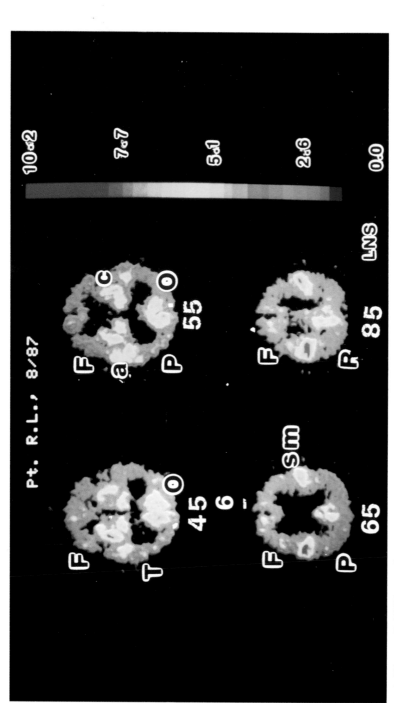

Figure 1 (*Chapter 6*). PET scans from severely demented patient with Alzheimer's disease. rCMR$_{glc}$, derived with a Scanditronix tomograph, in units of mg.100 g^{-1} min^{-1}. High metabolic rates are retained in the primary sensorimotor cortex (sm), primary visual cortex (o), primary auditory cortex (a), caudate and lenticular nuclei (c), but are reduced elsewhere in the brain. P; parietal lobe; F, frontal cortex; T, temporal cortex; O, occipital cortex. Numbers below scans are mm above inferior orbitomeatal line. (Laboratory of Neurosciences, National Institute on Aging)

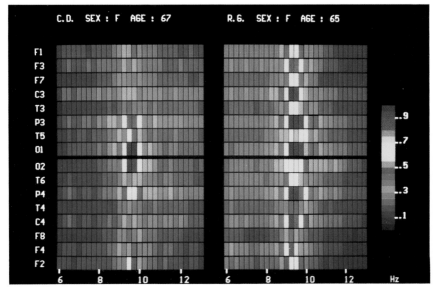

Figure 1 *(Chapter 9)*. HRSI of power (square root). Normal subjects (C.D., R.G.)

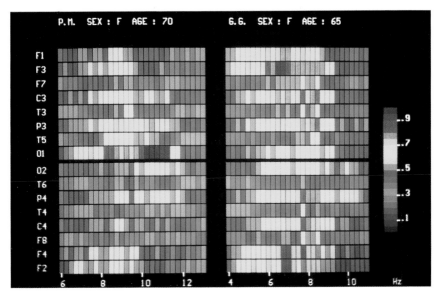

Figure 2 *(Chapter 9)*. HRSI of power (square root). SDAT patients (P.M., G.G.)

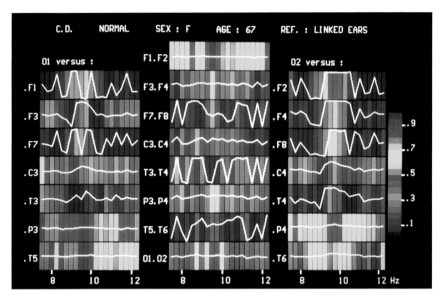

Figure 3 *(Chapter 9)*. HRSI of coherence and phase. Normal subject (C.D.)

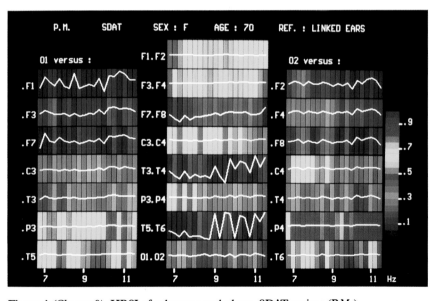

Figure 4 *(Chapter 9)*. HRSI of coherence and phase. SDAT patient (P.M.)

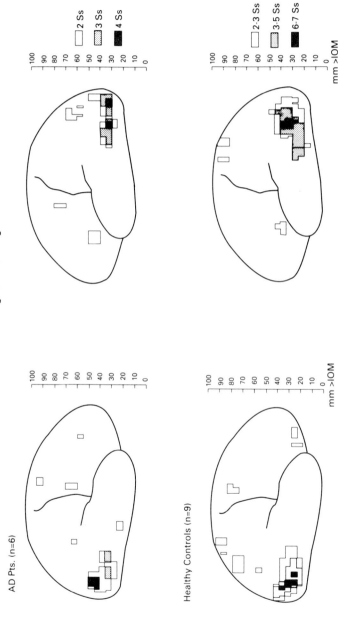

Figure 4. Cerebral blood flow activation patterns in Alzheimer's disease patients and healthy controls, on lateral hemispheric surfaces. Areas activated are identified if rCBF (normalized to whole brain rCBF) was 30% higher during face-matching task than in control sensorimotor task. Numbers of subjects in which this occurred are indicated. Scale gives level (mm) of brain region above inferior orbitomeatal (IOM) line. From Grady et al (12)

Many brain regions are too small to be readily visualized with PET. Nevertheless, postmortem studies of AD patients demonstrate neuropathology in many of these regions which are connected with the association neocortices, forming together an association 'system' (22-24). AD pathology is found in layers II and IV of the entorhinal cortex; the subiculum, CA1 region and outer two-thirds of the dentate gyrus of the hippocampal formation; the cortico-basolateral nuclear group of the amygdaloid complex; the nucleus basalis of Meynert; and midbrain-mesencephalic nuclear regions which project to the neocortex (9,22,23,26-30).

Thus, PET-derived measurements of resting $rCMR_{glc}$, when related to the topography of neuropathology post mortem, suggest that AD is a primary neurodegenerative disease which affects selectively regions of a brain association system — the association neocortices and subcortical regions with which they form direct and important reciprocal connections (31). As this association system has evolved markedly in higher primates and particularly in humans (22,24), its vulnerability to the AD process suggests that AD is a phylogenic disease, made likely by changes in the primate genome during evolution (22,23).

If this interpretation is correct, differences in gene expression between AD-vulnerable and AD-nonvulnerable regions of the human brain, and between the brains of human and nonhuman primates, should elucidate genetic factors which contribute to AD (22). In this regard, chromosome 21 may contain some of these differentially expressed genes. This chromosome has been implicated in some cases of early-onset familial AD (although not in other familial cases) (32-34), and brains of Down subjects older than 40 years exhibit neurochemical abnormalities, and neuropathology with the same densities, chemical and antigenic properties, and regional distributions as do brains of Alzheimer patients (25,26,35-37). Furthermore, as in AD, resting glucose metabolism is more abnormal in the association than in the sensory or motor neocortices of older, demented Down subjects (38,39).

REFERENCES

1. Huang S-C, Phelps ME, Hoffman EJ, Sideris K, Selin CJ, Kuhl DE. Am J Physiol 1980; 238: E69-82.
2. McKhann G, Drachman D, Folstein M, Katzman R, Price D, Stadlan EM. Neurology 1984; 34: 939-44.
3. Folstein MF, Folstein SE, McHugh PR. J Psychiat Res 1975; 12: 189-98.
4. Haxby JV, Grady CL, Duara R, Schlageter N, Berg G, Rapoport SI. Arch Neurol 1986; 43: 882-5.
5. Duara R, Grady CL, Haxby JV, Sundaram M, Cutler NR, Heston L, Moore A, Schlageter NL, Larson S, Rapoport SI. Neurology 1986; 36: 879-87.
6. Haxby JV, Duara R, Grady CL, Cutler NR, Rapoport SI. J Cereb Blood Flow Metab 1985; 5: 193-200.
7. Grady CL, Haxby JV, Schlageter NL, Berg G, Rapoport SI. Neurology 1986; 36: 1390-2.
8. Grady CL, Haxby JV, Horwitz B, Sundaram M, Berg G, Schapiro M, Friedland RP, Rapoport SI. J Clin Exp Neuropsychol 1988; 10: 576-96.
9. Arendt T, Bigl V, Tennstedt A, Arendt A. Neuroscience 1985; 14: 1-14.
10. Benton A. In Heilman KM, Valenstein E (eds) Clinical neuropsychology, 2nd edn. Oxford: Oxford University Press, 1985.
11. Haxby JV, Grady CL, Friedland RP, Rapoport SI. J Neural Trans 1987; 24 (suppl.): 49-53.

12. Grady C, Haxby J, Horwitz B, Schapiro M, Carson R, Herscovitch P, Rapoport SI. Soc Neurosci Abstr 1990; 16: 149.
13. Mishkin M, Ungerleider LG, Macko KA. Trends Neurosci 1983; 6: 414-17.
14. Haxby JV, Grady CL, Horwitz B, Schapiro MB, Carson RE, Ungerleider LG, Mishkin M, Herscovitch P, Friedland RP, Rapoport SI. Soc Neurosci Abstr 1988; 14: 750.
15. Brun A, Gustafson L. Arch Psychiatr Nervenkr 1976; 223: 15-33.
16. Pearson RC, Esiri MM, Hiorns RW, Wilcock GK, Powell TPS. Proc Natl Acad Sci (USA) 1985; 82: 4531-4.
17. Rogers J, Morrison JH. J Neurosci 1985; 5: 2801-8.
18. Lewis DA, Campbell MJ, Terry RD, Morrison JH. J Neurosci 1987; 7: 1799-1808.
19. Najlerahim A, Bowen DM. Acta Neuropathol (Berl) 1988; 75: 509-12.
20. DeCarli C, Atack JR, Ball MJ, Kaye JA, Grady CL, Fewster P, Katz D, Schapiro MB, Rapoport SI (in preparation).
21. Rapoport SI, Horwitz B, Grady CL, Haxby JV, DeCarli C, Schapiro MB. In 1st Toronto-Stockholm Symposium on perspectives in diabetes research, the nervous system and fuel homeostasis. New York: Plenum, in press.
22. Rapoport SI. Rev Neurol (Paris) 1988; 144: 79-90.
23. Rapoport SI. Med Hypotheses 1989; 29: 147-50.
24. Rapoport SI. Brain Res Revs (in press).
25. Ball MJ, Nutall K. Neuropath Appl Neurobiol 1981; 7: 13-20.
26. Mann DMA, Yates PO, Marcyniuk B. Neuropathol Appl Neurobiol 1984; 10: 185-207.
27. Mann DMA, Yates PO, Marcyniuk B. Neurosci Lett 1985; 56: 51-5.
28. Mann DMA, Marcyniuk B, Yates PD, Neary D, Snowden JS. Neuropathol Appl Neurobiol 1988; 14: 177-95.
29. Hyman BT, Van Hoesen GW, Kromer LJ, Damasio AR. Ann Neurol 1986; 20: 472-81.
30. Rapoport SI. In Rapoport SI, Petit H, Leys D, Christen Y (eds) Imaging, cerebral topography and Alzheimer's disease. Berlin: Springer, 1990; 1-17.
31. Rapoport SI, Horwitz B, Haxby JV, Grady CL. Can J Neurol Sci 1986; 13: 540-5.
32. St George-Hyslop PH, Tanzi RE, Polinsky RJ, Haines JL, Nee L, Watkins PC, Myers RH, Feldman RG, Pollen D, Drachman D, Growdon J, Bruni A, Foncin J-F, Salmon D, Frommelt P, Amaducci L, Sorbi S, Piacentini S, Stewart GD, Hobbs WJ, Conneally PM, Gusella JF. Science (Wash.) 1987; 235: 885-90.
33. Roses AD, Pericak-Vance MA, Haynes CS, Haines JL, Gaskell PA, Yamaoka LH, Hung W-Y, Clark CM, Alberts MJ, Lee JE, Siddique T, Heyman AL. Neurology 1988; 38 (suppl. 1): 173.
34. Schellenberg GD, Bird TD, Wijsman EM, Moore DK, Boehnke M, Bryant EM, Lampe TH, Nochlin D, Sumi SM, Deeb SS, Beyreuther K, Martin GM. Science (Wash.) 1988; 241: 1507-10.
35. Ball MJ, Fisman M, Hachinski V, Blume W, Fox A, Kral VA, Kirshen AJ, Fox H, Merskey H. Lancet 1985; i: 14-16.
36. Casanova MF, Walker LC, Whitehouse PJ, Price DL. Ann Neurol 1985; 18: 310-13.
37. Wiśniewski KE, Wiśniewski HM, Wen GY. Ann Neurol 1985; 17: 278-82.
38. Schapiro MB, Haxby JV, Grady CL, Rapoport SI. In Epstein CJ (ed.) The neurobiology of Down syndrome. New York: Raven Press, 1986: 89-108.
39. Schapiro MB, Rapoport SI. Brain Dysfunction 1988; 1: 2-11.

Address for correspondence:

Dr Stanley I. Rapoport,
Laboratory of Neurosciences,
National Institutes of Health, Bldg 10,
Rm 6C103, Bethesda, MD 20892, USA

7 Brain Energy Metabolism and its Significance for Alzheimer's Disease

SIEGFRIED HOYER

An adequate formation and turnover rate of energy in the form of ATP guarantees the maintenance of intracellular/extracellular ion homeostasis, axoplasmatic flux, synaptic function and structural integrity of any neuron. In the healthy, mature, nonstarved mammalian brain, 38 mol of ATP is formed from 1 mol of glucose. Glycolysis yields a total of 8 mol of ATP, 6 mol of which is derived from oxidation of $NADH_2$ generated in the glycerine aldehyde phosphate dehydrogenase reaction. Equivalents for the formation of another 30 mol of ATP are provided by mitochondrial oxidation via pyruvate dehydrogenase, isocitrate dehydrogenase, α-ketoglutarate dehydrogenase, succinate dehydrogenase, and malate dehydrogenase. Thus, although a total of 8 mol of ATP derives from glycolysis, only 2 mol of ATP (about 5%) is formed by other processes than oxidation (1). Nearly one half (47%) of the oxidation equivalents for ATP production are formed in the multienzyme complexes pyruvate dehydrogenase, isocitrate dehydrogenase and α-ketoglutarate dehydrogenase. These reactions can be activated by Ca^{2+} (2), and are capable of decarboxylation. In dementia of Alzheimer type (DAT), one prominent abnormality was found to be in the cerebral glucose metabolism (for review, see 3). In this chapter, the implications of a reduced cerebral metabolic rate (CMR) of glucose and of a diminished CMR of oxygen for energy production and related metabolism are discussed with respect to early-onset DAT and late-onset DAT (4).

BRAIN ENERGY METABOLISM IN DAT

In both suspected incipient early-onset DAT (EODAT) and suspected incipient late-onset DAT (LODAT), the CMR of glucose was found to be reduced by an average of 44% although the glucose supply to the brain was undisturbed. In EODAT, the CMR of oxygen was in the normal range, whereas in LODAT it was diminished by 20%. In EODAT, the lactate/glucose ratio increased from 0.06 (control) to 0.25, and in LODAT to 0.15, indicating an enhanced glycolytic breakdown of glucose (5,6). Recent findings documented an increased activity of lactate dehydrogenase in several brain areas in obvious EODAT (7). The oxidizable amount of glucose can thus be assumed to be decreased further. These findings may indicate a severe imbalance in the metabolic pathways of oxygen and glucose, and especially of glucose

Alzheimer's Disease: Basic Mechanisms, Diagnosis and Therapeutic Strategies
Edited by K. Iqbal, D. R. C. McLachlan, B. Winblad and H. M. Wisniewski
© 1991 John Wiley & Sons Ltd

leading to a lack of available neuronal glucose and thus giving rise to an energy deficit in the brain.

The ATP production in the brain can easily be calculated from the CMR of oxygen (measured) and the amount of oxidizable glucose calculated from the CMRs determined for glucose and lactate. Data recorded in healthy controls and in patients suffering from suspected incipient EODAT and LODAT are listed in Table 1. It becomes obvious that the ATP production decreases only slightly, by less than 10%, as normal aging progresses. In contrast, in the two dementia types considered here, ATP production solely from glucose oxidation is only 46% (EODAT) and 54% (LODAT) of that in age-matched controls. However, even these reduced levels are at least twice as high as those found in homogenates of freshly sampled cortical brain tissue in DAT patients in vivo (9).

It has been well established that glucose-C is rapidly transferred into amino acids, which are assumed to be compartmented in the brain: a metabolic compartment and a storage compartment from which amino acids can be released when glucose is lacking are assumed (10,11). Furthermore, a small compartment of free fatty acids may be assumed to be present in the brain (12). Thus, in the brain, the conditions are right for oxygen not necessarily used for glucose oxidation, as in the DAT brain, to oxidize substrates other than glucose, e.g. amino acids or free fatty acids (or both), to mitigate the severe energy deficit described above. The use of amino acids for oxidation could mean an additional 3.62 μmol/g.min ATP in EODAT, and an

Table 1. Cerebral metabolic rates (CMRs, measured and calculated) of oxygen (O_2), CO_2, oxidizable glucose ($Gluc_{ox}$), lactate (Lact) and ATP in normal elderly men (NEM) and patients with incipient early-onset (EODAT) and late-onset DAT (LODAT), and healthy age-matched controls (AMC)

	CMRs in μmol/g.min				
	O_2	CO_2	$Gluc_{ox}$	Lact	ATP
NEM (71 yr)					
(from Dastur, 8)					
measured	1.49		0.26*		
calculated	1.44		0.24		8.64 ~ 92% of AMC
balance	−0.05				
AMC (44 yr)					
measured	1.54	1.67	0.26	0.02	
calculated	1.56				9.36
balance	−0.02	+0.11			
EODAT (46 yr)					
measured	1.45	1.50	0.12	0.04	
calculated	0.72				4.32 ~ 46% of AMC
balance	+0.73	+0.78			
LODAT (66 yr)					
measured	1.27	1.24	0.14	0.02	
calculated	0.84				5.04 ~ 54% of AMC
balance	+0.43	+0.60			

*Inclusive Lact

additional 2.15 μmol/g.min ATP in LODAT, improving the ATP levels to 85% and 77%, respectively, of the values in age-matched controls. In the case of the oxidation of free fatty acids, the ATP deficit would be limited to give 77% in EODAT and 72% in LODAT, compared with age-matched controls. The utilization of these metabolic pathways, either alone or mixed, might explain the normal amount of CO_2 released, which was adapted to the CMR of oxygen (Table 1). The former was reported not to be reduced when studied in cortical brain tissue sampled from DAT patients in vivo (9). Furthermore, the ATP production rates calculated as described here are indeed in the same range as were found in vivo in the brain cortex of DAT patients (9). Thus, a permanent and presumably progressive energy deficit may be expected to be present in the brains of persons with incipient EODAT and incipient LODAT, giving rise to neuronal stress.

Glucose-related metabolism and consequences of energy deficit in DAT

There is evidence for the utilization of endogenous glutamate in the glucose-deprived EODAT brain. It is assumed that glutamate condenses with oxaloacetate to form α-ketoglutarate and aspartate in the aspartate aminotransferase reaction (13), the former being used for oxidation in the tricarboxylic acid cycle. Otherwise, the activities of lipases degrading phospholipids were found to be increased in cortex and hippocampus of DAT brain (14). This may indicate an enhanced formation of acetyl-CoA from β-oxidation rendering it possible for substrate to be oxidized in the tricarboxylic acid cycle. If this is so, the reduced formation of oxidation equivalents may be limited to glycerine aldehyde phosphate dehydrogenase and pyruvate dehydrogenase, and will not affect isocitrate dehydrogenase. Which of these catabolic pathways will be set in motion, to what degree, and in what sequence remains to be resolved.

In mixed cerebral cortical cell cultures, glucose deprivation induced disintegration in many neurons, whereas glial cells remained unchanged. Neuronal damage continued to increase for some hours after glucose deprivation had been reversed (15). Additional removal of extracellular glutamine potentiated the neuronal damage in a concentration-dependent manner (16). These data may be indicative not only of the nutrient effect of glutamine via glutamate, but also of the associated mediation of neurotoxic effects of glutamate/aspartate. Aspartate was found to accumulate in frontal and temporal brain cortex in antemortem DAT (17), and to be released in high concentrations from the EODAT brain (13). In glucose-deprived conditions, e.g. DAT, ammonia is generated endogenously in the brain (18), and the major source of it may be assumed to be glutamine (19).

Although the substitution of neuronal glucose deprivation by amino acids, preferentially glutamate and glutamine, may show some benefit for energy metabolism (see above), detrimental effects initiated subsequently may prevail. Reduced energy availability renders even a normal concentration of glutamate neurotoxic via the N-methyl-D-aspartate (NMDA) receptor (20). Increased aspartate binding to the NMDA receptor changes intracellular calcium homeostasis (21–23), and intracellular calcium was found to be enhanced after neuronal glucose deprivation (24).

Disturbances of neuronal calcium homeostasis contribute considerably to cellular damage and to cell death in vulnerable neuronal populations (25). In the presence of calcium, glutamate caused increases in the immunostaining of the microtubule-associated protein tau and of ubiquitin in a subpopulation of hippocampal neurons (26). Ammonia exerts detrimental effects on several important metabolic pathways in the brain (27). It may thus be concluded that the deprivation of neuronal glucose may induce metabolic abnormalities that can vary in severity but are always long-lasting, involving the energy state, the protein metabolism, and the calcium homeostasis of a cell. Hence, such a cell may succumb to a stress condition. Cellular stress is assumed to induce heat shock proteins (28), which are able to activate a promoter of the amyloid A4 precursor gene (29). Thus, the abnormality in neuronal glucose homeostasis occurring in incipient DAT may induce a cascade of self-propagating metabolic events (30) which may be regarded as the basis for the morphological abnormalities in DAT.

SUMMARY

The functional and structural integrity of a neuron is guaranteed by an adequate formation and turnover rate of ATP, which, in neuronal tissue, derives from glucose only. In suspected early-onset and late-onset DAT, a prominent disturbance was found in cerebral glucose metabolism in the early phase of the disorder. This metabolic abnormality may give rise to a reduced energy state of the brain, and it is accompanied by cerebral proteolysis of excitatory amino acids and ammonia; the former may be assumed to change neuronal calcium homeostasis. Altogether, these metabolic changes may represent a cellular stress capable of inducing the formation of heat shock proteins, which may activate the amyloid A4 precursor gene via its promoter. Severe metabolic abnormalities may thus precede morphological changes in DAT.

REFERENCES

1. Ereciska M, Silver IA. J Cereb Blood Flow Metab 1989; 9: 2–19.
2. Wan B, La Noue KF, Cheung JY, Scaduto RC Jr. J Biol Chem 1989; 264: 13430–9.
3. Hoyer S. Neuropsychopharmacol Biol Psychiat 1986; 10: 447–8.
4. Roth M. Brit Med Bull 1986; 42: 42–50.
5. Hoyer S, Oesterreich K, Wagner O. J Neurol 1988; 235: 143–8.
6. Hoyer S, Nitsch R, Oesterreich K. J Neural Transm (P-D sect) submitted for publication.
7. Liguri G, Taddei N, Nassi P, Latorraca S, Nediani C, Sorbi S. Neurosci Lett 1990; 112: 338–42.
8. Dastur DK. J Cereb Blood Flow Metab 1985; 5: 1–9.
9. Sims NR, Bowen DM, Neary D, Davison AN. J Neurochem 1983; 41: 1329–34.
10. Sacks W. J Appl Physiol 1965; 20: 117–30.
11. Wong KL, Tyce GM. Neurochem Res 1983; 8: 401–15.
12. Westerberg E, Deshpande JK, Wieloch T. J Cereb Blood Flow Metab 1987; 7: 189–92.
13. Hoyer S, Nitsch R. J Neural Transm 1989; 75: 227–32.

14. Farooqui AA, Liss L, Horrocks LA. Metabol Brain Dis 1988; 3: 19-35.
15. Monyer H, Goldberg MP, Choi DW. Brain Res 1989; 483: 347-54.
16. Monyer H, Choi DW. J Cereb Blood Flow Metab 1990; 10: 337-42.
17. Procter AW, Palmer AM, Francis PT, Low SL, Neary D, Murphey E, Doshi R, Bowen DM. J Neurochem 1988; 50: 790-802.
18. Hoyer S, Nitsch R, Oesterreich K. Neurosci Lett 1990; 117: 358-62.
19. Benjamin AM, Quastel JH. J Neurochem 1975; 25: 197-206.
20. Novelli A, Reilly JA, Lysko PG, Henneberry RC. Brain Res 1988; 451: 205-12.
21. Siesjö BK. J Cereb Blood Flow Metab 1981; 1: 155-85.
22. Rothman SM, Olney JW. Ann Neurol 1986; 19: 105-11.
23. Connor JA, Wadman WJ, Hockberger PE, Wong RKS. Science 1988; 240: 649-53.
24. Gibson GE, Manger T, Toral-Barza L, Freeman G. Neurochem Res 1989; 14: 437-43.
25. Khachaturian ZS. Aging 1989; 1: 17-34.
26. Mattson MP. Neuron 1990; 2: 105-17.
27. Cooper AJL, Plum F. Physiol Rev 1987; 67: 440-519.
28. Lindquist S. Ann Rev Biochem 1986; 55: 1151-91.
29. Salbaum JM, Weidemann A, Lemaire HG, Masters CL, Beyreuther K. EMBO J 1988; 7: 2807-13.
30. Hoyer S. Age 1988; 11: 158-66.

Address for correspondence:

Siegfried Hoyer,
Department of Pathochemistry and General Neurochemistry,
University of Heidelberg,
Im Neuenheimer Feld 220/221,
D-6900 Heidelberg, Germany

8 Regional Deficits in Cortical Metabolism in PET-Scanned Alzheimer Cases Correlate with Postmortem Indices of Gliosis, and not with Choline Acetyltransferase

P. L. McGEER, E. G. McGEER, H. AKIYAMA
AND R. HARROP

Correlations were sought between local cerebral metabolic rates (LCMRs) for glucose in various regions of the cortex, determined in premortem PET scans, with the regional activities of choline acetyltransferase (ChAT), acetylcholinesterase (AChE), β-glucuronidase (Gluc, a probable index of reactive gliosis) and phosphate-activated glutaminase (PAG, a possible index of the large pyramidal neurons) measured on postmortem tissue. Significant negative correlations between LCMRs and Gluc activities were found in six PET-scanned cases of Alzheimer disease (AD), and positive correlations of LCMRs with PAG were found in five. In contrast, a positive correlation with ChAT and AChE was found in only one. The results are consistent with the metabolic deficits in AD being primarily a reflection of local neuronal loss and gliosis. Similar data on two cases of Huntington's disease showed no significant correlations, while one patient with Parkinson dementia showed a significant (negative) correlation only with Gluc.

Work in a number of centers using ^{18}F-fluorodeoxyglucose (FDG) for positron emission tomography (PET) scans has shown that there are decreases in local cortical glucose metabolism (LCMR) in Alzheimer's disease (AD). Loss of tissue volume, as measured by CT or magnetic resonance imaging (MRI) scans, may play some role in the reduced cortical glucose metabolism but it is clearly not the most significant factor (1,2). Normal and AD cases with similar tissue shrinkage by these scanning techniques have dramatically different PET-FDG scans (3). Clearly, more specific factors are involved. It has been suggested in the literature by various groups that the reduced cortical glucose metabolism in AD may depend upon a loss of somatostatin (SOM) neurons in the cortex (4), on the decreased cholinergic innervation (5,6), or on tangle and plaque density and gliosis (7). However, there is little evidence available correlating premortem PET scan data with postmortem findings in individual cases. In our initial paper, on the first PET scanned AD case

Alzheimer's Disease: Basic Mechanisms, Diagnosis and Therapeutic Strategies
Edited by K. Iqbal, D. R. C. McLachlan, B. Winblad and H. M. Wisniewski
© 1991 John Wiley & Sons Ltd

to come to autopsy (8), we presented evidence that deficits in glucose metabolism seemed to reflect neuronal loss in the affected regions rather than simply plaque and tangle formation. The present study reports biochemical data on a number of further PET-scanned cases that have come to autopsy. These data are consistent with the hypothesis that the decreases in LCMR in AD reflect local neuronal loss and gliosis.

The enzymes chosen for the postmortem work were choline acetyltransferase (ChAT), β-glucuronidase (Gluc) and phosphate-activated glutaminase (PAG). ChAT was chosen because, of the known biochemical markers, it is the most reliably reduced in AD and, as mentioned above, it has been suggested that reductions in cholinergic activity may lead to reduced cortical glucose metabolism.

Gluc is a lysosomal enzyme found in reactive astrocytes and microglia (9), and its activity may therefore give some indication of the degree of gliosis. Elevated levels of Gluc have been reported in AD temporal cortex and Huntington's disease putamen (10). Work on rat and human tissue indicates it is probably not greatly affected by postmortem delay and confirms the elevated levels in AD cortex (11).

The rationale for studies on PAG is less explicit. Morphological data on the distribution of plaques and tangles in AD suggest that an important part of the pathology may be degeneration of the pyramidal neurons forming corticocortical association projections (12–14). There is considerable evidence that these neurons may use glutamate as their excitatory transmitter (15), and in both rat and human cortex (16–18) and in rat and guinea-pig hippocampus (19,20), these neurons stain immunohistochemically for PAG, a mitochondrial enzyme which catalyzes the hydrolysis of glutamine to glutamate and ammonia. PAG has therefore been suggested as a significant contributor to the synthesis of neurotransmitter glutamate. PAG also appears in other locations and may be sensitive to the antemortem state. However, in the absence of any really satisfactory marker of excitatory amino acid transmitter pools that can be used on postmortem tissue, and in view of the marked loss of PAG-positive pyramidal neurons seen in initial immunohistochemical studies on postmortem AD brains (18), a detailed biochemical study of the levels of this enzyme seemed worth while.

MATERIAL AND METHODS

PET studies

The methods used for obtaining the FDG PET scans and their analysis was as previously detailed (3,8,21). The problem of the extent of influence of cerebral atrophy was minimized by use of MRI scans in each case and analysis of a number of small regions of interest within a larger gyrus. The neuropathologist concerned in dissecting the postmortem brains (HA) was also actively involved in the PET analyses in order to ensure comparability.

Biochemical studies

Brains were obtained as soon as possible after death and small samples containing a full cortical thickness were dissected from multiple areas of the neocortex and frozen at $-70\,°C$ until assayed. The samples were weighed and homogenized in 10 volumes of ice-cold water and kept on ice. ChAT and acetylcholinesterase (AChE) were determined on portions of each homogenate by the previously reported radioactive methods (11,22). PAG was determined by a minor modification of the radioactive procedure of Kaneko et al (11,23). Studies in both rat and human tissue (18) indicated the method was reproducible, gave satisfactory results on frozen as well as fresh tissue samples and was linear with time and amount of tissue over the ranges used. Gluc activity was determined by a modification of the fluorometric method of Cross et al (10,11). Preliminary studies confirmed the applicability of the assay to frozen tissue and its linearity over the time and tissue concentrations used. Protein was determined by the method of Lowry et al (24) using bovine serum albumin as a standard and all enzyme activities were expressed on a protein basis.

Cases

Diagnosis of dementia in the AD cases was based upon the usual histopathological findings of multiple plaques and tangles in hippocampal and temporal cortex. The controls were persons dying without evidence of neurological disease and with no evident neuropathology. The two cases of Huntington's disease (HD) had familial and clinical histories, as well as pathology, consistent with the diagnosis. The single case of Parkinson dementia (PD) also showed the appropriate clinical and pathological signs. Data on the ages and sex of the PET-scanned cases are given in Table 1.

RESULTS

Table 1 gives the coefficients found for the correlations of LCMR with the various enzymes in the individual cases, while Table 2 lists the calculated equations which showed significant correlation.

In every AD case studied there was a significant negative correlation between the LCMR and Gluc activities. Moreover, the slopes and intercepts tended to be rather similar so that there was a significant correlation ($P < 0.001$, $r = 0.70$) if all the AD data were combined. Figure 1A shows a plot of the data for each individual and the overall line of correlation. In the single case of PD studied the LCMRs also correlated negatively with the regional Gluc activities, but no such correlation was found in the two HD cases (Tables 1 and 2).

In contrast to the negative correlations found for LCMR with Gluc, the correlations of the former with PAG tended to be positive and reached significance in 5 of the 6 AD cases. The slopes of 4 out of 5 of the significant lines of correlations were fairly similar to each other (Table 2) and to that of the line of correlation ($r = 0.52$) for the AD group as a whole (Figure 1B). No significant correlation between LCMRs and PAG activities was found in the three non-AD cases studied (Table 1).

Table 1. Age at death, sex, diagnosis, interval between PET scan and death, number of brain regions studied and correlations between LCMRs and enzyme activities found in various individuals

Case	Sex	Diagnosis	Age (years)	Interval (months)	Region number	Correlation coefficients (and *P* values) for LCMRs with				
						ChAT	AChE	AChE/ChAT	PAG	Gluc
270	F	AD	60	38	15	0.415 (n.s.)	0.396 (n.s.)	-0.187 (n.s.)	0.648 (0.009)	-0.718 (0.004)
278	F	AD	69	11	13	0.475 (n.s.)	0.338 (n.s.)	-0.325 (n.s.)	0.562 (0.046)	-0.702 (0.011)
310	M	AD	48	24	35	0.258 (n.s.)	0.332 (n.s.)	0.155 (n.s.)	0.376 (0.031)	-0.385 (0.027)
317	M	AD	81	51	17	0.241 (n.s.)	0.045 (n.s.)	-0.604 (0.010)	0.532 (0.028)	-0.589 (0.013)
332	M	AD	79	53	29	0.204 (n.s.)	0.130 (n.s.)	-0.154 (n.s.)	0.600 (<0.001)	-0.374 (0.045)
342	M	AD	80	43	39	0.360 (0.047)	0.453 (0.004)	-0.039 (n.s.)	0.186 (n.s.)	-0.562 (<0.001)
325	F	HD	65	51	34	-0.245 (n.s.)	-0.208 (n.s.)	-0.091 (n.s.)	-0.209 (n.s.)	-0.031 (n.s.)
338	M	HD	49	59	20	-0.088 (n.s.)	0.065 (n.s.)	0.079 (n.s.)	-0.230 (n.s.)	-0.177 (n.s.)
334	M	PD	84	20	37	0.260 (n.s.)	0.040 (n.s.)	-0.429 (0.008)	0.070 (n.s.)	-0.562 (<0.001)

Table 2. Equations showing significant correlations for the LCMRs in cortical regions with enzyme activities measured in the same regions*

Case	Equations		
AD			
270	Gluc = 11.81 − 0.192(LCMR)	PAG = 0.516(LCMR) − 2.028	
278	Gluc = 11.34 − 0.207(LCMR)	PAG = 0.407(LCMR) − 3.47	
310	Gluc = 9.17 − 0.138(LCMR)	PAG = 0.563(LCMR) + 4.47	
317	Gluc = 9.94 − 0.137(LCMR)	PAG = 0.539(LCMR) − 6.69	
332	Gluc = 10.46 − 0.176(LCMR)	PAG = 0.923(LCMR) − 16.35	AChE/ChAT = 766.91 − 15.98(LCMR)
342	Gluc = 12.01 − 0.234(LCMR)		ChAT = 0.028(LCMR) − 0.146
			AChE = 2.78(LCMR) + 1.676
PD			
334	Gluc = 8.43 − 0.172(LCMR)		AChE/ChAT = 759.35 − 22.30(LCMR)

*LCMR is in μmol/100 mg tissue.min; ChAT, AChE and PAG in μmol/100 g protein.h; and Gluc in nmol/mg protein.h.

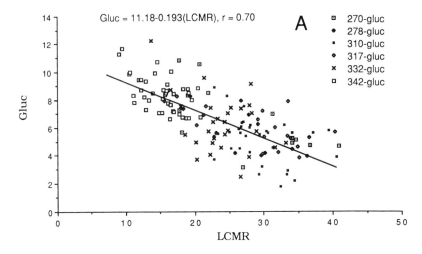

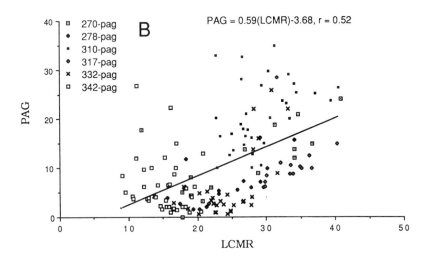

Figure 1. Overall plots of LCMR against Gluc (A) and PAG (B) for the six AD cases. The lines of correlations shown are calculated from the entire group of data. Units are as given in footnote to Table 2

Very few significant correlations were found between LCMR and any index of cholinergic function (Table 1) and the negative ones found with AChE/ChAT tended to have rather variable slopes (Table 2).

In attempting to interpret these findings, it is of interest to note that studies on a larger group of AD and control cases have confirmed the increases in Gluc in AD cortex and indicated that no significant abnormality in either Gluc or ChAT occurs in AD striatum (Figure 2). PAG seems to be decreased in both cortex and striatum, but the former is significantly more affected (Figure 2). The cortical deficits in PAG and ChAT in AD, and the increases in Gluc, involve most cortical regions with the exception of the cingulate gyrus (11, and further detailed data not shown).

DISCUSSION

The validity of trying to correlate postmortem data with PET scan LCMRs obtained many months previously may well be questioned. However, analyses of PET data on 32 regions of interest from serial scans on 13 AD cases suggest that, despite some regional variation in the rate of metabolic loss, the rank order of metabolism is fairly well maintained over time in the regions of interest of any individual (25). The time interval may have been a factor since, for the two serially scanned cases who have come to autopsy, the correlation coefficients calculated using the data from the second PET scan (shown) were somewhat higher than those using LCMRs from the first PET scan (not shown). However, an inspection of Table 1 suggests this time interval is not the major determining factor.

As indicated at the start of this chapter, it has been suggested that the reduced cortical glucose metabolism in AD may depend upon a loss of SOM neurons in the cortex, on the decreased cholinergic innervation, or on tangle and plaque density and gliosis. This last suggestion is based upon the finding in *different* groups of patients that the same parietal and temporal cortical regions which show the most

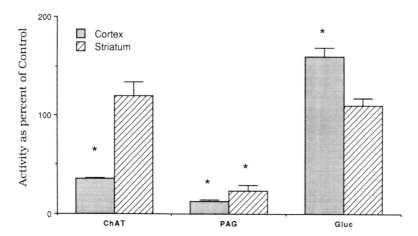

Figure 2. Mean (+SE) cortical and striatal ChAT, PAG and Gluc activities found for a group of 24 AD cases as a percentage of the means found in 10 controls. In each brain, 7–22 regions of cortex were analyzed and the average per brain used in calculating the group mean ± SE. Samples of mid-caudate and mid-putamen were averaged to get a striatal value for each brain. Control means in cortex and striatum, respectively, were: ChAT 0.51 ± 0.028, 12.0 ± 3.18; PAG 148.7 ± 8.28, 151.0 ± 28.8; and Gluc 4.82 ± 0.58, 4.81 ± 0.27. Units as defined in the footnote to Table 2. *Significantly different from control

severe metabolic defects are those which tend to be the most severely affected from a histopathological viewpoint (7). Our data do not bear directly upon this hypothesis.

The suggestion of a possible relation with cholinergic innervation is based upon the general finding — again in different patient populations — that the temporal and parietal regions tend to show the most severe decreases in ChAT activity in AD. It is supported to some extent by the reports that the cholinergic antagonist scopolamine (26) or lesions of the nucleus basalis (27–29) decrease cortical glucose metabolism in animals, especially in the parietal and temporal cortices (26); the effects of the lesions, however, seem to be slowly reversible over time (27–29), and not all groups find such significant effects (30). Administration of a cholinomimetic, arecoline (31) or oxotremorine (32), to rats is reported to increase cortical glucose metabolism. The work of Bowen's group (33), indicating that biopsied cortical tissue from AD cases shows a normal capacity to oxidize glucose in in-vitro studies, also suggests that the reduced metabolic rate seen in vivo may be due to a deficient subcortical driving mechanism rather than to intrinsic loss of the metabolic enzymes. Clearly, our data do not support this hypothesis since very few correlations between LCMRs and cholinergic indices were found. The possibility that a major factor is deficiency of some other subcortical drive — such as provided by the noradrenergic, serotonergic or histaminergic system — cannot be ruled out.

The suggestion that loss of cortical SOM neurons might underlie the decrease in glucose metabolism comes from Taminga et al (4), who found in postmortem studies (on 8 non-PET scanned AD cases) a relatively uniform loss of ChAT in the two frontal and two parietal regions measured, while SOM was decreased only in the parietal areas, where this group finds the significant losses of LCMR in AD. Moreover, they measured SOM levels in the CSF in 17 PET-scanned AD cases and 6 PET-scanned controls and found a positive correlation between the CSF peptide levels and the metabolic rates in the parietal ($r=0.54$) and temporal ($r=0.44$) cortices. A problem with this hypothesis, that the reduced metabolic rate depends solely (or mainly) upon the loss of SOM neurons, is that the literature on the extent of loss of SOM in AD is very controversial (e.g. 34–36) and it seems probable that SOM neurons are not lost, although their content of SOM is probably reduced (37–39). One report (40) of similar reductions in cortical cell cultures deprived of glucose suggests that the losses of SOM may be consequent upon, rather than causal to, the decreased glucose metabolic rates. Our data, however, do not bear directly upon this hypothesis.

A previous histochemical study on postmortem tissues from a single PET-scanned AD case suggested the metabolic deficits were related to local neuronal loss and reactive gliosis (8). The present data are consistent in as much as the LCMRs correlate negatively with Gluc (a presumptive index of reactive astrocytes and microglia which are known to proliferate in affected cortical regions in AD; cf. e.g. 41) and positively with PAG (a possible index for cortical pyramidal neurons). Work on postmortem human brain in our laboratory and in others (42,43) suggests, however, that premortem coma, postmortem delay or similar epiphenomena may have considerable influence on PAG in some brain regions. Butterworth et al (43) indicated that the PAG in subcortical regions is more sensitive to the agonal state than is the cortical

PAG. Thus, the relatively greater loss of this enzyme in AD cortex as compared to AD striatum (Figure 2), as well as the high levels found in controls suffering from chronic illnesses, suggest some other factor may be important to the losses seen in AD. The losses are, however, surprisingly large when one considers that PAG is also found in gabanergic neurons in the cortex (which are probably not greatly affected in AD) and may even occur in astrocytes (44). Clearly, further work on this enzyme in human tissue is needed, but the apparent correlation with premortem glucose metabolism in some types of patients should encourage such work.

The negative correlation of LCMRs with Gluc seen in the one PET-scanned case of PD that has come to autopsy, and the lack of any such correlation in the two HD patients, suggests the dementia of PD may be more closely akin to that of AD than either is to the dementia in HD. Little can be concluded, however, from so few cases, and this controversial question of cortical versus subcortical dementia requires much further work.

Acknowledgments

This research was supported by grants from the Medical Research Council of Canada, the American Health Assistance Foundation and the Alzheimer Society of BC, as well as donations from individual British Columbians. We thank Ms Kim Singh and the members of the UBC-TRIUMF PET team for technical assistance.

REFERENCES

1. Haxby JV, Rapoport SI. Neuropsychopharmacol Biol Psychiat 1986; 10: 427-38.
2. McGeer PL. Br Med Bull 1986; 42: 24-8.
3. McGeer PL, Kamo H, Harrop R et al. Can Med Assoc J 1986; 34: 597-607.
4. Taminga CA, Foster NL, Fedio P, Bird ED, Chase TN. Neurology 1987; 37: 161-5.
5. Rossor MR. Lancet 1983; ii: 465.
6. Najlerahim A, Bowen DM. Biochem J 1988; 251: 305-8.
7. Friedland RP, Brun A, Budinger TF. Lancet 1985; i: 228.
8. McGeer PL, Kamo H, Harrop R et al. Neurology 1986; 36: 1569-74.
9. Mackenzie IC, Bickenbach JR, Rittman BR. J Invest Dermatol 1982; 78: 239-42.
10. Cross AJ, Crow TJ, Dawson JM et al. J Neurochem 1986; 47: 882-9.
11. McGeer EG, McGeer PL, Akiyama H, Harrop R. Can J Neurol Sci 1989; 16: 511-15.
12. Lewis DA, Campbell MJ, Terry RD, Morrison JH. J Neurosci 1987; 7: 1799-808.
13. Pearson RCA, Esiri MM, Hiorns RW, Wilcock G, Powell T. Proc Natl Acad Sci USA 1985; 82: 4531-4.
14. Rogers J, Morrison JH. J Neurosci 1985; 5: 2801-8.
15. McGeer PL, Eccles JC, McGeer EG. Molecular neurobiology of the mammalian brain. New York: Raven Press, 1987: 180-6.
16. Donaghue JP, Wenthold RJ, Altschuler RA. J Neurosci 1985; 5: 2597-608.
17. Kaneko T, Mizuno N. J Comp Neurol 1988; 267: 599-602.
18. Akiyama H, McGeer PL, Itagaki S, McGeer EG, Kaneko K. Neurochem Res 1989; 14: 453-8.
19. Altschuler RA, Monaghan DT, Haser WG, Wenthold RJ, Curthoys NP, Cotman CW. Brain Res 1985; 330: 225-33.
20. Wolf G, Richter K, Schunzel G, Schopp W. Dev Brain Res 1988; 41: 101-8.
21. Akiyama H, Harrop R, McGeer PL, Peppard R, McGeer EG. Neurology 1989; 39: 541-8.

22. McGeer EG, Singh EA, McGeer PL. Alz Dis Assoc Disord 1987; 1: 50-63.
23. Kaneko T, Urade Y, Watanabe Y, Mizuno N. J Neurosci 1987; 7: 302-9.
24. Lowry OH, Rosebrough NJ, Farr AL, Randall R. J Biol Chem 1951; 193: 265-75.
25. McGeer EG, Peppard RP, McGeer PL et al. Can J Neurol Sci 1990; 17: 1-11.
26. Piercey MF, Vogelsang SD, Franklin SR, Tang AH. Brain Res 1987; 424: 1-9.
27. Kiyosawa M, Pappatas S, Duverger D et al. J Cerebr Blood Flow Metab 1987; 7: 812-17.
28. Kiyosawa M, Baron J-C, Hamel E et al. Brain 1989; 112: 435-55.
29. Orzi F, Diana G, Casamenti F, Palmobo E, Fieschi C. Brain Res 1988; 462: 99-103.
30. Lamarca MV, Fibiger HC. Brain Res 1984; 307: 366-9.
31. Soncrant TT, Holloway HW, Rapoport SI. Brain Res 1985; 347: 205-16.
32. Dam M, Wamsley JK, Rapoport SI, London ED. J Neurosci 1982; 2: 1072-8.
33. Sims NR, Bowen DM, Davison AN. Biochem J 1981; 196: 867-76.
34. Reinikainen KJ, Riekkinen PJ, Jolkkonen J, Kosma V-M, Soininen H. Brain Res 1987; 402: 103-8.
35. Whitford C, Candy JM, Edwardson JM, Perry R. J Neurol Sci 1988; 86: 13-18.
36. Arai H, Moroji T, Kosaka K. Neurosci Lett 1984; 52: 73-8.
37. Gaspar P, Duyckaerts C, Febvret A, Benoit R, Beck B, Berger B. Brain Res 1989; 490: 1-13.
38. Nakamura S, Vincent SR. Brain Res 1986; 370: 11-20.
39. Kowall NW, Beal MF. Ann Neurol 1988; 23: 105-14.
40. Robbins RJ. J Neurochem 1983; 40: 1430-4.
41. Itagaki S, McGeer PL, Akiyama H, Zhu S, Selkoe D. J Neuroimmunol 1989; 24: 173-82.
42. Procter AW, Lowe SL, Palmer AM et al. J Neurol Sci 1988; 84: 125-40.
43. Butterworth J, Yates CM, Reynolds GP. J Neurol Sci 1985; 67: 161-71.
44. Yudkoff M, Nisim I, Pleasures D. J Neurochem 1988; 51: 843-50.

Address for correspondence:

Dr Patrick L. McGeer,
Kinsmen Laboratory of Neurological Research,
University of BC,
2255 Wesbrook Mall, Vancouver, BC, V6T 1W5, Canada

9 New Techniques for the Visualization of EEG Fourier Analysis: Comparison of Power, Coherence and Phase Patterns Between Elderly Normals and SDAT Patients

C. BAGGIO, O. SCARPINO, M. MAGI, T. CENACCHI,
G. BOLCIONI AND F. ANGELERI

In spite of the recent diffusion of computerized EEG analysis techniques including fast Fourier transform (FFT) and brain mapping based on the availability of multi-channel electroencephalographic instrumentation and powerful microcomputers, electroencephalography has proven to be of questionable usefulness in the diagnosis of dementia.

The enormous quantity of data conveyed by FFT can hardly be interpreted by operators without a heavy investment of time and resources while, on the other hand, the synthesized image of brain mapping (1) necessarily results in a loss of information. There is therefore a need for a method to allow easy comprehension and an analytical separation of possibly useful information recorded by the spectral power elaboration. To this end computerized graphic programs performing high resolution spectra imaging (HRSI) have been developed (2), capable of visualizing simultaneously, with the same resolution as the FFT, power spectra as well as coherence and phase differences between pairs of electrodes. This method provides an immediate high resolution representation of all the information deriving from the frequency analysis.

The highly detailed description obtained via these specific procedures allows the observation of characteristic patterns, mainly related to the alpha band, which cannot be visualized by ordinary brain mapping systems. This seems to offer a promising possibility of interpreting collected data and perhaps identifying new additional parameters for discriminating between normal and pathological subjects.

To this end, we report the results of an investigation on power, coherence and phase patterns of the alpha band of representative subjects within a study comparing a group of normal subjects with a group of patients with senile dementia of Alzheimer type (SDAT). Obviously, given the limited size of our samples the study should be

Alzheimer's Disease: Basic Mechanisms, Diagnosis and Therapeutic Strategies
Edited by K. Iqbal, D. R. C. McLachlan, B. Winblad and H. M. Wisniewski
© 1991 John Wiley & Sons Ltd

considered a preliminary one. This report mainly refers to the analysis of the alpha band patterns of power coherence and phase which are, among normals, well-defined and stable, as a sort of 'fingerprint' for each individual. For these reasons alterations of such patterns could be of some interest in the evaluation of neurophysio-pathological conditions.

METHODS AND MATERIALS

A group of 12 healthy females (aged 61–72 years) was compared with 12 SDAT female patients (aged 58–73 years) with a score in the mini-mental state examination of between 12 and 23 and diagnosed according to the DSMIII-R criteria for dementia.

Artifact-free recording (for at least 5 minutes) of background EEG activity was obtained for each subject in the study. In order to maintain a high spectra resolution, power should be cumulated over epochs but not over frequencies, and therefore only a long EEG recording provides a sufficient number of degrees of freedom (i.e. epochs).

Background EEG was recorded with 16 electrodes placed laterally according to the IS 10–20 using linked earlobes reference. Fourier analysis of 4-second epochs was carried out using standard procedures (3–5) to obtain spectra of power, coherence and phase with a resolution of 0.25 Hz.

The HRSI method presents frequency–channel matrices of power spectra in a mosaic-like pattern: the value of each element of the matrix is represented by a color code. The leads are symmetrically positioned on the vertical axis. The occipital derivations are in the middle and the frontal ones are at the top and bottom. The left hemisphere is represented on the upper half of the figure while the right is on the lower.

Another application of the HRSI shows interhemispheric coherence between all pairs of homotopical derivations, and intrahemispheric coherence between a single electrode and the others in the same hemisphere.

A white line running across frequencies indicates positive (higher position) to negative (lower position) phase delay within pairs of leads.

RESULTS

The main results of our study are summarized as follows.

In normal subjects the alpha band power is typically distributed over the whole scalp close to the peak frequency. The maximum values of the power appear usually on the occipital leads.

In this ideal condition, which is also a common feature of young normals, some variation is even possible. A shift of maximum power from the occipital to the parietal regions and, for some channels, a dispersion of power near to the lower frequency side of the alpha band peak is observed. The interhemispheric coherence between homotopical derivations is particularly characterized by high values between the frontal polar derivations synchronized with the frequency peak of power and extending for a wider range of frequencies.

Consistent values are also observed between posterior leads. All these pairs of leads show complete phase concordance in the alpha band. The intrahemispheric coherence demonstrates high values synchronized with the power peak frequency.

High values of coherence are especially observed in the frontal to occipital derivations, sometimes with a complete phase opposition. Hypothetically, these phenomena could be due to a bias introduced by the transferring of the occipital power on the reference and/or a dipole effect: the phase opposition is typically found in the majority of young normals.

In the group of SDAT patients the distribution of the power in the alpha band appears substantially different from that of normal subjects. A fragmentation of the power on different frequencies and on different leads seems the main characteristic of the patient group. An increased asymmetrical distribution of the power is also frequently observed. A slowing of frequencies sometimes results in confounding of the alpha and the theta band.

The lower frequency peaks of power could be localized in the central and even frontal derivations. Both interhemispheric and intrahemispheric coherence reflect the poorly defined feature of power dispersion. Within a general decrease in coherence values the frontal-polar interhemispheric ones are relatively unchanged. In contrast, the frontal to occipital coherence is particularly reduced. From middle to high values of coherence, a phase concordance between leads could be usually observed.

We should note that, within the group, there is one case which shows a single peak alpha band, mainly occipital, with frontal to occipital coherence without phase opposition.

In order to illustrate the above, Figures 1-4 (see colour plate) show examples of HRSI of power in two normal subjects and in two patients; as well as the HRSI of coherence and phase for the first normal and the first patient. In these pictures the leads are specified on the vertical axis (pairs of leads respectively) and the frequency is specified on the horizontal axis with a resolution of 0.25 Hz. A vertical bar on the right side of the image displays the color code of the value of power (arbitrary scale) and coherence (absolute scale).

In the HRSI of coherence the phase relationship is represented by a white line across frequencies as previously explained.

Figure 1 shows the characteristic patterns of normal subjects, i.e. the alpha band power is distributed over the whole scalp close to the peak frequency. As a main difference between subjects the maximum power is on the occipital electrodes in subject C.D. while in subject R.G. there is a shift of power on parietal electrodes.

In Figure 2, the alpha band power of SDAT patient P.M. is clearly fragmented on different frequencies. Power is asymmetrically distributed with prevalence on the left hemisphere. Also patient G.G. shows fragmentation of alpha band power with a prevalent distribution from parietal to frontal regions. Due to the overall slowing of frequency, alpha and theta bands are confounded.

Figure 3, a normal subject, shows in the center the interhemispheric coherence between homotopical derivations, while on the left and on the right is represented the intrahemispheric coherence referred to the occipital leads. At the peak of the alpha band (9.5 Hz), high values of coherence (in phase) can be observed in the posterior as well as along the anterior derivations. The intrahemispheric coherence shows a similar pattern, although a complete phase opposition on the frontal derivation can be observed (white line).

In Figure 4 (SDAT patient), coherence reflects the dispersion of power across various frequencies. The anterior interhemispheric and the posterior intrahemispheric coherence is maintained and shows little relation to power. In the right hemisphere we observe (at 7.5 Hz) consistent values of frontal to occipital coherence resembling the pattern observed in normal subjects.

DISCUSSION

We have presented here the results of a new graphic technique for the quantitative analysis of the EEG. The power, coherence and phase of the EEG recording can be easily understood (at the same resolution allowed by the Fourier analysis) by means of a detailed visual representation of great intuitive efficacy. Examples drawn from a group of normal subjects, compared with a group of SDAT patients, are presented.

As far as the alpha band is concerned, a fragmentation of power over different frequencies and leads, together with a shift of the power peak from occipital to parietal or anterior regions, seem to be the major features which differentiate SDAT patients from normal subjects.

Some concomitant modifications of coherence and phase patterns seem also to be of subsidiary relevance in discriminating between the groups. More research on a larger sample of both normals and SDAT patients is needed before any firm conclusion about the possible diagnostic significance of such differences can be reached. Nevertheless, we would venture to formulate a criticism of the conventional evaluation of power of the whole alpha band. It is easy to see that the averaging over frequencies completely masks the major discriminating parameters.

In this study we focused our attention on the alpha band, mainly because in normal subjects it has a well-defined pattern. Using the same technique, similar results may possibly be obtained within other EEG bands. In addition, it should be pointed out that since a minor degree of fragmentation of the alpha band pattern can be present in the normal elderly population, statistical methods must be developed to evaluate these aspects of pattern deterioration.

REFERENCES

1. Duffy FH, Burchfiel JL, Lombroso CT. Ann Neurol 1979; 5: 309-21.
2. Bolcioni G, Baggio C. Electroenceph Clin Neurophysiol 1990; 75: 13p-14p.
3. Cooley VA, Tukey JW. Math Comput 1965; 19: 297-301.
4. Shaw JC. J Med Eng Tech 1981; 5: 279-88.
5. Shaw JC. Int J Psychophysiol 1984; 1: 255-66.

Address for correspondence:

Dr Gastone Bolcioni,
Clinical Research, Fidia S.p.A.,
Via Ponte della Fabbrica 3/A,
35031 Abano Terme, Padova, Italy

Part III

NEUROPATHOLOGY: STRUCTURAL AND BIOCHEMICAL

10 Validation of Diagnostic Criteria for Alzheimer's Disease

K. JELLINGER, H. LASSMANN, P. FISCHER AND
W. DANIELCZYK

A cohort of 27 prospectively evaluated elderly subjects and of 26 patients with Parkinson's disease with graded intellectual status were compared with their postmortem neuropathology, including senile plaque, neurofibrillary tangle and neuropil thread counts in standardized regions and using different morphologic criteria for the diagnosis of Alzheimer's disease (AD): Khachaturian, 1985 (K); Tierney et al, 1988 (T) (5,7). Among 12 nondemented elderly, 9 (2/3) met the K and 6 (50%) the T criteria; among 15 demented, 12 with probable clinical AD, postmortem confirmation was seen in 77% and 83%, respectively. Inclusion of two severely demented with AD lesions restricted to entorhinal cortex ('limbic type of AD') would have increased accuracy of clinical AD diagnosis to 88.9%.

Mental status in this group scored by MMSE showed significant correlations with tau positive plaques in frontal and temporal cortices, with neurofibrillary tangles and neuropil threads in frontal, parietal, temporal cortex and subiculum, but not with plaques containing chromogranin A or neurofilament protein.

Semiquantitative assessment of AD lesions in the cohort of PD subjects revealed that among 17 nondemented ones, only 7 (41%) met the K and 11 (65%) the T criteria for AD, while most of them had tangles in the entorhinal cortex. Among the 9 demented PD subjects, 7 met the K and all the T criteria of AD, thus indicating true combinations of PD and AD. In most PD cases, tangles and threads in entorhinal cortex correlated better with cognitive impairment than those in hippocampal sector CA1 or isocortex.

These and other recent data indicate that more specific criteria using standardized morphologic methods are necessary to separate demented from nondemented elderly subjects and to achieve a correct diagnosis of Alzheimer's disease and related disorders.

INTRODUCTION

In recent years there have been attempts to improve both the clinical and postmortem criteria for classifying the dementias in general (1-4) and to establish standardized

Alzheimer's Disease: Basic Mechanisms, Diagnosis and Therapeutic Strategies
Edited by K. Iqbal, D. R. C. McLachlan, B. Winblad and H. M. Wisniewski
© 1991 John Wiley & Sons Ltd

guidelines for the clinical and neuropathological assessment of Alzheimer's disease (AD) and related dementia disorders in order to improve diagnostic reliability (5-10). However, several retrospective and prospective studies on the accuracy of clinical diagnosis in elderly subjects with dementia using clinicopathologic correlations reported coincidence rates for AD ranging from 43% to 100% with an average of 80-85% (4,11,12), and the interrater reliability of both clinical and postmortem AD diagnosis needs to be further improved (13-15). In order to further validate the diagnostic criteria for AD, we compared clinical and neuropsychologic data in two cohorts of prospectively evaluated subjects with their postmortem neuropathology using standardized assessment methods. The study reports two sets of data: (a) validation of quantitative morphologic criteria for AD diagnosis in a cohort of elderly (group I) following those by Khachaturian (5) and Tierney et al (7); and (b) comparison of cognitive impairment with quantitative AD pathology and immunohistochemistry in this group and with semiquantitative AD pathology in a cohort of patients with Parkinson's disease (PD).

MATERIAL AND METHODS

Subjects

The material included two groups of elderly subjects of the Vienna Longitudinal Study on Dementia (16): group I consisted of 27 inpatients of a geriatric unit—5 males and 22 females (aged 57 to 97 years, mean 78); group II consisted of 26 cases of Parkinson's disease (PD) aged 65 to 92 years (mean 78.8) with duration of illness from 1 to 31 years (mean 10 years). Subjects from both cohorts were prospectively evaluated with repeated neurologic and psychometric examination, EEG, cranial CT and laboratory tests. Diagnosis of dementia, probable AD, multi-infarct dementia (MID), etc. was made using established criteria (1-3,6); severity of dementia was assessed by mini-mental state (MMS) study (17) at 6 to 12 months before death.

Pathology

Brains from both groups were studied on paraffin sections from standardized regions of frontal, temporal and parietal neocortex, hippocampus, subiculum, basal ganglia and cerebellum using routine stains, Bielschowsky and Bodian methenamine silver methods. Paraffin sections of group I were immunostained for tau, chromogranin A and B, synaptophysin and neurofilament protein (NFP) using monoclonal and polyclonal antibodies (for techniques see 18,19). Senile plaques (SP) were counted by means of Bielschowsky and immunostaining for tau, chromogranin A, synaptophysin and NFP; neurofibrillary tangles (NFT) and neuropil threads (NPT) (20) were counted using Bieschowsky silver technique and immunostaining for tau. We counted five contiguous fields of midfrontal, parietal, superior temporal cortex, subiculum and hippocampal fields CA1 and CA3 at $\times 200$ in a field measuring 1.4 mm^2, and then normalized to a 1 mm^2 area. In group II, postmortem diagnosis of PD of the Lewy body type followed current criteria (21). SP, NFT and NPT

Table 1. Age and sex of study subjects of group I

Clinical diagnosis	n	Age/yr (mean)	M/F	MMS	IS
No dementia (Co 1, PD 1, MIE 1, DAT 1)	4	66-97 (80)	0/4	24-30	3-16
Cognitive changes (Co 1, MID 3, DAT 2, PD/AD 2)	8	77-89 (82)	1/7	17-22	0-11
Moderate dementia (MID 2, DAT 1)	3	77-92 (85)	0/3	7-10	4-10
Severe dementia (AD 7; PD/AD 3, DU 1, MIXD 1)	12	57-87 (74)	4/8	0-3	0-10

Co, control; AD/DAT, probable Alzheimer's disease/dementia; PD/AD, Parkinson's plus Alzheimer's disease; DU, unclear dementia; MIE/MID, multi-infarct encephalopathy/dementia; IS, Hachinski ischemia score; MMS, mini-mental state score

were assessed semiquantitatively in three standardized regions of the isocortex in entorhinal cortex and hippocampal field CA1 using Gallyas and Bielschowsky silver methods (see 22).

RESULTS

Clinicopathologic validation of group I

Four subjects were cognitively normal, 8 had cognitive changes but no dementia, and 15 showed moderate dementia ($n=3$) or severe dementia ($n=12$). Of the nondemented subjects, 2 were considered normal; 3 each had clinical diagnoses of AD, PD and MID; 1 had a diagnosis of multi-infarct encephalopathy (MIE). Among the demented subjects, 16 had a clinical diagnosis of AD or PD/AD, 5 of MID and 1 of mixed type dementia (MIXD). Clinical data are listed in Table 1.

Figures 1 and 2 illustrate the total plaque counts in frontal, parietal, temporal and parahippocampal cortex of these cases. Three of 4 normal subjects met the Khachaturian (K) criteria for AD (5), with SP counts from $10/mm^2$ to $99/mm^2$ in frontal and parietal cortices and $8-32/mm^2$ in temporal and parahippocampal cortex. One female aged 66 with MMS of 28 was 'plaque-only type of AD' (23); another nondemented aged 97 years (MMS 30) showed multiple old infarcts of more than 100 ml volume with no SP and very few NFT in entorhinal cortex. None of these brains had SP in basal ganglia or cerebellum. Six of the 8 subjects with cognitive changes but no dementia met the K criteria for AD with total neocortical plaque counts ranging from $3/mm^2$ to $63/mm^2$ and in parahippocampus from $9/mm^2$ to $17/mm^2$. SP in basal ganglia and/or cerebellum were present in 3 such brains. Of the 15 demented subjects, 12 with a clinical diagnosis of AD or PD/AD, only 11 met the K criteria for AD, with neocortical SP counts ranging from $16/mm^2$ to $111/mm^2$ and from $10/mm^2$ to $47/mm^2$ in the subiculum. Widespread SP in basal ganglia and cerebellum were seen in 5 brains each.

Application of the criteria for AD by Tierney et al (T) using both plaque and tangle counts (7) gave somewhat different results. The counts of NFT and NPT are illustrated

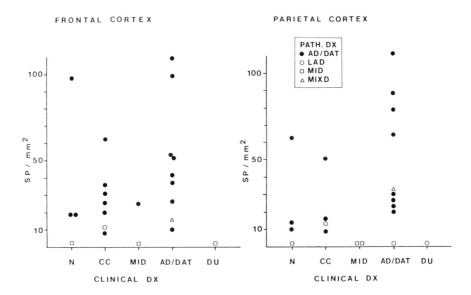

Figure 1. Total senile plaque (SP) count in frontal and parietal cortex. Subjects are grouped on the x-axis according to clinical diagnosis; different symbols denote different pathologic diagnoses. N, normal; AD/DAT, Alzheimer's disease/dementia of Alzheimer type; CC, cognitive change; LAD, limbic type of AD; MID, multi-infarct dementia; MIXD, mixed type dementia; DU, dementia type unspecified

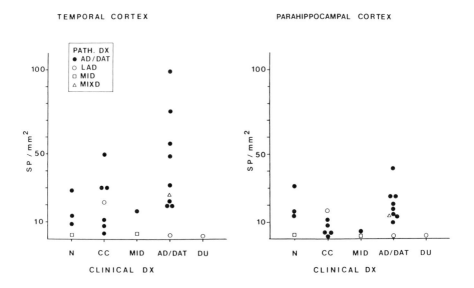

Figure 2. Total plaque count in temporal cortex and hippocampus

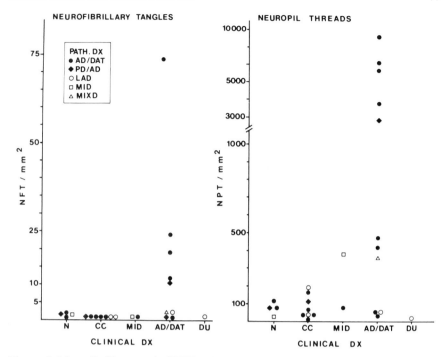

Figure 3. Neurofibrillary tangle (NFT) and neuropil thread (NPT) counts in frontal cortex

in Figures 3–6. No frontal and parietal NFT were found in nondemented subjects, but two of them showed between 10 and 46 NFT/mm^2 in temporal cortex and subiculum, thus meeting all T criteria for AD. No NFT in frontal and parietal cortex were seen also in subjects with cognitive changes but no dementia, but 4/8 or 50% of them had more than 3 NFT/mm^2 in temporal cortex (range 3–31/mm^2) and subiculum (range 2–83/mm^2) thus meeting some or all T criteria for AD. Seven of the 15 demented subjects had no frontal NFT, including 2 clinical MID cases and 5 cases with a clinical diagnosis of AD or PD/AD. No NFT in parietal cortex were seen in 3 cases of probable AD, while no NFT in temporal cortex and subiculum were present in one case each. On the other hand, 5 cases of clinical AD had frontal NFT counts ranging from 11/mm^2 to 73/mm^2; 6 had 10–65 NFT/mm^2 in parietal cortex, 8 showed between 8 and 52 NFT/mm^2 in temporal cortex, while all but two had NFT in subiculum ranging from 11/mm^2 to 134/mm^2. Thus, two-thirds of the demented cases met all T criteria for AD. Only a few neuropil threads were seen in frontal and parietal cortex of nondemented subjects or in cases of MID, while in temporal cortex and subiculum their density was usually much higher. Three of the demented subjects lacked NPT in frontal and parietal cortex, while most of them had large numbers in all cortical areas (Figures 5, 6). In summary, clinical diagnosis of AD in this cohort was confirmed at postmortem in 77.7% when using the Khachaturian criteria, and in 83.3% when using those of Tierney et al (7). Among the four demented subjects not meeting the K or T criteria for AD, one showed

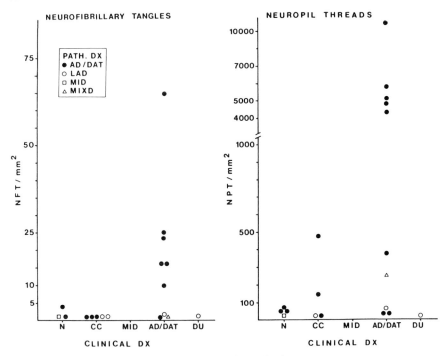

Figure 4. Tangle and neuropil thread counts in parietal cortex

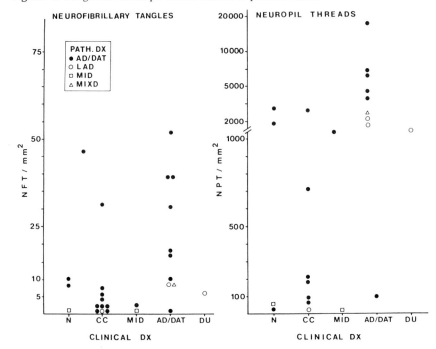

Figure 5. Tangle and neuropil thread counts in temporal cortex

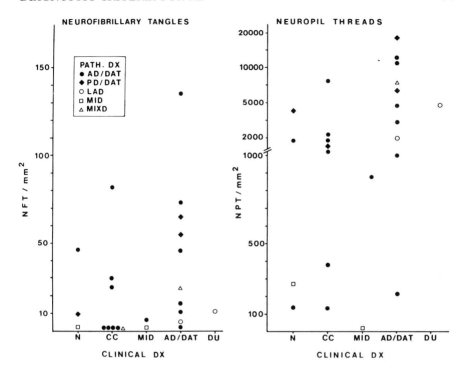

Figure 6. Tangle and neuropil thread counts in subiculum

only old striatal hemorrhage without other CNS pathology, one was Pick's disease, and two subjects aged 58 and 67 years respectively, whose clinical course met criteria for probable AD (MMS 2 and 0, respectively), had spongy changes, neuronal loss and large numbers of ghost tangles in entorhinal and parahippocampal cortex in the absence of neocortical SP. These cases were classified as *limbic type of AD*, recently described by Mizutani et al (24), that may represent a variant of AD or its initial stage (25). When including these criteria for diagnosis of AD, the clinicopathologic coincidence for AD in this series would have been 88.9%. Among the clinically suspected MID cases, only two were confirmed at postmortem, while four were AD with small lacunes or infarcts; one clinically suspected case of MIXD was confirmed at postmortem. A comparison of the clinical and postmortem findings in this series is given in Figure 7.

Relationship of mental status with morphologic changes

Comparison between the density of different types of SP in frontal and temporal cortex and of NFT and neuropil threads in neocortex and hippocampus with intellectual status scored by MMS examination gave the following results (Figures 8–10).

DEMENTED ELDERLY SUBJECTS
CLINICAL DX

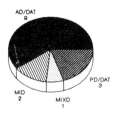

DEMENTED ELDERLY SUBJECTS
PATHOLOGIC DX

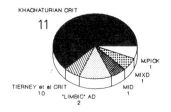

NON DEMENTED ELDERLY SUBJECTS
CLINICAL DX

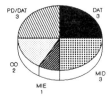

NON DEMENTED ELDERLY SUBJECTS
PATHOLOGIC DX

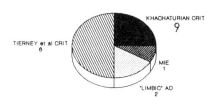

Figure 7. Comparison of clinical and pathological diagnoses in demented and nondemented subjects of group I

- Significant correlation between MMS and SP detected by Bielschowsky stain and tau was seen in the temporal cortex, while in the frontal cortex this correlation was only present for tau-positive plaques. Tau represents an end-stage marker sharing epitopes with Alz-50 and the AD protein A68 (26). No correlation was seen between MMS and the density of SP reacting with chromogranin A, NFP and synaptophysin (Figure 8).
- The density of NFT in frontal, parietal cortex and subiculum, less in hippocampal fields CA1 and CA3, showed significant correlation to cognitive impairment as scored by MMS examination (Figure 9).
- The density of NPT in all examined regions showed a significant correlation with MMS scored mental impairment (Figure 10). NPTs may occur in neurites both inside and outside of SP; they are suggested to be dendritic in origin and closely associated with NFT formation (20,27) and may play a role for cognitive changes (27).

Clinicopathologic evaluation in Parkinson's disease (group II)

All subjects of group II revealed the clinical picture of PD with or without dementia. Postmortem examination in all cases confirmed Parkinson's disease of the Lewy body type (21). Semiquantitative evaluation of AD lesions gave the following results (Table 2).

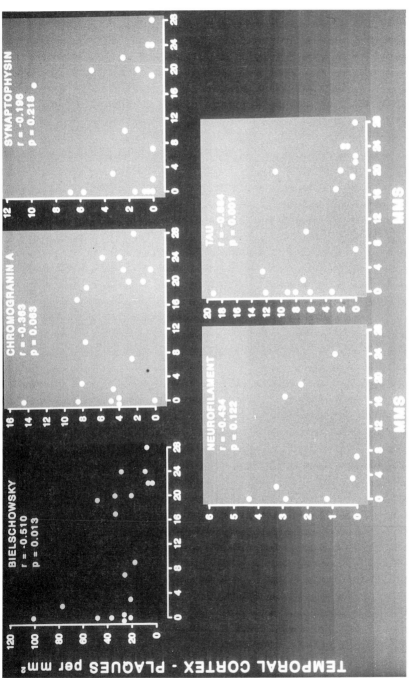

Figure 8. Comparison of plaque counts per/mm² in temporal cortex using Bielschowsky, chromogranin A, NFP, synaptophysin and tau immunoreactivity with cognitive state scored by MMS examination

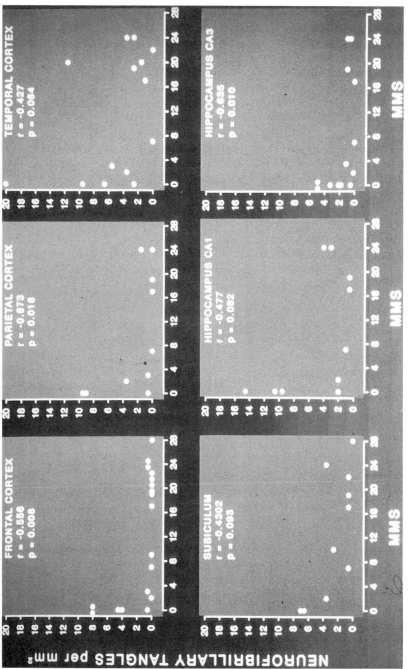

Figure 9. Comparison of tangle counts per/mm² in frontal, parietal, temporal cortex, subiculum, hippocampal fields CA1 and 3 with MMS

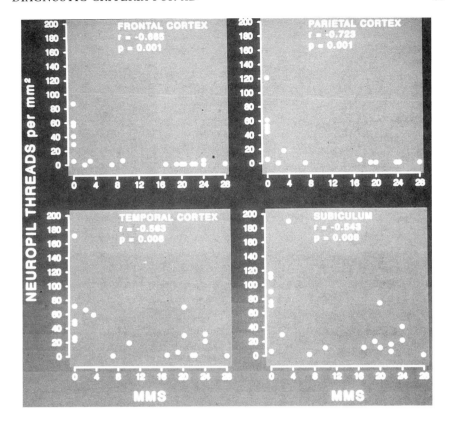

Figure 10. Comparison of neuropil threads per mm^2 in frontal, parietal, temporal cortex and subiculum with cognitive state scored by MMS examination

- Of the 5 nondemented subjects, only 2 had SP in neocortex entorhinal cortex and hippocampal field CA1; only 2 meeting the K criteria of AD. Two had few NFT in hippocampus, thus meeting the T criteria of AD, while 3 cases showed some NFT in the entorhinal cortex, almost entirely restricted to the pre-alpha(II) area (22); these cases did not meet the K and T criteria for AD (5,7), but were consistent with the 'limbic type of AD' (24).
- Almost all of the 12 PD subjects with cognitive changes but no dementia had neocortical plaques, only 5 of them meeting the K criteria for AD; 9 (75%) had NFT in neocortex and hippocampus, thus meeting some or all T criteria for AD. However, all such brains showed few to moderate numbers of NFT in the entorhinal cortex, often exceeding the pre-alpha(II) region, but only in 6 cases (50%) they were accompanied by entorhinal plaques.
- All of the 9 demented subjects showed large numbers of NFT, often ghost tangles, in entorhinal cortex with SP in 7 of them and less severe involvement of hippocampal field CA1 and isocortex. Only 2 of 4 cases with moderate dementia

Table 2. Cognitive state vs Alzheimer lesions in subjects with Parkinson's disease

Age, sex	Duration illness (years)	MMS	Entorhinal cortex				CA-hippocampus				Isocortex				
			ASP	NSP	NFT	NPT	ASP	NSP	NFT	NPT	ASP	NSP	NFT	NPT	AA
No dementia															
70F	6	28	0	0	±	±	0	0	±	0	0	0	0	0	0
79F	11	27	1+	±	1+	1+	1+	0	1+	±	1+	0	±	±	0
77F	10	26	1+	0	0	0	1+	0	0	0	2+	±	0	0	0
73M	20	24	0	0	0	0	0	0	0	0	±	0	0	0	0
83M	1	22	0	0	±	±	0	0	0	0	0	0	0	0	0
Cognitive changes															
72F	11	20	0	0	1+	1+	0	0	1+	±	0	0	0	0	0
73M	9	18	1+	0	1+	1+	0	1+	1+	1+	2+	±	±	±	0
92F	4	17	0	0	1+	±	0	0	±	0	±	0	0	0	0
70F	31	17	0	0	1+	±	0	0	0	0	2+	1+	±	0	0
77F	1	17	0	0	1+	0	0	0	±	±	±	±	0	0	0
70F	10	17	1+	1+	1+	1+	1+	1+	1+	1+	2+	2+	1+	1+	1+
75F	10	16	1+	0	1+	1+	0	0	1+	1+	1+	0	±	±	1+
81M	8	16	0	0	1+	1+	0	0	0	0	1+	0	±	±	0
81F	8	16	1+	1+	2+	1+	1+	1+	2+	2+	2+	1+	1+	1+	1+
90F	10	14	1+	0	2+	2+	0	0	1+	1+	1+	0	±	0	0
84M	4	12	0	0	2+	2+	0	0	1+	1+	1+	0	±	0	0
81F	17	10	1+	1+	2+	1+	1+	1+	2+	1+	2+	2+	2+	2+	1+
Dementia															
84F	4	08	2+	2+	3+	3+	2+	1+	2+	1+	1+	1+	±	1+	1+
83F	15	06	0	0	3+	3+	0	0	2+	2+	±	1+	1+	1+	0
85F	4	06	2+	0	3+	3+	2+	0	1+	1+	2+	1+	±	±	1+
81M	17	04	0	0	3+	3+	0	0	1+	1+	1+	0	1+	1+	1+
79F	10	03	2+	2+	3+	3+	2+	2+	2+	2+	3+	2+	2+	2+	2+
85F	8	02	2+	1+	3+	3+	1+	1+	2+	2+	3+	1+	1+	1+	2+
81M	10	00	2+	0	3+	3+	1+	1+	2+	2+	3+	1+	1+	1+	2+
79M	14	00	2+	1+	3+	3+	2+	2+	2+	2+	3+	3+	3+	3+	2+
65F	10	00	2+	1+	3+	3+	2+	2+	2+	2+	3+	3+	3+	3+	2+

ASP amyloid plaques; NSP neuritic plaques; NFT neurofibrillary tangles; NPT neuropil threads; AA amyloid angiopathy

would have met the K criteria, but all of them met the T criteria of AD, while all of the severely demented PD subjects met all current criteria for AD and thus revealed true combinations of PD and AD. Cases of diffuse Lewy body disease were not seen in this series.

DISCUSSION

The presented data confirm the current view that quantitative pathologic criteria of AD are age-dependent and indicate that some (or even numerous) neocortical $\beta A4$ or amyloid deposits and plaques in the absence of changes detectable by silver stains, tau or Alz-50 immunoreactivity may be part of normal aging without dementia (29-37). While neocortical SP are rare in nondemented subjects in their 60s, but occur in 75-80% of those in their 80s (34), the percentage of nondemented elderly showing no demonstrable SP by any of the employed techniques ranges from 10% to 45% (29-35). It was 16.6% in our group I and 40% of nondemented PD cases in group II. While neocortical SP associated with silver, tau or Alz-50 positive dystrophic neurites are rather rare in nondemented elderly (30-32, 35-37), 9/12 or three-quarters of the nondemented subjects in our group I and 6/9 (two-thirds) in that of Crystal et al (30) met the K criteria for AD based on age-related numbers of neocortical SP (5). Katzman et al (29) reported numerous neocortical SP in only one-third of their nondemented elderly, which is in line with the data in nondemented PD cases of group II (6 out of 17). In other series, the incidence of neocortical amyloid SP deposits in nondemented subjects over age 65 years ranged from 54% to 78% (28,33,35), while extensive AD type neurites immunoreactive to tau, Alz-50 or PHF are not found in normal aged humans (33-37). On the other hand, in our group I there were significant correlations between cognitive impairment and the density of neuritic or classic SP stained with silver methods and tau in frontal and temporal cortex, while no such correlation was seen for SP reactive with chromogranin A and NFP. These data are in broad agreement with those by others using thioflavin, silver, Alz-50 and tau methods (28-32,35,37).

While amyloid deposits in the brain appear to be a common feature of aging with no or little clinical significance, many nondemented elderly lack neocortical NFT (7,28,30-37). In our group I, no NFT were seen in frontal and parietal cortex of nondemented cases or those with mild cognitive changes, but few frontal NFT may occur in about one-third of the nondemented (30). By contrast, variable numbers of NFT in temporal cortex and subiculum were seen in at least 50% of our nondemented and those with cognitive changes, thus meeting some or all T criteria for AD (7). While about 30-37% of demented subjects with clinical AD and numerous SP may be devoid of neocortical NFT (23,30) and show only few NPT (38), representing the 'plaque-only' type of AD (23), in our group I, 5 of 12 demented subjects of clinically probable AD (41%) showed no frontal NFT, while 3 or 4 cases had no parietal and temporal NFT, i.e. only 83% met some or all T criteria for AD (7).

In a small number of severely demented subjects meeting clinical criteria of AD, large numbers of NFT and NPT with or without SP are restricted to the entorhinal and parahippocampal cortex, often without involvement of the neocortex. This 'limbic type of AD' (24) should be more considered in the future, since dense accumulation of NFT and NPT in the layer pre-alpha(II) of the entorhinal area (Brodmann 26) without sufficiently large numbers of neuritic SP or NFT in isocortex or Ammon's horn allowing AD diagnosis due to the K or T criteria have been seen in demented cases meeting clinical criteria of AD (25) and in demented PD subjects (22, our group II). Recent data on patients with Down's syndrome (37), AD (25,40,41) and PD (22, our group II) indicate that early neuronal alterations with deposition of NFT and NPT appear to occur in layer pre-alpha(II) of entorhinal cortex forming the anterior part of the parahippocampal cortex. It gives rise to major portions of the perforant pathway that communicates bidirectionally with the hippocampus and forms its major link with most of the isocortex (40,42). Bilateral destruction of these parts of the entorhinal cortex, as observed in the limbic type of AD (24), in a number of cases of fully developed AD (25,40) and of demented PD (Table 2) isolates the hippocampus from isocortical association areas and may cause severe cognitive impairment (22,25,39–42). In both AD and PD, neuritic SP and NFT appear to initially involve the entorhinal area, the neuritic lesions of which correlate much better with cognitive impairment than do those in hippocampal field CA1 and isocortex, while severely demented PD cases may show massive AD lesions both in entorhinal and isocortex, thus showing true association with AD.

In conclusion, the reported data in a cohort of 27 prospectively evaluated elderly subjects and in a group of 26 PD patients with graded intellectual status using different morphologic criteria for AD (5,7), in accordance with those of other recent studies, indicate that most of current histologic criteria for diagnosing AD cannot clearly distinguish between demented and nondemented subjects, and that βA4 immunohistochemistry or amyloid stains cannot be used alone for the diagnosis of AD without silver techniques and/or immunostaining for tau or Alz-50. In general, mental status shows significant correlations with tau-positive neuritic plaques in frontal and temporal cortex, and with NFT and NPT in frontal, parietal cortex and subiculum. While extensive neuritic AD lesions are not found in the neocortex of nondemented elderly, severe isolated or predominant involvement of the entorhinal area may contribute to cognitive disorders in both AD and PD subjects. Since normal brain aging and AD show a wide variety of lesions of differential distribution, more specific criteria using standardized qualitative and quantitative methods will be necessary to allow better correlations with cognitive changes and to achieve a more precise biopsy and postmortem diagnosis of AD.

REFERENCES

1. American Psychiatric Association. Diagnostic and statistical manual of mental disorders, 3rd ed. Washington, DC: APA, 1987.
2. Hachinski VC, Illif LD, Zilkha E et al. Arch Neurol 1975; 32: 632–7.
3. Bergener M, Reisberg B. Diagnosis and treatment of senile dementia. Berlin: Springer, 1989.
4. Jellinger K, Danielczyk W, Fischer P, Gabriel E. J Neurol Sci 1990; 95: 239–58.
5. Khachaturian Z. Arch Neurol 1985; 42: 1097–105.
6. McKhann G, Drachman D, Folstein M, Katzman R, Price D, Stadlan E. Neurology 1986; 34: 939–44.

7. Tierney MC, Fisher RW, Lewis AJ et al. Neurology 1988; 38: 359-64.
8. Wilcock GK, Hope RA, Brooks ND, Lantos PN et al. J Neurol Neurosurg Psychiat. 1989; 52: 693-700.
9. Lamy C, Duyckaerts C, Delaere P, Payan C, Fermanian J, Poulain V, Hauw JJ. Neuropathol Appl Neurobiol 1989; 15: 563-78.
10. Wisniewski HM, Rabe A, Zigman W, Silverman W. J Neuropathol Exp Neurol 1989; 48: 606-9.
11. Boller F, Lopez OL, Moossy J. Neurology 1989; 39: 76-9.
12. Risse SC, Raskind MA, Nochlin D et al. Am J Psychiat 1990; 147: 168-72.
13. Kukull WA, Larson EB, Reviler BV et al. Neurology 1990; 40: 257-60.
14. Chui HC, Tierney M, Zarow C et al. Neurobiol Aging 1990; 11: 268 (abstr. 64).
15. Duyckaerts C, Abbamondi-Pinto AL, Allen I et al. Neurobiol Aging 1990; 11: 268 (abstr. 65).
16. Fischer P, Gatterer G, Simanyi M, Jellinger K, Materer A, Danielczyk K, Danielczyk W. J Neural Transm (P-D Sect.) 1990; 2: 59-70.
17. Folstein M, Folstein S, McHugh PR. J Psychiatr Res 1975; 12: 189-98.
18. Bancher C, Brunner C, Lassmann H, Budka H, Jellinger K et al. Brain Res 1989; 477: 90-9.
19. Weiler R, Lassmann H, Fischer P, Jellinger K, Winkler H. FEBS Lett 1990; 263: 337-9.
20. Braak H, Braak E. Neuropathol Appl Neurobiol 1988; 14: 39-44.
21. Jellinger K. In Calne DB (ed.) Handbook of experimental pharmacology, vol. 88. Berlin: Springer, 1989: 47-112.
22. Braak H, Braak E. J Neural Transm (P-D Sect.) 1990; 2: 45-57.
23. Terry RD, Hansen LA, DeTeresa R, Davies P, Tobias H, Katzman R. J Neuropathol Exp Neurol 1987; 46: 262-8.
24. Mizutani T, Amano N, Sasaki H, Morimatsu Y, Mori H et al. Acta Neuropathol (Berl) 1990; 80: 575-80.
25. Braak H, Braak E. Acta Neuropathol (Berl) 1990; 80: 479-86.
26. Ksiezak-Reding KS, Binder LI, Yen S-H. J Neurosci Res 1990; 25: 412-30.
27. Yamaguchi H, Nakazato Y, Shoji M, Ihara Y, Hirai S. Acta Neuropathol (Berl) 1990; 80: 368-74.
28. Davies L, Wolska BV, Hilbich C, Multhaup G et al. Neurology 1988; 38: 1688-93.
29. Katzman R, Terry R, DeTeresa R, Brown T et al. Ann Neurol 1988; 23: 138-44.
30. Crystal H, Dickson D, Fuld P, Masur D et al. Neurology 1988; 38: 1682-7.
31. Delaere P, Duyckaerts C, Brion JP et al. Acta Neuropathol (Berl) 1989; 77: 645-53.
32. Delaere P, Duyckaerts C, Ho Y, Piette F. Acta Neuropathol (Berl) 1991: 81.
33. Mann DMA, Brown AMT, Prinja D, Jones D, Davies DA. Neuropathol Appl Neurobiol 1990; 16: 17-25.
34. Tomlinson BE. Neuropathol Appl Neurobiol 1989; 15: 491-512.
35. McKee AC, Kosik KS, Kowall NW. Neurobiol Aging 1990; 11: 283 (abstr. 124).
36. Dickson DW, Mattiace LA, Crystal H et al. Neurobiol Aging 1990; 11: 305.
37. Arriagada PV, Hyman BT. Neurobiol Aging 1990; 11: 324 (abstr. 297).
38. Joachim C, Morris J, Platt D, Mori H, Selkoe D. Neurobiol Aging 1990; 11: 282 (abstr. 123).
39. Hyman BT, Mann DMA. Neurobiol Aging 1990; 11: 267 (abstr. 61).
40. Van Hoesen GW, Kuljis RO, Damasio H, Damasio AR. Neurobiol Aging 1990; 11: 268 (abstr. 63).
41. Esiri MM, Pearson RCA, Steele JE, Bown DM, Powell TPS. J Neurol Neurosurg Psychiatr 1990; 53: 161-5.
42. Hyman BT, Kromer LJ, Van Hoesen GW. Brain Res 1988; 450: 392-7.

Address for correspondence:

Dr K. Jellinger, Ludwig Boltzmann Institute of Clinical Neurobiology, Lainz Hospital, 1 Wolkersbergenstrasse, A-1130 Vienna, Austria

11 Entorhinal Lesions in Dementia

HEIKO BRAAK AND EVA BRAAK

Many dementing disorders are associated with morphological changes in the antero-medial portions of the temporal lobe. Among these are Alzheimer's disease, Parkinson's disease, and the syndrome of dementia with argyrophilic grains. Alzheimer's disease certainly is the most important of these disorders (1). It accounts for approximately 60% of the cases of presenile and senile dementia. Parkinson's disease is not purely a disorder of the extrapyramidal system, since it is frequently associated with intellectual decline (2). Finally, it should be emphasized that numerous cases of clinically proven dementia fail to reveal the morphological features of known dementing disorders (3). Application of advanced silver methods revealed in quite a number of these cases hitherto unknown pathological changes in the form of small argyrophilic grains in the antero-medial portions of the temporal lobe (4-6).

Before going into details, it appears appropriate to recapitulate that the cerebral cortex in the mammalian brain is formed of two fundamentally different types of grey matter: the isocortex and the allocortex. The extended and more or less uniformly built isocortex represents the dominating structure in the human brain. The heterogeneous allocortex is small in comparison and comprises among other areas the hippocampal formation and the entorhinal region. The entorhinal region spreads over anterior portions of the parahippocampal gyrus and the gyrus ambiens. It exhibits a complex lamination pattern and numerous subareas. None of the entorhinal layers is matched by corresponding layers of the isocortex. The 'transentorhinal region' is located between the proper entorhinal region and the adjoining temporal isocortex. It is easily differentiated due to the conspicuous descent of the superficial entorhinal cellular layer (7-10).

When dissecting the brain for neuropathological examination, a piece of the hippocampal formation is usually cut out at the level of the lateral geniculate body. This provides the observer with the classical transversal section through the hippocampus but, unfortunately, this section will not contain any significant portions of the entorhinal region, since at this latitude the entorhinal cortex is either missing or present with only remnants of its posterior pole. This fact is frequently not taken into consideration and it might also explain why so little is known about the pathology of the entorhinal region in the various diseases of the human brain (8).

Alzheimer's Disease: Basic Mechanisms, Diagnosis and Therapeutic Strategies
Edited by K. Iqbal, D. R. C. McLachlan, B. Winblad and H. M. Wisniewski
©1991 John Wiley & Sons Ltd

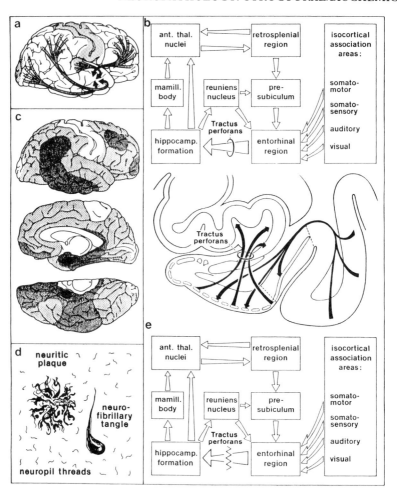

Figure 1. (a) (b): Fibre bundles from isocortical association areas converge upon the entorhinal cortex which in turn projects via the perforant path (thick arrow) to the hippocampal formation. (c) Distribution of Alzheimer-related cortical changes. The most severely affected area is seen in the entorhinal region (black spot). (d) Neurofibrillary changes consist of three kinds of lesions: neuritic plaques, neurofibrillary tangles, and neuropil threads. (e) The transport of information from isocortical association areas to the hippocampal formation is bilaterally interrupted by destruction of the cells of origin of the perforant tract. This also hampers the flow of information running within the limbic circuits (reuniens circuit and Papez circuit)

The highly differentiated entorhinal cortex serves as an association centre of the allocortex. This function gains more and more importance with phylogenetic advance and increasing predominance of the isocortex. This concept is corroborated by recent investigations in the primate brain showing that the entorhinal region receives a particularly dense input from all isocortical association areas providing it with abundant somatomotor, somatosensory, acoustic and visual information (Figure 1a) (11,12). Via the presubiculum there is also a strong input from limbic circuits such as the reuniens circuit and the Papez circuit (Figure 1b). The outer cellular layers of the entorhinal region generate the perforant path and via this fibre tract both the isocortical information and the limbic circuit data are transported to the hippocampal formation. This information transfer from isocortical association areas and limbic circuits via the entorhinal region to the hippocampal formation is of utmost significance for maintaining mnemonic functions.

All the territories under consideration—the isocortical association areas, the entorhinal region, the hippocampal formation and the relay stations of the limbic circuits—exhibit severe structural changes during the course of Alzheimer's disease. In Parkinson's disease, however, and in cases of dementia with argyrophilic grains, the cortical pathology is far more restricted and remains virtually confined to the entorhinal region.

ALZHEIMER'S DISEASE

Insoluble fibrous material is progressively accumulated during the course of Alzheimer's disease. This material is deposited in both extracellular and intraneuronal locations. The extracellular component is the A4 amyloid protein, while the intraneuronal deposits make up the neurofibrillary changes of the Alzheimer type. Highly selective and sensitive silver techniques are available for both the amyloid and neurofibrillary changes (13-15).

Amyloid deposits are seen in virtually all subdivisions of the cerebral cortex. Most amyloid patches turn out to be devoid of pathologically changed argyrophilic neurites. Amyloid deposits are even encountered in the white substance beneath the cortex.

Neurofibrillary changes (neuritic plaques, neurofibrillary tangles, neuropil threads, see Figure 1d) exhibit a distinct but varying distribution in different cortical areas (10,15). Figure 1c displays the severity of the cortical changes, as compiled from data available in the literature (16). In general, the isocortex is severely involved—in particular its association areas; nevertheless, the brunt of the pathology is borne by the entorhinal region (Figure 1c, black spot; Figure 2, upper row). The projection cells within the superficial layer of the entorhinal cortex are extremely susceptible to the development of tangles. The material available to us suggests that these cells are the first neurons in the brain showing the pathology. This is also indicated by cases of Down's syndrome ranging in age from 25 to 35 years exhibiting a cortex virtually devoid of neurofibrillary changes apart from an already severely affected superficial entorhinal cellular layer. The projection cells of the affected layer generate important portions of the perforant path. Accordingly, the bilateral pathological process will sooner or later lead to an impairment of the information transport from the entorhinal region to the hippocampal formation. The lamina-specific destructive process will ultimately cause a 'disconnection syndrome', in the sense of the late American neurologist Geschwind;

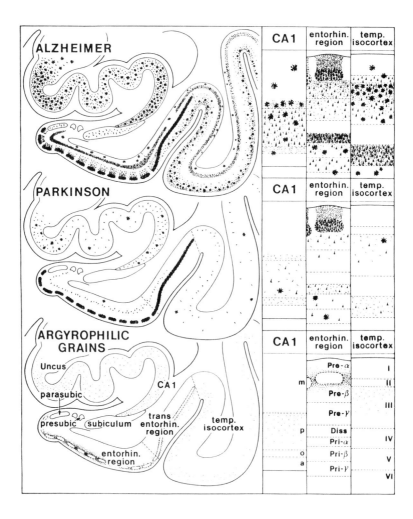

Figure 2. Summary diagram of neurofibrillary changes seen in cases of Alzheimer's disease (upper row), Parkinson's disease with cognitive decline (middle row), and dementia with argyrophilic grains (lower row). The distribution pattern of the neurofibrillary changes seen in Parkinson's disease differs markedly from that found in fully developed Alzheimer's disease. Neuritic plaques occur only rarely. Both the hippocampal formation and the isocortex display only a few tangles and neuropil threads. Severe destruction is virtually confined to the superficial cellular layer of the entorhinal region. Similarly, in cases of dementia with argyrophilic grains the pathologically changed processes can predominantly be found within the superficial layers of the entorhinal cortex. a, alveus; CA1, first sector of the Ammon's horn; Diss, lamina dissecans; entorhin. region, entorhinal region; m, molecular layer of CA1; p, pyramidal layers of CA1; parasubic, parasubiculum; Pre-α, superficial entorhinal layer; Pre-$\alpha\beta$, γ, sublayers of the lamina principalis externa; Pri-α, β, γ, sublayers of the lamina principalis interna; presubic, presubiculum proper; temp. isocortex, temporal isocortex; transentorhin. region, transentorhinal region; I-VI, isocortical layers (with kind permission from 20)

isocortex and allocortex become disconnected from each other and, in addition, the change will also disrupt the flow of information in the limbic circuits. The bilateral entorhinal pathology may, therefore, serve as an explanation for the early and severe impairment of intellectual capacities shown by individuals suffering from Alzheimer's disease (17,18).

PARKINSON'S DISEASE

Similar considerations can also be applied to Parkinson's disease with progressive cognitive decline. Previous studies have failed to disclose major Alzheimer-related changes in the cerebral cortex of the parkinsonian brain (19). Preparations processed with selective silver techniques, nevertheless, reveal a distinct set of cortical changes (9).

Amyloid patches are encountered in virtually all areas of the cerebral cortex. The density of cortical amyloid deposits is clearly above the level seen in mentally preserved, age-matched control cases and is similar to that seen in Alzheimer's disease. The hippocampal formation contains comparably small numbers of amyloid patches while the presubiculum, the entorhinal region and the isocortex turn out to be infested with amyloid deposits.

However, when focusing on neurofibrillary changes it becomes obvious that the parkinsonian isocortex remains almost devoid of intraneuronal changes. Neuritic plaques are extremely rare in Parkinson's disease. Both the hippocampal formation and the isocortex exhibit only a sparse number of neurofibrillary tangles and neuropil threads. Their numbers are by no means high enough to permit the diagnosis of a concomitant fully developed Alzheimer's disease. Only the entorhinal region and transentorhinal region show severe changes and these are virtually confined to the superficial cellular layer which appears to be infested with tangles and threads (Figure 2, middle row). The parkinsonian brain is obviously prone to develop circumscribed, layer-specific and particularly severe pathological changes in the entorhinal cortex. Initially, the change seems to begin in the transentorhinal region, then spreading to the proper entorhinal region. The bilateral circumscribed lesion destroys the perforant path and eventually hampers the transport of isocortical and limbic circuit information from the entorhinal region to the hippocampal formation (9).

DEMENTIA WITH ARGYROPHILIC GRAINS

A fair number of cases of clinically proven dementia remains uncorrelated with any of the known neuropathological changes even after thoroughgoing post-mortem examination (3). In quite a number of such cases it has been possible to demonstrate — with the use of advanced silver techniques — the presence of abundant argyrophilic grains scattered throughout the neuropil of a restricted number of cortical areas and subcortical nuclei (4,5). The grains occur predominantly in the hippocampal formation and the entorhinal region. A less dense distribution of grains is seen in the adjoining isocortical areas. The grains generally show an elongated body with cone-shaped poles frequently giving off filiform appendages. Size, shape, and pattern of distribution suggest the grains to be pathologically changed neurites. Grains of this type do not occur in the cortex of nondemented individuals of old age. Hence, these unusual structures cannot be considered typical age-related changes of the human brain.

The antero-medial portion of the temporal lobe is most severely affected. The highest density of grains is found within the superficial layers of the entorhinal region (Figure 2, lower row). The distinct distribution pattern again suggests an impairment of the nerve cells generating the perforant path. It may well be that even subtle lesions — provided that they are bilateral — cause severe disturbances in the information transfer from both the isocortex and the limbic circuits to the hippocampal formation, which will ultimately lead to a corresponding cognitive decline.

Acknowledgments

This work was kindly supported by the Deutsche Forschungsgemeinschaft, the Friedrich Merz Stiftung, Frankfurt and Degussa, Hanau. The authors would also like to gratefully acknowledge the support of the Alzheimer Association (USA) for their travel award.

REFERENCES

1. Von Braunmühl A. In Lubarsch O, Henke F, Rössle R (eds) Handbuch der speziellen pathologischen Anatomie und Histologie, Vol XIII/1A. Berlin: Springer, 1957: 337-539.
2. Cummings JL. Eur Neurol 1988; 28 (suppl. 1): 15-23.
3. Ulrich J, Probst A, Wüest M. J Neurol 1986; 233: 118-22.
4. Braak H, Braak E. Neurosci Lett 1987; 76: 124-7.
5. Braak H, Braak E. Neuropath Appl Neurobiol 1989; 15: 13-26.
6. Itagaki S, McGeer PL, Akiyama H, Beattie BL, Walker DG, Moore RW, McGeer EG. Ann Neurol 1989; 26: 685-9.
7. Braak H. Architectonics of the human telencephalic cortex. Berlin: Springer, 1980: 1-147.
8. Braak H, Braak E. Acta Neuropathol 1985; 68: 325-32.
9. Braak H, Braak E. J Neural Transm (P-D Sect.) 1990; 2: 45-57.
10. Braak H, Braak E. In Maurer K, Riederer P, Beckmann H (eds) Alzheimer's disease. Epidemiology, neuropathology, neurochemistry and clinics. Wien: Springer, 1990: 85-91.
11. Van Hoesen GW. Trends Neurosci 1982; 5: 345-50.
12. Van Hoesen GW, Pandya DN, Butters N. Science 1972; 175: 1471-3.
13. Campbell SK, Switzer RC, Martin TL. Soc Neurosci (abstr.) 1987; 13: 678.
14. Gallyas F, Wolff JR. J Histochem Cytochem 1986; 34: 1667-72.
15. Braak H, Braak E, Kalus P. Acta Neuropathol 1989; 77: 494-506.
16. Brun A. In Reisberg B (ed.) Alzheimer's disease. The standard reference. New York: Free Press, 1983: 37-47.
17. Hyman BT, van Hoesen GW, Damasio AR, Barnes CL. Science 1984; 225: 1168-70.
18. Hyman BT, van Hoesen GW, Kromer LJ, Damasio AR. Ann Neurol 1986; 20: 472-81.
19. Agid Y, Ruberg M, Dubois B, Pillon B, Cusimano G, Raisman R, Cash R, Lhermitte F, Javoy-Agid F. Clin Neuropharmacol 1986; 9 (suppl. 2): 22-36.

20. Braak H, Braak E. In Kostovic I, Knezevic S (eds) Neurodevelopment, aging, and cognition. Boston: Birkhäuser, 1990.

Address for correspondence:

Prof.Dr.med. Heiko Braak,
Zentrum der Morphologie,
Klinikum der J.W. Goethe Universität,
Theodor Stern Kai 7,
D-6000 Frankfurt/Main 70, Germany.
Tel. 069-6301-6900
Fax. 069-6301-6301

12 Diagnostic Difficulties in Kufs' Disease and Early Onset of Alzheimer's Disease

K. E. WISNIEWSKI, H. H. GOEBEL, E. KIDA AND K. RENKAWEK

We have studied seven cases with similar onset and progressive neurological symptoms starting between the ages of 30 to 40 years. They were all suspected for Kufs' disease, or adult form of neuronal ceroid lipofuscinosis (ANCL), but the diagnosis of Alzheimer's disease (AD) was also taken into consideration. Brain biopsy and/or postmortem studies allowed us to diagnose AD in 5/7 cases, and Kufs' disease in 2/7 cases. In all 7 cases brain atrophy associated with neuronal loss and aging lipopigment in the neurons was present. In AD cases neurofibrillary tangles and neuritic plaques were present, and in Kufs' disease cases storage lipopigment with fingerprints and curvilinear profiles in the lysosomes of neurons were present. In one case with Kufs' disease (age 53) neuritic plaques were found in the cortical mantle, but not neurofibrillary tangles. The small number of neuritic plaques in this case did not allow for the diagnosis of AD. The ultrastructural differences of the lipopigment in the lysosomes of neurons in these two conditions and the diagnostic difficulties are discussed.

INTRODUCTION

The adult form of neuronal ceroid lipofuscinosis (ANCL) or Kufs' disease (1-4) and early onset of familial Alzheimer's disease (AD) are rare, chronic and progressive neurodegenerative disorders of unknown etiology occurring in middle-aged persons. In both of these conditions progressive dementia, seizures, and motor disabilities leading to a vegetative stage associated with progressive brain atrophy are present. As the clinical course may be similar and there are no reliable diagnostic markers in either of these conditions the definite diagnosis may be difficult, and in some cases rests upon postmortem study. In both conditions neurons contain lipopigment within the lysosomes, which are increased in number and size and disclose autofluorescent positive granules. However, there are biochemical and immunocytochemical differences between lipopigment in AD and ANCL (5,6). Neuronal lipopigment is moreover incomparably more abundant in ANCL, usually visible also in proximal, distended segment of axons and reveals a typical pigmentoarchitectonic pattern (7).

Alzheimer's Disease: Basic Mechanisms, Diagnosis and Therapeutic Strategies
Edited by K. Iqbal, D. R. C. McLachlan, B. Winblad and H. M. Wisniewski
© 1991 John Wiley & Sons Ltd

At the ultrastructural level in ANCL brains, characteristic granular, fingerprint and/or curvilinear profiles are present. The extraneuronal tissue (skin punch, rectal biopsies, and buffy coat), however, may be negative for these lysosomal inclusion bodies. Alzheimer's disease has a much higher incidence than ANCL, but onset between 25–45 years is rare (8). Neuropathological diagnosis is established using morphological criteria (9,10) including the quantitative estimation of neurofibrillary tangles (NFT) and neuritic plaques (NP). However, in some cases even morphological study in these conditions may provide diagnostic difficulties, especially when lipopigment accumulation and senile changes coexist.

The following were observed in material collected at the Institute for Basic Research at the George A. Jervis Diagnostic and Research Clinic.

MATERIAL AND METHODS

Cases 1 and 2

Two siblings with signs of dementia, seizures (generalized and myoclonic) seen at the age of 35 years and motor difficulties since the age of 38 years were observed. The EEG showed slow background activity with periodic spikes and slow waves. CT scan and MRI revealed progressive brain atrophy. Intensive diagnostic work-up for metabolic diseases was negative. Lysosomal disease, leukodystrophies and mitochondrial disease were ruled out. In the younger sibling at the age of 39 years diagnostic brain biopsy was performed and showed neuronal loss, gliosis and accumulation of lipopigment in neurons. The latter at the ultrastructural level were without storage material in the neuronal lysosomes, such as curvilinear, fingerprint and/or granular profiles. In the cortical layers (mainly IIIth and Vth) many scattered NP were found. Also, NFT were also seen in some neurons. Diagnosis of AD was established. The patients are still alive at age 43 and 45 years respectively and are in a vegetative stage. Treatment for seizures, combinations of phenytoin, carbamazepine, clorazepate, barbiturates and valproic acid did not result in sustained improvement.

Cases 3, 4 and 5

Three siblings died aged 38, 46 and 48 years respectively. Clinically, all three siblings had a history of dementia, myoclonic seizures and motor disabilities from the age of 30 years. They were suspected for Kufs' disease. We received tissue only from a 38-year-old male sibling (buffy coat, skin punch biopsy and brain). The skin and buffy coat were nondiagnostic. The brain tissue showed neuronal loss that was replaced by glial proliferation and numerous neuritic plaques and NFT. At the ultrastructural level only aging lipopigment was found; no granular, fingerprint or curvilinear inclusions were noted. AD was diagnosed.

Case 6

This was a 53-year-old male who had progressive neurological dysfunction from the age of 30 (this case was published previously by Goebel et al, 11). Diagnosis of

Kufs' disease was made postmortem. A chronic subdural hematoma over both hemispheres and an old laceration over the left temporal lobe were noted. At the light microscopic level changes typical of Kufs' disease were found with storage of lipopigment present in hematoxylin (HE), periodic acid-Schiff technique (PAS), Luxol fast blue and at the ultrastructural level. However, when the case was first published (7,11), silver impregnation stainings were not performed. We performed both silver impregnation stainings and immunocytochemical studies using antibodies to some fragments (4G8) to the β-peptide of the amyloid beta precursor protein (ABPP) domain, and found the presence of neuritic plaques in the cortical mantle; however, their number was distinctly smaller than in AD cases. Immunoreactivity to different fragments of amyloid beta protein and to lectins, proteinase inhibitors to the neuritic plaques and neurons were described previously (5,12,13). No NFT could be detected in this case and the diagnosis of Kufs' disease was maintained.

Case 7

The onset of symptoms was at the age of 40 years. This patient had dementia, seizures, and motor disabilities and died at the age of 56 years. The skin punch biopsy and rectal biopsy were negative for storage disease. Postmortem showed storage lipopigment that was autofluorescent positive, and at the ultrastructural level fingerprints and curvilinear bodies were noted in addition to aging lipopigment. Diagnosis of Kufs' disease was made.

The pigmentoarchitectonic pattern described by Goebel and Braak (7,11) was present in cases 6 and 7.

DISCUSSION

Both AD and ANCL may present with similar neurological abnormalities; however, morphological changes are different. In all our seven cases similar onset and neurological presentation was observed, but only 5 of 7 cases were AD. Recently, it has been documented that in early onset of AD parietal lobe symptoms seem to predominate (14). ANCL is a rare disorder, and between 1925 and 1988 only about 100 cases were published; of these only 25% filled the clinicopathological criteria and 25% were not sufficiently documented (15). The diagnosis should be based on clinicopathological findings, especially the presence of typical pigmentoarchitectonic pathology, and characteristic lysosomal inclusion bodies (7,11,16,17). In the cases where a small quantity of tissue from brain biopsy is available, the proper diagnosis is usually very uncertain, as even the finding of lysosomal inclusion bodies can be misleading, as for example fingerprint profiles were described in metachromatic leukodystrophy (7). As we emphasized in all suspected cases, silver staining and immunocytochemistry may be useful as observed in cases 3, 4 and 5. It is important to notice that the presence of NP may be also the source of confusion, as we showed in case 6, representing unquestionable ANCL concomitant NP. It is of interest that in this case no NFT were found, which could confirm previous suggestions that NFT never occurs in ANCL (7), a finding of important diagnostic value if confirmed by future studies. The small number of NP in this case did not allow for diagnosis of ANCL/AD variant. The lack of NFT in case 3, however, could also hinder the diagnosis of early onset AD, but the presence of a large number of NP is conclusive. Clinical suspicion of ANCL could not be maintained on the pathological grounds that we did not observe typical storage material at both light and electron microscopic level in this case. Future biochemical and molecular genetic studies with specific diagnostic markers for these diseases will clarify the diagnosis of both of these conditions.

Acknowledgments

This work was supported by NIH Grant NS23717. The authors wish to express their appreciation to Madeline Tinney for excellent secretarial assistance and Mr Lawrence Black for bibliographical assistance.

REFERENCES

1. Kufs H. Über eine Spätform der amaurotischen Idiotie und ihre heredofamiliären Grundlagen. Zeit Ges Neurol Psychiat 1925; 95: 168-88.
2. Kufs H. Über die Bedeutung der optischen Komponente der amaurotischen Idiotie in diagnostischer und erbbiologischer Beziehung und über die Existenz 'spätester' Fälle bei dieser Krankheit. Zeit Ges Neurol Psychiat 1927; 109: 453-87.
3. Kufs H. Über einen Fall von Spätform der amaurotischen Idiotie mit atypischem Verlauf und mit terminalen schweren Störungen des Fettstoffwechsels im Gesamtorganismus. Zeit Ges Neurol Psychiat 1929; 122: 395-415.
4. Kufs H. Über einen Fall von spätester Form der amaurotischen Idiotie mit dem Beginn im 42 und Tod im 59. Lebensjahre in klinischer, histologischer und vererbungspathologischer Beziehung. Zeit Ges Neurol Psychiat 1931; 127: 432-48.
5. Wisniewski KE, Maslinska D, Kitaguchi T, Kim KS, Goebel HH, Haltia M. Topographic heterogeneity of amyloid b-protein epitopes in brains with various forms of neuronal ceroid lipofuscinoses suggesting defective processing of amyloid precursor protein. Acta Neuropathol 1990; 80: 26-34.
6. Kitaguchi T, Wisniewski KE, Maslinski S, Maslinska D, Wisniewski TM, Kim, KS. B-protein immunoreactivity in brains of patients with neuronal ceroid lipofuscinosis: ultrastructural and biochemical demonstration. Neurosci Lett 1990; 112: 155-60.
7. Goebel HH, Braak H. Review article: adult neuronal ceroid-lipofuscinosis. Clin Neuropathol 1989; 8: 109-19.
8. Rocca WA, Amaducci LA, Schoenberg BS. Epidemiology of clinically diagnosed Alzheimer's disease. Ann Neurol 1986; 19: 415-24.
9. Khachaturian ZS. Diagnosis of Alzheimer's disease. 1985; 42: 1097-105.
10. Lewis, AJ, Tierney, MC, Fisher RH, Zorzitto ML, Snow WG, Reid DW. Pathologic diagnosis of Alzheimer's disease. Neurology 1988; 38: 1660.
11. Goebel HH, Braak H, Seidel D, Doshi R, Marsden CD, Gullotta F. Morphologic studies on adult neuronal-ceroid lipofuscinosis (NCL). Clin Neuropathol 1982; 1: 151-62.
12. Wisniewski KE, Maslinska D. Lectin histochemistry in brains with juvenile form of neuronal ceroid-lipofuscinosis (Batten disease). Acta Neuropathol 1990; 80: 274-9.
13. Wisniewski KE, Kida E. Proteinase inhibitor α_1-antichymotrypsin has different expression in various forms of neuronal ceroid lipofuscinosis. Exp Neurol 1990; 110: 121-6.

14. Blennow K, Wallin A, Gottfries CG. Heterogeneity of 'probable Alzheimer's disease'. Neurobiol Aging 1990; 11: 254.
15. Berkovic, SF, Carpenter, S, Andermann F, Andermann E, Wolfe LS. Kufs' disease: a critical reappraisal. Brain 1988; 111: 27-62.
16. Carpenter S, Karpati G, Andermann F, Jacob JC, Andermann E. The ultrastructural characteristics of the abnormal cytosomes in Batten-Kufs' disease. Brain 1977; 100: 137-56.
17. Carpenter S. Morphological diagnosis and misdiagnosis in Batten-Kufs' disease. Am J Med Genet 1988; 5: 85-91.

Address for correspondence:

Dr K. E. Wisniewski,
New York State Office of Mental Retardation and Developmental Disabilities,
Institute for Basic Research in Developmental Disabilities,
Department of Pathological Neurobiology,
Staten Island,
NY 10314, USA

13 Alzheimer-Type Pathological Changes in Down's Syndrome Individuals of Various Ages

BRADLEY T. HYMAN AND DAVID M.A. MANN

Neurofibrillary tangles (NFT) and senile plaques (SP) are the characteristic morphological changes of Alzheimer's disease (AD). However, patients with Down's syndrome (DS) (trisomy 21) commonly are found to have developed NFT and SP in middle age, and to uniformly develop these changes over the age of 40 years. For example, in a large series Malamud found Alzheimer-type changes in 2.4% of DS individuals between the ages of 11 and 30 years, 30% of DS individuals between the ages of 31 and 40 years, and in 100% of individuals over the age of 41 years (1).

The degree to which the changes that occur in middle age in DS mimic those that occur in later years in AD has been investigated in depth (2-4; see 5 for review). NFT and SP appear to be morphologically and immunohistochemically indistinguishable between DS and AD. Neurochemical alterations are also analogous. These results, in combination with the age-prevalence data noted above, suggest that in Down's individuals over the age of 20 years there is a predictable accumulation of AD pathology proceeding inexorably from minimal alterations to full Alzheimer pathology. Thus a study of DS individuals across this age range provides a model for the identification of early and moderate changes in the disease process, in individuals in whom it can be safely assumed would have developed AD had they lived longer. This provides an approach to study the time course and regional hierarchical patterns of NFT and SP accumulation from cross-sectional data.

Initial studies of this issue in DS (6) and in normal aging and AD (7-9) suggest that a focus of early Alzheimer pathologic change is in the entorhinal cortex and hippocampal formation. Moreover, our previous studies of AD suggest that there is a stereotypic, hierarchical pattern of neuronal vulnerability according to certain anatomic areas, with certain cytoarchitectural regions and lamina affected earlier and more severely than others (10). Studies using the monoclonal antibody Alz-50 (11,12) suggest that this antibody recognizes neurons in an early state of neurofibrillary degeneration. We have now studied the distribution and degree of AD neuronal changes in the hippocampal formation of 20 individuals with Down's syndrome of various ages to test the hypotheses that Down's syndrome individuals would (a) develop NFT in a regionally specific and hierarchical fashion with

Alzheimer's Disease: Basic Mechanisms, Diagnosis and Therapeutic Strategies
Edited by K. Iqbal, D. R. C. McLachlan, B. Winblad and H. M. Wisniewski
©1991 John Wiley & Sons Ltd

increasing age, and (b) that Alz-50 immunoreactivity would occur specifically in these same cytoarchitectural fields, perhaps preceding the development of NFT. Analysis of the distribution of senile plaques will be presented separately (Hyman and Mann, in preparation).

METHODS

Twenty individuals with DS, ages 13–71 years, were studies (Table 1). Clinical history was supplied from hospital records or from observations of attending physicians, and patients were noted as demented or not demented regardless of baseline level of cognitive ability. Paraffin-embedded blocks of the hippocampal formation were available for study. Of the 20 cases, 11 included the hippocampal formation and anterior parahippocampal gyrus (entorhinal cortex), and the remainder were obtained at the level of the main body of the hippocampus and posterior parahippocampal gyrus. In one instance, 50-μm frozen sections were obtained from wet tissue blocks from throughout the hippocampus.

Thioflavin S and Alz-50 immunostaining were carried out as previously described (12). The number of neuronal alterations were assessed using a Leitz Aristoplan Variophot microscope with epifluorescence and bright field analysis. The number of lesions per 10× objective field was assessed in each cytoarchitectural region of the hippocampus. With the configuration of this microscope, this is a 1.8 mm^2 field.

Table 1. Characteristics of Down's syndrome individuals

	Age	Clinical status[1]	Neuropathology (NFT)	Alz-50:Thio-S[2]
DS-1	13	ND	None	NA
DS-2	31	ND	Mild	≥
DS-3	37	ND	Mild	>
DS-4	38	ND	Mild	>
DS-5	40	ND	Mild	=
DS-6	41	UNK	Mild	>
DS-7	42	ND	Mild	=
DS-8	47	ND	Moderate	>
DS-9	49	ND	Mild	>
DS-10	50	PD	Moderate	=
DS-11	52	UNK	Marked	<
DS-12	53	ND	Marked	>
DS-13	58	D	Marked	>
DS-14	59	D	Marked	>
DS-15	59	D	Marked	<
DS-16	60	D	Marked	=
DS-17	60	D	Marked	=
DS-18	64	D	Marked	>
DS-19	65	D	Marked	=
DS-20	71	D	Marked	>

[1]D, demented; ND, not demented; PD, probable dementia; UNK, unknown.
[2]Estimate of ratio of Alz-50 positive changes to thioflavin-S positive changes, as judged on adjacent sections. NA, not applicable.

A semiquantitative scale of 0 = no lesions, + = 1-10 lesions, + + = 11-25 lesions, + + + = 26-50 lesions, and + + + + = > 50 lesions was used (13). Based on the semiquantitative assessments, the amount of Alz-50 immunostaining of neuronal alterations was judged to be 'less than', 'equal to', or 'greater than' the degree of changes visualized with thioflavin S (Table 1). In addition, an overall assessment of 'none', 'mild', 'moderate', or 'severe' was also given to the degree of pathological changes in each case (Table 1). All histologic studies and assessments were performed without knowledge of age or clinical history.

RESULTS

Clinical pathological correlation

Of the 20 cases examined, 18 had available information from the attending physician to assign a clinical status of 'not demented' or 'demented'. Table 1 shows that none of the cases below age 49 years was considered to be demented, whereas all the cases above age 58 years were considered to be cognitively impaired. A comparison of age to clinical status shows that this relationship is highly significant ($P < 0.001$, Wilcoxon signed-rank test).

It is interesting to note that the degree of pathological change in the hippocampal formation was also related both to age and to clinical status. While 9 cases with available clinical histories had 'marked' pathological change, only 1 of these individuals was judged to be 'not demented'. In the 2 cases in which 'moderate' pathologic changes were noted, 1 was felt to be not demented and 1 was felt to be probably dementing. Of 7 instances in which pathologic changes were 'mild', all 6 for whom clinical history is available were felt to be nondementing.

NFT accumulate with increased age in a hierarchical fashion

Results of the semiquantitative assessment of neurofibrillary tangles are illustrated in Figure 1. The CA1/subicular zone is the most affected region of the hippocampus proper in DS. With increasing age, the number of NFT increases dramatically (Figure 1). The average number of NFT in this region is 0 in the 13-year-old individual, but after age 30 years begins to increase so that by the fourth decade there are, on average, more than 10 NFT per 1.8-mm^2 field, increasing to more than 50 NFT per 1.8-mm^2 field over the age of 50 years. The relationship to age is highly significant ($P < 0.001$, linear regression).

Other cytoarchitectural regions of the hippocampal formation were affected by NFT in a discrete, hierarchical fashion: CA1/subiculum $\gg$ CA4, CA3 > dentate gyrus, presubiculum. Of note, nearly a third of cases over age 61 years had > 10 NFT in the dentate gyrus granule cells (along with > 50 NFT in CA1/subiculum, etc.). As in AD, the granule cells appear to be extremely resistant to neurofibrillary degeneration, and NFT appear in this cytoarchitectural field only in instances with the most severe degree of overall pathological changes. The temporal neocortex also contained numerous NFT, SP and congophilic angiopathy in the moderate and markedly affected cases (Figure 2).

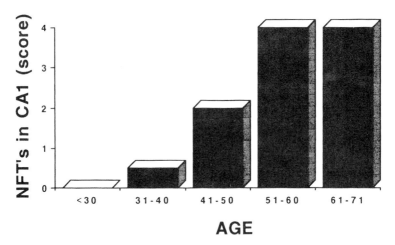

Figure 1. Number of neurofibrillary tangles in hippocampal field CA1 in Down's patients of various ages. The number of neurofibrillary tangles was assessed in a 1.8-mm^2 field using the fluorochrome thioflavin S. Semiquantitative scores were assigned as 0=no NFT, 1=1-10 NFT, 2=11-25 NFT, 3=26-50 NFT, and 4= >50 NFT per field. The averaged tangle score from all individuals in each age group is illustrated

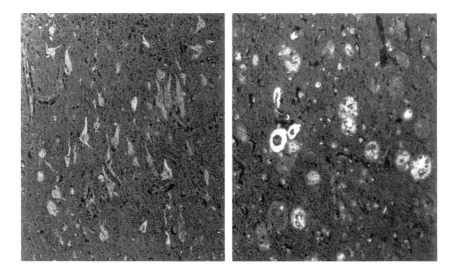

Figure 2. Thioflavin S staining of Alzheimer-related pathological changes in a 71-year-old patient with Down's syndrome. The left panel shows a cluster of neurons in layer II of entorhinal cortex, essentially all of which have undergone neurofibrillary degeneration in this individual. The right panel shows temporal neocortex (area 20) from the same individual, and demonstrates numerous senile plaques and amyloid (congophilic) vascular deposits. This individual was noted to have 'marked' pathological changes overall

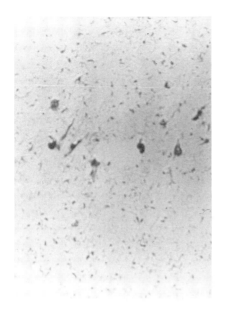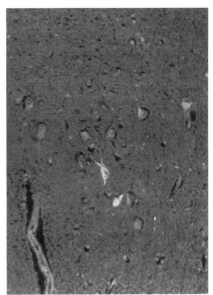

Figure 3. Entorhinal cortex changes in a 37-year-old individual with Down's syndrome. The left panel shows entorhinal cortex stained for Alz-50 immunocytochemistry, which reveals a cluster of well-stained neurons. The right panel is an equivalent area from the same individual stained with thioflavin S, showing two bright neurofibrillary tangles near the center of the photomicrograph. These may represent some of the initial manifestations of Alzheimer's disease pathology

The entorhinal cortex was examined in 11 cases. The large neurons of layer II were affected by NFT in every instance (Figure 2). Of interest, in three relatively young cases (ages 37, 41, and 49 years) the entorhinal NFT were either the sole or the most prominent neurofibrillary change of all fields examined, and may well represent some of the initial changes of the disease.

Relationship of Alz-50 immunoreactive neurons to NFT

Alz-50 staining revealed abnormal neurons, the neuritic component of neuritic plaques, and some neuropil threads in 19 out of 20 cases, the one exception being no staining in the 13-year-old. In 2 cases, Alz-50 staining was technically poor, which probably reflects a difference in original tissue fixation or embedding parameters. In both of these, thioflavin revealed many more lesions than Alz-50. In 5 cases, most of them with substantial disease, the thioflavin S and Alz-50 revealed a similar quantity of neuronal lesions, taking into account that Alz-50 does not recognize extraneuronal 'tombstone' tangles while thioflavin does so extremely well. In 12 instances, and especially prominently in the younger cases, Alz-50 revealed additional neuronal lesions compared to thioflavin S. Alz-50 showed not only lesions in a given

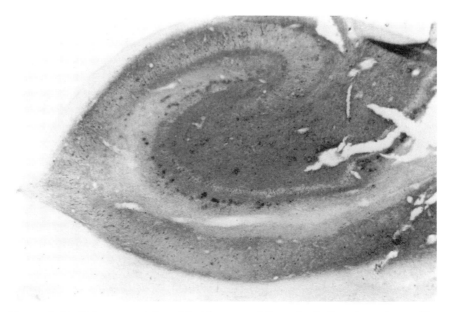

Figure 4. Alz-50 immunostaining of the hippocampal formation in Down's syndrome. This individual was 65 years old, and had marked neuropathological changes. The pattern of Alz-50 staining respects cytoarchitectural boundaries. For example, the CA1/subicular zone is heavily stained, while the mossy fiber zone in CA3 is nearly unstained. A prominent line of plaques is evident in the middle and outer portion of the molecular layer of the dentate gyrus, in an area that corresponds to the termination site of the perforant pathway

cytoarchitectural region, but a wider distribution over the 'hierarchy' noted above. For example, Figure 3 shows a cluster of neurons in layer II of the entorhinal cortex in the 37-year-old individual. There are relatively few thioflavin S positive neurons, and substantially more Alz-50 positive neurons.

Figure 4 shows a low-power view of the hippocampal formation stained with Alz-50 from a 65-year-old individual with DS. The section is a 50-μm thick frozen section. Immunoreactivity for neuropil threads is substantially improved in this type of preparation, and the level of neuronal and neuritic abnormality is striking. The most staining is seen in the CA1 and subicular regions, with far less in CA3 (mossy fiber zone). The hilus and CA4 neurons have a moderate degree of staining. A prominent line of deeply immunoreactive neuritic plaques is present in the middle and outer portions of the molecular layer of the dentate gyrus. This is a prominent finding in many cases, and corresponds anatomically to the terminal zone of the perforant pathway (14), which originates primarily in the neurons of layer II in entorhinal cortex.

DISCUSSION

Examination of neuronal changes in the hippocampal formation in DS individuals leads to several clear conclusions. The number of NFT increases monotonically with age. The pattern and quantity of NFT suggest a smoothly progressive illness during which NFT accumulate, rather than two pathological subgroups, one with mild changes, and the other with severe changes. Pathological changes begin in the patient's third decade and marked pathological changes are uniformly present over the age of 50 years.

Although a clinical impression of 'demented' or 'not demented' is not a sensitive instrument, it is nonetheless clear that there is a strong relationship between age, the accumulation of severe NFT and SP changes, and clinical dementia. This is in accord with previous clinical-pathological studies of dementia in DS (5,15–17) which form a consensus that the vast majority, if not all, patients with DS develop dementia in later middle age.

In some ways more interesting is the observation that approximately half of these individuals, those with 'mild' or 'moderate' accumulations of NFT, were not felt to be demented. In these individuals some NFT occur in layer II of entorhinal cortex or CA1 and subiculum of the hippocampal formation. Although these neurons subserve neural systems crucial for normal memory function, there is apparently sufficient 'reserve' in terms of redundancy of neural systems (18) or plasticity response (19,20) such that cognitive impairment is not manifested.

The topographic pattern of NFT in DS individuals also confirms the observation that certain neuronal populations such as the CA1/subicular zone are especially vulnerable to NFT formation while others, for example the presubiculum, are relatively spared. This is in accord with previous investigations in DS tissue (21), and is essentially identical to the hierarchical vulnerability patterns observed in AD (10,22) and normal aging (8).

The current study also highlights the universal and early changes in layer II of entorhinal cortex in DS (4,6,23). Again, this observation is paralleled by the finding of NFT in this population of neurons in AD (10,12,14,24) and in normal aging (7,8). These data strongly support the hypothesis that changes in the neurons of layer II of entorhinal cortex are one of the earliest manifestations of Alzheimer pathology.

Immunostaining with the Alz-50 antibody revealed neurofibrillary tangles, neuronal staining, neurities in SP, and in some cases 'neuropil threads'. The Alz-50 monoclonal antibody was developed against a homogenate of Alzheimer brain, and recognizes a protein referred to as A-68 (11). The microtubule-associated protein tau is also recognized by Alz-50 (25). NFT in DS are also recognized by Alz-50 (26), and it has been suggested that Alz-50 positive neurons appear prior to NFT in DS individuals (27). A recent study using sections from many of the same cases studied here showed a similar degree of staining using anti-tau antisera and the Palmgren silver method to visualize tangles (28). In our experience using anti-tau and Alz-50 immunostaining on optimally prepared tissue the two antibodies show similar results, but when using routinely prepared (i.e. formalin fixed) tissue Alz-50 appears to be a more sensitive marker for neuronal changes (Hyman et al, unpublished). The difference between Alz-50 and tau staining may be due to Alz-50 recognizing other Alzheimer-associated proteins as well as tau, or may simply reflect immunostaining properties of tissue fixed with formalin and paraffin embedded.

In any case, Alz-50 positive neurons are present in the same vulnerable neuronal populations, and in the same hierarchical distribution, as NFT. The fact that, especially in the younger cases, Alz-50 visualizes additional changes supports the hypothesis that Alz-50 recognizes early neuronal changes as neurons are developing NFT and further supports the idea that regions such as entorhinal cortex are among the first areas affected by Alzheimer neuronal pathology.

CONCLUSION

Down's syndrome individuals, presumably due to genetic factors linked to trisomy 21, appear to have an extremely strong predisposition to developing Alzheimer-type pathology and dementia by middle age. Because of this, study of individuals with Down's syndrome of various ages provides a unique opportunity to investigate the time course of Alzheimer-related pathology. Our studies on the development of neurofibrillary changes suggest that the neurons in layer II of entorhinal cortex, the perforant pathway, and the CA1/subicular zone of the hippocampus are early and consistent sites of neurofibrillary pathology. NFT appear to accumulate in a pattern that obeys hierarchical rules over perhaps 20 years, beginning in the third decade. During this time the number of lesions increases systematically from few to innumerable. The pattern and topographic specificity of these changes is identical to that described in Alzheimer's disease and, although in quantitatively fewer numbers, in normal aging.

Immunocytochemical investigation using the monoclonal antibody Alz-50 revealed a population of immunoreactive neurons that did not contain neurofibrillary tangles, but were in cytoarchitectural fields that were probably at high risk for tangle formation had the disease process continued. This result is consistent with the hypothesis that Alz-50 recognizes an alteration in neurons that precedes and accompanies neurofibrillary tangle formation.

Taken together, these results suggest that the study of patients with Down's syndrome of various ages may allow the identification of early sites and types of neuronal pathology that ultimately contribute to the pathophysiology of Alzheimer's disease itself.

Acknowledgments

We thank P. Davies, Albert Einstein College of Medicine, NY for the gift of Alz-50 and S. Melanson for typing the manuscript. Supported by NIH AG08487 and a Fellowship from the Brookdale Foundation.

REFERENCES

1. Malamud N. In CM Gaitz (ed), Ageing and the brain, vol. 3. New York: Plenum, 1972: 63-87.
2. Mann DMA, Yates PO, Marcyniuk B. Neuropath Appl Neurobiol 1984; 10: 185-207.
3. Mann DMA, Yates PO, Marcyniuk B. J Neurol Sci 1985; 69: 139-59.

4. Mann DMA, Yates PO, Marcyniuk B, Ravindra CR. Neuropath Appl Neurobiol 1986; 12: 447–57.
5. Mann DMA. Mech Age Develop 1988; 43: 99–136.
6. Mann DMA, Esiri MM, N Engl J Med 1988; 318: 789–90.
7. Ulrich J. Ann Neurol 1985; 17: 273–7.
8. Arriagada P, Hyman BT. J Neuropath Exp Neurol 1990; 49: 336 (abstr.).
9. Mann DMA, Tucker CM, Yates PO. Neuropathol Appl Neurobiol 1987; 13: 123–39.
10. Hyman BT, Damasio AR, Van Hoesen GW, Barnes CL. Science 1984; 225: 1168–70.
11. Wolozin B, Pruchnicki A, Dickson D, Davies P. Science 1986; 232: 648–50.
12. Hyman BT, Van Hoesen GW, Wolozin B, Davies P, Kromer LJ, Damasio AR. Ann Neurol 1988; 23: 371–9.
13. Kromer-Vogt LJ, Hyman BT, Van Hoesen GW, Damasio AR. Neurosci 1990; 37: 377–85.
14. Hyman BT, Van Hoesen GW, Kromer LJ, Damasio AR. Ann Neurol 1986; 20: 472–81.
15. Lai F, Williams RS. Arch Neurol 1989; 46: 849–53.
16. Ropper AH, Williams RS. Neurology 1980; 30: 639–44.
17. Wisniewski KE et al. Neurology 1985; 35: 957–61.
18. Hyman BT, Van Hoesen GW, Damasio AR. Neurology 1990; 40: 1721–30.
19. Geddes JW et al. Science 1985; 230: 1180–1.
20. Hyman BT, Kromer LJ, Van Hoesen GW. Ann Neurol 1987; 21: 259–67.
21. Ball M, Nuttall K. Neuropath Appl Neurobiol 1981; 7: 13–20.
22. Kemper TL. In Nandy K (ed.) Senile dementia, a biomedical approach. Amsterdam: Elsevier, 1978: 105–13.
23. Mann DMA, Yates PO. Ann Neurol 1987; 21: 613.
24. Braak H, Braak E. Acta Neuropathol 1985; 68: 325–32.
25. Nukina N, Kosik KS, Selkoe DJ. Neurosci Lett 1988; 87: 240–6.
26. Wolozin B, Scicutella A, Davies P. Proc Natl Acad Sci USA 1989; 85: 4885–8.
27. Mattiace LA, Dickson DW, Kress YS, Davies P. Neurosci Abstr 1989; 15: 1038.
28. Mann DMA, Prinja D, Davies CA, Ihara Y, Delacourte A, Defossez A, Mayer RJ, Landon MJ. Neurol Sci 1989; 92: 247–60.

Address for correspondence:

Dr Bradley T. Hyman,
Department of Neurology,
Massachusetts General Hospital,
Harvard Medical School,
Boston, MA 02114,
USA

14 Chromosome 21 Nondisjunction: Alzheimer's Disease Viewed as a Mosaic Form of Down's Syndrome

HUNTINGTON POTTER

It has been appreciated for some time that Alzheimer's disease has a complex etiology. At least 15% of the cases appear to be due to the inheritance of an autosomal dominant mutation, but the majority are 'sporadic', showing no clear association with any identifiable genetic or environmental factor (1-4). Even identical twins can show a large discordance in the age of onset of the disease (5). Yet despite this variation, Alzheimer's disease shows a uniform set of clinical and pathological features—progressive loss of memory and other intellectual functions beginning in middle to late life, coupled with neuronal cell loss in the higher centers of the brain (for review, see reference 6).

When examined by histochemical stains, Alzheimer's disease brains, particularly the hippocampus, neocortex, and amygdala, exhibit certain neuropathological protein deposits that serve as the defining characteristic of the disease. One such deposit, termed the neurofibrillary tangle, occurs inside neurons and is composed of paired helical protein filaments. Because they can be found in other neurodegenerative diseases, paired helical filaments are likely to be a common feature of dying neurons. The more definitive lesion of Alzheimer's disease is the 'neuritic' or 'senile plaque', which consists of a spherical, extracellular core of filamentous protein material surrounded by a halo of degenerating nerve cell processes. Extracellular protein filaments similar to those seen in the cores of neuritic plaques also accumulate in the walls of meningeal and intracortical blood vessels. The deposits of protein filaments in the cores of neuritic plaques and in blood vessels are referred to by the generic term 'amyloid'.

The first identified constituent of Alzheimer amyloid deposits was purified from meningeal blood vessels and its sequence determined by Glenner and Wong (7). This protein, termed β or A4, is a fragment about 42 amino acids long of a larger protein of uncertain function that is a normal constituent of the brain and other tissues. A second protein component of Alzheimer amyloid deposits was identified as the serine protease inhibitor α-antichymotrypsin (ACT) (8). In the last few years, much has been learned about the biochemistry and expression of the aberrant protein deposits that characterize Alzheimer's disease (for reviews see references 9-12).

Alzheimer's Disease: Basic Mechanisms, Diagnosis and Therapeutic Strategies
Edited by K. Iqbal, D. R. C. McLachlan, B. Winblad and H. M. Wisniewski
© 1991 John Wiley & Sons Ltd

However, no hypothesis has easily explained how both genetic and sporadic forms of Alzheimer's disease can be related by a common underlying mechanism. Perhaps the most interesting clue to the cause of Alzheimer's disease is the fact that Down's syndrome patients who live beyond the age of 30 or 40 years develop dementia and neuropathology essentially indistinguishable from classic Alzheimer's disease (13-15). The implication of this finding is that trisomy for chromosome 21—the pathogenetic cause of Down's syndrome—is also capable of causing Alzheimer's disease, possibly through the overexpression or duplication of a gene residing on chromosome 21 (for discussion see reference 16). On the other hand, almost all aged humans (and monkeys) develop some amyloid deposits which, by several criteria, appear to be identical to those that accumulate in much larger numbers and at an earlier time in Alzheimer's disease and Down's syndrome (17-19). Thus, any hypothesis for the pathogenesis of Alzheimer's disease must explain not only the relation between the familial and sporadic forms of the disease but also how these are related to Down's syndrome and to the 'normal' process of aging.

The association between Alzheimer's disease and chromosome 21 has been reinforced by a number of recent clinical and experimental findings. This review considers these and earlier results on the genetics, epidemiology, and cell biology of Alzheimer's disease, and, in particular, its association with Down's syndrome, and suggests that both the genetic and sporadic forms of Alzheimer's disease can be explained as arising from the accumulation of chromosome 21 trisomy cells during the life of the individual. That is, trisomy 21 cells, developing over time by unequal chromosome segregation during mitosis, may ultimately lead to Alzheimer's disease through the same (as yet unknown, and perhaps multistep) mechanism by which Down's syndrome patients get the disease, but at a later age due to the modulating effect of the mosaicism.

The first specific model linking Alzheimer's disease to Down's syndrome arose when the gene for the amyloid β-protein was cloned and found to be located on chromosome 21 (20-23). The implication of these results seemed clear—perhaps the accumulation of amyloid in Alzheimer's disease was caused by the overexpression of a mutant β-protein gene or by a duplication of the β-protein gene on chromosome 21 that mimicked the gene-dosage effect of Down's syndrome. The fact that some Alzheimer's disease families could be shown to harbor their autosomal dominantly inherited mutation on chromosome 21 further implicated the β-protein gene as a potential site for the disease locus (24). Very recently, a variant form of the β-protein gene encoding mutant β-protein *has* been found in families with hereditary cerebral hemorrhage with amyloidosis of Dutch origin, suggesting that the inherited defect in this disease may be in the β-protein gene (25,26). However, early studies suggesting that the β-protein gene existed in three copies in Alzheimer's disease patients were not confirmed. Furthermore, the actual location of a potential Alzheimer's disease mutation on chromosome 21 in some families was soon shown to be far from the β-protein gene itself and closer to the centromere (27-29). Then the finding of some families showing no linkage to any marker on chromosome 21, suggested that the inherited form of Alzheimer's disease is genetically heterogeneous (30). Chromosome 19 (31) and possibly the region of the ACT gene on chromosome 14 (32) have been proposed as candidate locations for the disease locus. These results have been interpreted as indicating that an aberrant biochemical pathway leading to the Alzheimer neuropathology can be initiated by mutation in a number of genes, including one on chromosome 21.

Chromosome 21 was further implicated in the etiology of Alzheimer's disease by the discovery that some families in which Alzheimer's disease is inherited as an autosomal dominant mutation produce a significantly higher-than-normal number of Down's syndrome children (33,34; but also see 35). In addition, mouse chromosome 16, which is partially homologous to human chromosome 21, including the β-protein gene, has been shown to result, when trisomic, in neurodegeneration similar to that seen in Alzheimer's disease (36). Although trisomy 16 mice suffer many developmental abnormalities and do not survive to term, the specific effect of this trisomy on the nervous system can be tested by transplanting embryonic brain tissue from a trisomy 16 embryo into the brain of a normal adult. When the brains of such host mice with their trisomy 16 grafts were examined, it was found that some of the neurons in the graft had accumulated aberrant proteins similar to those found in degenerating neurons in Alzheimer's disease.

Finally, there are two reports of women whose lymphocytes were found to be mosaic for trisomy 21 and who, though not mentally retarded, had developed Alzheimer-like dementia by age 40 (37,38; for discussion see 39). In one case the woman also had a Down's syndrome child. These patients demonstrate that it is not necessary for every cell of an individual to be trisomy 21 for the aberrant effects of this chromosome imbalance to result in early dementia.

If it is true that Alzheimer's disease and most Down's syndrome are the somatic and germline manifestations of the same problem of unequal chromosome 21 segregation, then much of the seemingly diverse data can be more easily understood. For instance, one immediate implication is that any genetic or environmental factor that increases the chances of forming chromosome 21 trisomic cells should increase the likelihood of developing Alzheimer's disease. Thus, in the families in which the disease is apparently inherited as an autosomal dominant mutation near the centromere of chromosome 21, perhaps the mutation resides in the centromere itself so as to cause an increased frequency of nondisjunction of chromosome 21. During mitosis, such nondisjunction would build up trisomy 21 somatic cells, eventually leading to Alzheimer's disease pathology, while during meiosis it would generate trisomy 21 germ cells and Down's syndrome offspring, as the epidemiological evidence suggests. Indeed, there are centromere mutations known in yeast that result in a 100-fold increase in chromosome nondisjunction (40).

Of course chromosome segregation is a complex process under the control of many gene products (for review, see 41), and an inherited disorder of chromosome segregation could be caused by mutations at a number of loci. In this light, the fact that familial Alzheimer's disease appears to be genetically heterogeneous is not surprising, since any one of several mutations could lead to the development of cells trisomic for chromosome 21, both somatic and germline, with the consequent development of Alzheimer's disease in the individual and an increased frequency of Down's syndrome offspring.

Although improper chromosome segregation can result from a genetic mutation, it can also be caused by environmental agents. Of the many exogenous factors that influence chromosome segregation, low doses of radiation, and microtubule-disrupting agents such as colchicine, are perhaps the best studied (see, for example, reference 42). Aluminum, the consumption of which shows a weak (but significant) association with the development of Alzheimer's disease (see, for example, reference 43), also binds to microtubules and, in the form of aluminum silicate, causes chromosome nondisjunction in cultured cells (44; for discussion see 45). Thus, the large proportion of Alzheimer's disease cases that arise in a sporadic manner not directly attributable to the inheritance of a genetic mutation can also be understood in the light of the chromosome 21 trisomy model.

An important prediction of this model is that it is the dividing cells in an individual that are most likely to develop chromosome 21 trisomy and lead to Alzheimer's disease. Extensive analysis by Rakic (46) has shown that the only dividing cells in the brains of adult monkeys exposed to ^{3}H-thymidine are glial cells and the endothelial cells lining blood vessels, while neurons, the cells most apparently affected by Alzheimer's disease, do not divide. The labeled glia were seen primarily in the hippocampus and the cerebral cortex. Thus cell division in adult primates occurs in those general brain regions that develop neuropathology in Alzheimer's disease, Down's syndrome, and normal aging. Interestingly, astroglia in the hippocampus and cortex are induced by brain disease or damage to overexpress the two proteins — ACT and the β-protein — that make up the Alzheimer amyloid deposits (47,48). Recently, two rapidly dividing peripheral tissues — skin and intestinal mucosa — have been reported to contain pre-amyloid deposits of β-protein in sporadic Alzheimer patients and some aged, normal subjects (49). Another region of active cell division, which has been shown to exhibit pathological changes in Alzheimer's disease, is the olfactory epithelium (50).

In sum, both genetic and sporadic forms of Alzheimer's disease can be explained as arising from the effects of trisomy 21 cells accumulating during the life of the individual. A propensity to develop such cells could be genetic in origin (either due to an aberrant chromosome 21 centromere, or to a mutation elsewhere in the genome affecting all chromosome segregation), or it could be caused by environmental factors. The combination of genetic and environmental influences on the formation of trisomic 21 cells could yield the observed variation in the age of onset of Alzheimer's disease in identical twins and in Alzheimer's disease families. In addition, the fact that almost 50% of the population over the age of 85 show some symptoms of Alzheimer's disease dementia (51), and an even larger proportion show some of the same neuropathological lesions, indicates that all individuals may, to some degree, be subject to stochastic events that lead to aberrant chromosome segregation with increasing age. The possibility that further biochemical or genetic events may be required before full Alzheimer neuropathology arises is indicated by the mature age (20s to 30s) that Down's syndrome patients begin to accumulate amyloid deposits.

Cytogenetic analysis of Alzheimer's disease patients has been carried out in a number of laboratories, with mixed reports of increased aneuploidy as measured directly (52–55). However, premature centromere division (PCD), a correlate and potential cause of improper chromosome segregation in vitro and in vivo, was found to be positively correlated with age, and to be increased in women with familial Alzheimer's disease (3.6% compared with 0.6% in age-matched controls), particularly affecting the X chromosome (55,56). Trisomy 21, and to a lesser extent trisomy 18, occurred in the lymphocytes and fibroblasts of a woman apparently prone to PCD, who also had three trisomy 21 conceptuses (57). The prevalence of trisomy 21, 18, and X cells arising in this case probably reflects differential cell viability. Indeed, lymphocyte cultures from trisomy 21 mosaic individuals often show a lower proportion of trisomy cells than do, for instance, fibroblast cultures, and some patients with a normal karyotype in lymphocytes can show mosaicism in fibroblasts (58,59). Thus, the fact that most cytogenetic studies on Alzheimer patients have relied on peripheral blood lymphocytes may explain why trisomy 21 mosaicism has not previously been linked to Alzheimer's disease. Further cytogenetic studies of Alzheimer patients, especially on dividing cells from affected areas of the brain—the olfactory epithelium, the meningeal and cortical vessels, and the glia—may establish a significant frequency of trisomy 21 in these regions.

Acknowledgments

I am grateful to the many colleagues who have read and commented on the manuscript, particularly Cynthia Morton, David Potter, John Cairns, David Dressler, and George Glenner. The work in the laboratory is supported by the NIH, the Alzheimer's Disease and Related Disorders Association, and the Freudenberger family. Stefan Cooke assisted in the preparation of the manuscript.

REFERENCES

1. Feldman RG, Chandler KA, Levy L, Glaser GH. Neurology 1963; 13: 811-24.
2. Heston LL, Mastri AR, Anderson VE, White J. Arch Gen Psychiat 1981; 38: 1084-90.
3. Terry RD. Aging 1973; 7: 377-82.
4. Jarvik LF, Matsuyama SS. (1986). In Scheibel AB, Wechslev AF (eds) The biological substrates of Alzheimer's Disease. Orlando; Academic Press, 1986.
5. Nee LE, Eldridge R, Sunderland T, Thomas CB, Katz D, Thompson KE, Weingartner H, Weiss H, Julian C, Cohen R. Neurology 1987; 37: 359-63.
6. Price DL. Ann Rev Neurosci 1986; 9: 489-512.
7. Glenner GG, Wong CW. Biochem Biophys Res Commun 1984; 122: 885-90.
8. Abraham CR, Selkoe DJ, Potter H. Cell 1988; 52: 487-501.
9. Abraham CR, Potter H. Biotechnology 1989; 7: 147-53.
10. Selkoe DJ. Ann Rev Neurosci 1989; 12: 493-520.
11. Müller-Hill B, Beyreuther K. Ann Rev Biochem 1989; 58: 287-307.
12. Neve RL, Potter H. In Brosius J, Fremeau R (eds) Molecular genetic approaches to neuropsychiatric disease. Academic Press (in press).
13. Olsson MI, Shaw CM. Brain 1969; 92: 147-56.
14. Glenner GG, Wong CW. Biochem Biophys Res Commun 1984; 122: 1131-5.
15. Wisniewski HM, Rabe A, Wisniewski KE. In Davies P, Finch C (eds) Molecular neuropathology of aging. Banbury Report. New York: Cold Spring Harbor Laboratory, 1988.
16. Schweber M. Ann NY Acad Sci 1985; 450: 223-38.

17. Wisniewski HM, Terry RD. In Ford DH (ed.) Progress in brain research, Vol. 40. Neurobiological aspects of maturation and aging. Amsterdam: Elsevier, 1973.
18. Selkoe DJ, Bell DS, Podlisny MB, Price DL, Cork LC. Science 1987; 235: 873-7.
19. Abraham CR, Selkoe DJ, Potter H, Price DC, Cork LC. Neurosci 1989; 32: 715-20.
20. Goldgaber D, Lerman MJ, McBride OW, Saffiotti V, Gadjusek DC. Science 1987; 235: 877.
21. Kang J, Lemaire HG, Unterback A, Salbaum JM, Masters CL, Grezeschik KH, Multhaup G, Beyreuther K, Muller-Hill B. Nature 1987; 325: 733.
22. Tanzi RE, Gusella JF, Watkins PC, Bruns GAP, St George-Hyslop P, Van Keuren ML, Patterson D, Pajan S, Kurnit DM, Neve RL. Science 1987; 235: 880.
23. Robakis NK, Ramakrishna N, Wolfe G, Wisniewski HM. Proc Natl Acad Sci USA 1987; 84: 4190.
24. St George-Hyslop PH, Tanzi RE, Polinsky RJ, Haines JL, Nee L, Watkins PC, Myers R, Feldman R, Pollen D, Drachman D, Growdon J, Bruni A, Foncin J-F, Frommelt P, Amaducci L, Sorbi S, Piacentini S, Stewart GD, Hobbs WJ, Conneally PM, Gusella JF. Science 1987; 235: 885-9.
25. Van Broeckhoven C, Hann J, Bakker E, Hardy JA, Van Hul, W, Wehnert A, Vegter-Van der Vlis M, Roos RAC. Science 1990; 248: 1120-2.
26. Levy E, Carman MD, Fernandez-Madrid IJ, Lieberburg I, Power MD, van Duinen SG, Bots GTAM, Luyendijk W, Frangione B. Science 1990 (in press).
27. Tanzi RE, St George-Hyslop PH, Haines JL, Polinsky RJ, Nee L, Foncin, J-F, Neve RL, McClatchey AI, Conneally PN, Gusella JF. Nature 1987; 329: 156-7.
28. Van Broeckhoven C, Genthe AM, Vandenberghe A, Horsthemke B, Backhovens H, Raeymaekers P, Van Hul W, Wehnert A, Gheuens J, Cras P, Bruyland M, Martin JJ, Salbaum M, Multhaup G, Masters CL, Beyreuther K, Gurling HMD, Mullan MJ, Holland A, Barton A, Irving N, Williamson R, Richards SJ, Hardy JA. Nature 1987; 329: 153-5.
29. Goate AM, Owen MJ, James LA, Mullan MJ, Rossor MN, Haynes AR, Farral M, Lai LYC, Roques P, Williamson R, Hardy JA. Predisposing locus for Alzheimer's disease on chromosome 21. Lancet 1989; i: 18: 352.
30. Schellenberg GD, Bird TD, Wijsman EM, Moore DK, Boehnke M, Bryant EM, Lampe TH, Nochlin D, Sumi SM, Deep SS, Beyreuther K, Martin GM. Science 1988; 241: 1505-10.
31. Roses AD, Pericak-Vance MA, Clark CM, Gilbert J-R, Yamaoka LH, Haynes CS, Speer MC, Gaskell PC, Hung WY, Trufatter JA et al. Linkage studies of late-onset familial Alzheimer's disease. Adv Neurol 1990; 51: 185-96.
32. Weitkamp LR, Nee L, Keats B, Polinsky RJ, Guttormsen S. Amer J Hum Genet 1983; 35: 443-53.
33. Heston LL, Mestri AR, Anderson VE, White J. Arch Gen Psychiat 1981; 38: 1084-90.
34. Heyman A, Wilkinson W, Hurwitz B, Schmechel D, Sigmon A, Weinberg T, Helms M, Swift M. Ann Neurol 1983; 14: 507-15.
35. Whalley LG, Buckton KE. In Glen AIM, Whalley LJ (eds) Alzheimer's disease: early recognition of potentially reversible deficits. Edinburgh: Churchill Livingstone, 1979.
36. Richards S-J, Waters JJ, Wischik CM, Abraham CR, Sparkman DR, White CL, Beyreuther K, Masters CL, Dunnett SB. Science 1990 (in press).
37. Schapiro MB, Kumar A, White B, Grady CL, Friedland RP, Rapoport SI. Neurology 1989; 39 (suppl. 1): 169.
38. Rowe IF, Ridler MAC, Gibberd FB. Lancet 1989; ii: 229.
39. Hardy J, Goate A, Owen M, Rossor M. Lancet 1989; ii: 743.
40. Gaudet A, Fitzgerald-Hayes M. Mol Cell Biol 1987; 7: 68-75.
41. Murray AW, Szostak JW. Ann Rev Cell Biol 1985; 1: 289-315.
42. Uchida IA, Lee CPV, Byrnes EM. Am J Hum Genet 1975; 27: 419-29.
43. Martyn CN, Osmond C, Edwardson JA, Barker DJP, Harris EC, Lacey RF. Lancet 1989; i: 59-62.

44. Palekar LD, Eyre JF, Most BM, Coffin DL. Carcinogen 1987; 8: 553-60.
45. Ganrot PO. Environ Health Persp 1986; 65: 363-441.
46. Rakic P. Science 1985; 227: 1054-6.
47. Pasternack JM, Abraham CR, Van Dyke B, Potter H, Younkin SG. Am J Pathol 1989; 135: 827-34.
48. Siman R, Card JP, Nelson RB, Davis LG. Neuron 1989; 3: 275-85.
49. Joachim CL, Mori H, Selkoe DJ. Nature 1989; 341: 226-30.
50. Talamo BR, Rudel RA, Kosik KS, Lee VM-Y, Neff S, Adelman L, Kauer JS. Nature 1989; 337: 736-9.
51. Evans DA, Funkenstein H, Albert MS, Scherr PA, Cook NR, Chown MJ, Hebert LE, Hennekens CH, Taylor JO. JAMA 1989; 262: 2551-6.
52. Ward BE, Cook RH, Robinson A, Austin JH. Am J Med Genet. 1979; 3: 137-44.
53. White BJ, Crandall C, Goudsmit J, Morrow CH, Alling DW, Gajdusek DC, Tjio, JH. Am J Med Genet 1981; 10: 77-89.
54. Buckton KE, Whalley LJ, Lee H, Christie JE. J Med Genet 1983; 20: 46-51.
55. Moorhead PS, Heyman A. Am J Med Genet 1983; 14: 545-6.
56. Fitzgerald PH, Pickering AF, Mercer JM, Miethke PM. Ann Hum Genet 1975; 38: 417-28.
57. Fitzgerald PH, Archer SA, Morris CM. Hum Genet 1986; 72: 54-62.
58. Pagon RA, Hall JG, Davenport SLH, Aase J, Norwood TH, Hoehn HW. Am J Hum Genet 1979; 31: 54-61.
59. Ford CE. In Burgio GR, Fraccaro M, Tiepolo, L, Wold U (eds) Trisomy 21. Berlin: Springer, 1981.

Address for correspondence:

Dr Huntington Potter,
Department of Neurobiology,
Harvard Medical School,
220 Longwood Avenue,
Boston, MA 02115, USA

15 Selective Alterations of Cerebellar Glutamate Receptor Subtypes in Alzheimer's Disease

D. DEWAR, D. T. CHALMERS, A. KURUMAJI, D. I. GRAHAM AND J. McCULLOCH

There are numerous reports of reductions in glutamate receptors in cortical and archicortical brain regions in Alzheimer's disease (1-5). In contrast, we have recently reported a marked and selective increase in the kainate subtype of glutamate receptors in frontal cortex (6). Using quantitative ligand binding autoradiography, we observed the increase in kainate receptor binding to be specifically localized to the deep layers (IV-VI) of the Alzheimer frontal cortex. Moreover, the level of kainate receptor binding was positively correlated with the local number of neuritic plaques.

Classical plaques comprising an amyloid core surrounded by degenerating neurites and glia are rarely observed in the cerebellum in Alzheimer's disease although there are reports of a distinct type of cerebellar plaque (7-11). In view of the prominent role played by glutamate in cerebellar neurotransmission (12-14), we have examined the status of glutamate receptor subtypes in the cerebellum of subjects with Alzheimer's disease. We have used quantitative autoradiography in order to examine the glutamate system in a brain region which is largely unaffected by the type of structural change commonly observed in cerebral cortex.

MATERIALS AND METHODS

Blocks of cerebellar cortex were obtained postmortem from six control subjects and six patients who had neuropathologically confirmed Alzheimer's disease. The two groups were matched for age, sex and postmortem delay. For receptor autoradiography, consecutive 20-μm cryostat sections mounted on glass slides were used for determination of [^{3}H]-kainate, [^{3}H]-amino-3-hydroxy-5-methylisoxazole-4-propionic acid (AMPA), NMDA-sensitive [^{3}H]-glutamate and strychnine-insensitive [^{3}H]-glycine binding according to previously described protocols (6). Receptor autoradiograms were analysed by computerized image analysis with reference to [^{3}H]-microscales. Sections adjacent to those used for receptor autoradiography

Alzheimer's Disease: Basic Mechanisms, Diagnosis and Therapeutic Strategies
Edited by K. Iqbal, D. R. C. McLachlan, B. Winblad and H. M. Wisniewski
© 1991 John Wiley & Sons Ltd

were fixed in 10% formalin and stained with King's amyloid stain to determine the presence of plaques. Additional sections were stained with cresyl violet and the number of Purkinje cells in each case was determined.

RESULTS

[³H]-AMPA binding to quisqualate receptors was markedly reduced in the molecular layer of the cerebellum in the Alzheimer subjects compared to controls (Figures 1 and 3). Scatchard analysis of [³H]-AMPA binding over the range 25–800 nM, in sections from all subjects revealed a significant reduction in the B_{max} value in the molecular layer of the Alzheimer group (107 pmol/g) compared to the controls (280 pmol/g). In the granule cell layer B_{max} values were similar in control (78 pmol/g) and Alzheimer (95 pmol/g) groups. K_d values were similar in control and Alzheimer groups in both cerebellar layers. In adjacent sections, [³H]-glycine receptor binding was increased in the granule layer of the Alzheimer cerebellar cortex (Figures 2 and 3). [³H]-Kainate and NMDA-sensitive [³H]-glutamate binding were no different in the Alzheimer group compared to control (Figure 3).

Determination of the number of Purkinje cells, expressed per mm of the cell line in each section, in both control (mean ± SEM = 2.3 ± 0.2) and Alzheimer (mean ± SEM = 2.0 ± 0.2) cerebellar cortices revealed no significant difference between the groups. Four of the six Alzheimer cases had plaques in the cerebellar cortex which were present predominantly in the molecular layer. These lesions had a diffuse, elongated appearance which was quite distinct from that of the classical plaque of

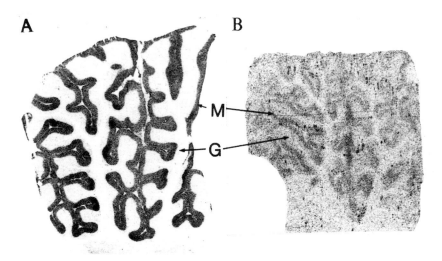

Figure 1. Representative autoradiograms showing binding of [³H]-AMPA to sections of cerebellar cortex from a control (A) and an Alzheimer (B) brain. The molecular (M) and granular (G) layers are indicated by arrows

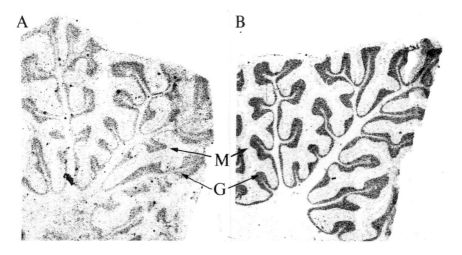

Figure 2. Representative autoradiograms showing strychnine-insensitive [^{3}H]-glycine binding to sections of cerebellar cortex from a control (A) and an Alzheimer (B) brain. The molecular (M) and granular (G) layers are indicated by arrows

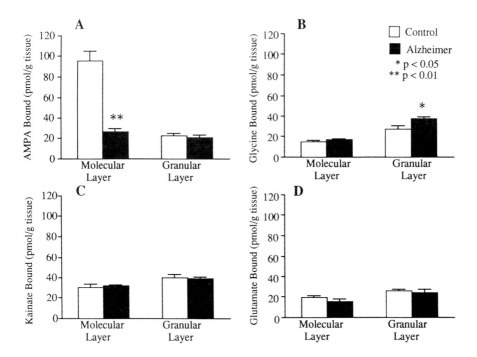

Figure 3. (A) [^{3}H]-AMPA (B) [^{3}H]-glycine (C) [^{3}H]-kainate and (D) NMDA-sensitive [^{3}H]-glutamate binding in control and Alzheimer cerebellar sections, derived from densitometric analyses of autoradiograms. Data are mean ± SEM, $n = 6$ for each group. Levels of significance determined by Student's t-test

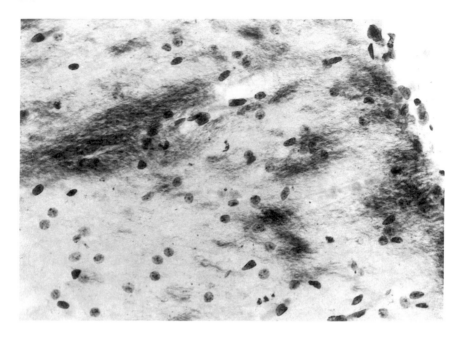

Figure 4. Photomicrograph of section of cerebellar cortex from an Alzheimer patient showing the characteristic diffuse, elongated appearance of cerebellar plaques (×315)

the cerebral cortex (Figure 4). Cerebellar plaques did not stain with congo red, thioflavin T or antisera to paired helical filaments. Cerebellar plaques were not observed in sections from control brains and neither Alzheimer nor control sections contained neurofibrillary tangles.

DISCUSSION

There is increasing evidence that the cerebellum is not spared in Alzheimer's disease. In addition to the numerous reports of cerebellar plaques we now report that this region also undergoes specific neurotransmitter receptor changes. The most striking finding of the present study is the massive and selective reduction of quisqualate (AMPA) receptors in the molecular layer of the Alzheimer cerebellar cortex. Autoradiographic studies of glutamate binding sites in the rodent cerebellum indicate that the majority of cerebellar quisqualate receptors are localized on the apical dendrites of Purkinje cells which extend into the molecular layer (15). In the Alzheimer cases in the present study, however, the reduction in the number of AMPA binding sites was not associated with a significant loss of Purkinje cells. We did not examine the dendritic arbor of these cells, and atrophic changes in the Purkinje cell tree, which pervades the cerebellar molecular layer, may account for the loss of quisqualate (AMPA) receptors in the Alzheimer brains. However, kainate receptor binding was unchanged in the molecular layer of the Alzheimer cerebellar cortex and there is electrophysiological evidence indicating the presence of these receptors on Purkinje cells (16). All Alzheimer subjects had significantly reduced AMPA binding in the molecular layer whether or not cerebellar plaques were observed. However, it was noted that the two subjects who did not have cerebellar plaques had slightly higher levels of AMPA binding than the other subjects in the Alzheimer group.

In adjacent sections, although there was no alteration in NMDA receptor binding in the Alzheimer subjects, there was a specific increase in granular layer glycine binding to a site on the NMDA receptor complex. The upregulation of a receptor commonly occurs in response to a loss of presynaptic input. However, it cannot be determined in postmortem brain whether cerebellar neuronal terminals were functioning normally in vivo, i.e. releasing and taking up normal levels of excitatory amino acids. There was no relationship between the presence of cerebellar plaques and the increase in glycine receptor binding in the granule cell layer of the Alzheimer group.

In conclusion, we have found significant and selective alterations in quisqualate (AMPA) and glycine receptor binding in the cerebellum in Alzheimer's disease. It is uncertain, at present, whether these receptor alterations result from the pathophysiological process of the disease itself or whether they are the consequences of morphological and neurochemical abnormalities in anatomically related brain regions. However, it may be significant that receptor alterations of such magnitude (AMPA) and direction (glycine) occur in the absence of gross neuronal loss.

Acknowledgments

This work was entirely funded by the Wellcome Trust. D.D. gratefully acknowledges the award of an Alzheimer Association (USA) Junior Travel Fellowship.

REFERENCES

1. Greenamyre JT, Penney JB, Young AB, D'Amato CJ, Hicks SP, Shoulson I. Science 1985; 227: 1496-9.
2. Greenamyre JT, Penney JB, D'Amato CJ, Young AB, J Neurochem 1987; 48: 543-51.
3. Maragos WF, Chu DCM, Young AB, D'Amato CJ, Penney JB Jr. Neurosci Lett 1987; 74: 371-6.
4. Cowburn R, Hardy J, Roberts P, Briggs R. Neurosci Lett 1988; 86: 109-13.
5. Ninomiya H, Fukunaga R, Taniguchi T, Fujiwara M, Shimohama S, Kameyama M. J Neurochem 1990; 54: 526-32.
6. Chalmers DT, Dewar D, Graham DI, Brooks DN, McCulloch J. Proc Natl Acad Sci USA 1990; 87: 1352-6.
7. Cole G, Williams P, Alldryck D, Singharo S, Clin Neuropathol 1989; 8: 188-91.
8. Joachim CL, Morris JH, Selkoe DJ. Am J Pathol 1989; 135: 309-19.
9. Yamaguchi H, Hivai S, Morimatsu M, Shoji M, Nazakato Y. Acta Neuropathol 1989; 77: 320-8.
10. Braak H, Braak E, Bohl J, Lang W. J Neurol Sci 1989; 93: 277-87.
11. Suenaga T, Hirano A, Llena JF. J Neuropath Exp Neurol 1990; 49: 31-40.
12. Foster GA, Roberts PJ. Neurosci 1983; 8: 277-84.
13. Freeman ME, Lane JD, Smith JE, J Neurochem 1983; 40: 1441-7.
14. Hudson BD, Valcana T, Bean G, Timiras PS. Neurochem Res 1976; 1: 73-81.

15. Olson JMM, Greenaway JT, Penney JB, Young AB. Neurosci 1987; 22: 913-23.
16. Garthwaite J, Garthwaite G, Hajos F. Neurosci 1986; 18: 449-60.

Address for correspondence:

Dr D. Dewar,
Wellcome Neuroscience Group,
Wellcome Surgical Institute & Hugh Fraser Neuroscience Laboratories,
University of Glasgow,
Garscube Estate, Bearsden Road,
Glasgow, Scotland, UK

16 Decreased α-Adrenergic Receptors at the Blood-Brain Barrier in Alzheimer's Disease

PAULA GRAMMAS, ALEX E. ROHER AND MELVYN J. BALL

STRUCTURAL AND FUNCTIONAL ABNORMALITIES OF THE BLOOD-BRAIN BARRIER IN ALZHEIMER'S DISEASE

Major histopathologic features of Alzheimer's disease (AD) include the deposition of intracellular neurofibrillary tangles and extracellular amyloid proteins in the neuritic plaques and around cerebral blood vessels (1-4). While the source of amyloid has yet to be identified, evidence for a blood-borne or vascular origin includes the presence of 'amyloidic' capillaries within senile plaques and the similarity of vascular amyloid deposition to other systemic amyloidosis with a known blood-borne amyloid source (5-7). Furthermore, the possibility of blood-borne amyloid is supported by studies that describe demonstrable ultrastructural abnormalities of brain capillaries, i.e. the blood–brain barrier (BBB), in AD. In this regard, structural changes that have been described include thickening and reduplication of capillary basement membrane, endothelial cell swelling and the loss of perivascular innervation (8,9).

The leakage of immunoglobulins, albumin and other serum proteins across the BBB implicates (10-12) functional changes of cerebral endothelium. Support for the concept that there may be selective functional abnormalities at the BBB in AD is provided by Kalaria and Harik (13) who demonstrated impaired glucose transport in microvessels from AD patients with no change in the cerebrovascular $(Na^+ + K^+)ATPase$ or other marker enzymes.

REGULATION OF THE BIOCHEMICAL BLOOD-BRAIN BARRIER

The factors that regulate the biochemical events at the BBB have not been completely elucidated, although several studies suggest the involvement of adrenergic receptors. Stimulation of these cell surface receptors leads to activation of phosphoinositol hydrolysis (via α-adrenergic receptors) and activation of adenylate cyclase (via β-adrenergic receptors) in a variety of cell types. The notion that adrenergic receptors may be important in controlling functions at the BBB is supported by studies demonstrating that adrenergic neurotransmitters from the locus ceruleus control cerebrovascular permeability and transport (14-17). Previous work in this laboratory

Alzheimer's Disease: Basic Mechanisms, Diagnosis and Therapeutic Strategies
Edited by K. Iqbal, D. R. C. McLachlan, B. Winblad and H. M. Wisniewski
© 1991 John Wiley & Sons Ltd

has shown that adrenergic receptors in cerebral endothelium regulate GTP-mediated binding, τ-glutamyltranspeptidase activity and cAMP generation (18,19). Furthermore, preliminary data have recently shown that stimulation of α or β-adrenergic receptors on cerebral microvessels could increase the uptake of small neutral amino acids via the Na^+-dependent A system of amino acid transport (20).

It has been proposed that adrenergic control of the cerebral microcirculation is diminished in aging and AD. Mann (21) has suggested that cell loss from the locus ceruleus, a nucleus that innervates the cerebral microcirculation, contributes to the pathogenesis of neuronal degeneration and death in AD. Therefore, the purpose of this study was to examine whether neurohumoral control of the BBB, at the level of adrenergic receptors, is altered in AD.

METHODS

Brains from seven patients who died as the result of AD and four age-matched controls from subjects whose neuropathology showed no neurological or psychiatric disease were studied. The right cerebral hemispheres were immediately frozen and stored at $-70\,°C$ until use. The left cerebral hemispheres were histologically processed for diagnostic and morphometric studies.

The clinical diagnosis of primary degenerative dementia of Alzheimer type was confirmed by neuropathological examination and accepted quantitative criteria. Each case met the diagnostic criteria for neuritic plaques and neurofibrillary tangles recommended by the National Institutes of Health Neuropathology Panel (22).

In a survey of 19 404 microscopic fields from ten standardized neocortical regions of each brain (superior, middle, inferior temporal; middle frontal gyrus; precentral and postcentral gyri; inferior parietal; calcarine; and cingulate), no plaques or tangles could be found in any of the controls, whereas the AD cases showed neocortical plaque densities ranging from $156/mm^3$ to as much as $4701/mm^3$, and neurofibrillary tangle indices from $2.3/mm^3$ up to as high as $528/mm^3$.

The procedure utilized for the isolation of cerebral microvessels from human brain is a modification of our previously described procedure for microvessel isolation from rat brain (23) as shown in Figure 1.

Radioligand binding assays to determine α and β-adrenergic receptor binding parameters were performed using [^{3}H]-prazosin (PZ) and [^{125}I]-iodocyanopindolol (ICYP), respectively, according to published methods (24,25).

RESULTS

After microvessels were removed from the Percoll gradient (26) they were essentially free of neuronal and other nonvascular debris (Figure 2).

Examination of the microvessels from Alzheimer patients and nondemented elderly controls using the β-receptor antagonist ICYP in the concentration range of 10 pM to 160 pM indicated that the binding is specific and saturable (Figure 3). The saturation binding isotherm demonstrated that the specific binding of ICYP was comparable in microvessels from Alzheimer patients when compared to the

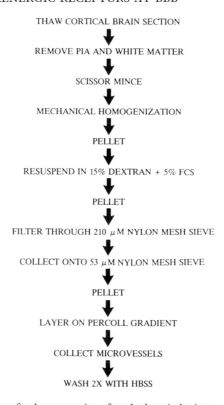

THAW CORTICAL BRAIN SECTION
↓
REMOVE PIA AND WHITE MATTER
↓
SCISSOR MINCE
↓
MECHANICAL HOMOGENIZATION
↓
PELLET
↓
RESUSPEND IN 15% DEXTRAN + 5% FCS
↓
PELLET
↓
FILTER THROUGH 210 μM NYLON MESH SIEVE
↓
COLLECT ONTO 53 μM NYLON MESH SIEVE
↓
PELLET
↓
LAYER ON PERCOLL GRADIENT
↓
COLLECT MICROVESSELS
↓
WASH 2X WITH HBSS

Figure 1. Isolation scheme for the preparation of cerebral cortical microvessels from human brain

microvessels obtained from nondemented elderly controls. Scatchard analysis of the saturation binding data indicated that microvessels from Alzheimer patients exhibited a K_d and a binding capacity (B_{max}) that were not statistically different from the data obtained from microvessels from nondemented elderly controls (Table 1).

In contrast to the β-adrenergic receptors, α-adrenergic receptors were significantly decreased in microvessels from Alzheimer patients relative to control microvessels. A composite binding curve, using the data from four or five separate experiments, is shown in Figure 4. Examination of [^{3}H]-prazosin (0.05–0.4 nM) binding to microvessels from Alzheimer patients indicated a significant decrease ($P < 0.001$) at each concentration measured relative to nondemented elderly control microvessels (Figure 4). Scatchard analysis of the composite saturation isotherms showed a twofold decrease in the binding capacity of microvessels from Alzheimer patients (13.5 fmol/mg protein) relative to controls (30.3 fmol/mg protein) with a slight but not significant decrease in the affinity of the α-receptor (Figure 5).

DISCUSSION

The results of this study indicate that brains from Alzheimer patients and nondemented elderly controls obtained at autopsy can be used to isolate cerebral

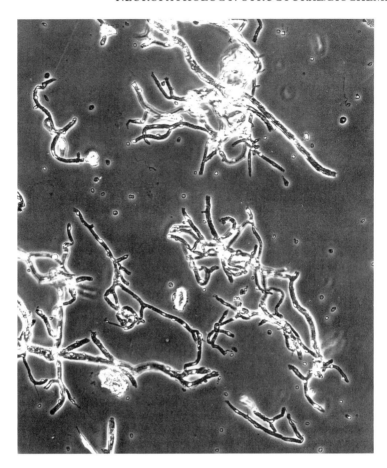

Figure 2. Phase-contrast micrograph of isolated microvessel segments from control human brain (×550)

cortical microvessels and assess adrenergic receptor alterations by radioligand binding techniques. The data indicated that there is no difference in the β-adrenergic receptor binding parameters, i.e. receptor affinity (K_d) or binding capacity (B_{max}), in microvessels from Alzheimer brains compared to controls. In contrast, examination of the α-adrenergic receptor yielded a significant decrease in the number of receptors present in microvessels from Alzheimer brains relative to controls, with a small but not significant change in receptor affinity.

The role of BBB abnormalities in AD has not been clearly defined. Scheibel (9) has presented evidence of structural alterations including ultrastructural thickening and reduplication of endothelial cell basement membrane, endothelial cell swelling and loss of perivascular neural plexus. These changes could underlie a failing BBB in AD, and in fact Scheibel has described AD as a 'capillary dementia' (27). Several studies have observed a close correlation between senile plaques and capillaries that

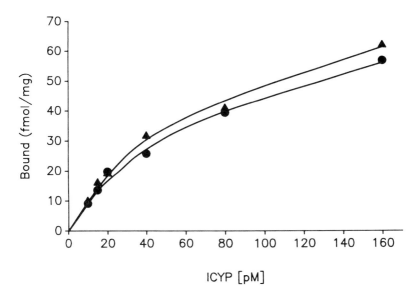

ICYP [pM]

Figure 3. Specific binding of ICYP to microvessels isolated from Alzheimer patients (▲) and nondemented elderly controls (●) as a function of ICYP concentration. 50 μg of protein was incubated at 37 °C for 60 min in 0.5 ml of assay buffer with various concentrations of ICYP. Each point represents the mean of three separate experiments

Table 1. Binding of ICYP to microvessels from Alzheimer and control brains

	Control	Alzheimer
B_{max} (fmol/mg)	55.5 ± 5.5	57.2 ± 8.7
K_d (nM)	0.033 ± 0.007	0.038 ± 0.008
r	0.97 ± 0.009	0.93 ± 0.03

Values are mean ± SEM determined from 3 experiments performed in triplicate.

have undergone amyloid angiopathy (5,6). It has been suggested that in AD deposits of β-amyloid occur in diffuse, non-fibrillar form prior to the development of dystrophic neurites and that such deposits may represent the earliest structural abnormality detected in AD brain (28-30). In a recent review, Selkoe has suggested these deposits could have a vascular origin (7). This possibility of a defective BBB in AD is supported by the presence of immunoglobulins and other serum proteins within senile plaques (10-12).

There are selective *functional* alterations in the BBB in AD. Reduced glucose transport and hexokinase activity at the BBB have been shown in this type of dementia (13,31). Although the role of vascular amyloid in the pathogenesis of AD is controversial, lack of vascular amyloid does not rule out an important role for

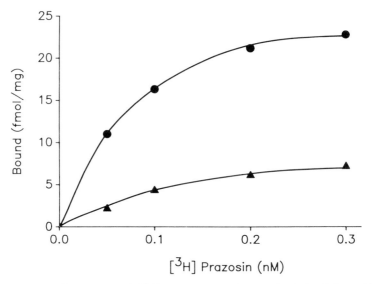

Figure 4. Specific binding of [³H]-prazosin to microvessels isolated from Alzheimer patients (▲) and controls (●) as a function of [³H]-prazosin concentration. 100 μg protein was incubated at 25 °C for 30 min in 0.2 ml assay buffer with various concentrations of [³H]-prazosin. Each point represents the mean of 4 or 5 separate experiments

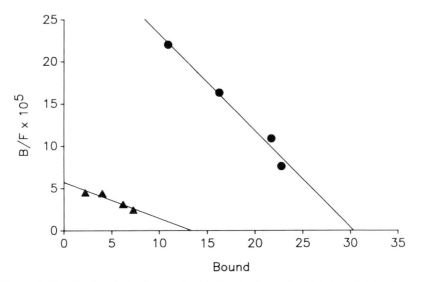

Figure 5. Scatchard analysis of saturation binding isotherms for Alzheimer (▲) and control (●) derived microvessels shown in Figure 4

a damaged BBB in the pathogenesis of AD. Mann has theorized that a defective functioning of the cerebral vasculature may lead to focal leakage of a 'neurotoxic' factor from the circulation into the brain and that this factor may or may not be β-amyloid (32).

The notion that changes in adrenergic receptors may be important in aging and dementia is highlighted by a recent examination of α_1-receptor in the brains of aged and Alzheimer patients where the binding of an α_1-antagonist [^{125}I]-HEAT— [^{125}I]-2-(β-4-hydroxyphenylamino-ethyltetralone)—was significantly decreased in prefrontal cortex (33).

Adrenergic receptor changes in aging and AD in the cerebral endothelium may be important since it has been demonstrated that noradrenergic innervation of the microvasculature helps preserve the integrity of the BBB, arguing for neuronal control of the brain microvasculature (14-17). Cerebral capillaries constitute the portion of the BBB that limits the transendothelial transport of molecules and ions from blood to brain and from the CSF to the plasma. Therefore the regulation of these active processes is important to the maintenance of the ionic and nutrient milieu of the brain. Work in this laboratory has shown that adrenergic receptors modulate adenylate cyclase, guanylate cyclase and amino acid uptake (18,20,34). Since adrenergic neurotransmitters appear to play a role in overall homeostasis of transport at the BBB, Mann has suggested that cell loss in the locus ceruleus initiates a cascade of cellular disturbances at the BBB leading to failure of homeostasis and ultimately forms the basis of the dementia characteristic of AD (32). The data presented here support the possibility of a selective abnormality at the BBB in AD by demonstrating alterations in the first step in adrenergic responsiveness, namely the binding of labelled prazosin to α_1-receptors. Although the function of these adrenergic receptors has not been delineated, our data showing a selective reduction in the number of α_1-receptors at the BBB in AD suggest that this deficiency may underlie perturbations in functions such as permeability that are thought to be mediated by these receptors. In contrast to the results reported in the present study, Kalaria and Harik (35) reported a significant increase in β_2 and α_2-receptors and no change in the α_1-receptor subtype in cerebral microvessels isolated from AD brains. These differences may be attributable, at least in part, to differences in microvessel preparation and specific ligands utilized.

Pardridge has shown that intraparenchymal microvessels can be isolated in pure form and in high yield from autopsy human brain (26) even if the brain is obtained up to 36 hours post mortem, although the functional integrity of this preparation with regard to specific enzymes, receptors and transport systems remains to be elucidated. The results of the present study confirm the validity of using isolated cerebral microvessels from autopsy brains to evaluate receptors and receptor-mediated functional properties of the BBB. Thus, this in-vitro preparation could be used to unravel the biochemical basis of BBB dysfunction in AD that may contribute to the multistep pathogenesis of neuronal cell death in this neuro-degenerative disorder.

Acknowledgments

The authors thank L. Mrock, D. Bessert, J. MacGregor, E. Ojalvo-Rose and S. Griffin-Brooks for technical assistance. Supported in part by a grant from the American Health Assistance Foundation (P.G.) and the Atkinson Charitable Foundation of Toronto (M.J.B.).

REFERENCES

1. Kidd M. Nature 1963; 197: 192-3.
2. Wisniewski HM, Ghetti B, Terry RD. J Neuropath Exp Neurol 1973; 32: 566-84.
3. Glenner GC, Wong CN. Biochem Biophys Res Comm 1984; 120: 885-90.
4. Price DL. Ann Rev Neurosci 1986; 9: 489-512.
5. Miyakawa T, Uehara Y. Acta Neuropathol 1979; 48: 153-6.
6. Miyakawa T, Shimoji A, Kuramoto R, Higuchi Y. Virch Arch 1982; 40: 121-9.
7. Selkoe DJ. Neurobiol Aging 1989; 10: 387-95.
8. Bell M, Ball MJ. Acta Neuropathol 1981; 53: 299-318.
9. Scheibel AB. In Wertheimer J, Narois M (eds) Senile dementia: outlook for the future. New York: Alan R Liss Inc. 1984: 137-49.
10. Wisniewski HM, Kozolowski PB. Ann NY Acad Sci 1982; 396: 119-29.
11. Coria F, Castano E, Prelli F, Larrondo-Lillo M, Van Duinen S, Shelanski M, Frangione B. Lab Invest 1988; 58: 454-8.
12. Abraham CR, Selkoe DJ, Potter H. Cell 1988; 52: 487-501.
13. Kalaria RN, Harik SI. J Neurochem 1989; 53: 1083-8.
14. Raichle ME, Hartman BK, Eichling JO, Sharpe LG. Proc Natl Acad Sci USA 1975; 72: 3726-30.
15. Abraham WC, Delanoy RL, Dunn AJ, Zorneter SF. Brain Res 1979; 172: 387-92.
16. Harik SI, McGunigal T. Ann Neurol 1984; 15: 568-74.
17. Kobayashi H, Magnoni MS, Govoni S, Izumi F, Wada A, Trabucchi M. Experientia 1985; 41: 427-34.
18. Grammas P, Diglio CA, Giacomelli F, Wiener J. J Neurochem 1985; 44: 1732-5.
19. Grammas P, Caspers ML, Diglio CA, Giacomelli F, Wiener J. Biochem Pharmacol 1985; 34: 4177-9.
20. Grammas P, Kwaiser TM, Caspers ML. Soc Neurosci 1989; 15: 1025 (abstr.).
21. Mann DMA. Mech Aging Develop 1983; 23: 73-94.
22. Khachaturian ZS. Arch Neurol 1985; 42: 1097-105.
23. Diglio CA, Grammas P, Giacomelli F, Wiener J. Lab Invest 1982; 46: 554-63.
24. Skomedal T, Aass H, Osnes JB. Biochem Pharmacol 1984; 33: 1897-906.
25. Palmer KC, Grammas P. Lab Invest 1987; 56: 329-34.
26. Pardridge WM, Yang J, Eisenberg J, Tourtellottee WW. J Neurosci Res 1987; 18: 352-7.
27. Scheibel AB, Duong T, Jacobs R. Ann Med 1989; 21: 103-7.
28. Probst A, Brunnschweiler H, Lautenschlager C, Ulrich J. Acta Neuropathol 1988; 74: 133-41.
29. Ikeda SI, Allsop D, Glenner GG. Lab Invest 1989; 60: 113-22.
30. Mann DMA, Brown AMT, Prinja D, Jones D, Davies CA. Neuropath Appl Neurobiol 1990; 16: 17-31.
31. Marcus DL, DeLeon MJ, Goldman J, Logan J, Christman DR, Wolf AP, Fowler JS, Hunter K, Tsai J, Pearson J, Freedman ML. Ann Neurol 1989; 26: 91-4.
32. Mann DMA. Mech Aging Develop 1985; 31: 213-55.
33. Kalaria RN. Brain Res 1989; 501: 287-94.
34. Grammas P, Giacomelli F, Diglio CA, Wiener J. Soc Neurosci 1988; 14: 1031 (abstr.).
35. Kalaria RN, Harik SI. Neurosci Lett 1989; 106: 233-8.

Address for correspondence:

Dr Paula Grammas,
Department of Pathology,
University of Oklahoma Health Sciences Center,
940 Stanton L. Young Blvd,
Oklahoma City, OK 73104, USA

17 Stability of Dendritic Extent in Neurons of the Vertical Limb of the Diagonal Band of Broca in Alzheimer's Disease

DOROTHY G. FLOOD, SHARON B. STECHNA
AND STEVEN D. HANKS

Although the cholinergic basal forebrain is not the only site of lesion in Alzheimer's disease (AD), its importance as a site of major pathology in the disease has permitted it to remain as one of the most studied regions or systems in the field of AD research. Deficits in cholinergic markers of neurotransmission in both the basal forebrain and in its projection areas of the cerebral cortex and hippocampus have been well documented in AD (e.g. 1,2). Similarly, there have been numerous studies of neuronal number in the cholinergic basal forebrain in AD, all showing neuronal loss and/or shrinkage of the cholinergic neurons (for review, see reference 3). Despite the massive attention these cholinergic basal forebrain neurons have received in AD research on their cell bodies, axonal projections, and neurotransmitter system, only one report has appeared on the dendrites of these neurons (4). In this report (4) it was found that both cell body area and total dendritic extent increased in the AD group compared with an age-matched control group. Additionally, in spite of some obvious degenerative changes in some of the basal forebrain neurons, the occurrence of filopodial extensions was reported on both the cell bodies and dendrites in the AD subjects but never in the control subjects, suggesting the existence of dendritic plasticity in AD in this brain region (4). There was increased dendritic extent in the AD subjects without the inclusion of the filopodial extensions, but the increased dendritic extent was more marked with their inclusion. However, since decreases (rather than increases) in cell body size are generally reported for subjects with AD (for review, see 3), and since cell body size and dendritic extent are often positively correlated (5), it seemed that this question of possible dendritic growth in AD should be reinvestigated. Thus, we have undertaken a study of dendritic extent in the cholinergic forebrain nucleus, the vertical limb of the diagonal band of Broca.

Nine cases obtained at autopsy through the Rochester Alzheimer's Disease Project (RADP) and one case obtained earlier were placed into one of two groups: an Alzheimer's disease (AD) group and an age-matched control (CON) group. Information

Alzheimer's Disease: Basic Mechanisms, Diagnosis and Therapeutic Strategies
Edited by K. Iqbal, D. R. C. McLachlan, B. Winblad and H. M. Wisniewski
©1991 John Wiley & Sons Ltd

Table 1. Subject details

Group & case no.	Age at death[1]	Sex	PMD[2] (hr)	Clinical severity	Pathological severity	Duration of illness (yr)
Alzheimer's disease (AD) group						
A-156-85	74	M	5.00	Severe	Moderate	5–6
A-205-85	75	M	2.50	Severe	Severe	15
A-018-86	76	F	3.00	Moderate	Not available	11
A-041-86	81	F	5.50	Severe	Not available	9–10
A-020-85	83	F	4.50	Moderate	Severe	2
A-104-86	87	F	2.25	Severe	Not available	3–4
Mean	79.3		3.79			
SEM	2.3		0.62			
Control (CON) group						
R-007-81	73	F	23.00		Not available	
A-102-85	80	M	5.00		Minimal	
A-195-84	81	M	3.50		Minimal	
A-144-84	82	M	10.20		Minimal	
Mean	79.0		10.43			
SEM	2.4		5.12			

[1]Age at death, t (2-tailed)=0.10, d.f.=8, NS.
[2]PMD (postmortem delay), t (2-tailed)=1.86, d.f.=8, p>0.10.

regarding age at death, sex, postmortem delay (PMD), clinical and pathological severity of dementia, and duration of illness is provided in Table 1. All cases in the AD group had a clinical history of progressive dementia which proved to be AD at autopsy. These cases were free from other neurological and psychiatric illnesses and from other neuropathological findings at autopsy. All cases in the control group had a clinical history lacking in any neurological or psychiatric abnormality, and showed no significant neuropathology. The pathological severity of Alzheimer's changes, when present at all in the CON cases, was within established age-adjusted criteria for normal elderly subjects (6). The clinical histories of the CON cases and two of the AD cases (A-041-86 and A-104-86) were obtained retrospectively from health care workers, medical records, and family members. The remaining AD cases were followed clinically prior to their deaths by the RADP.

At autopsy blocks of the basal forebrain from either hemisphere were dissected fresh and placed into Golgi–Cox fixative (7). Following impregnation, dehydration, and embedding in celloidin, alternate coronal sections were cut at 200 μm or 80 μm and further processed (7). The 80 μm-thick sections were counterstained with cresyl violet and aided in delineation of the basal forebrain nuclei. Each case was given a code number so that analysis was performed blind to the subject's identity. Low-power camera lucida maps were drawn of Ch2 (vertical limb of the diagonal band of Broca), as defined by Mesulam and Geula (8), from two or three 200-μm thick sections per case. On these maps the Golgi-impregnated neurons were marked and numbered. Fifteen neurons per case that were located in the middle one-third of the section thickness and that were not overly obscured by nonspecific stain deposits, were randomly chosen by drawing numbers and were drawn using a 40× objective and a camera lucida attachment. Cell body size and appearance of the dendritic tree were not selection criteria. The drawings of the dendritic trees and cell bodies were then digitized and measured using an Apple II+ microcomputer with attached graphics tablet. Student's *t*-tests (two-tailed) were performed to compare the AD and CON groups, with *n* equal to the number of subjects.

Figure 1 shows low-power photomicrographs of neurons in Ch2. Figure 1A shows a typical staining pattern, with many impregnated neurons and the large, presumably cholinergic neurons being quite apparent. Also evident are fine axonal processes and scattered glia that have been impregnated. Figure 1B is a particularly nice example of dendritic staining since axons and glia did not stain as heavily in this portion of Ch2. Although Figure 1A is from an AD case and Figure 1B is from a CON case, both patterns of staining occurred in both subject groups and within the same subject. However, it was generally more common to have some axonal and glial staining.

CON and AD cases were qualitatively indistinguishable. Dendritic staining was excellent in cases from both groups, with the majority of neurons having large dendritic trees. Occasional atrophic neurons were observed in all cases. Although there have been previous reports of cell body shrinkage of neurons in the basal forebrain (3,9–11), the difference in cell size between the AD and CON groups was not qualitatively apparent, as for example between Figure 1A and B.

Filopodia arising from cell bodies and dendrites, as described previously on basal forebrain neurons (4), were not apparent in our Golgi–Cox stained material. Fine processes, with a filopodial-like appearance, did occasionally appear associated with cell bodies and dendrites, but these could usually be identified as axons, sometimes forming synapses en passant, or as glial processes. Some filopodial-like processes were axonal in appearance and formed terminal boutons on dendrites and cell bodies. These most closely resembled the processes described by Arendt et al (4), but because they looked like processes that were clearly axonal, they were not considered to be filopodia. These processes, which we felt were most likely axonal terminals, were seen on neurons in both the AD and CON groups; and they were not included in our analysis of dendritic extent.

Quantitative data on the 15 sampled neurons per case and averaged by case are presented in Figure 2 for cell body area (A) and total dendritic length (B). Cell body area for the AD cases was lower than for all of the CON cases (Figure 2A). The group averages and standard errors of the mean (SEM) for cell body area were $405.0 \pm 17.6 \mu m^2$ for the AD group and $581.8 \pm 17.9 \mu m^2$ for the CON group. Cell body area was significantly reduced in the AD group by 30% ($t = 7.53$, d.f. $= 8$, $P < 0.01$). Reports of reductions in cell body area in AD cases compared with CON cases have ranged from 25% (9,10) to 30% (11) for the nucleus basalis of Meynert. Although reported in a different manner, cell shrinkage was fairly comparable in the nucleus basalis (Ch4) and in the vertical limb of the diagonal band of Broca (Ch2) (3). Thus, it would seem that our random sample of 15 Golgi–Cox impregnated neurons per case is representative of the population of Ch2 neurons in AD and CON cases in terms of the degree of cell body shrinkage seen in the diseased subjects.

Total dendritic length for these same neurons was comparable between the AD and CON cases, except for one AD case (A-041-86), in which dendritic extent was markedly reduced (Figure 2B). There was nothing remarkable about the clinical or neuropathological history of A-041-86; and the dendritic extent of neurons from this case in other regions of the cholinergic basal forebrain was comparable to that of the CON cases. Means±SEM for total dendritic length were 1216.9±167.8 μm for the AD group and 1375.6±123.2 μm for the CON group. The groups did not differ significantly in total dendritic length ($t=0.76$, d.f.$=8$, NS).

In summary we found a shrinkage of the cell bodies of Ch2 neurons, consistent with the cell counting studies (3,9–11), but a maintenance of dendritic extent of these neurons in the AD group compared with the CON group. These findings contrast with the report of Arendt et al (4), who found increases in both cell body size and dendritic extent in their AD subjects. They also found filopodial processes

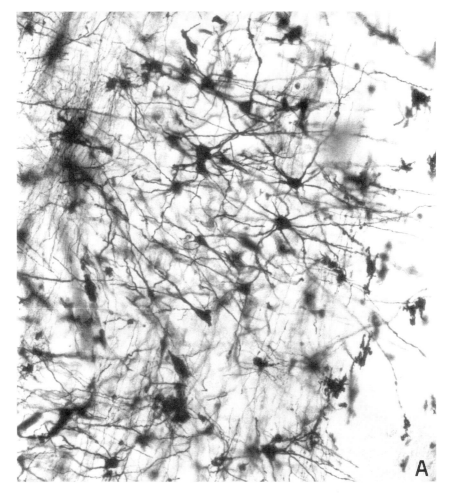

Figure 1. (*caption opposite*)

on the neurons of these subjects, which further suggested to them that there was dendritic growth in basal forebrain cholinergic neurons in AD. There are several differences between our study and that of Arendt et al (4); some are relevant and others are likely to be irrelevant. First, the subjects in the Arendt et al (4) study were younger at death (55–68 years old) and the AD subjects had a shorter duration of illness (2–5 years) than the subjects of our study. This could be a factor of some

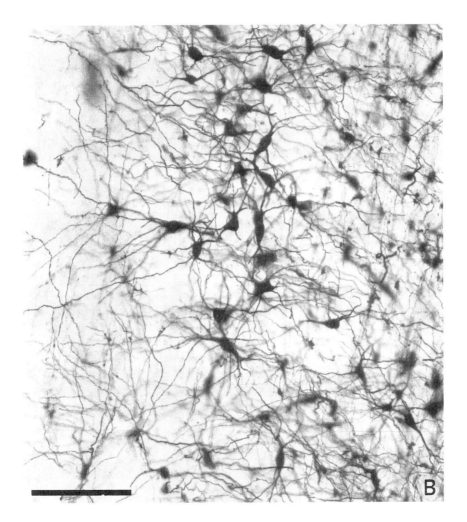

Figure 1. Low-power photomicrographs of Ch2 (vertical limb of the diagonal band of Broca) from A-018-86, an AD case (A), and from A-102-85, a CON case (B). Numerous well-impregnated neurons are present in both cases. The additional staining of axons and glia seen in A is more characteristic of the majority of our case material. In B, which lacks axonal and glial staining in this field, the dendritic processes of Ch2 neurons are more easily seen. Scale bar 200μm

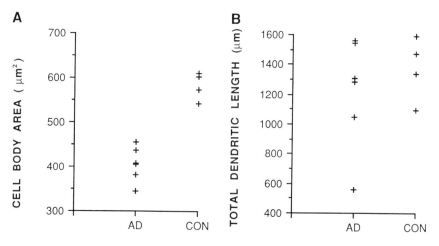

Figure 2.   (A) Cell body area (μm^2) and (B) total dendritic length (μm) presented for Alzheimer disease (AD) and control (CON) cases. Each point represents a subject and the mean of 15 neurons sampled at random from Ch2

importance and one about which our data cannot provide any information. Thus, we are currently expanding our study to include younger subjects and AD subjects with shorter durations of illness. Another difference is our use of the mercuric Golgi-Cox technique, and their use of the silver rapid Golgi method. The Golgi methods may have differentially stained the filopodial processes, but equally possible is the difference in interpretation between the studies of similar appearing structures. Lastly, and most likely to have produced the differing quantitative results, are differences in neuronal sampling procedures between the studies, that were probably exacerbated by the differences in Golgi methods used. Arendt et al (4) excluded from quantitative analysis cells with degenerative changes since it was impossible for them to distinguish poorly impregnated neurons from degenerating neurons in their material. Unfortunately, the rapid Golgi method is particularly sensitive to fixation factors, including postmortem delay (12,13), making the likelihood of observing poorly impregnated neurons high. Because impregnations with the Golgi-Cox method are consistently good in human postmortem tissue, this sampling bias has never been necessary in our studies. Thus, here and in other studies, we sampled any neuron, regardless of cell body size or appearance of dendritic staining. This difference is the most probable source of the varying results. Since our sampling procedure was unbiased and since our finding of 30% cell body shrinkage in the AD cases represents a finding comparable to those of cell count studies, we believe that the finding of stability of dendritic extent in AD is the more accurate result. Our data showing stability of dendritic extent have encouraging implications since they suggest that in spite of alterations in AD to the axonal field and cell bodies of cholinergic neurons, the afferent surfaces, the dendrites, of these neurons remain intact.

Acknowledgments

We wish to thank the members of the Rochester Alzheimer's Disease Project (RADP) for the clinical and neuropathological diagnosis of nine of the cases used in this study and for making this tissue available. This work has been supported by NIH grant AG 03644.

REFERENCES

1. Coyle JT, Price DL, DeLong MR. Science 1983; 219: 1184-90.
2. Araujo DM, Lapchak PA, Robitaille Y, Gauthier S, Quirion R. J Neurochem 1988; 50: 1914-23.
3. Vogels OJM, Broere CAJ, Ter Laak HJ, Ten Donkelaar HJ, Nieuwenhuys R, Schulte BPM. Neurobiol Aging 1990; 11: 3-13.
4. Arendt T, Zvegintseva HG, Leontovich TA. Neuroscience 1986; 19: 1265-78.
5. Sholl DA. J Anat 1953; 87: 387-406.
6. Khatchaturian ZS. Arch Neurol 1985; 42: 1097-105.
7. Van der Loos H. Mschr Psychiat Neurol 1956; 132: 330-4.
8. Mesulam M-M, Geula C. J Comp Neurol 1988; 275: 216-40.
9. Pearson RCA, Sofroniew MV, Cuello AC, Powell TPS, Eckenstein F, Esiri MM, Wilcock GK. Brain Res 1983; 289: 375-9.
10. Rinne JO, Paljärvi L, Rinne UK. J Neurol Sci 1987; 79: 67-76.
11. Allen SJ, Dawbarn D, Wilcock GK. Brain Res 1988; 454: 275-81.
12. Morest DK, Morest RR. Amer J Anat 1966; 118: 811-32.
13. Williams RS, Ferrante RJ, Caviness VS Jr. J Neuropath Exp Neurol 1978; 37: 13-33.

Address for correspondence:

Dr Dorothy G. Flood,
Department of Neurology, Box 673,
School of Medicine and Dentistry,
University of Rochester,
601 Elmwood Avenue,
Rochester, NY 14642, USA

18 Autopsy Alzheimer's Brains Show Increased Peroxidation to an In-Vitro Iron Challenge

J. STEVEN RICHARDSON, KALA V. SUBBARAO
AND LEE C. ANG

Oxygen free radicals, any compound containing an oxygen atom with an unpaired electron in the outer shell, are highly reactive and can initiate the peroxidation of a variety of substrates that are essential to the survival of living cells. Free radicals are formed during many normal metabolic processes involving electron transport (1) and rather efficient defense systems have evolved to contain the effects of free radicals generated by enzymes such as cytochrome P-450, monoamine oxidase, cyclo-oxygenase and many other oxidase or reductase enzymes. In addition to these metabolic sources, free radical formation is also catalyzed by free ions of transition metals such as iron, copper or manganese (2). Free ferric or ferrous iron ions have been shown to catalyze the production of free radicals and to initiate the in-vitro peroxidation of neural tissue (3,4). The peroxidation products of numerous substrates such as lipids, fatty acids, proteins, and nucleic acids will give a characteristic color reaction with thiobarbituric acid (5) and the formation of these thiobarbituric acid reactive products (TBAR) is a reliable index of peroxidation activity.

Generally, there is a good balance between the generation of free radicals and the activity of the protective factors so that little harm is done to the cell. However, if the capacity of the free radical defense system is exceeded, then tissue destruction and cell death can occur. Many of the abnormal biochemical observations in Alzheimer's disease, such as increased membrane permeability, disrupted protein structure and function, and altered gene expression, are consistent with the expected effects of excess free radicals (6). Free radicals attack membrane free fatty acids and proteins, disrupt ion channels and increase cell membrane permeability. Free radicals alter protein cross-linking, conformation and function and change enzyme activity and the cellular cytoskeleton. Free radicals affect the structure of DNA, leading to a misreading of genes and reduced mRNA formation. As a preliminary step in studying the role of free radicals in the etiology of Alzheimer's disease, we investigated free radical induced peroxidation, measured as TBAR formation, in autopsy samples from clinically and histologically verified Alzheimer's patients, from normal controls and from nondemented people with plaque and tangle densities below the criteria

Alzheimer's Disease: Basic Mechanisms, Diagnosis and Therapeutic Strategies
Edited by K. Iqbal, D. R. C. McLachlan, B. Winblad and H. M. Wisniewski
©1991 John Wiley & Sons Ltd

level set by the NIH-AARP workshop (7). The data from the Alzheimer's patients and the normal controls have been reported previously (8).

METHODS

Sample collection

Autopsy was performed 6 to 24 hours post mortem on donors with or without premortem evidence of dementia. The brains were removed, sectioned in half sagitally and one half was placed in 10% buffered formalin for histological study. The other half was sectioned coronally into 10-15 mm thick slices, frozen immediately and stored at $-80°C$ until assay. The samples used in this study (Table 1) came from six verified Alzheimer's disease patients, three nondemented people with a senile plaque and tangle density below the NIH-AARP criterion level (NDSP-nondemented subthreshold plaques) and six normal controls.

Biochemical studies

On the day of the assay, comparable samples of frontal cortex and cerebellum were cut from the coronal slices of the brains, weighed while frozen and homogenized separately in 10 volumes of ice-cold normal saline at a pH of 7.0, that had been bubbled with nitrogen for 10 minutes just prior to use. Aliquots of the frontal cortex and cerebellum homogenates were used with concentrations of ferric chloride from 0-200 μM dissolved in double-distilled water in an iron-induced peroxidation dose response study. Aliquots of frontal cortex homogenates were used in a dose response study of the effects of the 21-aminosteroid U-74500A on the peroxidation induced by 200 μM ferric chloride. TBAR formation was measured after 30 minutes incubation at 37°C in all tubes, and protein, total glutathione, RNA and DNA levels in each sample were determined as described previously (4,8).

Table 1. Characteristics of tissue donors

Group	Age	Sex	Postmortem delay (hr)	Cause of death
Control	68.3 (53 to 78)	6M	10.9 (6 to 24)	1 traumatic transection of the aorta 5 complications of ischemic heart disease
AD	68.5 (50 to 79)	2M, 4F	15.1 (6 to 24)	1 pulmonary embolism 1 subarachnoid hemorrhage 4 acute bronchopneumonia
NDSP	77.6 (67 to 91)	1M, 2F	15.3 (10 to 19)	2 myocardial infarct 1 during heart surgery

Numbers in parentheses indicate range of values.

Table 2. Basal TBAR formation and the levels of DNA, RNA, protein and total glutathione in autopsy brains

Region	TBAR formation (nmol)[a] /g tissue	/mg protein	/mg DNA	DNA[b] (mg)	RNA[b] (mg)	Protein[b] (mg)	Total GSH[b] (μmol)
Frontal cortex							
Control	70 ± 7^{c}	0.76 ± 0.07	26.6 ± 2.6	2.6 ± 0.04	2.4 ± 0.10	92 ± 6	2.4 ± 0.24
NDSP[d]	$178 \pm 46^{*}$	1.63 ± 0.40	71.8 ± 21.2	2.6 ± 0.14	2.6 ± 0.24	101 ± 8	2.0 ± 0.23
Alzheimer	$168 \pm 32^{*}$	$1.96 \pm 0.40^{*}$	$63.3 \pm 12.2^{*}$	2.7 ± 0.26	2.2 ± 0.16	87 ± 5	2.0 ± 0.21
Cerebellum							
Control	78 ± 12	0.90 ± 0.12	14.0 ± 1.6	5.3 ± 0.35	2.6 ± 0.11	85 ± 3	2.5 ± 0.49
NDSP	132 ± 39	1.53 ± 0.43	23.3 ± 6.2	5.6 ± 0.22	2.7 ± 0.16	89 ± 6	1.8 ± 0.09
Alzheimer	132 ± 39	1.50 ± 0.40	25.0 ± 7.3	5.2 ± 0.21	2.4 ± 0.16	84 ± 6	1.8 ± 0.21

[a] in 30 minutes incubation at 37 °C.
[b] per g tissue wet weight.
[c] all data entries are mean $\pm$ SEM for 6 tissue samples, or 3 for NDSP, run in duplicate.
[d] NDSP stands for nondemented subthreshold plaque.
[*] $P < 0.05$ compared to controls.

Statistical analyses

All data were analysed for statistical significance by appropriate ANOVAs, MANOVAs and posthoc tests using the SPSS-X statistical package for the VAX mainframe computer.

RESULTS

Basal TBAR formation, expressed as nmol TBAR formed in 30 minutes per g of tissue wet weight, per mg protein or per mg DNA, is significantly higher in homogenates of Alzheimer's frontal cortex than in control frontal cortex (Table 2). Basal TBAR formation in NDSP frontal cortex is closer to the Alzheimer's values than to the controls but because of the high standard deviation, it is not significantly different from either control or Alzheimer's cortex. In the cerebellum, there are no significant differences in basal TBAR formation in any of the groups. Nor do the groups differ significantly on the amounts of DNA, RNA, protein or glutathione per g of wet weight (Table 2).

Figure 1 presents TBAR formation and total glutathione levels in Alzheimer's and control frontal cortex as related to the length of time from death to placing the brain samples in the $-80°C$ freezer. Postmortem delay had no effect on TBAR formation (Figure 1A), but total glutathione levels tended to decrease with increasing postmortem delay times (Figure 1B). The effects on TBAR formation of adding 50 μM to 200 μM ferric chloride to aliquots of the sample homogenates are shown in Figure 2. Iron produced a dose-dependent increase in TBAR formation in samples from all three groups that was significantly higher in Alzheimer's frontal cortex than in controls at all concentrations of iron tested. Iron-induced TBAR formation

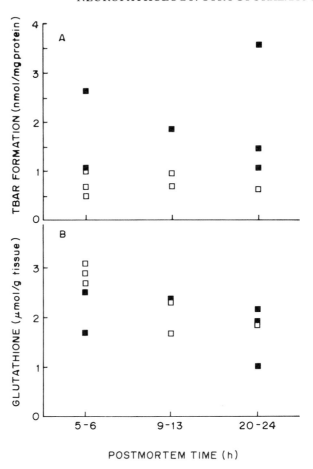

Figure 1. Effects of postmortem delay on TBAR formation (A) and total glutathione levels (B) in Alzheimer's (■) and normal control (□) frontal cortex. Each data point represents a single donor

in the NDSP samples fell midway between that of the Alzheimer's and that of the control frontal cortex (Figure 2A). Iron produced a dose-dependent increase in TBAR formation in the cerebellum samples but there were no differences between the groups at any concentrations of iron tested (Figure 2B).

The ability of the 21-aminosteroid U-74500A to reduce TBAR formation induced by 200 μM iron is shown in Figure 3. U-74500A gave significantly less protection to Alzheimer's frontal cortex (IC$_{50}$ 10 μM) than to control frontal cortex (IC$_{50}$ 2.5 μM) at all doses of U-74500A tested, and the NDSP samples (IC$_{50}$ 10μM) were almost identical to the Alzheimer's samples. Compared to controls, the NDSP samples received significantly less protection at all concentrations of U-75400A.

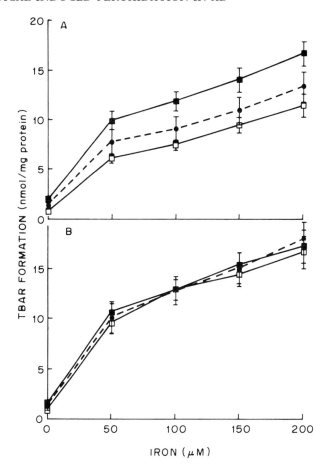

Figure 2. Iron dose response effects on TBAR formation in homogenates of Alzheimer's (■), NDSP (●) and normal control (□) frontal cortex (A) and cerebellum (B). Each data point represents the mean ± SEM of 3 to 6 samples run in duplicate. All of the Alzheimer's values are significantly different from the corresponding controls in the case of frontal cortex (Student/Newman-Keuls': $P < 0.05$). No other group differences are significant

DISCUSSION

Free radicals seem to play a causal role in the neural destruction following central nervous system trauma or ischemia (9,10) and have been implicated in a variety of other brain disorders involving neuron degeneration (11). While the data from the present study do not indicate that free radicals are responsible for the biochemical abnormalities and the characteristic pattern of cell death seen in Alzheimer's disease, they are consistent with such a mechanism. The increased basal TBAR formation compared to controls in Alzheimer's frontal cortex but not in the cerebellum suggests that there is some innate difference in factors related to peroxidation in Alzheimer's

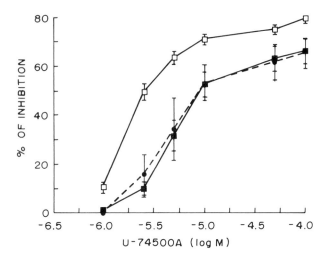

Figure 3. Dose response study of the effects of U-74500A on inhibiting TBAR formation induced by 200 μM ferric chloride in frontal cortex homogenates from Alzheimer's (■), NDSP (●) and control (□) subjects. Each data point represents the mean ± SEM of 3 to 6 samples run in duplicate. Each individual value was calculated as the percentage of the TBAR formation in the absence of U74500A of the respective groups. For the Alzheimer's group this was 16.5 nmol TBAR per mg protein; for the NDSP, 18 nmol; and for the controls, 12.5 nmol. At each concentration, the Alzheimer's values are significantly different from the corresponding controls (Student/Newman-Keuls': $P < 0.05$). The NDSP values for all concentrations are also significantly different from the corresponding controls (Student/Newman-Keuls': $P < 0.05$). No significant differences were found between the AD and NDSP groups

frontal cortical tissue that is either not present in Alzheimer's cerebellar tissue or present to a much smaller degree. Since there is considerable tissue degeneration in the frontal cortex but relatively little change in the cerebellum in Alzheimer's disease, the observed regional differences in TBAR formation correlate very nicely with the regional differences in tissue damage. Nor do our data indicate whether the increased cortical TBAR formation is related to excessive production of free radicals or to deficient free radical defenses, or both. In the statistical analysis of our data, the MANOVA condition by iron interaction was not significant. This indicates that the samples of Alzheimer's cortex did not show increased sensitivity to the concentrations of iron used in this study. Andorn and coworkers reported excess iron in Alzheimer's tissue (12), but the only reports in the literature concerning brain free radical defenses in Alzheimer's disease (13) support our present observation that total glutathione in Alzheimer's cortex and cerebellum appears to be normal. However, the results of the U-74500A dose response study suggest both that there is an abnormality in the way that tissue homogenates of Alzheimer's frontal cortex handle iron and that there is some difference in the endogenous free radical generation or defense systems. In the presence of any of the concentrations of U-74500A used, 200 μM iron produced more peroxidation in Alzheimer's tissue than in controls; and it takes four times more U-74500A to supplement the endogenous free radical defenses to reach the IC_{50} in Alzheimer's tissue than in controls. Although it must be left to future research to delineate the exact nature and the causes of the peroxidation differences between Alzheimer's and control frontal cortex, these data provide some support for the hypothesis that the neural degeneration in Alzheimer's disease is due to the action of free radicals.

There has been continuing controversy as to whether the presence of plaques and tangles in the brain is indicative of Alzheimer's disease (14). Our observations with frontal cortex homogenates from the NDSP samples support the idea that it is. Although our NDSP donors had no premortem evidence of dementia, their tissue samples were very similar to those of the Alzheimer's patients in both the iron-induced TBAR and the U-74500A studies. That these people were symptom free indicates that at the time of death they still had enough surviving neurons to compensate for those neurons that had been lost. Had these people not died from cardiovascular causes when they did but rather had they lived long enough, they would have developed dementia when the neural degeneration had progressed to the stage where there were not enough surviving neurons to maintain normal function. This situation is also seen in Parkinson's disease where it has been estimated that future patients remain symptom free until over 80% of the dopamine cells in the substantia nigra have been destroyed. As long as at least 20% of the original number of dopamine cells survive, normal function can be maintained. Although it has not yet been reported in Alzheimer's disease, it is likely that future patients remain symptom free as long as some critical number of neurons remain active. If free radicals are responsible for the neural degeneration in Alzheimer's disease, identification of these covert, presymptomatic people would allow interventions to prevent futher cell loss, to maintain brain function at its current levels and to prevent the development of the symptoms and the disabilities of this disease.

Acknowledgments

The secretarial assistance of Mrs N. N. Johnson is greatly appreciated. Supported in part by Saskatchewan Health Research Board, Saskatchewan Alzheimer's Society, Alzheimer's Society of Regina and Alzheimer's Society of Canada.

REFERENCES

1. Byczkowski JZ, Gessner T. Int J Biochem 1988; 20: 569-80.
2. Halliwell B, Gutteridge JMC. Biochem J 1984; 219: 1-14.
3. Braughler JM, Chase RL, Pregenzer JF. Biochim Biophys Acta 1987; 921: 457-64.
4. Subbarao KV, Richardson JS. J Neurosci Res 1990; 26: 224-32.
5. Gutteridge JMC. Int J Biochem 1982; 14: 649-53.
6. Subbarao KV, Richardson JS (in preparation).
7. Khachaturian ZS. Arch Neurol 1985; 42: 1097-105.
8. Subbarao KV, Richardson JS, Ang LC. J Neurochem 1990; 55: 342-5.
9. Braughler JM, Hall ED. Free Radical Biol Med 1989; 6: 289-301.
10. Hall ED, Braughler JM. Free Radical Biol Med 1989; 6: 303-13.
11. Jesberger JA, Richardson JS. Int J Neurosci 1990 (in press).
12. Andorn AC, Britton RS, Bacon BR. Neurobiol Aging 1990; 11: 316.

13. Perry TL, Yong VW, Bergeron C, Hansen S, Jones K. Ann Neurol 1987; 21: 331-6.
14. Jones AWR, Richardson JS. Int J Neurosci 1990; 50: 147-68.

Address for correspondence:

Dr J. Steven Richardson,
Department of Pharmacology,
College of Medicine,
University of Saskatchewan,
Saskatoon, SK S7N 0W0,
Canada

Part IV

MECHANISMS OF NEURONAL DEGENERATION: CYTOSKELETAL PATHOLOGY AND OTHER MECHANISMS

19 Signal Transduction and the Pathobiology of Alzheimer's Disease

SAMUEL E. GANDY, JOSEPH D. BUXBAUM AND
PAUL GREENGARD

Protein phosphorylation is one of the major biochemical mechanisms by which extracellular stimuli regulate cell function (1,2). Protein phosphorylation systems have the necessary specificity and flexibility to control a great number of physiological functions in mammalian tissues (1,2). Numerous signal molecules are known to activate specific protein kinases, one of the best characterized being the 'second messenger' cAMP (3,4). Many of the intracellular actions of other second messengers, including cGMP (3), Ca^{2+} (5) and diacylglycerol (6) are also mediated by protein kinases. In addition, a variety of agents, including the insulin receptor, oncogenic viruses, growth factors, steroid hormones and interferon regulate protein phosphorylation without the apparent involvement of second messengers (1,7).

There are three distinct functional units in any protein phosphorylation system. One component is a protein kinase which catalyzes the transfer of a phosphoryl group from a donor molecule (usually adenosine triphosphate) to a second component, a protein substrate to which phosphate is covalently bound in phosphoester linkage to the hydroxyl group of a specific serine, threonine or tyrosine residue. A third component is a phosphoprotein phosphatase which catalyzes the removal of the phosphoryl group from the substrate. The state of phosphorylation of a specific substrate results from the relative activities of protein kinases and phosphatases. The phosphorylation state of the protein determines certain physical properties of the protein, and these properties, in turn, determine its functional state.

PROTEIN PHOSPHORYLATION IN THE NERVOUS SYSTEM

Protein phosphorylation plays a prominent role as a regulatory mechanism in the nervous system (1,2). Mammalian brain contains very high amounts of cAMP-, cGMP-, Ca^{2+}/calmodulin- and Ca^{2+}/diacylglycerol-dependent protein kinases (1,2) as well as a large number of neuron-specific phosphoproteins (8,9). A variety of neurotransmitters and hormones, as well as the nerve impulse itself, alter the intracellular concentrations of second messengers and the state of phosphorylation

Alzheimer's Disease: Basic Mechanisms, Diagnosis and Therapeutic Strategies
Edited by K. Iqbal, D. R. C. McLachlan, B. Winblad and H. M. Wisniewski
© 1991 John Wiley & Sons Ltd

156

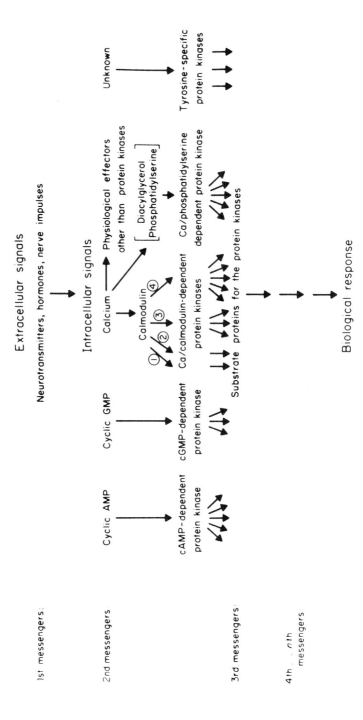

Figure 1. Signal transduction in the nervous system. Extracellular signals (first messengers) produce specific biological responses in target neurons via a series of intracellular signals (second, third, and other messengers). Second messengers in the brain include cyclic AMP, cyclic GMP, diacylglycerol, and calcium. Cyclic AMP and cyclic GMP produce many of their second messenger actions through the activation of virtually one type of cyclic AMP-dependent protein kinase and one type of cyclic GMP-dependent protein kinase, respectively. The former enzyme exhibits a broad substrate specificity and the latter a more restricted specificity. Calcium exerts certain second messenger actions through the activation of calcium-dependent protein kinases and other second messenger actions through the activation of physiological effectors other than protein kinases. Calcium activates protein kinases in conjunction with calmodulin or with diacylglycerol plus phosphatidylserine. These various cyclic nucleotide-dependent and calcium-dependent protein kinases phosphorylate proteins specifically at serine and threonine residues. Another important class of serine/threonine protein kinases, the casein kinases (not shown), has been recently recognized to play an important role in neuronal function. There is also a class of protein kinases that phosphorylate proteins specifically at tyrosine residues (protein tyrosine kinases). The activation of individual protein kinases causes the phosphorylation of specific substrate proteins in target neurons. In some cases these substrate proteins, or third messengers, represent the immediate effector for the biological response. In other cases they produce the biological response indirectly through fourth, fifth, sixth and other messengers (from Greengard P. 1987; Mol Neurobiol 1: 81–119; reproduced by permission of the Humana Press)

of proteins in neurons (for review, see 1,2). In addition, direct evidence for a role of protein phosphorylation in nerve cells has been obtained following the intracellular injection of various individual protein kinases into several types of neurons (for review, see 10; for summary, see Figure 1). Based on these and other studies it has been suggested (for review, see 1) that protein phosphorylation is involved in regulating such diverse processes as neurotransmitter biosynthesis, axoplasmic transport, neurotransmitter release, generation of postsynaptic potentials, ion channel conductance, neuronal shape and motility, elaboration of dendritic and axonal processes, and development and maintenance of differentiated characteristics of neurons. These biochemical events may also underlie various aspects of neuronal plasticity (e.g. 11,12). The molecular basis of short-term memory may involve the phosphorylation-dependent regulation of proteins that are directly involved in presynaptic or postsynaptic components of synaptic transmission (13). The phosphorylation of proteins that play a part in the regulation of gene expression, which would result in more permanent modifications of synaptic transmission, may contribute to the process of long-term memory (13).

PROTEIN PHOSPHORYLATION IN DISEASE

Recently, abnormalities in signal transduction via protein phosphorylation have been shown to be associated with several disease processes. For example, cystic fibrosis (CF) is a disease characterized by abnormal chloride ion transport. Our research group, in collaboration with others, demonstrated that in normal airway epithelia cells, protein phosphorylation caused the activation of transmembrane chloride transport (14,15). When cells from CF patients were used, this response of chloride transport to phosphorylation could not be induced although the channels were present (14,15). The CF gene (16–18) may encode a protein that regulates the ion channel for chloride. It seems likely that the physiological defect present in the channel complex from CF patients involves either direct loss of its phosphorylatability or loss of the proper conformational shift upon phosphorylation (14,15).

Aberrant protein-tyrosine phosphorylation is likely to play a role in oncogenesis, as many of the identified oncogenes are protein-tyrosine kinases (7). In addition, a population of patients suffering from diabetes mellitus appear to possess insulin receptors which lack the normal protein-tyrosine kinase activity associated with the receptor (19,20). This results in a cell-surface receptor which binds insulin normally but fails to transduce the appropriate signal to the intracellular compartment.

PROTEIN PHOSPHORYLATION IN ALZHEIMER'S DISEASE

Because the brain is the richest tissue source of protein kinase and protein phosphatase activity, derangements in signal transduction via protein phosphorylation may be expected to play primary or secondary roles in many diseases of the brain. Evidence has accumulated that signal transduction abnormalities are a hallmark of Alzheimer's disease (21–27), a progressive encephalopathy of late life. Alzheimer's disease is initially characterized by amnesia for recent events. Over the ensuing 6 to 20 years, much or all of cerebral cortical function is lost, leading to loss of independent function and ultimately to loss of content of consciousness (vegetative state) and death. Pathologically, Alzheimer's disease is invariably characterized by the accumulation of poorly soluble structures within neurons, in the neuropil and surrounding cerebral vessels (28).

Neurofibrillary tangles (NFTs) develop inside neurons. NFTs have not yet been fully characterized, but they have been shown, by primary sequencing and by immunochemistry, to contain cytoskeletal proteins—microtubule-associated proteins (MAPs) tau (29) and MAP1B (30)—and ubiquitin (31). They may also contain the β/A4 amyloid protein, the major component of plaques and vascular deposits (discussed in detail below) (32). Of note, the cytoskeletal proteins present in NFTs appear to be phosphorylated in an unusual or aberrant manner, and evidence from several laboratories implicates calcium/calmodulin-dependent protein phosphorylation in the pathogenesis of NFTs. The binding to NFTs of antibodies specific for the dephospho-form of certain cytoskeletal proteins is dramatically enhanced if Alzheimer brain sections are preincubated with phosphatase, while normal brain sections do not demonstrate this phenomenon (21,22). On polyacrylamide gels, the microtubule-associated protein tau extracted from NFTs migrates in an aberrant manner when compared to normal tau. Normal tau may be induced to assume the Alzheimer-type mobility if the preparation is pretreated with calcium/calmodulin-dependent protein kinase, but not with protein kinase C (24). Chronic treatment of primary hippocampal neurons in culture, with either calcium ionophore or glutamate, induces NFT-like immunoreactivity (25). Calcium/calmodulin-dependent protein kinase II immunoreactivity has been reported to be enhanced in hippocampal neurons in Alzheimer's disease (26).

NFTs are not specific to Alzheimer's disease. Cytochemically similar tangles have been observed in the apparently unrelated conditions of progressive supranuclear palsy, Hallervorden–Spatz disease, Guam parkinsonism dementia complex, and dementia pugilistica (33,34), suggesting a common pathological response to several, albeit a limited number of, different insults. The relationship of the aberrant phosphorylation of NFT proteins to the pathogenesis of tangle formation is unclear. Techniques of molecular biology, such as preparation of transgenic mice overexpressing various protein kinases, may permit exploration of this particular question.

In Alzheimer's disease, deposits of amyloid protein accumulate outside the cell and around the cerebral and meningeal vessels. These precipitates are also poorly soluble but, unlike NFTs, have been successfully solubilized using either guanidine hydrochloride or hot formic acid (35,36). Surprisingly, the amyloid deposits were discovered to be remarkably homogeneous, composed almost exclusively ($>90\%$) of β/A4 amyloid. Other components, such as α_1-antichymotrypsin (37) and cathepsins D and B (38), have recently been reported. The biochemical homogeneity of parenchymal amyloid (plaques) and vascular amyloid suggests that Alzheimer's disease is either caused, or accompanied, by a brain 'protein storage disorder'. One group has suggested that the presence of β/A4 amyloid may also be detectable in other organs of Alzheimer's patients (39).

Unlike NFTs, β/A4 amyloid deposition is detected only in the related conditions of Alzheimer's disease, Down's syndrome (trisomy 21), hereditary cerebral hemorrhage with amyloidosis (Dutch type), and, to a lesser degree, normal aging. Alzheimer's disease has therefore been likened to an acceleration of brain aging. Down's syndrome provides a curious insight into Alzheimer's disease. The gene encoding the precursor of β/A4 amyloid is localized on chromosome 21 (40), and so Down's patients possess a 1.5-fold higher than normal gene dosage for the Alzheimer's β/A4 amyloid precursor protein (APP). Since Down's patients invariably develop typical Alzheimer's pathology by the late fourth decade of life (41), APP overexpression may be responsible.

The role of APP in the pathogenesis of Alzheimer's disease is unclear. A locus for certain familial cases of Alzheimer's disease also lies on chromosome 21 (42), but this locus is distinct from the coding region of APP. Analysis of APP mRNA expression in normal and Alzheimer's brain has yielded conflicting results, complicated by the existence of at least five APP-related alternate transcripts, containing either 770, 751, 714, 695 or 563 amino acids (40, 43–49). It is clear, however, that aberrant APP disposition, leading to β/A4 amyloid accumulation, is a constant feature of Alzheimer's disease. The prominence of amyloid deposition in Alzheimer's disease, and the central role in the nervous system of signal transduction mediated via protein phosphorylation, make it attractive to study the interaction of APP with neuronal protein phosphorylation systems.

Alzheimer β/A4 Amyloid Precursor Protein (APP)

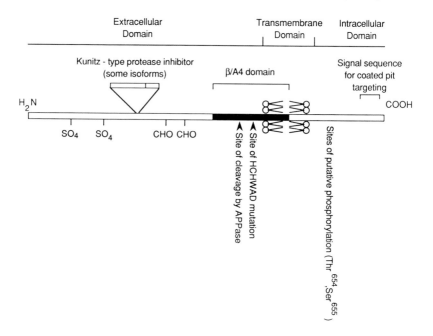

Figure 2. Domain model of APP

$\beta/A4$ AMYLOID PRECURSOR PROTEIN AND ITS PROTEOLYTIC PROCESSING

Amyloidogenic isoforms of APP are integral transmembrane proteins, each with a single membrane-spanning domain (40, 43-49, Figure 2). The biological function of APP in the brain is unknown. Glycosylation sites and tyrosine sulfation sites are contained in the large extracellular domain (ectodomain). Some isoforms (APP_{770}, APP_{751} and APP_{563}, references 46-49) contain a Kunitz protease inhibitor sequence in the ectodomain but the 695 amino acid isoform, lacking this sequence, predominates in brain. The ~ 40 residue $\beta/A4$ portion of APP, which is deposited in the brain in aging and Alzheimer's disease, lies at the predicted junction of the ectodomain and transmembrane domain with 28 residues outside the cell, and 14-15 residues embedded in the membrane. In transfected cells expressing certain populations of APP molecules, much of the ectodomain is cleaved and released from the cell surface (50), probably via a lysosomal pathway (51). Detailed analysis of this cleavage and its regulation is the subject of intense study by several laboratories. The evidence currently available (52,53) indicates that, in cultured transfected cells, the primary constitutive cleavage occurs within the $\beta/A4$ domain, hence precluding amyloidogenesis. Therefore, the failure of this cleavage is a potentially abnormal event which may form the biochemical basis of cerebral amyloidosis. Failure of the cleavage may be due to defective regulation of protease activity (either diminished activity of the 'normal' enzyme or increased activity of an 'alternate' enzyme), or to altered proteolytic sensitivity of APP, possibly due to post-translational modification of APP. APP processing in the brain (and more specifically in the nerve terminal, believed to be a site of origin for amyloid which is deposited) has not yet been characterized.

Some clues already exist which may aid in distinguishing among these possibilities and allow us to identify possible sites for biochemical lesions which could underlie amyloidogenesis. One particularly fruitful line of inquiry has focused on hereditary cerebral hemorrhage with ($\beta/A4$) amyloidosis, Dutch type (HCHWAD), in which there is a genetic mutation (glutamate to glutamine) in the coding region of the APP gene (54). The mutation lies only a few residues COOH-terminal to the site of intra $\beta/A4$ cleavage (Figure 2) and probably alters the binding of APP to the protease—'APP secretase' (53), 'APPase' or 'normal APPase' (our terminology)—responsible for making the normal proteolytic cut. This suggests that APP conformation plays a crucial role in its normal proteolytic processing. Inefficient APP cleavage by normal (intra $\beta/A4$) APPase could conceivably lead to increased processing via an alternate pathway, i.e. via an alternate APPase, which cleaves NH_2-terminal to the normal (intra $\beta/A4$) APPase site. Such an alternate pathway may generate the NH_2-terminus of amyloidogenic $\beta/A4$ (Figure 3). The observation that trisomy 21, possibly via APP gene dosage effect, also leads to cerebral amyloidosis, supports the idea that normal APPase may be relatively easily saturated.

APP processing pathways may be regulated either qualitatively, quantitatively, or both. As discussed above, protein phosphorylation critically regulates many physiological processes. Within the cytodomain of isoforms APP_{770}, APP_{751},

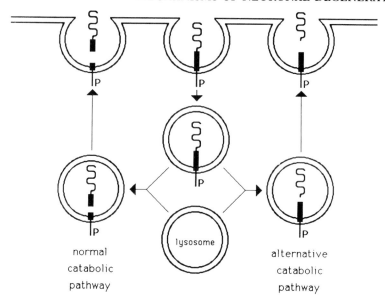

Figure 3. Schematic representation of possible APP processing pathways, including normal intra β/A4 APPase (left) and possible alternative APPase (right). Solid boxed domain is β/A4; top of figure is extracellular space

APP_{714} and APP_{695}, Thr^{654}/Ser^{655} (according to Kang et al numbering scheme for APP_{695}, reference 44) have been identified as candidate sites for rapid phosphorylation by protein kinase C and calcium/calmodulin-dependent protein kinase II (55; Table 1, Figures 2 and 4). Recent extension of these studies using the synthetic peptide $APP^{645-694}$ suggests that these are the major sites of APP phosphorylation. Other investigators have confirmed that immunoprecipitable mature APP holoprotein is phosphorylated (56). The *Drosophila* homologue of APP, known as APP-like (APPL), is homologous with APP in this region, maintaining a phosphorylation consensus site near the plasma membrane (57). In addition, a phosphorylatable tyrosine residue is present in the cytoplasmic domains of APP

Table 1. Kinetics of phosphorylation of the synthetic peptide $APP^{645-661}$ by various protein kinases (residues numbered according to ref. 44 for APP_{695})

Protein kinase	V_{max} μmol/min. mg	K_m μM	Catalytic efficiency $V_{max}/K_m \times 10^3$
Protein kinase C	7.3	132	55.3
Ca^{2+}/CaM kinase II	1.3	24	54.2
cAMP-dependent protein kinase	0.02	170	0.1
cGMP-dependent protein kinase	<0.01	—	—
Casein kinase II	<0.01	—	—
Insulin receptor	<0.01	—	—

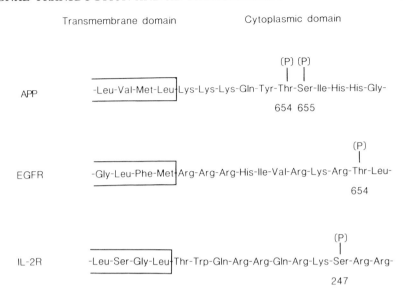

Figure 4. Location of phosphorylatable residues in the putative cytoplasmic domains of APP, epidermal growth factor receptor (EGFR), and interleukin-2 receptor (IL-2R). In each case, the PKC phosphorylation site is within 10 residues of the plasma membrane (reproduced by permission of the National Academy of Sciences, USA)

and APPL (58). If APP phosphorylation is important in regulating the synthesis, processing, or action of APP, therapeutic intervention in Alzheimer's disease could potentially be targeted to phosphorylation-mediated events.

PROTEIN PHOSPHORYLATION AND MODULATION OF APP PROCESSING

Recent evidence demonstrates that protein phosphorylation plays an important role in regulating APP processing (59). In pulse-chase studies using PC12 cells, phorbol esters (drugs which stimulate protein kinase C) dramatically diminished recovery of mature $APP_{751/770}$ while enhancing recovery of a COOH-terminal fragment of approximately 15 kDa (Figures 5-7). Okadaic acid (a drug which inhibits protein phosphatases 1 and 2A) had similar effects (Figures 5-7). When both phorbol ester and okadaic acid were applied to the cells, in addition to the effects on mature $APP_{751/770}$ and the 15-kDa COOH-terminal fragment, a larger ($\sim$ 19-kDa) COOH-terminal fragment was generated in elevated amounts (Figure 5). In other experiments, H-7 (an inhibitor of protein kinases including protein kinase C) led to an apparent decrease in the basal rate of processing of APP (Figure 6), supporting the physiological significance of modulation of APP processing by protein kinase C. These results provide the first direct evidence for the regulation of APP processing by protein phosphorylation, and raise the possibility of regulated and/or qualitatively

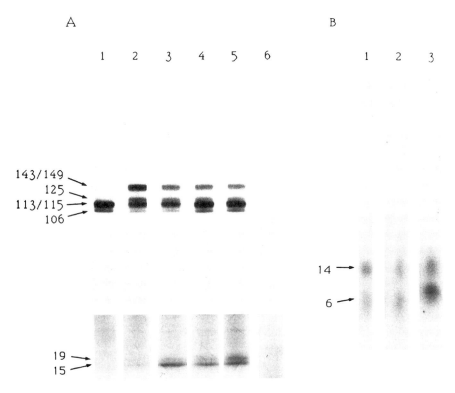

Figure 5. Identification of APP and APP-derived peptides in PC12 cells and regulation of processing by phorbol ester and okadaic acid. (A) Immunoprecipitation of APP and APP-derived peptides by using anti-APP[645-694] antibodies—numbering according to Kang et al (44) for APP$_{695}$. Cells were prelabeled with [^{35}S]methionine for 20 min and either immediately harvested (lane 1) or chased for 45 min with unlabeled methionine and then harvested (lanes 2-6). Vehicle alone or a test substance was added at the start of the chase period (time zero). After cell lysis, extracts were subjected to immunoprecipitation, SDS-PAGE, and autoradiography. (Upper) Large molecular mass region of a 6-18% gradient gel; arrows indicate the positions of the six protein bands of 106, 113, 115, 125, 143, and 149 kDa. (Lower) A longer exposure of low molecular mass region of the gel; arrows indicate the positions of the 15- and 19-kDa peptides. Levels of the 106-kDA band and the 113/115-kDa doublet were maximal at time zero and decreased thereafter with a half-life of 30-40 min. Levels of the 125-kDa band and the 143/149-kDa doublet were minimal at time zero, increased to a maximum by 45 min of chase, and decreased thereafter (lanes 1 and 2). The 15- and 19-kDa peptides were detectable by 15 min of chase and the levels of these peptides remained elevated throughout the 135 min of chase (lanes 1 and 2; see also Figure 7). These data suggest a precursor–product relationship between the doublets of 113/115 and 143/149 kDa, as well as between the bands of 106 and 125 kDa. Based on these observations and on the results of Wiedemann et al (50), we made the following tentative assignments: 106-, 113-, and 115-kDa bands represent the immature (N-glycosylated) forms of APP$_{695}$, APP$_{751}$, and APP$_{770}$, respectively; 125-, 143-, and 149-kDa bands represent the mature (sulfated, and N- and O-glycosylated) forms of APP$_{695}$, APP$_{751}$, and APP$_{770}$ respectively. Since the antibodies used were prepared against COOH-terminal regions of APP, we concluded that the 15- and 19-kDa peptides were COOH-terminal fragments of APP. Lanes: 1, 2, vehicle; 3, 1 μM phorbol ester (PDBu); 4, 1 μM okadaic acid; 5 and 6, 1 μM PDBu and 1 μM okadaic acid. For lane 6,

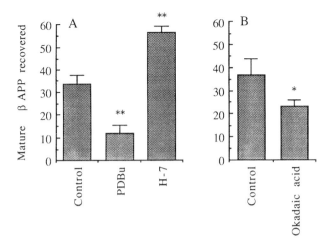

Figure 6. Regulation of levels of mature $APP_{751/770}$ by PDBu, by H-7, and by okadaic acid. PC12 cells were incubated with the indicated agents and processed as described in the legend to Figure 5. Mature $APP_{751/770}$ was quantified by densitometric scanning of the 143/149-kDa doublet of the autoradiogram. The results shown are the means ± SEM of four experiments. Data were normalized to the total $APP_{751/770}$ recovered (100 units) at time zero. Data were corrected for the amount of mature $APP_{751/770}$ present at time zero (10 units in A, 6 units in B). PDBu, 1 μM; H-7, 100 μM; okadaic acid, 1 μM. *$P < 0.05$ compared to control; **$P < 0.01$ compared to control (reproduced by permission of the National Academy of Sciences, USA)

different alternative pathways of APP processing. One possible interpretation of these observations is that the 15-kDa COOH-terminal fragment represents 'normal' constitutive intra-β/A4 cleavage while the 19-kDa COOH-terminal fragment represents processing via an alternative and potentially amyloidogenic pathway, perhaps by cleavage at or near the β/A4 NH_2-terminus (Figure 3). Although we favor the idea that phorbol esters and okadaic acid increase the formation of the 15-kDa and 19-kDa peptides, we cannot exclude the possibility that the effects observed are due to decreased degradation of these peptides. Resolution of COOH-terminal fragments of APP into a low molecular mass doublet has also been observed by others (60,61). Identification of potentially amyloidogenic pathways and elucidation of how these pathways are regulated will be crucial to our understanding of the pathogenesis of amyloidosis.

Figure 5 (*continued*) 100 μM $APP^{645-694}$ peptide (ref. 44) was present during immunoprecipitation. (B) Limited proteolysis of the putative APP isoforms in PC12 cells and of human APP_{695}. The 113/115-kDa doublet (from A, lane 1) and the 143/149-kDa doublet (from A, lane 2) were excised, subjected to limited proteolytic digestion with V8 protease, electrophoresed, and compared with similarly treated in-vitro transcribed and translated human APP_{695}. Lanes: 1, 113/115-kDa doublet; 2, 143/149-kDa doublet; 3, human APP_{695}. Arrows indicate the positions of 14- and 6-kDa digestion products (reproduced by permission of the National Academy of Sciences, USA)

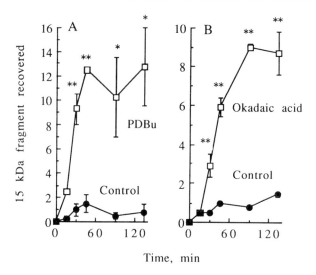

Time, min

Figure 7. Regulation of levels of 15-kDa putative COOH-terminal fragment of APP by PDBu and by okadaic acid. PC12 cells were metabolically labeled for 20 min with [^{35}S] methionine followed by a chase with complete medium for periods ranging from 0 to 135 min. After cell lysis, extracts were subjected to immunoprecipitation, SDS-PAGE, and autoradiography. The 15-kDa fragment was quantified by densitometric scanning of the autoradiogram. Data were normalized as described in the legend to Figure 6. Incubation was carried out in the presence of vehicle alone (Control), 1 μM PDBu (A) or 1 μM okadaic acid (B). Test substances were added at the start of the chase period. Results are the means ± SEM of four experiments. *$P < 0.05$ compared to control; **$P < 0.01$ compared to control (reproduced by permission of the National Academy of Sciences, USA)

Studies of other integral transmembrane proteins offer insights which may be applicable to the study of APP. Certain cell-surface receptors are phosphorylated in their cytodomains as a mechanism of modifying sensitivity to ligand-induced effects (62). Cell adhesion molecules and extracellular matrix receptors (integrins) are phosphorylated in their cytodomains: the entire sequence of molecular events and interactions is not yet clear, but phosphorylation may regulate interactions with and binding to elements of the cytoskeleton. The cleavage of the ectodomain is a feature of APP that is also observed in the biology of certain other transmembrane proteins, such as the interleukin-2 receptor (IL-2R) (63), the growth hormone receptor (64), and the cell adhesion molecule(s) L1 and NILE (65). Both IL-2R and L1/NILE are phosphoproteins, but the relationship of phosphorylation to ectodomain cleavage is unknown.

Regulation of trafficking of cell surface molecules is another important consequence of their phosphorylation. Endocytosis of the EGF and the IL-2 receptors is regulated by protein kinase C-mediated phosphorylation in their respective cytodomains, at residues near the transmembrane domain (66–70). Of note, an APP phosphorylation site lies in a homologous location (Figure 4), within 10 residues of the plasma membrane. This provides a basis for establishing a model to examine the biological consequence of APP phosphorylation.

Protein phosphorylation may also play a role in APP expression. At the transcriptional level, signal transduction has been shown to regulate APP mRNA expression. Interleukin-1 induces APP transcription in endothelial cells in culture (71). This induction is prevented by H-7, a protein kinase inhibitor, and mimicked by phorbol ester, a protein kinase C activator (71). Further, several ontogenetic transcription factors, such as the homeoprotein hox 1.3 (72), bind the APP promoter, suggesting that APP may be a nonhomeoprotein target gene for homeoprotein regulation. Hox 1.3 (73), hox 2.2 (74), and *engrailed* (75) are phosphoproteins, and in several other instances, protein phosphorylation has been shown to regulate the activities of transcription factors, e.g. CREB (76) and Myb (77). This may also be the case for homeoproteins and the APP promoter.

SOME MODELS OF HOW PROTEIN PHOSPHORYLATION MIGHT MODULATE APP PROCESSING

Studies of signal transduction via protein phosphorylation are likely to illuminate the pathogenesis of Alzheimer's disease and suggest avenues of potential therapy. An abnormality in either a protein kinase, or a protein kinase regulator (e.g. cytosolic Ca^{2+}), or in a protein phosphatase or a protein phosphatase regulator, might alter the phosphorylation state of APP or of a substrate protein involved in APP processing (Figure 8). Several models exist for APP trafficking and catabolism, and can be used to illustrate how signal transduction via protein phosphorylation might play a regulatory role.

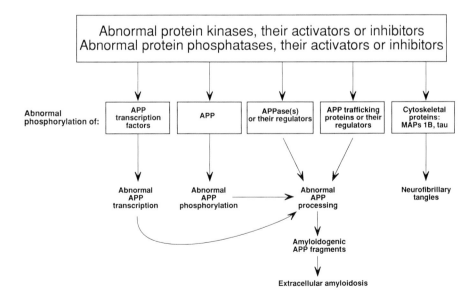

Figure 8. Some possible mechanisms by which abnormalities in protein phosphorylation might induce Alzheimer-type cerebral pathology

Model 1

Altered phosphorylation of an APP-regulating transcription factor could lead to increased expression of APP in Alzheimer's disease. Perhaps at the normal low concentrations of APP, it is processed via a high affinity (low K_m), low capacity (low V_{max}) protease pathway, which cleaves within β/A4 (52,53). In the situation of elevated APP concentrations, an alternate processing pathway having low affinity (high K_m) might be important. This alternative pathway, theoretically, could cleave at the NH_2-terminus of β/A4, rather than intra-β/A4, thus generating amyloidogenic fragments.

Model 2

Posttranslational modification of APP, such as a change in the phosphorylation state of the cytodomain, could induce a conformational change in APP. Intra-β/A4 cleavage by normal APPase (53) might then be relatively decreased and cleavage at the β/A4 NH_2-terminus, by an alternate APPase, could then be relatively increased. Phosphorylation-state regulation of the protease sensitivity of phosphoproteins has been documented (78–80). Dephosphorylation of neurofilament enhances its degradation by calpain (79), and, in epidermis, dephosphorylation of the structural protein profilaggrin is apparently required for its proteolytic processing to filaggrin (80). The hereditary skin disease harlequin ichthyosis, characterized by extensive accumulation of profilaggrin, appears to result from a defect in the dephosphorylating enzyme profilaggrin phosphatase.

Model 3

Current cell biological concepts of the trafficking of transmembrane proteins would suggest that there is an obligate endocytotic step in amyloidogenesis, regardless of the proteolytic pathway involved in the initial processing of APP. Thus, although the degradative fate of transmembrane domains in general is poorly understood, it is suggested that proteins containing transmembrane domains are endocytosed and that the endosome is engulfed by a 'giant' vacuole (multivesicular body) surrounding all sides of the endosome. All intraluminal components are then digested by the activation of lipases and proteases. Such events would release amyloidogenic proteins from the lipid bilayer, which could, in turn, be released into the extracellular space by fusion of the vacuole with the plasma membrane. Once outside the cell, other proteins, such as α_1-antichymotrypsin, might associate with the β/A4 domain (81), protecting it from extracellular proteolysis, and further promoting amyloid accumulation. The identification of a coated pit targeting signal sequence in APP (82; Figure 2) and the immunocytochemical localization of APP to lysosomes (83) further support the existence of an endocytotic step in the biology of APP.

If amyloidogenesis proceeds via such an endocytotic pathway, identification of signals regulating APP endocytosis could form the basis for rational antiamyloidogenic therapy to inhibit APP endocytosis and/or prevent release of APP from the lipid bilayer. As we have described (55), there exists a striking homology between an APP phosphorylation site and phosphorylation sites of EGF receptor and IL-2 receptor (55,66-70). In both of the latter cases, phosphorylation at this homologous site induces endocytosis of those proteins in the presence of the appropriate ligand. As a further analogy, protein kinase C is implicated in regulating the phosphorylation of the juxtamembrane sites in EGFR, IL-2R and APP (55,66-70). Acceleration of APP endocytosis and processing, perhaps mediated via APP phosphorylation, could lead to saturation of normal APPase and alternative processing via an alternate APPase. Quantitative studies of APP metabolites in the cerebrospinal fluid of normal (young and old) and demented (Alzheimer) aged individuals are consistent with acceleration of APP turnover in aging and to a greater extent in AD (84). If APP endocytosis and subsequent processing are regulated by phosphorylation, the regulation of APP phosphorylation might be an effective target for antiamyloid therapy.

SUMMARY

Proper regulation of protein phosphorylation is vital to the normal physiology of neurons. Alzheimer's disease is characterized by the intracellular accumulation of cytoskeletal phosphoproteins and the extracellular deposition of a portion of an integral membrane phosphoprotein. The apparent modulatory effect of protein phosphorylation on APP processing, together with observations from Alzheimer's disease, Down's syndrome and Dutch cerebrovascular β/A4 amyloidosis, suggest that an abnormality of protein phosphorylation may be involved in the pathogenesis of Alzheimer-type cerebral β/A4 amyloidosis. Although the precise role, if any, of abnormal protein phosphorylation in the pathobiology of Alzheimer's disease is not yet known, some testable hypotheses have been proposed. Testing these model mechanisms should offer insights which may have clinical and therapeutic relevance.

Acknowledgments

We thank Carol Ebbecke for secretarial assistance with this manuscript. This work was supported by US Public Health Service Grants NS-01095 to S.E.G., and MH-39327, MH-40899 and NS-21550 to P.G. J.D.B. was the recipient of a postdoctoral fellowship from the Rothschild Foundation and is the recipient of Individual National Research Award NS-08523.

REFERENCES

1. Nestler EJ, Greengard P. Protein phosphorylation in the nervous system. New York: Wiley, 1984.
2. Nairn AC, Hemmings HC Jr, Greengard P. Ann Rev Biochem 1985; 54: 931-76.
3. Nathanson JA, Kebabian JW. Handbook of experimental pharmacology. New York: Springer, 1982.
4. Beebe SJ, Corbin JD. Enzymes 1986; XVII: 44-113.
5. Schulman H. Adv Cyclic Nucleotide Protein Phosphorylation Res 1988; 22: 39-112.
6. Kikkawa U, Nishizuka Y. Ann Rev Cell Biol 1986; 2: 149-78.

7. Hunter T, Cooper JA. Ann Rev Biochem 1985; 54: 897-930.
8. Walaas SI, Nairn AC, Greengard P. J Neurosci 1983; 3: 291-301.
9. Walaas SI, Nairn AC, Greengard P. J Neurosci 1983; 3: 302-11.
10. Hemmings HC Jr, Nairn AC, McGuinness TL, Huganir RL, Greengard P. FASEB J 1987; 3: 1583-92.
11. Castellucci VF, Kandel ER, Schwartz JH, Wilson FD, Nairn AC, Greengard P. Proc Natl Acad Sci USA 1980; 77: 7492-6.
12. Hu G-Y, Hvalby O, Walaas SI, Albert KA, Skjeflo P, Anderson P, Greengard P. Nature 1987; 328: 426-9.
13. Greengard P, Kuo JF. Adv Biochem Psychopharmacol 1970; 3: 287-306.
14. Li M, McCann JD, Liedtke CM, Nairn AC, Greengard P, Welsh MJ. Nature 1988; 331: 358-60.
15. Li M, McCann JD, Anderson MP, Clancy JP, Liedtke CM, Nairn AC, Greengard P, Welsh MJ. Science 1989; 244: 1353-6.
16. Rommens JM, Iannuzzi MC, Kerem BS, Drumm ML, Melmer G, Dean M, Rozmahel R, Cole JL, Kennedy D, Hidaka N, Zsiga M, Buchwald M, Riordan JR, Tsui LC, Collins FS. Science 1989; 245: 1059-65.
17. Riordan JR, Rommens JM, Kerem BS, Alon N, Rozmahel R, Grzelczak Z, Zielenski J, Lok S, Plavsic N, Chou JL Drumm ML, Iannuzzi MC, Collins FS, Tsui LC. Science 1989; 245: 1066-73.
18. Kerem BS, Rommens JM, Buchanan JA, Markiewicz D, Cox TK, Chakravarti A, Buchwald M, Tsui LC. Science 1989; 245: 1073-80.
19. Taira M, Taira M, Hashimoto N, Shimada F, Yoshifumi S, Kanatsuka A, Nakamura F, Ebina Y, Tatibana M, Makino H, Yoshida S. Science 1989; 245: 63-6.
20. Odawara M, Kadowaki T, Yamamoto R, Shibasaki Y, Tobe K, Accili D, Bevins C, Mikami Y, Matsuura N, Akanuma Y, Takaku F, Taylor SI, Kasuga M. Science 1989; 245: 66-8.
21. Sternberger NH, Sternberger LA, Ulrich J. Proc Natl Acad Sci USA 1985; 82: 4274-6.
22. Grundke-Iqbal I, Iqbal K, Tung Y-C, Quinlan M, Wisniewski HM, Binder LI. Proc Natl Acad Sci USA 1986; 83: 4913-17.
23. Selkoe DJ. Ann Rev Neurosci 1989; 12: 463-90.
24. Baudier J, Cole RD. J Bio Chem 1987; 262: 17577-83.
25. Mattson MP. Neuron 1990; 2: 105-17.
26. McKee AC, Kosik KS, Kennedy MB, Kowall NW. J Neuropath Exp Neurol 1990; 49: 49-63.
27. Saitoh T, Iiomoto DS. In Boller F, Katzman R, Rascol A, Signoret JL, Christen Y (eds) Biological markers of Alzheimer's disease. New York: Springer, 1989; 105-17.
28. Tomlinson BE, Corsellis JAN. In Adams JH, Corsellis JAN, Duchen LW (eds) Greenfield's neuropatholgy. London: Arnold, 1984; 951-1025.
29. Ihara Y, Nukina N, Miura R, Ogawarra M. J Biochem 1986; 99; 1807-10.
30. Hasegawa M, Arai T, Ihara Y. Neuron 1990; 4: 909-18.
31. Mori H, Kondo J, Ihara Y. Science 1987; 235: 1641-4.
32. Masters CL, Multhaup G, Simms G, Pottigiesser J, Martins RN, Beyreuther K. EMBO J 1985; 4: 2757-63.
33. Joachim CL, Morris JH, Kosik KS, Selkoe DJ. Ann Neurol 1987; 22: 514-20.
34. Selkoe DJ, Duffy LK, Nukina N, Podlisny MB, Abraham C, Kosik KS. In Miner GD, Richter RW, Blass JP, Valentine JL, Winters-Miner LA (eds) Familial Alzheimer's disease. New York: Dekker, 1989; 137-151.
35. Glenner GG, Wong CW. Biochem Biophys Res Comm 1984; 122: 885-90.
36. Masters CL, Simms G, Weinmann NA, Multhaup G, McDonald BL, Beyreuther K. Proc Natl Acad Sci USA 1985; 82: 4245-9.
37. Abraham CR, Selkoe DJ, Potter H. Cell 1988; 52: 487-501.
38. Cataldo AM, Nixon RA. Proc Natl Acad Sci USA 1990; 87: 3861-5.
39. Joachim CL, Mori H, Selkoe DJ. Nature 1989; 341: 226-30.

40. Goldgaber D, Lerman MI, Mcbride OW, Saffioti U, Gajdusek DC. Science 1987; 235: 877-80.
41. Wisniewski KE, Dalton AJ, Crapper McLachlan DR, Wen GY, Wiesniewski HM. Neurology 1985; 35: 957-61.
42. St George-Hyslop PH, Tanzi RE, Polinsky RJ, Haines JL, Nee L, Watkins PC, Myers RH, Feldman RG, Pollen D, Drachman D, Growdon J, Bruni A, Foncin JF, Salmon D, Frommelt P, Amaducci L, Sorbi S, Piacentini S, Stewart GD, Hobbs WJ, Connelly PM, Gusella JF. Science 1987; 235: 885-9.
43. Tanzi R, Gusella JF, Watkins PC, Bruns GAP, St George-Hyslop P, Van Keuren ML, Patterson D, Pagan S, Kurnit DM, Neve RL. Science 1987; 235: 880-4.
44. Kang J, Lemaire HG, Unterbeck A, Salbaum JM, Masters CL, Grzeschik KH, Multhaup G, Beyreuther K, Muller-Hill B. Nature 1987; 325: 733-6.
45. Robakis NK, Ramakrishna N, Wolfe G, Wisniewski HM. Proc Natl Acad Sci USA 1988; 84: 4190-4194.
46. Tanzi RE, McClatchey AI, Lamperti ED, Komaroff LV, Gusella JF, Neve RL. Nature 1988; 331: 528-30.
47. Ponte P, Gonzales-DeWhitt P, Schilling J, Miller J, Hsu D, Greenberg B, Davis K, Wallace W, Lieberburg I, Fuller F, Cordell B. Nature 1988; 331: 525-7.
48. Kitaguchi N, Takahashi Y, Tokushima Y, Shiojiri S, Ito H. Nature 1988; 331: 530-2.
49. De Sauvage F, Octave J-N. Science 1989; 245: 651-3.
50. Weidemann A, Konig G, Bunke D, Fischer P, Salbaum JM, Masters CL, Beyreuther K. Cell 1989; 57: 115-26.
51. Cole GM, Tuan HV, Saitoh T. Neurochem Res 1989; 14: 933-9.
52. Sisodia SS, Koo EH, Beyreuther K, Unterbeck A, Price DL. Science 1990; 248: 492-5.
53. Esch FS, Keim PS, Beattie EC, Blacher RW, Culwell AR, Oltersdorf T, McClure D, Ward PJ. Science 1990; 248: 1122-4.
54. Levy E, Carman MD, Fernandez-Madrid IJ, Power MD, Lieberburg I, Van Duinen SG, Bots GT, Luyendijk W, Frangione B. Science 1990; 248: 124-6.
55. Gandy SE, Czernik, AJ Greengard P. Proc Natl Acad Sci USA 1988; 85: 6218-21.
56. Oltersdorf T, Ward PJ, Henriksson T, Beattie EC, Neve R, Lieberburg I, Fritz LC. J Biol Chem 1990; 265: 4492-7.
57. Rosen DR, Martin-Morris L, Luo L, White K. Proc Natl Acad Sci USA 1989; 86: 2478-82.
58. Bunke D, Kypta RM, Mönning U, Courtneige SA, Masters CL, Beyreuther KT. Neurobiol Aging 1990; 11: 284.
59. Buxbaum JD, Gandy SE, Cicchetti P, Ehrlich ME, Czernik AJ, Fracasso P, Ramabhadran TV, Unterbeck A, Greengard P. Proc Natl Acad Sci USA 1990; 87: 6003-6.
60. Selkoe DJ. Neurobiol Aging 1989; 10: 387-95.
61. Wolf D, Quon D, Wang Y, Cordell B. EMBO J 1990; 9: 2079-84.
62. Huganir RL, Greengard P. Trends Pharmacol Sci 1987; 8: 472-7.
63. Robb RJ, Kutny RM. J Immunol 1987; 139: 855-62.
64. Leung DS, Spencer SA, Cachianes G. Nature 1987; 330: 537-43.
65. Prince JT, Milona N, Stallcup WB. J Neurosci 1988; 9: 1825-34.
66. Hunter T, Ling N, Cooper JA. Nature (Lond.) 1984; 311: 450-3.
67. Gallis B, Lewis A, Wignall J, Alpert A, Mochizuki DY, Cosman D, Hopp T, Urdal D. J Biol Chem 1986; 5075-80.
68. Beguinot L, Hanover JA, Ito S, Richert ND, Willingham MC, Pastan I. Proc Natl Acad Sci USA 1985; 82: 2774-8.
69. Lin CR, Chen WS, Lazar CS, Carpenter CD, Gill GN, Evans RM, Rosenfeld MG. Cell 1986; 44: 839-48.
70. Shackelford DA, Trowbridge IS. J Biol Chem 1986; 261: 8334-41.
71. Goldgaber D, Harris HW, Hla T, Maciag T, Donnelly RJ, Jacobsen JS, Vitek MP, Gajdusek DC. Proc Natl Acad Sci USA 1989; 86: 7606-10.
72. Goldgaber D, Schmechel DE, Odenwald WF. Soc Neurosci Abstr 1989; 5: 23.

73. Odenwald WF, Garbern J, Arnheiter H, Tournier-Lasserve E, Lazzarini RA. Genes Dev 1989; 3: 158-72.
74. Fienberg AA, Belting H-G, Nordstedt C, Schughart K, Gandy SE, Elting J, Nairn AC, Greengard P, Ruddle F. Cold Spring Harbor Laboratory Press 1990 (in press).
75. Gay NJ, Poole SJ, Kornberg TB. Nucleic Acids Res 1988; 16: 6637-47.
76. Yamamoto KK, Gonzales GA, Biggs WH III, Montminy MR. Nature 1988; 334: 494-8.
77. Lüscher B, Christenson E, Litchfield DW, Krebs EG, Eisenman RN. Nature 1990; 344: 517-22.
78. Laumas S, Abdel-Ghany M, Leister K, Resnick R, Kandrach A, Racker E. Proc Natl Acad Sci USA 1989; 86: 3021-5.
79. Pant HC. Biochem J 1988; 256: 665-8.
80. Dale BA, Holbrook KA, Fleckman P, Kimball JR, Brumbaugh S, Sibert VP. J Invest Dermatol 1990; 94: 6-18.
81. Potter H, Abraham CR, Dressler DH. Neurobiol Aging 1990; 11: 312.
82. Chen W-J, Goldsten JL, Brown MS. J Biol Chem 1990; 265: 3116-23.
83. Benowitz LI, Rodriguez PP, Mufson EJ, Schenk D, Neve RL. Exp Neurol 1989; 106: 237-50.
84. Palmert MR, Usiak M, Mayeux R, Raskind R, Tourtellotte WW, Younkin SG. Neurology 1990; 40: 1028-34.

Address for correspondence:

Dr Samuel E. Gandy,
Laboratory of Molecular and Cellular Neuroscience,
The Rockefeller University,
1230 York Avenue,
New York, NY 10021, USA

20 Alzheimer's Disease: From Cytoskeletal Protein Pathology to Neuronal Degeneration

KHALID IQBAL AND INGE GRUNDKE-IQBAL

At present, neither the etiology nor the pathogenesis of Alzheimer's disease (AD) is understood. An understanding of the basic mechanism(s) of degeneration of neurons in this neurodegenerative disorder will help in development of rational therapeutic approaches to reverse or arrest the progression of the disease.

Cytoskeletal protein pathology in the form of neurofibrillary tangles is one of the most characteristic brain lesions of AD. Many of these affected neurons may be only partially functional and in some areas of the brain such as neocortex many of them may eventually die, leaving behind the appropriately named 'tombstones' or 'ghost tangles'. However, two points ought to be clarified: (a) that all neuronal degenerations which occur in AD may not necessarily involve neurofibrillary changes, and (b) that in certain areas of the brain such as some of the hypothalamic nuclei (see Chapter 21), neurons affected by cytoskeletal protein alterations may undergo minimal degeneration or even display no measurable functional deficit.

In this review (an update of reference 1) we have attempted to identify a sequence of some key molecular changes that may constitute a major mechanism of neuronal degeneration, i.e. neurons undergoing neurofibrillary degeneration, in AD.

NEUROFIBRILLARY CHANGES

Microtubules and neurofilaments are the two principal fibril components of the cytoskeleton of a normal mature neuron. In the brain of patients with AD the cytoskeleton of many neurons is progressively disrupted and displaced by the appearance of bundles of paired helical filaments (PHF) (2), which are morphologically unlike any of the normal neurofibrils (3). These Alzheimer neurofibrillary tangles (ANT) of PHF are most prominent in the neuronal perikarya, filling almost all the cytoplasm of the affected cells. Accumulations of PHF are also seen in the dystrophic neurites surrounding wisps or a core of extracellular amyloid in the neuritic (senile) plaques. Thus, both the tangles and the plaques, which are the two histopathological hallmarks of Alzheimer's disease, contain

Alzheimer's Disease: Basic Mechanisms, Diagnosis and Therapeutic Strategies
Edited by K. Iqbal, D. R. C. McLachlan, B. Winblad and H. M. Wisniewski
© 1991 John Wiley & Sons Ltd

PHF. PHF are also found as bundles in neurites in the neuropil of the telencephalic cortex. At this third location, PHF occur in small, inconspicuous profiles as neuropil threads scattered throughout both allocortical and isocortical areas (4).

Neither the ANT nor the plaques are unique to AD. ANT are also found in great abundance in Guam–Parkinsonism dementia complex, dementia pugilistica, postencephalitic Parkinsonism and adults with Down's syndrome, and in small number in a few cases of subacute sclerosing panencephalitis, Hallervorden–Spatz disease and neurovisceral lipid storage disease (for review, see references 5,6). The neuritic (senile) plaques are also seen in Down's syndrome, in aged humans and in some species of animals. Unlike the tangles, which are present in only very small numbers in nondemented elderly and absent in animals, the plaques are seen frequently in both aged human and animal brains. The numbers of plaques in nondemented aged humans are sometimes similar to those seen in AD cases (e.g. 7). Recent studies have shown that unlike in AD most of the plaques found in nondemented elderly are free of PHF in the dystrophic neurites (8,9).

Both ANT and amyloid are congophilic and because of this common staining property a close relationship between the two lesions has been suggested. However, it has been shown that this property is most likely due to β-pleated sheet structure (10) and this conformation can be induced in many unrelated polypeptides. PHF and amyloid are different ultrastructurally and biochemically and in several staining properties other than those observed with congo red and thioflavin S.

ANT are heterogeneous in both morphology and solubility. Most of the ANT are composed of PHF. Only occasionally tangles of 15-nm straight filaments or these filaments admixed with PHF have been observed in a few AD cases (11,12). PHF are stable in both fresh and frozen autopsy tissue and are resistant to solubilization in aqueous buffer in the absence of detergents or denaturants. Two general populations of ANT, ANT I and ANT II, have been identified on the basis of their solubility and insolubility, respectively, in 2% SDS at room temperature for 3–5 minutes (13). However, ANT II are solubilized on repeated extractions in SDS and β-mercaptoethanol at 90–100 °C or, more effectively, by ultrasonication followed by heating in 1% each of SDS and β-mercaptoethanol. Although native PHF are resistant to proteolysis, PHF isolated by SDS treatment are digested by proteases (14). In agreement with the biochemical studies, ultrastructural studies of PHF have revealed that there are indeed two general populations of PHF, i.e. PHF with right-handed helices and PHF with left-handed helices (15). The right-handed PHF are larger than the left-handed PHF, both in diameter and in periodicity of the helices.

POLYPEPTIDE COMPOSITION OF PHF

Different approaches to isolate PHF have been based on the sparing solubility of PHF in detergents or their resistance to proteolysis, or both (13,14,16–19). Highly purified PHF are isolated from autopsied tissue by a combination of sucrose density gradient centrifugation and SDS treatment of neuronal cell body-enriched preparations at room temperature (13). Because native PHF are resistant to proteolysis, PHF have also been isolated from crude tissue fractions without detergents by a combination of protease digestion and centrifugation on sucrose and/or $CsCl_2$ gradients (19,20). Although PHF isolated by the protease treatment are highly purified, fragments of PHF polypeptides are lost due to proteolysis in the fibrils prepared by this technique (19). PHF prepared by any of the above methods are contaminated to a certain degree with amyloid, lipofuscin and some amorphous or granular tissue debris.

Unlike the brain amyloid in AD, which has been shown to be composed of a 40–42 amino acid peptide, the β-peptide (21,22), the biochemistry of the PHF has not been completely established. On SDS-polyacrylamide gels the protein composition of the highly purified PHF bulk isolated from AD brain is complex. The major polypeptides are in the 45–62 kDa region (13,14). In addition a varying number of low molecular weight polypeptides are found in each PHF preparation. The third component of PHF are high molecular weight aggregates, which stay at the top of the gel during electrophoresis (13,14). Immunostaining of the 45–62 kDa polypeptides with antibodies to PHF and immunoabsorption of the tangle staining antibodies with these polypeptides have determined their PHF origin (23–25). Immunochemical crossreactivity and coelectrophoresis on SDS-polyacrylamide gels of the 45–62 kDa PHF polypeptides with microtubule-associated polypeptide tau and the labeling of isolated PHF and of PHF in tissue sections with antibodies to tau have suggested that tau is a major component of PHF (26–29). The immunocytochemical labeling of PHF in tissue sections with antibodies to tau has been confirmed by several other laboratories (30–34). The presence of tau in PHF has also been confirmed by amino acid sequencing of tau fragments isolated from highly purified PHF (19,35).

A group of investigators has also reported sequences of amyloid β-protein in preparations enriched in neurofibrillary tangles both from patients with Alzheimer's disease and with Guam–Parkinsonism dementia (36,37). However, neither data on yields of the protein obtained from the PHF preparations nor data on the percentage of protein sequenced were reported. Furthermore, no definitive immunostaining of PHF with antibodies to amyloid protein or of amyloid with antibodies to PHF has been shown to date. On the other hand, both the mRNA (38) for the amyloid β-peptide precursor and β-peptide immunoreactivity (39) have been demonstrated to be present intraneuronally. Unlike the fibrillar tangles the amyloid reactivity in both Alzheimer and normal cases is localized mainly to lipofuscin in different types of neurons, including the neurons with the neurofibrillary tangles (39,40). Some of the ghost tangles are labeled with antibodies to β-amyloid (41). This immunoreactivity might be caused by the adherence of the β-protein and the β-protein precursor present in the extracellular space. It thus remains to be determined whether the amyloid peptide is actually a component of the PHF or a contaminant of the PHF preparations employed for sequencing.

ABNORMAL PHOSPHORYLATION AND UBIQUITINATION OF PHF POLYPEPTIDES

In addition to tau the presence of ubiquitin peptides in isolated PHF (42) and the immunostaining of PHF with antibodies to ubiquitin (42,43) have been demonstrated.

Ubiquitin, a protease itself (44), is believed to be a part of the cellular defense system that tags abnormal proteins for the action of ATP-dependent nonlysosomal proteases (45). Monoclonal antibodies 3–39 and 5–25 raised against PHF (46) have been shown to recognize ubiquitin. These antibodies, the epitopes of which reside in the amino acid residues 50–65 and 64–76 of the ubiquitin sequence, respectively (47), label PHF polypeptides with the same molecular weights as tau on Western blots. However, they do not react with tau from normal and Alzheimer brain cytosol (28). Furthermore, the monoclonal antibodies to PHF react much more strongly with PHF polypeptides than with free ubiquitin (28). It thus appears that some of the tau in PHF might be ubiquitinated.

One of the modifications of tau in PHF is its abnormal phosphorylation (27,29). Unlike normal tau, in PHF this protein is inaccessible to both monoclonal antibody Tau-1 (27,48), the epitope of which resides in amino acid residues 196–214 (49) of the cDNA-derived sequence (50) of bovine tau, and to an antiserum to a synthetic peptide, the amino acid sequence of which is highly homologous to residues 28–46 of bovine tau (27,29). Both on tissue sections and on immunoblots of PHF, the labeling of PHF polypeptides with these antibodies is markedly increased when the sections or blots have been treated with alkaline phosphatase before immunolabeling. This effect is specific and most probably due to the action of the phosphatase and not that of any contaminating protease, since it is not seen in the presence of phosphatase inhibitors like chelating agents, nor in high concentrations of phosphate or pyrophosphate. Similarly, in cytosol treated for in-vitro assembly of microtubules from Alzheimer brains but not from control brains tau is abnormally phosphorylated, and this is most prominent in the case of the molecular species of tau with the slowest electrophoretic mobility (27,51). The presence of the abnormally phosphorylated tau in AD brain has also been confirmed in another laboratory (52). The aberrant phosphorylation in AD brains might be selective to a few neuronal proteins, and not the result of a generalized hyperphosphorylation. Levels of both total free phosphate and phosphoprotein phosphate are normal in AD brain (53). At present, neither the nature of the phosphorylation site(s) nor the protein phosphorylation/dephosphorylation system responsible for the abnormal phosphorylation of tau in AD is known. Preliminary studies have revealed the presence of phosphoserine, phosphothreonine and phosphotyrosine in isolated PHF, suggesting that more than one protein kinase might be involved in the phosphorylation of PHF (Murthy and Iqbal, in preparation).

The abnormal phosphorylation of tau appears to represent one of the earliest changes leading to Alzheimer neurofibrillary pathology. Tau-1 reactivity is seen after dephosphorylation in a number of apparently morphologically normal neurons of the neocortex in the nondemented aged and in cases with AD, but not in normal young brains (54). At the electron microscopic level the immunoreactivity is found associated with granular material and a few scattered PHF and 15–20 nm straight filaments. This 'embryonic' stage of tangles is neither stained with silver impregnation nor labeled by antibodies to ubiquitin or to cytoskeletal proteins other than tau. Furthermore, abnormally phosphorylated tau isolated biochemically from AD brain cytosol does not contain ubiquitin immunoreactivity as tested by Western blots (55). Thus both immunocytochemical and biochemical studies indicate that the accumulation of abnormally phosphorylated tau precedes the incorporation of ubiquitin in neurofibrillary tangles.

ROLE OF ALTERED TAU IN NEURONAL DEGENERATION

One of the vital functions of the neuron is the transport of materials between the cell body and the nerve endings. Microtubule assembly, which is necessary for this intracellular transport, might be defective in AD (51,56). Microtubules can be assembled in vitro from the cytosol of normal fresh autopsy brain obtained within 5 hours post mortem. In AD brain the microtubule assembly is defective and no assembly of microtubules is observed. The in-vitro assembly of microtubules from the AD tissue, however, is induced by the addition of DEAE dextran, a polycation that mimics the effect of tau for microtubule assembly. Tau stimulates microtubule assembly by polymerizing with tubulin, and maintains the microtubule structure. Since tau in Alzheimer brain cytosol is abnormally phosphorylated (27,51) and phosphorylation of tau depresses its ability to promote microtubule assembly (57), it appears that this alteration of tau in the Alzheimer brain might contribute to the microtubule assembly defect. Binding of guanosine triphosphate (GTP) to the β-subunit of tubulin which initiates microtubule assembly is stimulated by tau. Lack of functional tau in AD brain might lead to decreased GTP binding and consequently decreased assembly of microtubule (58).

The concentrations of tubulin may decrease with age (59). As is the case in vitro, a critical concentration of brain tubulin is probably required for in-vivo microtubule assembly. Any change in tubulin or in microtubule-associated proteins that would decrease the efficiency of microtubule assembly, would therefore be critical in the aged brain. The presence of abnormally phosphorylated tau might thus mean that this threshold is reached in AD, the result being reduced microtubule assembly and consequently impaired axoplasmic flow and in the case of some neurons, cell death. Since tau in PHF is abnormally phosphorylated, it seems that the altered tau might be catabolized inefficiently, thereby accumulating as PHF in the affected neurons. A disturbance in axoplasmic flow, both anterograde and retrograde, should lead to accumulations of components of the axoplasmic flow in both the perikaryon and the nerve terminals. PHF accumulate at both of these locations, i.e. ANT and plaque neurites. The amount of accumulation of the affected proteins depends on the rate of their transport, synthesis and the rate of their degradation by the cell. Thus several neuronal components that are normally transported between the cell body and the terminals and not rapidly degraded can be expected to accumulate in the affected neurons. However, only one or a few of these polypeptides may be capable of polymerizing into PHF. Immunocytochemical staining of ANT has been shown with antibodies to several proteins (60-70). However, these proteins—except tau and ubiquitin (see above)—have not been observed in PHF treated with detergents/denaturants to remove nonspecific proteins trapped between the fibrils. Discoveries of the abnormal phosphorylation of tau in AD brain and of the presence of abnormal tau and of ubiquitin in PHF and the failure to induce microtubule assembly in vitro in AD brain cytosol lead us to hypothesize (a) that the protein phosphorylation-dephosphorylation system is defective in AD brain, leading to abnormally phosphorylated tau and some other neuronal proteins, and (b) that the abnormal phosphorylation of tau contributes to a microtubule assembly defect and consequent impairment of axoplasmic flow and neuronal degeneration.

Protein phosphorylation is one of the major mechanisms for regulation of cellular function (for review, see reference 71). The state of phosphorylation of substrate proteins depends on the relative activities of protein kinases and phosphoprotein phosphatases. Our studies (27,29,53) showing the dephosphorylation of the abnormally phosphorylated sites of tau on treatment with alkaline phosphatase in vitro suggest that the protein phosphorylation/dephosphorylation defect might be in part the result of a deficiency of a protein phosphatase system (or systems) in the affected neurons in AD.

Acknowledgments

Studies from our laboratories reviewed in this article were conducted by postdoctoral fellows Dr S. Khatoon, Dr E. Koepke-Secundo and Dr G. P. Wang and research assistants Tanweer Zaidi, Yunn-Chyn Tung, Sadia Shaikh, Nasim Ali and Debbie Devine. Secretarial support was provided by Concetta Veneziano and Kathleen Case. Maureen Stoddard Marlow made many useful editorial suggestions. This work was supported in part by funds from the New York State Office of Mental Retardation and Developmental Disabilities, National Institutes of Health Grants AG 05892, NS 18105 and NS/AG 04220 and a grant from the Alzheimer's Disease Research Program of the American Health Assistance Foundation (Rockville, Maryland).

REFERENCES

1. Iqbal K, Grundke-Iqbal I. In Miyatake T, Selkoe DJ, Ihara Y (eds) Molecular biology and genetics of Alzheimer's disease. Amsterdam: Elsevier 1990: 47–56.
2. Kidd M. Brain 1964; 87: 307–20.
3. Wisniewski HM, Merz PA, Iqbal K. J Neuropath Exper Neurol 1984; 43: 643–56.
4. Braak H, Braak E, Grundke-Iqbal I, Iqbal K. Neurosci Lett 1986; 65: 351–5.
5. Wisniewski K, Jervis GA, Moretz RC, Wisniewski HM. Ann Neurol 1979; 5: 288–94.
6. Iqbal K. Wisniewski HM. In Reisberg B (ed.) Alzheimer's disease. The standard reference. New York: Free Press, 1983: 48–56.
7. Katzman R, Terry RD, DeTeresa R, Brown R, Davies P, Fuld P, Renbing X, Peck A. Ann Neurol 1988; 23: 138–44.
8. Dickson DW, Farlo J, Davies P, Crystal H, Fulld P, Yen SH. Am J Pathol 1988; 132: 86–101.
9. Barcikowska M, Wisniewski HM, Bancher C, Grundke-Iqbal I. Acta Neuropathol (Berl) 1989; 78: 225–231.
10. Glenner GG, Eanes EG, Bladen HA, Linke RP, Termine JD. J Histochem Cytochem 1974; 22: 1141–58.
11. Shibayama H, Kitoch J. Acta Neuropathol (Berl) 1978; 48: 27–30.
12. Yagishita S, Itoh Y, Nan W, Amano N. Acta Neuropathol (Berl) 1981; 54: 239–46.
13. Iqbal K, Zaidi T, Thompson CH, Merz PA, Wisniewski HM. Acta Neuropathol (Berl) 1984; 62: 167–77.

14. Iqbal K, Grundke-Iqbal I, Zaidi T, Ali N. Life Sci 1986; 38: 1695-700.
15. Wisniewski HM, Wen GY, Wang KC, Iqbal K, Rubenstein R. In Metuzals J (ed.) Electron microscopy and Alzheimer's disease. San Francisco: San Francisco Press, 1986: 21-4.
16. Ihara Y, Abraham C, Selkoe DJ. Nature 1983; 304: 727-30.
17. Masters CL, Multhaup G, Sims G, Pottgiesser J, Martins RN, Beyreuther K. EMBO J 1985; 4: 2757-63.
18. Rubenstein R, Kascsak RJ, Merz PA, Wisniewski HM, Carp RI, Iqbal K. Brain Res 1986; 372: 80-8.
19. Wischik CM, Novak M, Thogersen HC, Edwards PC, Runswick MJ, Jakes R, Walker JE, Milstein C, Roth M, Klug A. Proc Natl Acad Sci USA 1988; 85: 4506-10.
20. Grundke-Iqbal I, Vorbrodt AW, Iqbal K, Tung Y-C, Wang GP, Wisniewski HM. Molec Brain Res 1988; 4: 43-52.
21. Glenner GG, Wong CW. Biochem Biophys Res Comm 1984; 120: 855-90.
22. Masters CL, Simms G, Weinman NA, Multhaup G, McDonald BL, Beyreuther K. Proc Natl Acad Sci USA 1985; 82: 4245-9.
23. Grundke-Iqbal I, Iqbal K, Tung YC, Wang GP, Wisniewski HM. Acta Neuropathol (Berl) 1984; 62: 259-67.
24. Grundke-Iqbal I, Iqbal K, Tung YC, Wang GP, Wisniewski HM. Acta Neuropathol (Berl) 1985; 66: 52-61.
25. Grundke-Iqbal I, Wang GP, Iqbal K, Tung YC, Wisniewski HM. Acta Neuropathol (Berl) 1985; 68: 279-83.
26. Grundke-Iqbal I, Iqbal K, Quinlan M, Tung Y-C, Zaidi MS, Wisniewski HM. J Biol Chem 1986; 261: 6084-9.
27. Grundke-Iqbal I, Iqbal K, Tung Y-C, Quinlan M, Wisniewski HM, Binder LI. Proc Natl Acad Sci USA 1986; 83: 4913-17.
28. Grundke-Iqbal I, Vorbrodt AW, Iqbal K, Tung Y-C, Wang GP, Wisniewski HM. Mol Brain Res 1988; 4: 43-52.
29. Iqbal K, Grundke-Iqbal I, Smith AJ, George L, Tung Y-C, Zaidi T. Proc Natl Acad Sci USA 1989; 86: 5646-50.
30. Brion JP, Passareiro H, Nunez J, Flament-Durand J. Arch Biol (Brux) 1985; 95: 229-35.
31. Kosik KS, Joachim CL, Selkoe DJ. Proc Natl Acad Sci USA 1986; 83: 4044-8.
32. Wood JG, Mirra SS, Pollock NJ, Binder LI. Proc Natl Acad Sci USA 1986; 83: 4040-3.
33. Delcourte A, Defossez A. J Neurol Sci 1986; 76: 173-86.
34. Yen SY, Dickson DW, Crowe A, Butler M, Shelanski ML. Am J Pathol 1987; 126: 81-91.
35. Kondo J, Honda T, Mori H, Hamada Y, Miura R, Ogawara M, Ihara Y. Neuron 1988; 1: 817-25.
36. Masters CL, Multhaup G, Sims G, Pottgiesser J, Martins RN, Beyreuther K. EMBO J 1985; 4: 2757-63.
37. Guiroy DC, Miyazaki M, Multhaup G, Fischer P, Garruto RM, Beyreuther K, Masters CL, Simms G, Gibbs CJ, Gajdusek DC. Proc Natl Acad Sci USA 1987; 84: 2073-7.
38. Bahmanyer S, Higgins GA, Goldgaber D, Lewis DA, Morrison JH, Wilson MC, Shankar SK, Gajdusek DC. Science 1987; 237: 77-80.
39. Grundke-Iqbal I, Iqbal K, George L, Tung Y-C, Kim KS, Wisniewski HM. Proc Natl Acad Sci USA 1989; 86: 2853-7.
40. Bancher C, Grundke-Iqbal I, Iqbal K, Kim KS, Wisniewski HM. Neurobiol Aging 1989; 10: 125-32.
41. Hyman BT, Van Hoesen GW, Beyreuther K, Masters L. Neurosci Lett 1989; 101: 352-5.
42. Mori H, Kondo J, Ihara Y. Science 1987; 235: 1641-4.
43. Perry G, Friedman R, Shaw G, Chau V. Proc Natl Acad Sci USA 1989; 84: 3033-6.
44. Fried VA, Smith HT, Hildebrandt E, Weiner K. Proc Natl Acad Sci USA 1987; 84: 3685-9.
45. Hershko A, Ciechanover A. Ann Rev Biochem 1982; 51: 335-64.
46. Wang GP, Grundke-Iqbal I, Kascsak RJ, Iqbal K, Wisniewski HM. Acta Neuropathol (Berl) 1984; 62: 268-75.

47. Perry G, Mulvihill P, Fried VA, Smith HT, Grundke-Iqbal I, Iqbal K. J Neurochem 1989; 52: 1523-8.
48. Binder LI, Frankfurter A, Rebhun LI. J Cell Biol 1985; 101: 1371-8.
49. Kosik KS, Orecchio LD, Binder L, Trojanowski JQ, Lee VM-Y, Lee G. Neuron 1988; 1: 817-25.
50. Himmler A, Dreschsel D, Kirschner MW, Martin DW Jr. Mol Cell Biol 1989; 9: 1381-8.
51. Iqbal K, Grundke-Iqbal I, Zaidi T, Merz PA, Wen GY, Shaikh SS, Wisniewski HM, Alafuzoff I, Winblad B. Lancet 1986; ii: 421-6.
52. Flament S, Delacourte A, Hemon B, Defossez A. J Neurol Sci 1989; 92: 133-41.
53. Iqbal K, Grundke-Iqbal I. Neurobiol Aging 1990; 11: 277 (abstr.).
54. Bancher C, Brunner C, Lassmann H, Budka H, Jellinger K, Winche G, Seitelberger F, Grundke-Iqbal I, Iqbal K, Wisniewski HM. Brain Res 1989; 477: 90-9.
55. Koepke-Secundo E, Grundke-Iqbal I, Iqbal K. Neurobiol Aging 1990; 11: 281 (abstr.).
56. Iqbal K, Grundke-Iqbal I, Wisniewski HM. Lancet 1987; i: 102.
57. Lindwall G, Cole RD. J Biol Chem 1984; 259: 5301-5.
58. Khatoon S, Iqbal K, Grundke-Iqbal I. Neurobiol Aging 1990; 11: 279 (abstr.).
59. Yan S-C, Hwang S, Rustan TD, Frey WH. Neurochem Res 1985; 10: 1-18.
60. Ishii T, Haga S, Tobutake S. Acta Neuropathol (Berl) 1979; 48: 105-12.
61. Anderton BH, Breinburg D, Downes MJ, Green PJ, Tomlinson BE, Ulrich J, Wood JN. Nature 1982; 298: 84-6.
62. Dahl D, Selkoe DJ, Pero RT, Bignami A. J Neurosci 1982; 2: 113-19.
63. Gambetti P, Shecket G, Ghetti B, Hirano A, Dahl D. J Neuropathol Exp Neurol 1983; 42: 69-79.
64. Yen SH, Gaskin F, Fu SM. Am J Pathol 1983; 113: 373-81.
65. Grundke-Iqbal I, Iqbal K, Wisniewski HM. J Neuropath Exp Neurol 1985; 44: 368.
66. Kosik KS, Duffy LK, Dowling MM, Abraham C, McCluskey A, Selkoe DJ. Proc Natl Acad Sci USA 1984; 81: 7941-5.
67. Perry G, Rizzuto N, Autilio-Gambetti L, Gambetti P. Proc Natl Acad Sci USA 1985; 82: 3916-20.
68. Roberts GW, Crow TJ, Polak JM. Nature 1985; 314: 92-4.
69. Sternberger NH, Sternberger LA, Ulrich J. Proc Natl Acad Sci USA 1985; 82: 4274-6.
70. Nukina N, Ihara Y. J Biochem (Tokyo) 1986; 99: 1541-4.
71. Nairn AC, Hemmings HC Jr, Greengard P. Annu Rev Biochem 1985; 54: 931-76.

Address for correspondence:

Dr Khalid Iqbal,
New York State Institute for Basic Research in Developmental Disabilities,
1050 Forest Hill Road,
Staten Island, NY 10314, USA.
Tel: 718-494-5259
Fax: 718-494-5269

21 Cytoskeletal Alterations in the Hypothalamus During Aging and in Alzheimer's Disease are not Necessarily a Marker for Impending Cell Death

D. F. SWAAB, P. EIKELENBOOM, I. GRUNDKE-IQBAL,
K. IQBAL, H. P. H. KREMER, R. RAVID AND J. A. P. VAN DE NES

CYTOSKELETAL CHANGES IN ALZHEIMER'S DISEASE

Alzheimer's disease is histopathologically characterized by extracellular amyloid deposits and abundant cytoskeletal abnormalities. By means of classical histochemical staining, especially silver staining, these abnormalities can be visualized in the perikaryon (the neurofibrillary tangle) and in neurites (dystrophic neurites). These latter phenomena may be associated with extracellular amyloid depositions, to form neuritic plaques, or they may lie outside the plaques, in which case they have been termed neuropil threads (1,2). The formation of these altered cytoskeletal constituents is a dynamic process, and silver staining offers but a restricted view of the final stages of these alterations. New vistas are offered by the use of antibodies directed against specific cytoskeletal structural proteins, e.g. microtubule-associated protein tau or ubiquitin (see below). At present, however, it seems difficult to fit all the old and new data into one mode of neuronal alterations in Alzheimer's disease.

A limited number of immunoreactive neurons may also be found in the brains of nondemented individuals and of patients suffering from some other neurological diseases (3,4), which complicates the diagnostic specificity of such antibodies for Alzheimer's disease. Moreover, the cytoskeletal alterations are distributed in a very heterogeneous way over cortical areas and layers, subcortical nuclei and different neuron populations. In the literature several hypothetical explanations for the different staining patterns have been given. It has been proposed that cytoskeletal staining preferentially takes place in cortical neurons or neurons projecting to the cortex (5). Diffuse labeling of the perikaryon of neurons lacking tangles has been considered to precede the formation of tangles (6,7). Cytoskeletal staining is thought to be a sign of impending neuronal death, not only in Alzheimer's disease (7-9), but also in normal brain development (9,10). A causal relationship between the

Alzheimer's Disease: Basic Mechanisms, Diagnosis and Therapeutic Strategies
Edited by K. Iqbal, D. R. C. McLachlan, B. Winblad and H. M. Wisniewski
©1991 John Wiley & Sons Ltd

occurrence of dystrophic neurites and deposition of amyloid has been presumed, but not confirmed (11).

THE HUMAN HYPOTHALAMUS

The human hypothalamus is a unique structure for testing the different hypotheses on the pathophysiological meaning of the cytoskeletal markers in Alzheimer's disease. In the first place it contains both neurons that project to the cortex, e.g. the nucleus basalis of Meynert (NBM), and neurons that do not project to the cortex, e.g. the supraoptic nucleus (SON), the paraventricular nucleus (PVN), the suprachiasmatic nucleus (SCN) and probably the sexually dimorphic nucleus (SDN) and the nucleus tuberis lateralis (NTL), so that the hypothesis that mainly systems connected to the cortex are affected (5) can be tested in this structure. The human hypothalamus also offers the possibility of testing hypotheses on the relation between cytoskeletal changes and the fate of neurons in aging and dementia. The NBM is generally assumed to degenerate in aging and even more so in Alzheimer's disease (see below). In the SCN, which is the clock of the hypothalamus, a decrease in cell number occurs in normal aging, which is even more pronounced in Alzheimer's disease (12). The sexually dimorphic nucleus (SDN) shows a decrease in cell number which is similar in aging and in Alzheimer's disease (13,14). On the other hand, no cell loss is found in the SON, PVN and NTL either in Alzheimer patients or in controls (15,16).

METHODS

Cytoskeletal alterations in aging and Alzheimer's disease were related to cell counts in the different hypothalamic nuclei by using the following four antibodies:

60e, a polyclonal antibody raised against isolated neurofibrillary tangles which was also used following pretreatment of the sections with formic acid in order to uncover epitopes on tangles (17). This antiserum contains antibodies to normal tau and to an abnormal form of tau, but is not phosphatase-sensitive and does not react with ubiquitin (18).

tau-1, a monoclonal antibody to the microtubule-associated protein tau (19). Dephosphorylation of the tissue sections with alkaline phosphatase (86 μg/ml) was performed prior to immunocytochemistry, since it increases the number of tangles and plaques recognized by the antibody (20). Without dephosphorylation no staining was obtained with tau-1 in the hypothalamic nuclei of Alzheimer patients or controls.

3-39, a monoclonal antibody raised against isolated neurofibrillary tangles and directed against ubiquitin (7,21–23).

Alz-50, a monoclonal antibody which reacts with tau and A68 (24–27).

For the present study 6-μm paraffin sections of formalin-fixed hypothalami were used from 13 neuropathologically confirmed Alzheimer patients and 13 age-

and sex-matched controls. The age of the controls ranged from 47 to 91 years and that of the Alzheimer patients from 46 to 94 years.

RESULTS (Figures 1, 2)

The nucleus basalis of Meynert (NBM) is an origin of the cholinergic innervation of the neocortex. It is as yet unclear whether the degenerative changes in the NBM in Alzheimer's disease contribute to the memory disturbance in this condition (28) and whether neuronal loss in the NBM occurs during normal aging (29,30). The number of large cholinergic neurons is generally reported to decrease in Alzheimer's disease (29–31). However, since at the same time the proportion of small neurons is increasing (32,33), many of the large cells in the NBM may be shrunken instead of dead. NBM neurons of Alzheimer patients showed abundant staining, compared to those of controls, with antibodies 60e (even more so after pretreatment with formic acid), anti-tau-1 (after dephosphorylation) and 3-39. After dephosphorylation, tau-1 visualized dystrophic neurites as well as neuritic plaques. The most obvious difference between Alzheimer patients and controls was observed with Alz-50 staining. In controls, NBM neurons are generally unstained, except for some neurons in a 63-year-old man, and some neurons and dystrophic neurites in a 90-year-old woman. In Alzheimer patients the NBM was generally full of diffusely staining perikarya, tangles and dystrophic neurites. Therefore, the NBM is a very suitable brain structure for an immunocytochemical validation of the neuropathological diagnosis of Alzheimer's disease. The NBM changes are compatible with the various pathophysiological hypotheses mentioned before.

The supraoptic nucleus (SON) can be regarded in many respects as the opposite of NBM. The neurosecretory neurons of the SON produce the neuropeptides vasopressin and oxytocin, which are released into the circulation in the neurohypophysis. They form a population of extremely stable cells. Neither in the course of normal aging nor in Alzheimer's disease was any significant loss in neurons or total cell number observed (15). None of the four antibodies mentioned earlier revealed any cytoskeletal staining in the SON. The differences between the cytoskeletal alterations observed in the NBM, which is affected in Alzheimer's disease, and those observed in the SON, which is spared in this condition, are in agreement with the various hypotheses on the possible meaning of cytoskeletal staining mentioned in the introduction. However, results obtained from other hypothalamic nuclei (see below) are inconsistent with most of these hypotheses.

The paraventricular nucleus (PVN) contains neurosecretory neurons that project to the neurohypophysis and median eminence. In this nucleus no loss of total cell number was observed either in aging or in Alzheimer's disease (15). Yet, both in controls and in Alzheimer patients diffuse cytoplasmic staining was regularly observed with 60e following formic acid pretreatment, with tau-1 following dephosphorylation, with 3-39 and, most clearly, with Alz-50. This staining was also present in young controls (Figure 1F).

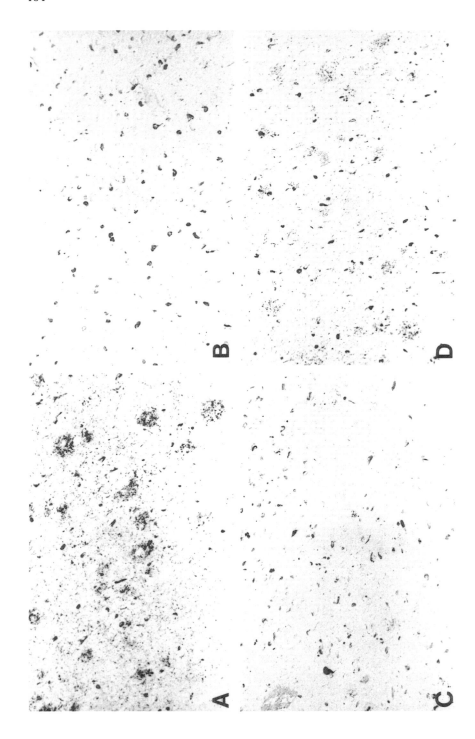

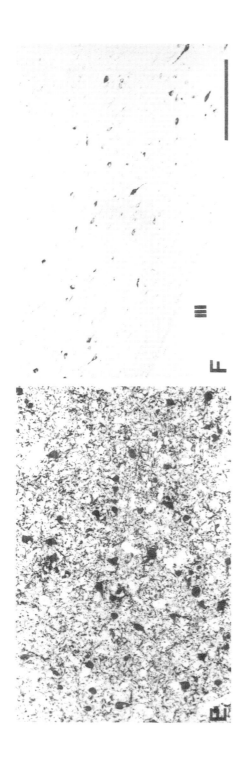

Figure 1. (A–D) Nucleus basalis of Meynert of a 45-year-old male Alzheimer patient (no. 86.3645.2) stained with (A) Alz-50 — note plaques, tangles and dystrophic neurites; (B) 60e, directed against neurofibrillary tangles, following pretreatment with formic acid; (C) 3-39, raised against tangles and directed against ubiquitin; (D) tau-1 following dephosphorylation; note plaques, tangles and dystrophic neurites. (E) Nucleus tuberalis lateralis, stained with Alz-50. Note tangles and dystrophic neurites (female Alzheimer patient no. 88.325, 64 years of age). (F) Paraventricular nucleus of a 47-year-old male control (no. 87.271). Note the cytoplasmatic staining of the neurons. Scale bar 200 μm; III, third ventricle

186

Figure 2. (A,B) Suprachiasmatic nucleus of 64-year-old female Alzheimer patient (no. 87.494.2) stained with anti-vasopressin (A; note the few positive cells in the degenerated nucleus indicated by arrows) and with the anti-ubiquitin 3-39 (B); III, third ventricle. (C,D) Sexually dimorphic nucleus of 70-year-old female Alzheimer patient no. 8560 stained with tau-1 following dephosphorylation (C) and with 60e following formic acid pretreatment (D); note the cell body staining (C,D) and dystrophic neurites (D). Scale bar 200 μm

Therefore, in PVN diffuse perikaryal labeling of neurons may not be indicative of intraneuronal abnormalities preceding the formation of tangles and impending cell death. Interestingly enough, Alz-50 positive neuropil threads were observed only in the PVN of Alzheimer patients and not in that of controls, except for the presence of some neuropil threads in one 90-year-old female control.

The lateral tuberal nucleus (NTL) is supposed to be present only in humans and higher primates. In adulthood it contains 60 000 neurons, whereas in Huntington's disease this number may be reduced to less than 10 000 (34). Pathological changes in the NTL have also been described in dementia with argyrophilic grains throughout the neuropil and silver-staining coiled bodies, containing straight filaments (35). In both Alzheimer's disease and Huntington's disease, dementia is associated with severe loss of weight despite normal or even increased food intake. In the condition described by Braak and Braak (35), the severe NTL pathology is also accompanied by cachexia (H. Braak, personal communication). Therefore, the NTL may play a role in feeding behavior and metabolism.

In Alzheimer's disease, no alteration in the number of NTL neurons was found. Neurofibrillary tangles were rare in conventional silver stains. Yet, immuno-cytochemical staining by Alz-50 showed such an abundant reactivity of both perikaryal and dystrophic neurites that the NTL of Alzheimer patients could even be recognized with the naked eye (34). It seems, therefore, that the NTL represents a brain area in which Alzheimer's disease affects the neurons in a limited way, without progression toward the classical silver staining tangles or neuronal loss. The observations in this nucleus show that even a very strong Alz-50 staining does not predict impending neuronal death, since in Alzheimer's disease neuron counts in the NTL did not show any decline in numbers. The other three antibodies have not been applied to the NTL.

The sexually dimorphic nucleus (SDN) of the preoptic area was first described by Gorski et al (36) in the rat. In the rat the SDN is three to eight times larger in the male than in the female, due to differences in perinatal steroid levels (37). The SDN is involved in aspects of male sexual behavior (e.g. mounting), not only in male, but also in female rats (38,39). In the human brain the SDN is twice as large in males as in females and contains twice as many cells (40). The SDN is identical to the 'intermediate nucleus' described by Braak and Braak (41). Cell numbers in the male SDN decrease sharply after 50 years of age, while in females a phase of marked cell loss sets in approximately around the age of 70 (13,14). The decrease in cell numbers in this nucleus later in life might be related to the hormonal changes which accompany both male and female senescence (14), and to the decrease in male sexual activity. Yet it is not clear whether the hormonal changes would be the cause or effect of the observed cell loss in this nucleus. Cell numbers in the SDN of Alzheimer's patients were found to be within the normal range for age and sex so that this condition does not seem to affect the SDN in any specific way (13).

Some positive cell bodies were found in the SDN of a small number of Alzheimer patients with 60e, tau-1 and 3-39 staining. Alz-50 staining revealed some positive SDN neurons and dystrophic neurites in Alzheimer patients, whereas controls were negative for all four antibodies (except for a few Alz-50 positive neurons in one control patient, a 63-year-old male). Since the SDN cell numbers decrease in a similar way in Alzheimer patients and controls, cytoskeletal staining cannot be related in a simple way to cell death in the SDN.

The suprachiasmatic nucleus (SCN) is considered to be the major circadian pacemaker of the mammalian brain, coordinating hormonal and behavioral circadian rhythms (42). Age-related changes in circadian rhythms have been reported in humans as well as in animals (43). Among the most prominent changes is a fragmentation of sleep–wakefulness patterns in senescence, a phenomenon that is even more pronounced in Alzheimer's disease (44). Sleep disturbances often lead to hospital admission of the elderly (45). Total SCN cell numbers and numbers of vasopressin-expressing neurons were, therefore, determined during aging and in Alzheimer's disease. A marked decrease was found in total SCN cell numbers and in the number of vasopressin neurons in subjects of 80–100 years of age, while in Alzheimer's disease these changes were still more dramatic (46,47).

In spite of the pronounced SCN changes in Alzheimer's disease, the cytoskeletal alterations were generally only minimal, with the exception of one 64-year-old female Alzheimer patient, whose entire SCN was stained with tau-1 and 3-39 but not with 60e or Alz-50. Several Alzheimer patients had few positive SCN cells with 60e following formic acid treatment, with tau-1 after dephosphorylation, and with 3-39, but the stainings were far from impressive. Alz-50 showed some positive perikarya, whereas dystrophic neurites were hardly seen at all.

CONCLUSIONS

Some diffuse cytoplasmatic staining was also observed in young nondemented controls, raising doubts about the specificity of the antibodies for Alzheimer's disease. This phenomenon was most conspicuous in PVN neurons with Alz-50. However, Alz-50 staining of dystrophic neurites was clearly observable only in Alzheimer patients, so staining of dystrophic neurites seems to be more specific for the histopathological diagnosis of Alzheimer's disease than perikaryal staining.

Perikaryal staining is not necessarily indicative of neuronal abnormalities preceding the formation of tangles or impending cell death, as is clear from the PVN staining in young controls and the NTL staining in Alzheimer patients. Bondareff et al (48), using thioflavin-S staining, also came to the conclusion that the appearance of tangles does not necessarily herald the demise of a neuron in Alzheimer's disease.

The very strong Alz-50 staining in the NTL, from which no direct cortical connections are known, raises doubts about the idea that cytoskeletal changes would be restricted to cortical areas or nuclei projecting to the cortex. The same can be said about the SCN and SDN staining observed in some Alzheimer patients, since these nuclei are not considered to be directly connected to the cortex either.

Consequently, the pathophysiological meaning of cytoskeletal staining in Alzheimer's disease is at present far from clear.

Acknowledgments

Brain material was obtained from the Netherlands Brain Bank (Amsterdam, The Netherlands). Alz-50 was kindly donated by Abbott Laboratories (Abbott Park, IL, USA). Tau-1 was generously supplied by Dr L. Binder (University of Alabama, Birmingham, USA). The authors wish to thank Mr B. Fisser and Ms Y.-C. Tung for their technical assistance, Mr G. Van der Meulen for his photographical work, and Ms O. Pach and Mr A. Janssen for their secretarial assistance. The study was supported by Stimuleringsprogramma Gezondheidsonderzoek (SGO) of the Ministry of Science and Education in The Netherlands, by New York State Office of Mental Retardation and Developmental Disabilities, and by NIH grants AG 05892, NS 18105 and AG 04220. D.F. Swaab and I. Grundke-Iqbal were recipients of Senior Travel Fellowships of Alzheimer Society of Canada and Alzheimer's Association, USA, respectively, to participate in the Second International Conference on Alzheimer's Disease, Toronto, Canada, 1990.

REFERENCES

1. Braak H, Braak E, Grundke-Iqbal K. Neurosci Lett 1986; 65: 351-5.
2. Braak H, Braak E. Neuropath Appl Neurobiol 1988; 14: 39-44.
3. Iqbal K, Wisniewski HM, Grundke-Iqbal I, Terry RD. In Nandy K, Sherwin L (eds) The aging brain and senile dementia. New York: Plenum, 1977: 209-27.
4. Love S, Saitoh T, Quijada S, Cole GM, Terry RD. J Neuropath Exp Neurol 1988; 47: 393-405.
5. German DC, White CL III, Sparkman DR. Neurosci 1987; 21: 305-12.
6. Joachim CL, Morris JH, Selkoe DJ, Kosik KS. J Neuropath Exp Neurol 1987; 46: 611-22.
7. Bancher C, Brunner C, Lassmann H, Budka H, Jellinger K, Wiche G, Seitelberger F, Grundke-Iqbal I, Iqbal K, Wisniewski HM. Brain Res 1989; 477: 90-9.
8. Ulrich J, Probst A, Anderton BH, Brion JP. The neuronal cytoskeleton in senile dementia of Alzheimer type and other types of dementia. In Von Hahn HP (ed.) Interdisciplinary topics in gerontology, vol. 25. Basel: Karger, 1988: 101-5.
9. Wolozin B, Scicutella A, Davies P. Proc Natl Acad Sci USA 1988; 85: 6202-6.
10. Al-Ghoul WM, Miller MW. Brain Res 1989; 481: 361-7.
11. Tabaton M, Mandybur TI, Perry G, Onorato M, Autilio-Gambetti L, Gambetti P. Ann Neurol 1989; 26: 771-8.
12. Swaab DF, Fliers E, Partiman TS. Brain Res 1985; 342: 37-44.
13. Swaab DF, Hofman MA. Dev Brain Res 1988; 44: 314-18.
14. Hofman MA, Swaab DF. J Anat 1989; 164: 55-72.
15. Goudsmit E, Hofman MA, Fliers E, Swaab DF. Neurobiol Aging 1990; 11: 529-36.
16. Kremer HPH, Swaab DF, Bots GTAM, Fisser B, Ravid R, Roos RAC. Ann Neurol 1990; 29 (in press).
17. Grundke-Iqbal I, Iqbal K, Tung Y-C, Wisniewski HM. Acta Neuropathol (Berl) 1984; 62: 259-67.
18. Grundke-Iqbal I, Vorbrodt AW, Iqbal K, Tung Y-C, Wang GP, Wisniewski HM. Mol Brain Res 1988; 4: 43-52.
19. Binder LI, Frankfurter A, Rebhun LI. J Cell Biol 1985; 101: 1371-8.
20. Grundke-Iqbal I, Iqbal K, Tung Y-C, Quinlan M, Wisniewski HM, Binder LI. Proc Natl Acad Sci USA 1986; 4913-17.
21. Wang GP, Grundke-Iqbal I, Kascsak RJ, Iqbal K, Wisniewski HM. Acta Neuropathol (Berl) 1984; 62: 268-75.
22. Grundke-Iqbal I, Wang, GP, Iqbal K, Tung Y-C, Wisniewski HM. Acta Neuropathol (Berl) 1985; 68: 279-83.
23. Perry G, Mulvihill P, Fried VA, Smith HT, Grundke-Iqbal I, Iqbal K. J Neurochem 1989; 52: 1523-8.

24. Ksiezak-Reding H, Binder LI, Yen S-H. J Biol Chem 1988; 263: 7948-53.
25. Ksiezak-Reding H, Davies P, Yen S-H. J Biol Chem 1988; 263: 7943-7.
26. Wolozin BL, Pruchnicki A, Dickson DW, Davies P. Science 1986; 232: 648-50.
27. Nukina N, Kosik KS, Selkoe DJ. Neurosci Lett 1988; 87: 240-6.
28. Candy JM, Perry EK, Perry RH, Court JA, Oakley AE, Edwardson JA. Prog Brain Res 1986; 72: 105-32.
29. Mann DMA, Yates PO, Marcyniuk B. Mech Ageing Dev 1984; 25: 189-204.
30. Coleman PD, Flood DG. Neurobiol Aging 1987; 8: 521-45.
31. Lowes-Hummel P, Gertz H-J, Ferszt R, Cervos-Navarro J. Arch Geront Geriatr 1989; 8: 21-7.
32. Rinne JO, Paljärvi L, Rinne UK. J Neurol Sci 1987; 79: 67-76.
33. Allen SJ, Dawbarn D, Wilcock GK. Brain Res 1988; 454: 275-81.
34. Kremer HPH, Roos RAC, Dingjan G et al. J Neuropath Exp Neurol 1990; 49: 371-82.
35. Braak H, Braak E. Neuropath Appl Neurobiol 1989; 15: 13-26.
36. Gorski RA, Gordon JH, Shryne JE, Southam AM. Brain Res 1978; 148: 333-46.
37. Jacobson CD, Shryne JE, Shapiro F, Gorski RA. J Comp Neurol 1980; 193: 541-8.
38. Turkenburg JL, Swaab DF, Endert E, Louwerse AL, Van de Poll NE. Brain Res Bull 1988; 21: 215-24.
39. De Jonge FH, Louwerse AL, Ooms MP, Evers P, Endert E, Van de Poll NE. Brain Res Bull 1989; 23: 483-92.
40. Swaab DF, Fliers E. Science 1985; 228: 1112-15.
41. Braak H, Braak E. Anat Embryol 1987; 176: 315-30.
42. Rusak B, Zucker I. Physiol Rev 1979; 59: 449-526.
43. Van Gool WA, Mirmiran M. Prog Brain Res 1986; 70: 255-79.
44. Witting W, Kwa IH, Eikelenboom P, Mirmiran M, Swaab DF. Biol Psychiatry 1990; 27: 563-72.
45. Sanford JRA. Br Med J 1975; 3: 471-3.
46. Swaab DF, Fliers E, Partiman TS. Brain Res 1985; 342: 37-44.
47. Swaab DF, Roozendaal B, Ravid R, Velis DN, Gooren L, Williams RS. Prog Brain Res 1987; 72: 301-10.
48. Bondareff W, Mountjoy CQ, Roth M, Hauser DL. Neurobiol Aging 1989; 10: 709-15.

Address for correspondence:

Dr D.F. Swaab,
Netherlands Institute for Brain Research,
Meibergdreef 33,
1105 AZ Amsterdam,
The Netherlands

22 Possible Involvement of Calcium and Inositol Phospholipid Signaling Pathways in Neurofibrillary Degeneration

MARK P. MATTSON, B. RYCHLIK AND M. G. ENGLE

Although studies of nonviable postmortem human tissue have provided important data on the histological and molecular alterations in Alzheimer's disease (AD) and related disorders, the events underlying neuronal degeneration and neurofibrillary tangle (NFT) formation remain unknown. In order to fully understand the dynamics of NFT formation, it seems important to directly examine living human neurons in an *experimental system*. In the study described here we used cultured human cerebral cortical neurons to test the hypothesis that alterations in the calcium and inositol phospholipid signaling systems are involved in NFT formation. Experimental elevation of intracellular calcium levels caused ultrastructural and antigenic changes in the neuronal cytoskeleton similar to those seen in NFT. A loss of microtubules, the accumulation of 8–15 nm straight filaments, and an increased antigenicity towards tau antibodies occurred within hours to days under conditions that caused sustained elevations in intracellular calcium levels. Paired helical filament (PHF)-like structures were occasionally observed but were not developed to the extent seen in AD NFT suggesting that PHF formation occurs late in the process of neurofibrillary degeneration. Specific activation of protein kinase C (PKC) also caused NFT-like antigenic changes. Taken together, these findings suggest the involvement of calcium-dependent kinase(s) and PKC in neurofibrillary degeneration and indicate that in-vitro approaches may provide a valuable complement to studies of AD pathology in situ.

INTRODUCTION

Nfts are a histological feature of AD (1,2) as well as many other neurodegenerative conditions ranging from dementia pugilistica (3) to Down's syndrome (4) to subacute sclerosing panencephalitis (5). A loss of microtubules, the formation of PHF and 8–15 nm straight filaments, and alterations in microtubule-associated proteins are characteristic features of NFTs (1,6). Valuable information on the molecular composition of NFTs has been obtained from analyses of postmortem tissue (1). For

Alzheimer's Disease: Basic Mechanisms, Diagnosis and Therapeutic Strategies
Edited by K. Iqbal, D. R. C. McLachlan, B. Winblad and H. M. Wisniewski
© 1991 John Wiley & Sons Ltd

example, two components of NFTs that have been positively identified are the microtubule-associated protein tau (7-10) and ubiquitin (11,12). It has, however, proved difficult to retrace the events leading to NFTs. Thus, the cause(s) of NFT formation and the relationship of NFTs to neuronal death remain unclear. A major impediment to understanding the process of NFT formation has been the lack of direct experimental studies of living human neurons that are vulnerable to NFT formation.

One useful approach to studies of neurodegenerative disorders is to first understand the cellular and molecular mechanisms that normally regulate neuronal cytoarchitecture adaptively, and then apply this knowledge to the pathological condition. This approach is based upon the idea that abnormalities in control systems for adaptive plasticity underlie neurodegenerative disorders. The calcium and inositol phospholipid systems are two signaling mechanisms that play important roles in the development of neuroarchitecture (13,14), as well as in adaptive plasticity in the mature nervous system (15,16). Beyond their adaptive roles in regulating the neuronal cytoskeleton, the calcium and inositol phospholipid pathways have been implicated in neurodegenerative processes (17-20). Interestingly, tau in NFTs has been shown to be abnormally phosphorylated (21-23), an observation consistent with a role for altered kinase activity in NFT formation. In the present study we used cultured human cerebral cortical neurons to make an initial experimental test of the hypothesis that overactivation of the calcium and/or inositol phospholipid pathways can lead to neurofibrillary degeneration.

ELEVATED INTRACELLULAR CALCIUM LEVELS CAUSE NEUROFIBRILLARY-LIKE CHANGES IN CULTURED HUMAN CEREBRAL CORTICAL NEURONS

Dissociated cell cultures of embryonic (12-14 week gestation) human cerebral cortex were established and maintained as described previously (24). Neurons in these cultures contain tau and the low molecular weight (68 kDa) neurofilament protein (24; G. Perry and M. Mattson, unpublished). The majority of neurons elaborate one long process which contains tau (the axon), and one or more minor processes which are dendrite-like (24).

In order to test the hypothesis that altered calcium homeostasis can lead to NFT formation, we exposed cultures to conditions that increased intracellular calcium levels and then processed the cells for either ultrastructural examination or immunocytochemical localization of tau at the light microscope level (25). In untreated control cultures the neuronal cytoskeleton was dominated by microtubules which were particularly abundant in the axons where they were oriented parallel to the long axis (Figure 1A). Neurofilaments (10 nm) and microfilaments (6 nm) were very sparse in these embryonic neurons but growth cones did contain abundant microfilaments in their periphery. Exposure of neurons to calcium ionophore A23187 (2 μM) resulted in a fivefold to eightfold rise in intracellular calcium levels (measured with the calcium indicator dye fura-2) and quite striking changes in the neuronal cytoskeleton. Within 1 hour of exposure to A23187, microtubules were greatly

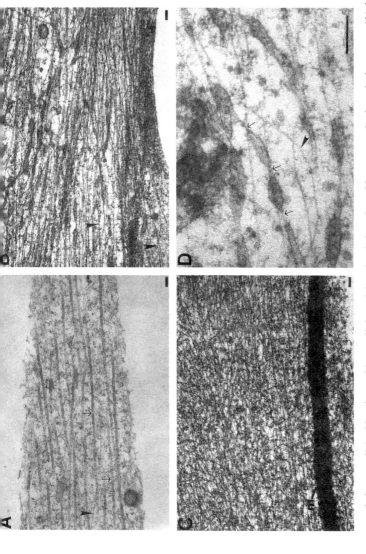

Figure 1. Ultrastructural changes elicited by elevated intracellular calcium levels in cultured human cerebral cortical neurons. (A) Axon of an untreated neuron. Microtubules (arrows) oriented with the long axis of the axon are the major cytoskeletal feature. A few 10 nm neurofilaments are present (arrowhead). (B) After exposure to 2 μM calcium ionophore A23187 for 1 hr, microtubules are greatly reduced and filaments of diameters ranging from 8–15 nm have accumulated (e.g. arrowheads). (C) Incubation of neurons in a medium with a reduced level of Na$^+$ (10%), which elevated intracellular calcium levels for 24 hr, resulted in the massive accumulation of filaments that often filled the axoplasm (m, mitochondrion). (D) Structures that appeared to be twisted pairs of filaments were observed in neurons that had been exposed to an elevated level of intracellular calcium (in this case, 2 μM A23187 for 1 hr). Arrows point to sites of constriction and the arrowhead points to a single filament. Scale bars 100 nm

reduced in numbers and there was a marked accumulation of filaments of variable diameter (8-15) nm) which often occurred in bundles (Figure 1B). Occasionally, paired twisted filaments were present (Figure 1D), but these structures were not identical to the PHF seen in AD in situ, as their apparent twist periodicities and diameters were highly variable. After 4 hours in the presence of A23187, the neuronal membranes became fragmented and most neurons had detached from the culture substrate by 8 hours post-treatment. A more prolonged calcium-induced neuronal degeneration was caused by exposure of cultures to a medium containing a reduced level of extracellular Na^+ (90% of the NaCl was replaced with N-methyl-D-glucamine). This procedure reduces the efficacy of the Na^+-Ca^{2+} exchanger and resulted in a twofold to threefold elevation in the intracellular calcium level over a 24-48 hour period. Neurons maintained under these conditions showed massive accumulations of 8-15 nm filaments in their somata and neurites (Figure 1C), and occasional paired twisted filaments were observed which were similar to those elicited by A23187 (Figure 1D).

Three monoclonal antibodies that recognize the microtubule-associated protein tau in NFT were used to further examine the NFT-like properties of neurons exposed to elevated intracellular calcium levels: Alz-50, raised against AD tangle material (26,27); tau-1, raised against bovine brain tau (8); and 5E2 raised against human fetal tau (9). In control cultures, neurons showed weak immunoreactivity with 5E2 (Figure 2A) and Alz-50 (not shown) antibodies. Exposure of neurons to A23187 or a reduced Na^+ medium resulted in a striking increase in 5E2 immunoreactivity in the somata and axons (Figure 2B and C). Alz-50 immunoreactivity was also increased in response to calcium influx, while tau-1 staining was not increased (not shown). Thus, antigenic changes similar to those seen in AD NFT were induced by an elevation in the intracellular calcium level.

PROTEIN KINASE C AND NEUROFIBRILLARY-LIKE CHANGES IN HUMAN CORTICAL NEURONS

In an earlier study of cultured rat hippocampal pyramidal neurons we noted that micromolar levels of phorbol activators of PKC were neurotoxic (20). Since overactivation of the calcium system can cause neurodegeneration and elicit several features of NFTs, we tested the possibility that overactivation of PKC might also result in NFT-like changes in the human neuronal cytoskeleton (28). A specific activator of PKC (PMA; phorbol 12-myristate 13-acetate), an inactive phorbol (PDD; 4œ-phorbol 12,13-didecanoate), and an inhibitor of PKC (H-7; 1-[5-isoquinolinyl-sulfonyl]-2-methylpiperazine) were used to manipulate PKC in cultured human cortical neurons. PDD (5 μM) affected neither neuronal survival nor tau immunoreactivity (Figure 2D). In contrast, PMA (1-5 μM) caused neurodegeneration and greatly increased tau immunoreactivity over a period of several hours (Figure 2E). The effects of PMA were blocked by H-7 (Figure 2F) indicating that the neurofibrillary-like degeneration caused by PMA was due to specific activation of PKC. The increased tau immunoreactivity elicited by PMA was not the result of enhanced calcium influx since the increase was seen in cultures incubated in medium

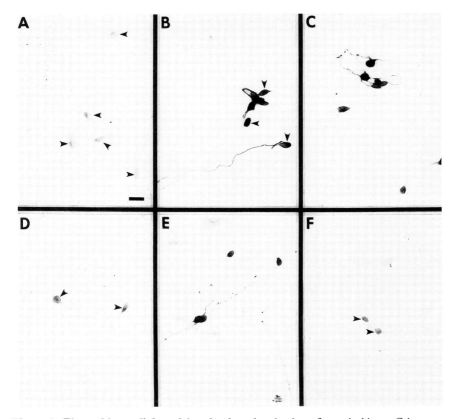

Figure 2. Elevated intracellular calcium levels and activation of protein kinase C increase neuronal immunoreactivity with antibodies that recognize tau in NFT. All pictures are bright-field light micrographs of cultures processed using the biotin-avidin-peroxidase procedure (arrowheads point to neuronal somata). (A) Staining with monoclonal antibody 5E2 in an untreated control culture. (B) Staining with 5E2 in a culture exposed for 2 hr to 2 μM A23187. (C) Staining with 5E2 in a culture exposed for 24 hr to medium with a reduced level (10%) of Na$^+$. (D) Staining with monoclonal antibody Alz-50 in a culture exposed for 2 hr to 5 μM of the inactive phorbol PDD. (E) Staining with Alz-50 in a culture exposed for 2 hr to 5 μM PMA, an activator of PKC. (F) Staining with Alz-50 in a culture exposed for 2 hr to the PKC inhibitor H-7 plus PMA (5 μM each). Scale bar 20 μm

lacking calcium and containing 1 mM EGTA. Thus, activation of PKC can cause antigenic changes in human cortical neurons similar to those seen in AD and related disorders.

IS EXCESS KINASE ACTIVITY INVOLVED IN NEUROFIBRILLARY DEGENERATION?

When taken together with previous work by others, our observations in cultured human cortical neurons suggest that overactivation of the calcium and/or inositol phospholipid signaling pathways may be involved in neurodegeneration in AD and

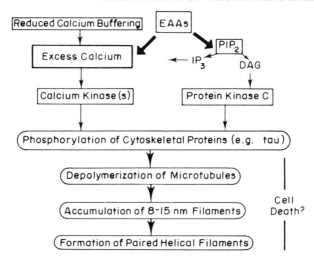

Figure 3. Proposed roles for the calcium and inositol phospholipid systems in the formation of neurofibrillary tangles. Excess levels of intracellular calcium can arise from enhanced influx (due, for example, to exposure to excitatory amino acids, EAAs) or reduced calcium buffering (due to faulty plasma membrane extrusion systems or calcium binding proteins). Calcium (through intermediary proteins such as calmodulin) then activates calcium-dependent protein kinases. Overactivation of receptors linked to the inositol phospholipid pathway results in a breakdown of phosphatidylinositol-4,5-bisphosphate (PIP$_2$) to diacylglycerol (DAG) and inositol triphosphate (IP$_3$). DAG activates protein kinase C (PKC), while IP$_3$ causes the release of calcium from intracellular stores. Calcium-dependent kinases and PKC catalyze the phosphorylation of cytoskeletal proteins. Excess phosphorylation results in a breakdown of the normal cytoskeletal organization and the formation of abnormal structures such as 8-15 nm straight filaments and paired helical filaments. Phosphorylation of tau can cause the depolymerization of microtubules and may therefore play a key role in the cascade of events that lead to neurofibrillary degeneration. The points in this series of events at which the damage to the cell becomes irreversible and cell death occurs are not known.

related disorders (Figure 3). Although the neurodegenerative actions of calcium are well established (17–19), the specific events leading to the disruption of the cytoskeleton are unclear. We suggest that at least the early events in cytoskeletal disruption are mediated by protein kinase(s). Consistent with this possibility are previous findings demonstrating the abnormal phosphorylation of tau in AD NFT (21–23), and a shift in the electrophoretic mobility of tau caused by calcium/calmodulin-dependent kinase in vitro identical to that observed in NFT-associated tau (29). Furthermore, neurons that are vulnerable in AD (e.g. hippocampal CA1 neurons) contain high levels of calcium/calmodulin-dependent kinase (30).

A role for PKC in neurodegenerative processes has only recently begun to be examined. Alterations in the subcellular distribution of PKC occur in rat brain following ischemia (31), and the PKC inhibitor H-7 can reduce ischemia-induced neurodegeneration in an animal model of stroke (32). We found that H-7 could prevent neurodegeneration and NFT-like alterations in the cytoskeleton of cultured human cortical neurons. These kinds of data suggest that activation of PKC may be a common intracellular event in neurodegenerative processes. Of course, studies of the inositol phospholipid pathway in AD will be required in order to relate the findings obtained in experimental systems to the pathology of AD in situ.

Excitatory amino acids (EAAs) have been implicated in the neurodegeneration that occurs in disorders ranging from AD to stroke (18,19,33,34). EAAs have been shown to activate both the calcium (35) and inositol phospholipid (36) pathways. We found that overactivation of either of these systems can cause neurodegeneration and neurofibrillary-like changes in the cultured human cortical neurons. Previous work in cultured rat hippocampal neurons showed that glutamate could elicit antigenic changes similar to those seen in NFT by a calcium-mediated mechanism (37). More chronic exposure of cultured human spinal neurons to glutamate resulted in the formation of PHF (38). Thus, neurofibrillary degeneration may be a consequence of altered cellular signaling resulting in a loss of homeostasis in the calcium and inositol phospholipid systems and excess activation of calcium-dependent kinases and PKC (Figure 3). Loss of control in these signaling systems might arise from overactivation of receptors or alterations in subsequent regulatory systems. In the calcium system, for example, excess levels of intracellular calcium might arise from deficient calcium-buffering systems (e.g. plasma membrane Ca^{2+} ATPase or Na^+-Ca^{2+} exchanger, or calcium binding proteins).

The sequence of events that lead to the formation of NFT are not clear. Based upon studies of tangles presumed to be at different stages of formation in situ, Bancher et al provided evidence that the accumulation of abnormally phosphorylated tau precedes the formation of PHF (23). Our findings support this sequence. Increased immunoreactivity with tau antibodies was a very early change in the cultured neurons, occurring within the first 10–30 min of calcium elevation. Early changes at the ultrastructural level included a loss of microtubules and the accumulation of 8–15 nm filaments. Later (1–2 days), large bundles of the 8–15 nm filaments filled the cytoplasm. Occasionally we observed PHF-like structures. Our findings are therefore consistent with a scenario in which PHFs form in the later stages of neurofibrillary degeneration (Figure 3) as previously suggested (6,38,39). The specific molecular changes underlying the different stages of NFT formation, and the relationship of these changes to cell death, are important questions that remain to be answered.

Acknowledgments

We thank Drs W. R. Markesbery, G. Perry, J. E. Sisken, and D. L. Sparks for critical comments on portions of this work. Drs L. Binder, P. Davies, and K. Kosik were very generous in their contribution of antibodies. L. Nguyen and C. Wright provided technical assistance. Supported by PSP and BRSG awards, the Alzheimer's Disease and Related Disorders Association, and the International Life Sciences Institute.

REFERENCES

1. Terry RD. J Neuropath Exp Neurol 1963; 22: 629-41.
2. Selkoe DJ. Ann Rev Neurosci 1989; 12: 463-90.

3. Wisniewski HM, Narang HK, Corsellis JAN. J Neuropath Exp Neurol 1976; 35: 367-78.
4. Olson MI, Shaw CM. Brain 1969; 92: 147-56.
5. Wisniewski K, Jervis GA, Moretz RC, Wisniewski HM. Ann Neurol 1979; 5: 288-94.
6. Metzuls J et al. Cell Tiss Res 1988; 252: 239-48.
7. Grundke-Iqbal I, Iqbal K, Quinlan M, Tung Y-C, Zaidi MS, Wisniewski HM. J Biol Chem 1986; 261: 6084-9.
8. Wood JG, Mirra SS, Pollock NJ, Binder LI. Proc Natl Acad Sci USA 1986; 83: 4040-4.
9. Kosik KS, Orecchio LD, Binder L, Trojanowski JQ, Lee VM-Y, Lee G. Neuron 1988; 1: 817-25.
10. Perry G, Mulvihill P, Manetto V, Autilio-Gambetti L, Gambetti P. J Neurosci 1987; 7: 3736-8.
11. Perry G, Friedman R, Shaw G, Chau V. Proc Natl Acad Sci USA 1987; 84: 3030-6.
12. Mori H, Kondo J, Ihara Y. Science 1987; 235: 1641-4.
13. Kater SB, Mattson MP, Cohan CS, Connor JA. Trends Neurosci 1988; 11: 315-21.
14. Mattson MP. Current Aspects of the Neurosciences. London: Macmillan, 1990: 1-45.
15. Malenka RC, Kauer JA, Zucker RS, Nicoll RA. Science 1988; 242: 81-4.
16. Routtenberg A. Prog Brain Res 1986; 69: 211-34.
17. Siesjo BK, Bengtsson F, Grampp W, Theander S. Ann NY Acad Sci 1989; 568: 234-51.
18. Choi DW. Neuron 1988; 1: 623-34.
19. Mattson MP. Mech Ageing Dev 1989; 50: 103-57.
20. Mattson MP, Guthrie PB, Kater SB. J Neurosci Res 1988; 21: 447-64.
21. Grundke-Iqbal I et al. Proc Natl Acad Sci USA 1986; 83: 4913-17.
22. Ihara Y, Nukina N, Miura, R, Ogawara M. J Biochem 1986; 99: 1807-10.
23. Bancher C et al. Brain Res 1989; 477: 90-9.
24. Mattson MP, Rychlik B. Brain Res 1990; 522: 204-14.
25. Mattson MP, Engle MG, Rychlik B. Neurobiol Aging (submitted for publication).
26. Wolozin BL, Pruchnicki A, Dickson DW, Davies P. Science 1986; 232: 648-50.
27. Nukina N, Kosik KS, Selkoe DJ. Neurosci Lett 1988; 87: 240-6.
28. Mattson MP, Exp Neurol (in press).
29. Baudier J, Cole RD. J Biol Chem 1987; 36: 17577-83.
30. McKee AC, Kosik KS, Kennedy MB, Kowall NW. J Neuropath Exp Neurol 1990; 49: 49-63.
31. Louis J-C, Magal E, Yavin E. J Biol Chem 1988; 263: 19282-5.
32. Joo F, Tosaki A, Olah Z, Koltai M. Brain Res 1989; 490: 141-3.
33. Rothman SM, Olney JW. Ann Neurol 1986; 19: 105-11.
34. Greenamyre JT, Young AB. Neurobiol Aging 1989; 10: 593-602.
35. Mattson MP, Guthrie PB, Hayes BC, Kater SB. J Neurosci 1989; 9: 1223-32.
36. Nicoletti F, Meek JL, Iadarola MJ, Chuang DM, Roth BL, Costa E. J Neurosci 1986; 46: 40-6.
37. Mattson MP. Neuron 1990; 4: 105-17.
38. DeBoni U, Crapper-McLachlan DR. J Neurol Sci 1985; 68: 105-18.
39. Alzheimer A. Ges Neurol Psych 1911; 4: 356-85.

Address for correspondence:

Dr M. P. Mattson,
Sanders-Brown Research Center on Aging,
University of Kentucky,
Lexington, KY 40536-0230, USA

23 Post-Translational Modifications of a Tau-Related Protein Present in Paired Helical Filaments

I. CORREAS, J. DÍAZ-NIDO AND J. AVILA

Senile dementia of Alzheimer type is a neurodegenerative disease of unknown etiology which affects several neuronal populations in the central nervous system. Two types of aberrant structures—senile plaques and neurofibrillary tangles—appearing within the brains of the patients serve as histopathological hallmarks of the disease. Senile plaques are made up of extracellular amyloid deposits. Neurofibrillary tangles are derived from intraneuronal inclusions, constituted by the aggregation of paired helical filaments (PHFs), which become eventually located extracellularly upon neuronal death. Studies on the composition of both types of structures suggest that their major constituents may correspond to abnormally processed neuronal proteins. The major component of amyloid seems to be a fragment of an integral membrane protein which usually interacts with the extracellular matrix (1). On the other hand, PHFs appear to contain as a major component a protein which has been identified as a modified form of the microtubule-associated tau protein (2-7).

We have focused our attention on the modifications affecting tau protein. The binding of tau protein to tubulin seems to stabilize neuronal microtubules (8,9); however, tau phosphorylation by different protein kinases reduces its binding to tubulin (10,11) and also may modulate its sorting between the somatodendritic and the axonal compartments of nerve cells (12-14). It remains to be established whether or not such modifications play a role in the association of tau with PHFs within the neuron, although the presence of hyperphosphorylated forms of tau in Alzheimer's disease supports this view (15-17). A proper understanding of this question requires a detailed knowledge of the main features of tau phosphorylation both in vitro and in vivo under normal and pathological conditions. Previous analyses have already been carried out on the phosphorylation of tau protein by cAMP-dependent protein kinase, Ca^{2+}/calmodulin-dependent protein kinase and protein kinase C (10,11,18-23). Now we have further analyzed the in vitro phosphorylation of microtubule-associated tau protein by these protein kinases as well as by casein-kinase II and compared it with the phosphorylation of a tau-related protein present in Alzheimer's PHF fractions.

Alzheimer's Disease: Basic Mechanisms, Diagnosis and Therapeutic Strategies
Edited by K. Iqbal, D. R. C. McLachlan, B. Winblad and H. M. Wisniewski
© 1991 John Wiley & Sons Ltd

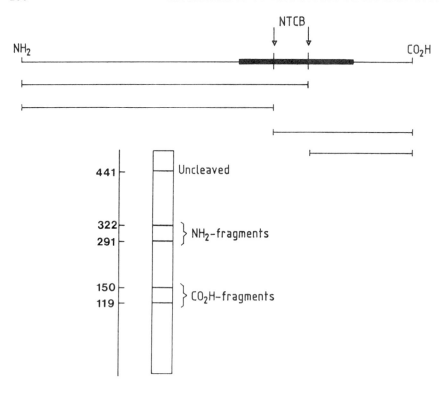

Figure 1. Schematic representation of human tau protein cleaved with NTCB. Arrows indicate NTCB cleavage sites at Cys residues on tau molecule. Numbers represent amino acid residues corresponding to the uncleaved protein and to the amino-terminal and carboxy-terminal fragments of tau. Lane represents an SDS polyacrylamide gel electrophoresis of NTCB-treated tau protein

STUDIES ON THE IN-VITRO PHOSPHORYLATION OF MICROTUBULE-ASSOCIATED TAU PROTEIN

Tau protein isolated from bovine or rat brain microtubules (24) was used as substrate for the different kinases. Sequences of cDNAs isolated from different sources have revealed the existence of several isoforms of tau sharing a main feature: the presence of three or four repetitive motifs containing one or two cysteines, respectively (4,25). Thus, treatment of tau with 2-nitro-5-thiocyanobenzoic acid (NTCB), a chemical reagent which cleaves at cysteine residues, splits the molecule into two halves: one containing the amino-terminal fragment and the other one containing the carboxy-terminal fragment (Figure 1). This allows the localization of the tau regions which are phosphorylated in vitro by different kinases upon cleaving phosphorylated tau molecules with NTCB. Here we will focus on the phosphorylation of one tau polypeptide. The results obtained for other tau polypeptides are identical. However, different tau polypeptides render one or two amino-terminal phosphorylated

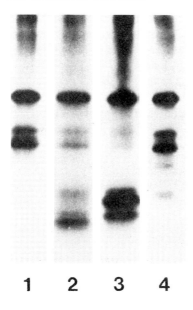

1   2   3   4

Figure 2. NTCB phosphopeptide patterns of microtubule-associated tau protein phosphorylated in vitro by cAMP-dependent protein kinase (lane 1), protein kinase C (lane 2), Ca^{2+}/calmodulin-dependent protein kinase (lane 3) and casein-kinase II (lane 4)

fragments. This may be explained by the presence of one or two cysteines in the molecule.

The first enzyme assayed in this study was the cAMP-dependent protein kinase. This protein kinase has been found associated with microtubules (26,27), and the association appears to be mediated by the microtubule-associated protein MAP2 (27). Our results indicate (Figure 2, lane 1) that phosphorylation of tau by cAMP-dependent protein kinase takes place at the amino-terminal region of the tau molecule. The second kinase assayed in this study was the protein kinase C. There is no evidence for an association between this protein kinase and microtubules; however, due to the possible role of calcium in different aspects of neural regulation, the implication of this kinase in tau phosphorylation has been previously analyzed (22). We have found that the phosphorylation of tau by this kinase occurs at both halves of the molecule, as indicated in Figure 2 (lane 2). Third, we have assayed tau phosphorylation by Ca^{2+}/calmodulin-dependent protein kinase. This kinase has been found associated to microtubules (28) and phosphorylation of tau by this enzyme results in a decrease in its electrophoretic mobility (21). This could be correlated with the presence of hyperphosphorylated forms of tau with decreased electrophoretic mobilities in brain extracts of patients with Alzheimer's disease (AD) (15–17,21). Phosphorylation of tau by Ca^{2+}/calmodulin-dependent protein kinase takes place at the carboxy-terminal half of the tau molecule. Slower migration of the C-terminal phosphorylated peptides was observed (Figure 2, lane 3), a similar shift to that described for the intact phosphorylated tau protein (21). Finally, we have studied the phosphorylation of tau by casein-kinase II, since this kinase has also been found associated with microtubules (29). Casein-kinase II phosphorylates tau at the amino-terminal half of the molecule (Figure 2, lane 4).

All these results allow us to distinguish phosphorylation of tau by different protein kinases, except for the cases of casein-kinase II and cAMP-dependent protein kinase since both of them phosphorylate tau at the amino-terminal half of the molecule. It is interesting to note that only those kinases which depend on calcium ions phosphorylate the carboxy-terminal region of tau protein.

STUDIES ON THE PHOSPHORYLATION OF A TAU-RELATED PROTEIN PRESENT IN ALZHEIMER'S PHF FRACTIONS

The mechanisms leading to PHF formation in AD remain unknown. We have found that a 33-kDa tau-related protein is one of the main components of PHF preparations isolated from brains of Alzheimer's disease patients (7). Amino-terminal sequencing of this protein (Nieto et al, submitted for publication) indicates that its first residue corresponds to amino acid 71 of the human tau sequence (4). Interestingly, this region corresponds to a possible cleavage site for calpain. Calpain is a Ca^{2+}-activated protease which is present in high concentrations in brain and degrades some cytoskeletal proteins (30,31), including tau protein (32). The preferred substrates for calpain are those calmodulin-binding proteins containing sequences enriched

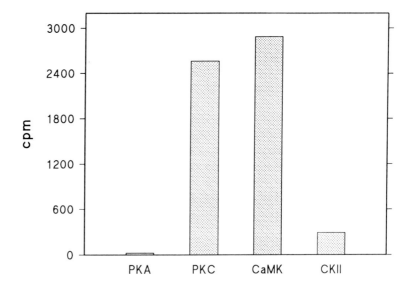

Figure 3. Quantitation of phosphate incorporation into 33-kDa tau-related protein present in PHFs phosphorylated in vitro by different kinases. The following kinases were assayed: cAMP-dependent protein kinase (PKA), protein kinase C (PKC), Ca^{2+}/calmodulin-dependent protein kinase (CaMK) and casein-kinase II (CKII)

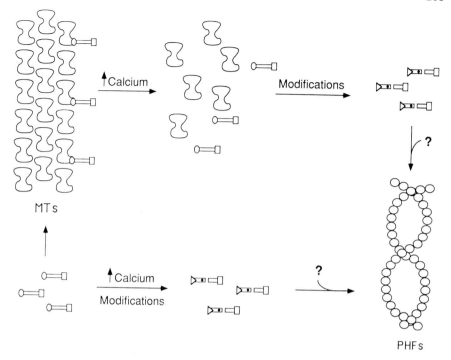

Figure 4. Proposed mechanism for tau incorporation into PHFs in Alzheimer's disease. Tau protein is normally bound to microtubules (MTs). Increased levels of intraneuronal calcium ions induce microtubule depolymerization. Unbound tau could be phosphorylated by Ca^{2+}-dependent protein kinases and proteolyzed by Ca^{2+}-dependent proteases. The resulting modified tau could then be accumulated into PHFs. Question mark indicates other possible still-unknown modifications of tau or binding to other components

in proline, glutamic acid, serine and threonine residues which are flanked by basic residues (the so-called PEST regions) (33). The presence of these high-affinity recognition sites for calpain in the tau molecule (33) together with the existence of a cleavage site at amino acid 70 supports the notion that the 33-kDa tau-related protein present in PHF fractions could be generated upon calpain proteolysis. Furthermore, it has previously been reported that tau cleavage by calpain originates a resistant fragment of approximately this size (32). The fact that tau protein isolated from Alzheimer's disease patient brain microtubules is mainly intact whereas the PHF-associated 33-kDa tau-related protein is proteolyzed (34) argues against a nonspecific postmortem degradation, thus suggesting that calpain proteolysis of tau protein may be a prior step to PHF formation.

We have analyzed whether or not the 33-kDa tau-related protein is post-translationally modified by phosphorylation. The same exogenous kinases used for the study of tau phosphorylation have been assayed with the 33-kDa tau-related protein. Interestingly, the 33-kDa tau-related protein is susceptible of phosphorylation preferentially by Ca^{2+}/calmodulin-dependent protein kinase and by protein kinase

C (Figure 3), the two kinases whose activation is Ca^{2+}-dependent and that mainly phosphorylate the carboxy-terminal regions of tau molecules.

In view of these data, we propose a hypothetical model to explain the origin of the 33-kDa tau-related protein in AD pathology and its implication in PHF formation (Figure 4). Under physiological conditions, tau protein would become associated with tubulin and sorted into axonal microtubules. Under pathological conditions, an increase in the intracellular levels of calcium ions, possibly due to imbalance in glutamate neurotransmission (35), could induce calpain to cleave tau protein. On the other hand, Ca^{2+}/calmodulin-dependent protein kinase, highly enriched in hippocampal neurons (36), and protein kinase C could phosphorylate the calpain-resistant tau proteolytic fragment. Also, the tubulin-binding domain of tau may be further modified to completely prevent associations between tubulin and modified tau. Modified tau could self-assemble or co-assemble with still unknown components to accumulate into PHFs within the somatodendritic compartment of pathological nerve cells. Further studies are required to completely characterize all the possible post-translational modifications of tau protein in AD as well as their influence in both cytoskeleton disruption and PHF formation.

Acknowledgments

We greatly appeciate Dr P.J. González and Dr M. García-Rocha for providing us with PHF preparations and Ca^{2+}/calmodulin-dependent protein kinase, respectively. We also acknowledge Dr A. Nieto and Dr J.E. Domínguez for their valuable comments on various aspects of this work.

REFERENCES

1. Schubert D, Schroeder R, La Corbiere M, Saitoh T, Cole G, Science 1988; 241: 223–6.
2. Grundke-Iqbal I, Iqbal K, Quinlan M, Tung YC, Zaidi MS, Wisniewski HM. J Biol Chem 1986; 261: 6084–9.
3. Wischik CM, Novak M, Edwards PC, Klug A, Tichelaar W, Crowther RA. Proc Natl Acad Sci USA 1988; 85: 4884–8.
4. Goedert M, Wischik CM, Crowther RA, Walker JE, Klug A. Proc Natl Acad Sci USA 1988; 85: 4051–5.
5. Kosik KS, Joachim CL, Selkoe DJ. Proc Natl Acad Sci USA 1986; 83: 4044–8.
6. Nukina N, Ihara Y. J Biochem 1986; 99: 1541–4.
7. Nieto A, Correas I, Montejo E, Avila J. Biochem Biophys Res Comm 1988; 154: 660–7.
8. Drubin DG, Kirschner MW. J Cell Biol 1986; 103: 2739–46.
9. Kanai Y, Takemura R, Oshima T, Mori H, Ihara Y, Yanagisawa M, Masaki T, Hirokawa N. J Cell Biol 1989; 109: 1173–84.
10. Lindwall G, Cole RD. J Biol Chem 1984; 259: 5301–5.
11. Yamamoto H, Fukunaga K, Tanaka E, Miyamoto E. J Neurochem 1983; 41: 1119–25.
12. Binder LI, Frankfurter A, Rehbum LI. J Cell Biol 1985; 101: 1371–8.
13. Papasozomenos SC, Binder LI. Cell Motil Cytoskel 1987; 8: 210–6.
14. Kosik KS. Curr Op Cell Biol 1990; 2: 101–4.
15. Flament S, Delacourte A. FEBS Lett. 1989; 2: 213–16.
16. Grundke-Iqbal I, Iqbal K, Tung YC, Quinlan M, Wisniewski HM, Binder LI. Proc Natl Acad Sci USA 1986; 83: 4913–17.
17. Ihara Y, Nukina N, Miura R, Ogawara M. J Biochem 1986; 99: 1807–10.

18. Lindwall G, Cole RD. J Biol Chem 1984; 259: 12241-5.
19. Pierre M, Nunez J. Biochem Biophys Res Comm 1983; 115: 212-19.
20. Butler M, Shelanski ML. J Neurochem 1986; 47: 1517-22.
21. Baudier J, Cole RD. J Biol Chem 1987; 262: 17577-83.
22. Baudier J, Lee SH, Cole RD. J Biol Chem 1987; 262: 17584-90.
23. Ishiguro K, Ihara Y, Uchida T, Imahori K. J Biochem 1988; 104: 319-21.
24. Herzog W, Weber K. Eur J Biochem 1978; 92: 1-8.
25. Goedert M, Spillantini MG, Potier MC, Ulrich J, Crowther RA. EMBO J 1989; 8: 393-9.
26. Sloboda RD, Rudolph SA, Rosenbaum JL, Greengard P. Proc Natl Acad Sci USA 1975; 72: 177-81.
27. Theurkauf WE, Vallee RB. J Biol Chem 1983; 258: 7883-6.
28. Larson RE, Goldering JR, Vallano ML, DeLorenzo RJ. J Neurochem 1985; 44 1566-72.
29. Serrano L, Hernandez MA, Díaz-Nido J, Avila J. Exp Cell Res 1989; 181: 263-72.
30. Nixon RA, Brown BA, Marotta CA. Brain Res 1983; 275: 384-8.
31. Malik MN, Sheikh AM, Fenko MD, Wisniewski HM. Life Sci 1986; 29: 1335-43.
32. Johnson GVW, Jope RS, Binder LI. Biochem Biophys Res Comm 1989; 163: 1505-11.
33. Wang KKW, Villalobo A, Roufogalis BD. Biochem J 1989; 262: 693-706.
34. Nieto A, Montejo de Garcini E, Correas I, Avila J. Neuroscience 1990; 37: 163-70.
35. Mattson MP. Neuron 1990; 2: 105-17.
36. McKee AC, Kosik KS, Kennedy MB, Kowall NW. J Neuropath Exp Neurol 1990; 49: 49-63.

Address for correspondence:

Dr I. Correas,
Centro de Biología Molecular,
Universidad Autónoma, Cantoblanco,
28049 Madrid, Spain

24 Indiana Kindred of Gerstmann-Sträussler-Scheinker Disease: Neurofibrillary Tangles and Neurites of Plaques with PrP Amyloid Share Antigenic Determinants with Those of Alzheimer's Disease

GIORGIO GIACCONE, FABRIZIO TAGLIAVINI, LAURA VERGA,
BLAS FRANGIONE, MARTIN R. FARLOW, ORSO BUGIANI
AND BERNARDINO GHETTI

Gerstmann-Sträussler-Scheinker (GSS) disease is an hereditary disorder clinically characterized by ataxia, pyramidal signs and dementia, and neuropathologically by the presence of amyloid deposits in the brain parenchyma (1,2). The amyloid of GSS disease does not immunoreact with antibodies against the β-protein of Alzheimer's disease (AD), whereas it is immunoreactive to antisera against the PrP protein 27-30 (3,4), a structural component of the scrapie-associated fibrils (5).

An Indiana family of GSS disease has been previously described (6,7). In four patients studied neuropathologically, neurofibrillary tangles (NFT) composed of paired helical filaments (PHF) were numerous, widespread, and consistently present in the cerebral cortex and several subcortical structures (4). Amyloid plaques immunoreactive with anti-PrP antibodies are present in the cerebrum and cerebellum. Furthermore, many of the plaques showed a prominent neuritic component. In view of the fact that anti-PrP immunoreactive amyloid plaques and NFT with PHF coexist, the disease of the Indiana kindred appears to be an atypical form of GSS disease, at least from the neuropathological standpoint. This contention is also supported by recent molecular genetic data. In fact, unlike other cases of GSS disease, where sequencing of the PrP gene open-reading-frame (ORF) have shown mutations (8), the PrP gene ORF in three patients of the Indiana kindred revealed no mutation (9,10).

NFT of AD are recognized by antibodies against tau (11-13), MAP2 (14), neurofilament proteins (15), ubiquitin (16,17) and by Alz-50, a monoclonal antibody which recognizes a 68-kDa protein present in large amounts in AD brains (18).

Alzheimer's Disease: Basic Mechanisms, Diagnosis and Therapeutic Strategies
Edited by K. Iqbal, D. R. C. McLachlan, B. Winblad and H. M. Wisniewski
© 1991 John Wiley & Sons Ltd

In addition to NFT, these antibodies stain the neuritic component of senile plaques; anti-tau and Alz-50 antibodies also detect numerous, short, slightly thickened neurites randomly dispersed in the cortical neuropil, i.e. neuropil threads (19–21).

Since the antigenic profile of the NFT found in the affected members of the Indiana kindred has not been established, the aims of the present study were to determine whether (a) antibodies known to recognize the NFT of AD also label the NFT in this atypical form of GSS disease and (b) the NFT in this Indiana kindred are associated with more diffuse cytoskeletal changes.

Blocks of frontal and temporal lobes, basal forebrain, brainstem and cerebellum were obtained from two patients of the Indiana kindred of GSS disease (ages at death 49 and 58 years), from three patients with sporadic AD (ages at death 63, 69 and 75 years) and from one patient with familial AD (age at death 40 years). The specimens were fixed in 4% formaldehyde and embedded in Paraplast. Serial 7-μm thick sections were stained with haematoxylin-eosin, thioflavine S, and silver salts (Bodian's and Gallyas' methods). Adjacent sections were immunostained with Alz-50 (1:10), with a monoclonal antibody to ubiquitin (1:200, Chemicon), and with rabbit polyclonal antibodies to PrP 27-30 purified from scrapie-infected hamster brain (1:100) (22), to a 28-residue synthetic peptide homologous to the NH$_2$-terminal region of the β-protein (1:50) (23), to PHF isolated from AD brains (1:100) (24). Before anti-PrP, anti-β-protein and anti-PHF immunohistochemistry, the sections were treated with 98% formic acid for 30 min (3). Since the anti-PHF antiserum immunoreacted with tau (B. Frangione, unpublished observation), additional sections were incubated with anti-PHF antiserum absorbed with tau. For immunodetection the peroxidase-antiperoxidase (PAP) method was used, with rabbit antimouse immunoglobulins and monoclonal mouse PAP complex (Dako, Denmark) for Alz-50 and antiubiquitin antibodies; as well as swine antirabbit immunoglobulins and rabbit PAP complex (Dako, Denmark) for the polyclonal antibodies. Peroxidase substrates were 3,3'-diaminobenzidine (DAB) and 0.015% H$_2$O$_2$. Double immunohistochemical labeling of the neuritic plaques was carried out using anti-PrP or anti-SP28 antibodies for the demonstration of the amyloid and Alz-50 antibodies for the demonstration of the neuritic component. The demonstration of anti-PrP or anti-SP28 antibodies by the PAP method with DAB as chromogen was followed by the demonstration of Alz-50 immunoreactivity with biotinyl-antimouse serum (Amersham, 1:200), streptavidin-biotinylated alkaline phosphatase complex (Amersham, 1:100) and naphthol-AS-MX-phosphate/fast blue BB salt/levamisole as chromogen. The immunocytochemical controls were done using nonimmune IgG mouse and rabbit sera as primary antibodies.

In the GSS patients of the Indiana kindred, PrP-positive, β-protein immunonegative amyloid deposits were distributed in most regions of the cerebrum, cerebellum, midbrain and pons. In the cerebral cortex and the hippocampus, numerous amyloid deposits were surrounded by dystrophic neurites. NFT were abundant in the cingulate gyrus, insular cortex, parahippocampal gyrus, hippocampus, basal nucleus of Meynert, substantia nigra and periaqueductal gray (4).

In the patients with GSS disease a large number of nerve cell bodies were strongly immunolabeled by Alz-50 and two patterns of perikaryal staining were

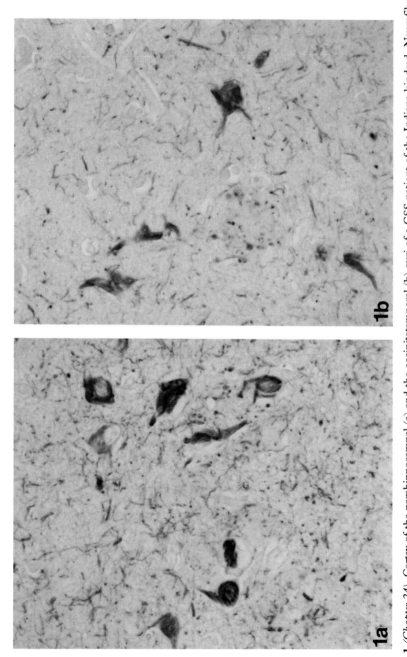

Figure 1 (*Chapter 24*). Cortex of the parahippocampal (a) and the occipitotemporal (b) gyri of a GSS patient of the Indiana kindred. Neurofibrillary tangles and neuropil threads are immunolabeled by Alz-50 (a,b) (×450)

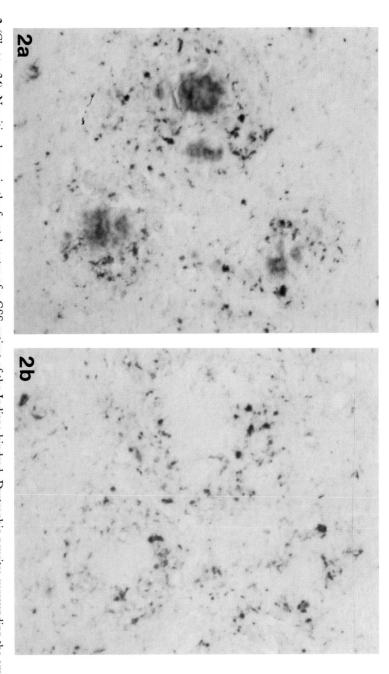

Figure 2 (*Chapter 24*). Neuritic plaques in the frontal cortex of a GSS patient of the Indiana kindred. Dystrophic neurites surrounding the amyloid deposits are immunolabeled by Alz-50 (a,b). The amyloid cores are immunoreactive to antisera against the PrP protein (a) and not to antisera against the β-protein (b) (×450)

recognized. In most labeled neurons the reaction product was circumscribed in a portion of the cytoplasm and showed a globular or flame-shaped fibrillary appearance (Figure 1, see colour plate). In adjacent sections, stained with thioflavine S, Bodian or Gallyas, cytoplasmic areas of similar shape were found to contain NFT. On the other hand, in a few neurons the cytoplasm was diffusely immunolabeled; however, in adjacent sections, stained with thioflavine S, Bodian or Gallyas, such cells failed to show NFT.

Anti-PHF, anti-PHF absorbed with tau and antiubiquitin antibodies also immunostained NFT in the GSS patients; however, the NFT recognized with these antibodies were fewer than those labeled by Alz-50 and their labeling was less intense.

All these antibodies revealed the neuritic component of the plaques present in the cerebral hemispheres (Figure 2, see colour plate). Moreover, Alz-50 labeled numerous neuropil structures, most probably processes of neuronal origin, scattered throughout the cerebral cortex. These neuropil threads were not spatially associated with plaques or tangles, and were particularly abundant in the parahippocampal gyrus (Figure 1a). Double anti-PrP/Alz-50 and anti-SP28/Alz-50 immunohisto-chemical staining clearly demonstrated that anti-PrP positive and anti-SP28 negative amyloid deposits in the cerebral cortex were surrounded by Alz-50 positive dystrophic neurites (Figure 2). With regard to the cerebellum, no immunolabeling with Alz-50 and anti-PHF antibodies was detected around the amyloid deposits.

In AD patients, Alz-50, anti-PHF and antiubiquitin antibodies decorated NFT and the enlarged neurites around senile plaques. As observed in the GSS patients, Alz-50 revealed the greatest number of NFT and, in addition, labeled some neurons without NFT as well as numerous neuropil threads.

This study shows that neurofibrillary tangles of GSS patients of the Indiana kindred share antigenic determinants with those of AD, being recognized by Alz-50, by an antiserum raised against PHF isolated from AD brains (either with or without absorption with tau protein) and by an antiubiquitin antibody. NFT are also selectively stained by Gallyas' silver impregnation technique, a method known to detect structures containing tau (25). This finding is consistent with a previous observation that anti-tau antibodies labeled NFT in one case of GSS disease (26).

Alz-50 is, at present, one of the most effective antibodies recognizing cytoskeletal changes in AD and other neurodegenerative disorders. In Alzheimer brains, it labels not only the NFT and the neuritic component of senile plaques, but also neuropil threads and neurons considered to be at an early stage of NFT formation (18,21,27). On the other hand, Alz-50 decorates NFT of Guam parkinsonism dementia complex (21,28) as well as Pick bodies (28) and NFT composed of straight filaments in progressive supranuclear palsy (27).

Nukina and co-workers have shown that Alz-50 recognizes both phosphorylated and dephosphorylated forms of rat and normal human tau proteins (29). These authors speculated that the proteins detected in increased amount in AD brains by Alz-50 are modified and/or aggregated forms of tau, and that in AD tau undergoes post-translational modifications important in the genesis of PHF.

To our knowledge, this GSS family represents the first instance of the coexistence of NFT and neuritic plaques with PrP amyloid. The chemical composition of NFT of patients of the Indiana kindred needs to be further investigated. The composition of NFT of AD is not completely known; in particular it is still debated whether β-protein is a constituent of PHF (30). The fact that, in patients of the Indiana kindred, NFT indistinguishable from those of AD are present does not necessarily mean that their chemical composition is identical to that of the tangles seen in AD.

Another abnormality, evidenced by Alz-50 in GSS brains, consisted of short, randomly oriented neurites dispersed in the cortical neuropil. They were indistinguishable from the neuropil threads of AD, decorated by Gallyas' silver method (19), and by anti-tau (20) and Alz-50 antibodies (21). Wolozin and Davies (21) reported that the extensive staining of neuropil threads was the most characteristic feature of Alz-50 immunohistochemistry in AD, since this abnormality was not observed in other disorders such as Guam parkinsonism dementia complex, progressive supranuclear palsy or Pick's disease, in spite of the presence of Alz-50 positive perikaryal inclusions.

The finding of antigenically identical neuropil threads in AD and GSS disease leads us to speculate that this diffusely distributed abnormality of neurites might be related to widespread amyloid deposition in the cortical neuropil, regardless of the chemical composition of amyloid.

Acknowledgment

The authors are grateful to Dr Paul Brown (Laboratory of Central Nervous System Studies, NINDS, NIH, Bethesda, MD) for providing antisera against the PrP protein.

REFERENCES

1. Gerstmann J, Sträussler E, Scheinker I. Z Ges Neurol Psychiatr 1936; 154: 736-62.
2. Masters CL, Gajdusek DC, Gibbs CJ Jr. Brain 1981; 104: 559-88.
3. Kitamoto T, Ogomori K, Tateishi J, Prusiner SB. Lab Invest 1987; 57: 230-6.
4. Ghetti B, Tagliavini F, Masters CL, Beyreuther K, Giaccone G, Verga L, Farlow MR, Conneally PM, Dlouhy SR, Azzarelli B, Bugiani O. Neurology 1989; 39: 1453-61.
5. Prusiner SB, McKinley MP, Bowman KA, Bolton DC, Bendheim PE, Groth DF, Glenner GG. Cell 1983; 35: 349-58.
6. Azzarelli B, Muller J, Ghetti B, Dyken M, Conneally PM. Acta Neuropathol 1985; 65: 235-46.
7. Farlow MR, Yee RD, Dlouhy SR, Conneally PM, Azzarelli B, Ghetti B. Neurology 1989; 39: 1446-52.
8. Hsiao K, Baker HF, Crow TJ, Poulter M, Owen F, Terwilliger JD, Westaway D, Ott J, Prusiner SB. Nature 1989; 338: 342-5.
9. Hsiao K, Cass C, Conneally PM, Dlouhy SR, Hodes ME, Farlow MR, Ghetti B, Prusiner SB, Neurobiol Aging 1990; 11: 302.
10. Hsiao K, Cass C, Conneally PM, Dlouhy SR, Hodes ME, Farlow MR, Ghetti B, Prusiner SB (in preparation).
11. Brion JP, Passareiro H, Nunez J, Flament-Durand J. Arch Biol 1985; 95: 229-35.
12. Grundke-Iqbal I, Iqbal K, Tung Y-C, Quinlan M, Wisniewski HM, Binder LI. Proc Natl Acad Sci USA 1986; 83: 4913-17.
13. Kosik KS, Joachim CL, Selkoe DJ. Proc Natl Acad Sci USA 1986; 83: 4044-8.

14. Kosik KS, Duffy LK, Dowling MM, Abraham C, McCluskey A, Selkoe DJ. Proc Natl Acad Sci USA 1984; 81: 7941-5.
15. Gambetti P, Schecket G, Ghetti B, Hirano A, Dahl D. J Neuropath Exp Neurol 1983; 42: 69-79.
16. Manetto V, Perry G, Tabaton M, Mulvihill P, Fried VA, Smith HT, Gambetti P, Autilio-Gambetti L. Proc Natl Acad Sci USA 1988; 85: 4501-5.
17. Mori H, Kondo J, Ihara Y. Science 1987; 235: 1641-4.
18. Wolozin BL, Pruchnicki A, Dickson DW, Davies P. Science 1986; 232: 648-50.
19. Braak H, Braak E, Grundke-Iqbal I, Iqbal K. Neurosci Lett 1986; 65: 351-5.
20. Joachim CL, Morris JH, Selkoe DJ, Kosik KS. J Neuropath Exp Neurol 1987; 46: 611-22.
21. Wolozin B, Davies P. Ann Neurol 1987; 22: 521-6.
22. Bendheim PE, Barry RA, DeArmond SJ, Stites DP, Prusiner SB. Nature 1984; 310: 418-21.
23. Castaño EN, Ghiso J, Prelli F, Gorevic PD, Migheli A, Frangione B. Biochem Biophys Res Comm 1986; 141: 782-9.
24. Gorevic PD, Goni F, Pons-Estel B, Alvarez F, Peress NS, Frangione B. J Neuropath Exp Neurol 1986; 45: 647-64.
25. Iqbal K, Grundke-Iqbal I, Wisniewski HM. J Neuropath Exp Neurol 1987; 46: 333.
26. Joachim CL, Morris JH, Kosik KS, Selkoe DJ. Ann Neurol 1987; 22: 514-20.
27. Tabaton M, Whitehouse PJ, Perry G, Davies P, Autilio-Gambetti L, Gambetti P. Ann Neurol 1988; 24: 407-13.
28. Love S, Saitoh T, Quijada S, Cole GM, Terry RD. J Neuropath Exp Neurol 1988; 47: 393-405.
29. Nukina N, Kosik KS, Selkoe DJ. Neurosci Lett 1988; 87: 240-6.
30. Selkoe DJ. Neurobiol Aging 1989; 10: 387-95.

Address for correspondence:

Dr Bernardino Ghetti,
Department of Pathology,
Indiana University School of Medicine,
635 Barnhill Drive,
Indianapolis, IN 46202-5120, USA

25 Aberrant Neurofilament Phosphorylation Produced in Neuronal Degeneration by a Glutamate Agonist

J. HUGON, J. M. VALLAT, P. SINDOU,
C. YARDIN AND P. COURATIER

Kainic acid is an excitatory amino acid agonist which produces neuronal degeneration, after systemic or intracerebral injection in experimental animals (1). When kainic acid is intrathecally injected in rats, it induces acute and delayed neuronal changes; the latter is essentially characterized by a 'chromatolytic'-like aspect of neuronal cells with eccentric nucleus, swollen cytoplasm, progressive accumulations of neurofilaments and lipid vacuolizations (2). These pathological storages of cytoskeletal components are diffuse in the cytoplasm or can take the form of a round neurofilament inclusion surrounded by a peripheral membrane. Accumulations of neurofilaments or their immunoreactive products are observed in various neuropathological lesions of degenerative disorders: neurofibrillary tangles in Alzheimer's disease (3), Lewy bodies in Parkinson's disease (4), Pick bodies (5), abnormal motoneurons and axonal spheroids in amyotrophic lateral sclerosis (6,7). These neurofilament inclusions react to antibodies which recognize phosphorylated epitopes. The goal of this study is to determine the antigenicity of the cytoskeletal anomalies produced in neurons by kainic acid after intrathecal administration.

Several lines of evidence are consistent with the involvement of the excitatory amino acid neurotransmitters aspartate and glutamate in the degeneration of selective areas of the central nervous system. Abnormal glutamate metabolism has been reported in patients with amyotrophic lateral sclerosis (8). Cellular glutamate dehydrogenase activity was found to be decreased in those patients also (9). Excitatory amino acids of exogenous or endogenous origin have also been implicated in the pathogenesis of Huntington's disease (10,11), Alzheimer's disease (12), status epilepticus (13), stroke (14) and Guam amyotrophic lateral sclerosis–Parkinsonism dementia complex (15).

MATERIAL AND METHODS

Male Wistar rats (200–250 g body weight) were divided into two groups: isotonic saline injected rats ($n=12$) and kainic acid injected rats ($n=12$). The animals were

Alzheimer's Disease: Basic Mechanisms, Diagnosis and Therapeutic Strategies
Edited by K. Iqbal, D. R. C. McLachlan, B. Winblad and H. M. Wisniewski
© 1991 John Wiley & Sons Ltd

anesthetized with barbitone sodium (30 mg/kg IP) and intrathecally injected in the lumbar region with 20 μl of a sterile aqueous solution of isotonic saline alone or containing kainic acid (10^{-4} mol). A 26/0 needle with a hand-held microsyringe was inserted between the L4 and L5 vertebrae. Two hours, 1, 3, 6, 10 and 14 days after injections animals were reanesthetized and systematically perfused via the aortic arch with fixative chemicals. The lumbar spinal cord was excised and prepared for histological procedures.

Semithin sections and electron microscopy

Animals were perfused with 4% paraformaldehyde (30 s) followed by 5% glutaraldehyde (10 min). Sections of the spinal cord were post-fixed in 2% Dalton's chrome osmium solution, dehydrated stepwise and infiltrated with expoxy resin. Semithin and ultrathin sections were prepared from selected blocks.

Light microscopic immunohistochemistry

Animals were perfused with a mixture containing 4% paraformaldehyde and 0.3% glutaraldehyde. Sections of the lumbar cord 40 μm thick were cut on a Vibratome and processed for immunocytochemistry.

For 1 μm-thick cryosections, the tissue was cryoprotected with 2.3 M sucrose and 30% polyvinyl pyrrolidine. The tissue pieces were mounted on specimen stubs, frozen in liquid nitrogen and cut at $-75°C$ with an ultracryomicrotome. Cryosections were mounted on polylysine-coated glass slides rinsed in PBS and processed for immunocytochemistry.

Immunostaining was carried out using a monoclonal antibody (Amersham) against 200-kDa phosphorylated neurofilaments by the peroxidase-antiperoxidase procedure. Cerebellar sections of normal rats were utilized as positive controls.

RESULTS

Intrathecal injections of kainic acid in rats immediately produced spasms of the tail and hind limbs for a period of 1–2 hours. In the following days 50% of the rats displayed a paraplegia with definitive bilateral spastic extension.

On light microscopic examination the lumbar spinal cord of saline-injected animals did not reveal abnormal neuropathological features. In kainic-acid injected rats striking morphological changes were observed. Early changes (2 and 24 hours) were predominantly located in the grey matter of the ventral horns. The perikarya of neurons were shrunken and hyperchromatic, or swollen and vacuolated. The oedema of the neuropil was quite constant. Delayed changed occurred 3 to 14 days after injection. At 3 days many neurons of the ventral horns had a condensed and vacuolated cytoplasm with displacement of the nuclei and dispersion of Nissl bodies. Fourteen days after injection affected neurons had a chromatolytic aspect with diffuse round inclusions of lipids. Proximal enlargements of axons were seen randomly dispersed in the dorsal and ventral horns of the spinal cord. Accumulations of

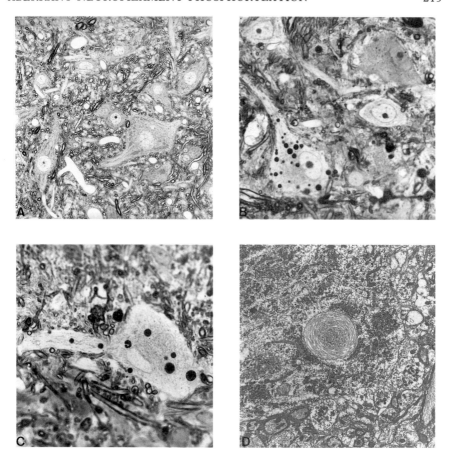

Figure 1. Lumbar spinal cord. (A) Saline-injected rat: absence of morphological lesions (×340). (B) Kainic acid-injected rat (10 days): spinal neurons with eccentric nucleus and round lipid accumulations (×860). (C) Kainic acid-injected rat (10 days): this affected neuron displays a proximal neurite enlargement (×900). (D) Kainic acid-injected rat (10 days) electron micrograph: cytoplasmic filament inclusion surrounded by a membrane (×5000)

neurofilaments were observed in degenerating neurons, either scattered in the cytoplasm or surrounded by a membrane (Figure 1).

Immunohistochemical studies were carried out 2 and 10 days after intrathecal injections. In saline-injected rats, immunolabelling of phosphorylated neurofilaments was observed in axons of the white and grey matter, and in small dorsal horn neurons. Ventral horn neurons of all sizes were mostly not marked. A morphometric study revealed that 12.0±0.9% of ventral horn neurons were immunostained.

In kainic acid-injected rats, similar features were observed accompanied by an intense labelling of ventral horn neurons. The percentage of positive ventral horn neurons was maximal (82.3±6.8%) 2 days after kainic acid administration. At 10 days, the value was 68.3±7.2%. The immunolabelling was mostly spread in the

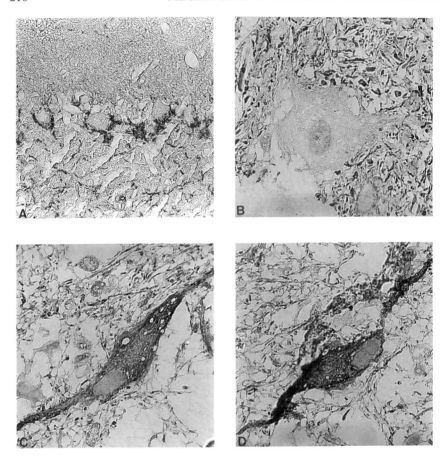

Figure 2. (A) Saline-injected rat cerebellum (Vibratome sections): positive staining observed in basket cell fibres (×270). (B) Saline-injected rat lumbar spinal cord 1-μm cryosections: absence of cytoplasmic labelling of spinal neurons (×900). (C,D) Kainic acid-injected rat lumbar spinal cord 1-μm cryosections, two sections of the same neuron: intense immunostaining of the cytoplasm and proximal neurites (200-kDa phosphorylated neurofilaments) (×860)

cytoplasm of degenerating neurons and was often but not constantly associated with the chromatolytic aspect of the cells (Figure 2).

DISCUSSION

These findings suggest that delayed neuronal damage due to the cytotoxic action of a glutamate receptor agonist, kainic acid, is associated with the presence of an abnormal distribution of phosphorylated neurofilaments within the cytoplasm. Additionally abnormal accumulation of phosphorylated neurofilaments is observed in neurites of the spinal grey matter.

Neurofilaments, microtubules and microfilaments are major components of the neuronal cytoskeleton. They are carried by slow axonal transport and play a major role in determining neuronal shape and axon diameter (16). Previous studies have indicated that certain nerve cell bodies and proximal axons possess nonphosphorylated neurofilaments and that long fibres including terminal axons possess phosphorylated neurofilaments (17). The delayed action of kainic acid after two days was marked by an abnormal phosphorylation of neurofilaments in the perikarya of vulnerable neurons detected by increased neuronal immunolabelling. This abnormal distribution was seen in morphologically normal and in degenerating neurons. Similar findings are also produced after aluminium intoxication (18), after acrylamide intoxication (19) and after axonal injury (20). The presence of phosphorylated epitopes in the perikarya of neurons after kainic acid administration could result from two possible mechanisms. Neurofilament protein may become abnormally phosphorylated in the perikarya, and/or a defect in the slow axonal transport could prevent them from being loaded in the axon. The proximal axonal enlargement seen in kainic acid-induced pathology is in favour of an altered axonal transport. Phosphorylation of the 200-kDa protein side arms may play a role in regulating the crosslinking of neurofilaments to other cytoskeletal components of neurons (18). This crosslinking may be involved in the compactness and intracellular movement of neurofilaments. An abnormal phosphorylation could disturb this cytoplasmic movement.

Finally, in-vitro studies have also focused on cytoskeletal protein anomalies produced by excitatory amino acids. Glutamate and aspartate could induce the appearance of paired helical filaments of Alzheimer type in cultured human neurons (21). A recent study has shown that glutamate and Ca^{++} influx can elicit antigenic changes similar to those seen in neurofibrillary tangles, producing tau protein and ubiquitin accumulations (22).

The abnormal cellular mechanism at the origin of the aberrant distribution of phosphorylated neurofilaments after kainic acid administration is presently unknown. The delayed cytotoxicity produced by excitatory amino acid is Ca^{++} mediated (23). Massive calcium influx into the cells could certainly be at the origin of a proteolysis of neurofilaments (14).

Taken in concert, clinical, in-vivo and in-vitro experimental studies suggest that excitatory amino acid toxicity could represent one of the possible mechanisms at the origin of the neuropathological changes observed in some neurodegenerative disorders, such as amyotrophic lateral sclerosis.

Acknowledgments

This work was supported by grants from the Association Française contre les Myopathies and the INSERM (CRE), no. 901002.

REFERENCES

1. Olney JW, Rhee V, Ho OL. Brain Res 1974; 74: 507–12.
2. Hugon J, Vallat JM, Spencer PS, Leboutet MJ, Barthe D. Neurosci Lett 1989; 104: 758–63.

3. Sternberger NH, Sternberger LA, Ulrich J. Proc Natl Acad Sci USA 1985; 82: 4274-6.
4. Forno LS, Sternberger LA, Sternberger NH, Streifling AM, Swanson K, Eng LF. Neurosci Lett 1986; 64: 253-8.
5. Rasool CG, Selkoe DJ. N Engl J Med 1983; 312: 700-5.
6. Munoz DG, Greene C, Perl DP, Selkoe DJ. J Neuropath Exp Neurol 1988; 47: 9-18.
7. Manetto V, Sternberger NH, Perry G, Sternberger LH, Gambetti P. J Neuropath Exp Neurol 1988; 47: 642-53.
8. Plaitakis A, Caroscio JT. Ann Neurol 1987; 22: 575-9.
9. Hugon J, Tabaraud F, Rigaud M, Vallat JM, Dumas M. Neurology 1989; 39: 956-8.
10. Coyle JT, Schwarcz R. Nature 1976; 263: 244-6.
11. McGeer EG, McGeer PL. Nature 1976; 263: 517-19.
12. Maragos WF, Greenamyre JT, Penney JB, Young AB. Trends Neurosci 1987; 10: 65-8.
13. Sloviter RS. Brain Res Bull 1983; 10: 675-97.
14. Rothman SM, Olney JW. Ann Neurol 1986; 19: 105-11.
15. Spencer PS, Nunn PB, Hugon J, Ludolph AC, Ross SM, Roy DN, Robertson RC. Science 1987; 237: 517-22.
16. Hoffman PN, Griffin JW, Price DL. J Cell Biol 1984; 99: 705-14.
17. Sternberger LA, Sternberger NH. Proc Natl Acad Sci USA 1983; 80: 6126-30.
18. Troncoso JC, Sternberger NH, Sternberger LA, Hoffman PN, Price DL. Brain Res 1986; 364: 295-300.
19. Gold BC, Price DL, Griffin JW, Rosenfeld J, Hoffman PN, Sternberger NH, Sternberger LA. J Neuropath Exp Neurol 1988; 47: 145-57.
20. Rosenfeld J, Dorman ME, Griffin JW, Sternberger LA, Sternberger NH, Price DL. J Neuropath Exp Neurol 1987; 46: 269-82.
21. De Boni U, Crapper-McLachlan DR. J Neurol Sci 1985; 68: 105-18.
22. Mattson MP. Neuron 1990; 2: 105-17.
23. Choi DW. Neurosci Lett 1985; 55: 89-94.

Address for correspondence:

Dr J. Hugon,
Departments of Neurology and Histology,
University Hospital,
87042 Limoges, France

26 Differential Distribution of Lactoferrin and Alz-50 Immunoreactivities in Neuritic Plaques and Neurofibrillary Tangles in Alzheimer's Disease

ALEXANDER P. OSMAND AND ROBERT C. SWITZER III

The biochemical characterization of the protein components of the senile (neuritic and amyloid) plaques and neurofibrillary tangles of the brain in Alzheimer's disease (AD) has been a major focus of research in recent years. The distinctive amyloid β-protein (AβP) of the plaques in AD brain has been extensively studied, and the deposition of this protein in diffuse plaque-like zones may be one of the earliest events in the formation of plaques, as reviewed in (1). The amyloid β-protein has been shown to be derived from a membrane protein precursor by abnormal proteolytic processing (2–4). Although earlier studies had suggested that AβP was also a major component of the paired helical filaments of the neurofibrillary tangles, it is now considered that these are composed primarily of modified tau and tau fragments (5–7). It has been further shown that a monoclonal antibody, Alz-50, that is reactive with an epitope uniquely expressed in susceptible neurons, neurofibrillary tangles, and neurites in AD brain appears to react with a modified form of tau, designated A68, that may transiently appear in neurons during processing of the neuronal cytoskeleton (8,9).

Numerous additional biochemical abnormalities have been identified both generally within the neuropil in AD and in association with the specific lesions, and there is considerable speculation as to the extent to which such changes are primary factors in the pathophysiology of AD. Certain changes may be secondary to neuronal damage, such as the accumulation of immunoglobulin and complement components, while others, for example the focal increase in α_1-antichymotrypsin (10), may play a role in the abnormal extracellular processing of the amyloid precursor. During studies on the potential role of iron as a pathogenetic factor in AD, we detected significant immunoreactivity for the iron-binding protein, lactoferrin, in association with certain neurofibrillary tangles and plaques in AD brain (11). This reactivity was found in regions of the temporal lobe that are primarily and most extensively involved in AD, namely the hippocampal formation, amygdala, and entorhinal cortex. Several investigators have drawn attention to the neuroanatomic correlation of these

Alzheimer's Disease: Basic Mechanisms, Diagnosis and Therapeutic Strategies
Edited by K. Iqbal, D. R. C. McLachlan, B. Winblad and H. M. Wisniewski
© 1991 John Wiley & Sons Ltd

areas with projections of the olfactory system, leading to the suggestion that in AD the olfactory system may be a primary pathway or site of involvement (12). That lactoferrin is a major protein of mucous secretions and is uniformly absent from normal or uninvolved brain tissue prompted us to speculate that the protein may have derived from the olfactory mucosa where it is present at relatively high concentration (13), although local synthesis or transport from another site could not be excluded.

The functions of lactoferrin purportedly include an antimicrobial activity through chelation of iron and a role in iron transport. Although lactoferrin has been reported to inhibit free radical formation in xanthine–xanthine oxidase-dependent systems (14-16), several model systems provide evidence for some promotion of oxidative damage (17-19). Such damage has been advocated as one of the basic processes in aging (20,21) and indirect evidence for the presence of oxidative stress in AD has been found (22-24). Particularly relevant is the consistent development of AD pathology in aging individuals with Down's syndrome where the primary genetic defect may be the presence of an extra copy of the gene for Cu/Zn superoxide dismutase located on the long arm of chromosome 21 (25). An imbalance in the production of hydrogen peroxide could presumably be responsible for excessive oxidative damage.

We report here further definition of the localization of lactoferrin in AD brain tissue, and describe a marked difference in the relative distribution of Alz-50 immunoreactivity. The anatomical and morphological distribution of lactoferrin appears, in involved regions, to more closely parallel amyloidogenesis and neurofibrillary tangle formation than the neuritic changes that appear to be associated with the generation and transient appearance of the Alz-50 reactive epitope. In addition, we provide preliminary evidence for focal oxidative stress by demonstrating the selective accumulation of immunoreactivity for superoxide dismutase isoenzymes and glutathione peroxidase in various components of the plaques in AD. We further hypothesize that the amyloid protein precursor may be uniquely sensitive to oxidative damage.

MATERIALS AND METHODS

Brains from AD, control and other neurological disease cases were perfused at autopsy and stored at 4 °C in buffered 10% formalin. Diagnosis of AD was based on a premortem history of dementia and established neuropathological criteria. Freeze-cut coronal sections (40 μm) of brain, taken at a region between the mamillary body and anterior commissure, were examined routinely and for the presence of lactoferrin and other proteins using sensitive immunohistochemical procedures as described previously (13) or as recently described by Armstrong and colleagues (26). The following primary antisera were used at the indicated dilution: affinity purified rabbit antihuman lactoferrin (Jackson ImmunoResearch), 1:1000; Alz-50 monoclonal antibody, as a culture supernatant, 1:10; rabbit antiserum to a synthetic peptide corresponding to the first 28 residues of AβP (27), 1:1000; immunocytochemical grade immunoglobulin fractions of sheep antisera (The Binding Site): antihuman superoxide dismutase (Cu/Zn enzyme), 1:5000; antihuman superoxide dismutase (Mn enzyme), 1:1500; antihuman glutathione peroxidase, 1:1000; and antihuman lactoferrin, 1:1000. Following incubation for 24 hr in primary antisera, sections were washed, and bound primary antibody detected with the Vectastain 'Elite' ABC method (Vector Laboratories) using nickel-enhanced diaminobenzidine substrate to detect peroxidase. Sections were mounted on gelatin-coated glass slides and processed for light microscopy. Immunochemical specificity was implied by the sensitivity and selectivity of the reactivity of antisera at high dilution.

RESULTS AND DISCUSSION

Distribution of lactoferrin immunoreactivity in AD

The presence of lactoferrin immunoreactivity has been examined in over 75 cases of AD and 22 controls (Table 1). Some level of lactoferrin was detected in all but 2 cases in both AD plaques and neurofibrillary tangles in discrete locations. Immunochemical reactivity was highly variable as to the density of product and extent of involvement, both of which appeared unrelated to duration of history of dementia, postmortem interval before autopsy, or numbers of neurofibrillary tangles (NFTs) or senile plaque density. The majority of cases, however, confirmed the presence of lactoferrin in plaques in amygdala, hippocampus, and parahippocampal gyrus, and in NFTs in these regions and in the nucleus of Meynert (Figures 1 and 2). Lactoferrin was frequently also seen in plaques in scattered regions of temporal and insular cortex, typically at the base of sulci. Although the increased sensitivity in the immunohistochemical procedure of Armstrong et al (26) has enabled detection of a more extensive reactivity, most plaques and NFTs in these cortical regions were unreactive. Lactoferrin immunoreactivity can be considered a reasonably consistent and unique marker of AD lesions in the limbic system.

Relative distribution of lactoferrin, Sp28 and Alz-50 immunoreactivity

Enumeration of plaques by staining for amyloid with rabbit antiserum to Sp28 (data not shown) frequently, but not invariably, corresponded to the number of lactoferrin-positive plaques, particularly in the amygdala; the distribution of lactoferrin within plaques however was clearly distinguishable from amyloid. Thin sections (not shown)

Table 1. AD cases and controls

Patient group	No.	Age (yr)	Time to autopsy
AD			
Male	34	75.15 ± 7.46	14.90 ± 8.34
Female	41	75.98 ± 8.81	15.29 ± 9.84
Non-AD			
Male	11	72.18 ± 6.63	14.42 ± 7.67
Female	11	74.36 ± 11.62	11.64 ± 7.99

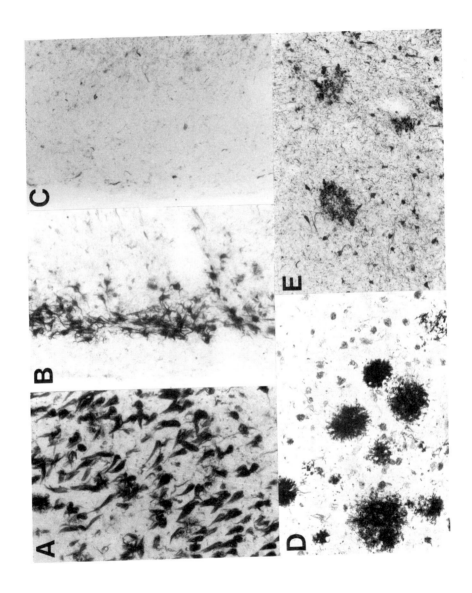

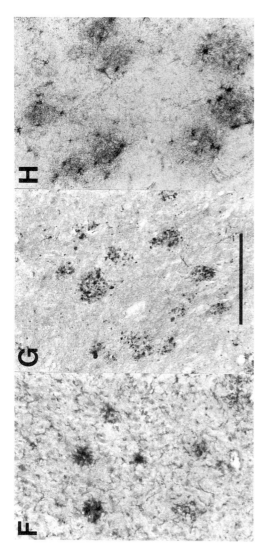

Figure 1. Immunohistochemical localization in AD brain tissue of lactoferrin (A, B, D), Alz-50 (C, E), glutathione peroxidase (F), and superoxide dismutases [Cu/Zn enzyme] (G) and [Mn enzyme] (H). Intense lactoferrin immunoreactivity is generally limited to the hippocampal formation, particularly the subiculum (A), stellate cells in layer II of entorhinal cortex (B), and AD plaques and tangle-containing neurons in amygdala (D). Alz-50 reactivity is seen in neurites in the molecular layer of entorhinal cortex and in deeper layers, but rarely in layer II (C), and in neurons and neurites in the amygdala (E). The oxygen protecting enzymes are detected in numerous plaques in cortex and, shown here, in amygdala; glutathione peroxidase immunoreactivity is seen in cells with the morphological appearance of microglia both throughout the neuropil and as dense accumulations in plaques (F); superoxide dismutase [Cu/Zn] is seen as accumulations in structures resembling dystrophic or degenerating nerve terminals (G); superoxide dismutase [Mn] has a punctate distribution within astroglial cells enveloping plaques (H); additional weak reactivity was seen in glia throughout the neuropil and in certain cortical pyramidal neurons. Scale bar (G) 200 μm

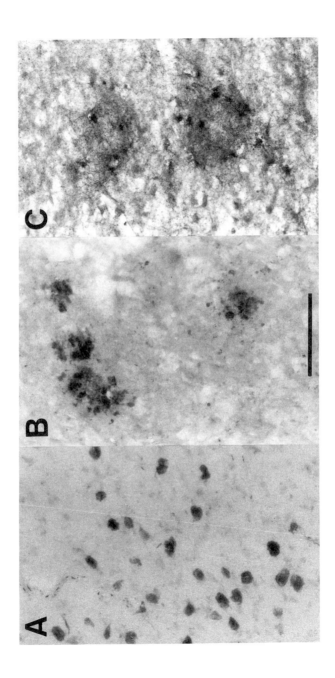

Figure 2. (A) Lactoferrin immunoreactivity is frequently found in tangled neurons in nucleus basalis of Meynert in AD brain. (B) Focal immunoreactivity for superoxide dismutase (Cu/Zn) is seen in neuritic plaques in amygdala, in the absence of definitive staining for cellular elements. (C) Superoxide dismutase (Mn) in the mitochondria of astroglia around plaques is distributed throughout their processes in plaques and (data not shown) along blood vessel walls. Scale bar (B) 100 μm

revealed that lactoferrin was associated with the extracellular matrix of both diffuse and amyloid plaques and decorated both intracellular and extracellular tangles. The relative distribution of Alz-50 and lactoferrin reactivities were found to be disparate in over 22 cases thus far examined. Alz-50 reactivity is seen both in neurons and neurites in characteristic layers throughout involved regions of neocortex, while in association with plaques it is confined to the same intracellular compartment of reactive neurites (Figure 1E).

Oxygen protecting enzymes in AD brain

Based on gross estimates of enzyme activities in homogenates of brain, the oxygen protecting enzymes have been reported to be unaltered in AD relative to normal aging (22). Since lactoferrin has been suggested to be involved in the oxidative mechanisms of neutrophils, evidence that the presence of this protein in AD lesions might be contributing to oxidative damage would be provided by the local detection of oxygen protecting enzymes. As shown in Figures 1 and 2, glutathione peroxidase and the superoxide dismutase isoenzymes were found to be dramatically increased in numerous neuritic plaques, providing an indication that an oxidative stress response is indeed a component of numerous plaques. Surprisingly each enzyme was characteristically and independently distributed. The superoxide dismutase (Cu/Zn) encoded on chromosome 21 was found to accumulate in structures resembling dystrophic nerve terminals; the Mn isoenzyme was found highly elevated in the mitochondria of reactive astroglia surrounding plaques. The location of these enzymes would be expected to generate freely diffusible hydrogen peroxide from intracellular superoxide anion. The induction of the primary salvage enzyme for hydrogen peroxide, glutathione peroxidase, appeared at a separate site in microglia within plaques. There exists therefore the potential for the development of significant extracellular concentrations of hydrogen peroxide.

Aromatic amino acids, in particular the indole ring of tryptophan and the imidazole ring of histidine, are highly sensitive to oxidative damage by free radicals; however, under mild acidic conditions the thioether group of methionine can be selectively oxidized by H_2O_2 (28). As suggested in Figure 3, the Alzheimer's amyloid precursor protein contains several methionine residues that might be susceptible to oxidation such that oxidized derivatives may have a modified protease inhibitory function and an altered catabolism, profoundly influencing both the functions of the precursor and its amyloidogenic potential.

SUMMARY

A substantial difference must exist between the modest reactions that lead to the widespread deposition of amyloid in the diffuse plaques that accompany the normal aging process (29) and the extensive amyloidosis and neuritic changes associated with AD. The presence of lactoferrin in those regions of the brain that are characteristically involved early in AD suggests a possible role for this protein in such processes. Alz-50 and lactoferrin reactivities are found at autopsy to be present

226

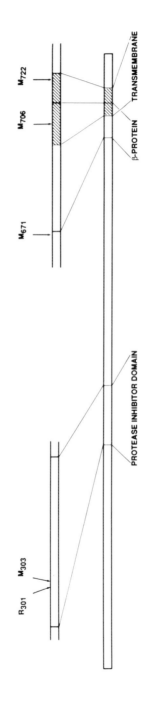

Figure 3. Potential sites of hydroperoxidation in the Alzheimer's amyloid precursor protein. The putative active site arginine residue (R_{301}) in the protease inhibitor domain is close to a methionine residue (M_{303}) that may be exposed in the active site; a methionine residue in the active site of the unrelated inhibitor, α_1-antitrypsin, has been shown to be exquisitely sensitive to oxidation, reviewed in (32). A methionine residue (M_{671}) immediately precedes the amyloid fragment; oxidation of this residue would provide a cleavage site for a methionine sulfoxide specific peptidase. The transmembrane domain of the precursor is unusual in containing two methionine residues (M_{706}, M_{722}); oxidation of these residues by lipid peroxidation reactions within cells expressing this protein would be expected to drastically alter the processing of this domain. The methionine residue at 706 is within the β/A4 amyloid fragment and has been found to be oxidized in the extracted amyloid protein; oxidation during extraction cannot be excluded at this time.

in different structures, although it is not possible to determine whether Alz-50 reactivity precedes the appearance of lactoferrin. We have also shown for the first time that oxygen protective enzymes are selectively increased focally in plaques in AD. Lactoferrin may function either to potentiate or to initiate oxidative damage; the hypothetical model presented here indicates a mechanism whereby such oxidative reactions could play an important role in the processing of the amyloid precursor protein and in the pathological deposition of amyloid in AD.

Acknowledgments

The authors are grateful to Dr Peter Davies, Albert Einstein College of Medicine, for generous supplies of the monoclonal antibody, Alz-50 (30), and to Dr Blas Frangione, New York University School of Medicine, for rabbit antiserum, anti-Sp28 (31). Supported by grants from the Alzheimer's Research Program of the American Health Assistance Foundation, the NIH (NS-23634), and the Robert H. and Monica Cole Foundation.

REFERENCES

1. Selkoe DJ. Science 1990; 248: 1058-60.
2. Esch FS, Keim PS, Beattie EC, Blacher RW, Culwell AR, Oltersdorf T, McClure D, Ward PJ. Science 1990; 248: 1122-4.
3. Oltersdorf T, Ward PJ, Henriksson T, Beattie EC, Neve R, Lieberburg I, Fritz LC. J Biol Chem 1990; 265: 4492-7.
4. Weidemann A, König G, Bunke D, Fischer P, Salbaum JM, Masters CL, Beyreuther K. Cell 1989; 57: 115-26.
5. Wischik CM, Novak M, Thogerson HC, Edwards PC, Runswick MJ, Jakes R, Walker JE, Milstein C, Roth M, Klug A. Proc Natl Acad Sci USA 1988; 85: 4506-10.
6. Kosik KS, Joachim CL, Selkoe DJ. Proc Natl Acad Sci USA 1986; 83: 4044-8.
7. Bancher C, Lassmann H, Budka H, Grundke-Iqbal I, Iqbal K, Wiche G, Seitelberger F, Wisniewski HM. Acta Neuropathol 1987; 74: 39-46.
8. Ksiezak-Reding H, Binder LI, Yen S-H. J Neurosci Res 1990; 25: 420-30.
9. Ksiezak-Reding H, Davies P, Yen S-H. J Biol Chem 1988; 263: 7943-7.
10. Abraham CR, Selkoe DJ, Potter H. Cell 1988; 52: 487-501.
11. Osmand AP, Switzer RC III. In Goldstein AL (ed.) Biomedical advances in aging. New York: Plenum, 109-24.
12. Pearson RCA, Esiri MM, Hiorns RW, Wilcock GK, Powell TPS. Proc Natl Acad Sci USA 1985; 82: 4531-4.
13. Masson PL, Heremans JF, Dive CH. Clin Chim Acta 1966; 14: 735-9.
14. Gutteridge JMC, Paterson SK, Segal AW, Halliwell B. Biochem J 1981; 199: 259-61.
15. Britigan BE, Rosen GM, Thompson BY, Chai Y, Cohen MS. J Biol Chem 1986; 261: 17026-32.
16. Baldwin DA, Jenny ER, Aisen P. J Biol Chem 1984; 259: 13391-4.
17. Nakamura M. J Biochem (Tokyo) 1990; 107: 395-9.
18. Vercellotti GM, Sweder van Asbeck B, Jacob HS. J Clin Invest 1985; 76: 956-62.
19. Ambruso DR, Johnston RB Jr. J Clin Invest 1981; 67: 352-60.
20. Harman D. Mol Cell Biochem 1988; 84: 155-61.
21. Harman D. Age 1984; 7: 111-31.
22. Marklund SL, Adolfsson R, Gottfries CG, Winblad B. J Neurol Sci 1985; 67: 319-25.
23. Martins RN, Harper CG, Stokes GB, Masters CL. J Neurochem 1986; 46: 1042-5.
24. Halliwell B. Acta Neurol Scand Suppl 1989; 126: 23-33.

25. Delabar JM, Sinet PM, Chadefaux B, Nicole A, Gegonne A, Stehelin D, Fridlansky F, Créau-Goldberg N, Turleau C, de Grouchy J. Hum Genet 1987; 76: 225-9.
26. Armstrong DM, Benzing WC, Evans J, Terry RD, Shields D, Hansen LA. Neuroscience 1989; 31: 663-71.
27. West CD. Complement 1989; 6: 49-64.
28. Brot N, Weissbach H. Arch Biochem Biophys 1983; 223: 271-81.
29. Mann DMA, Brown AMT, Prinja D, Jones D, Davies CA. Neuropathol Appl Neurobiol 1990; 16: 17-25.
30. Wolozin BL, Pruchnicki A, Dickson DW, Davies P. Science 1986; 232: 648-50
31. Tagliavini F, Giaccone G, Frangione B, Bugiani O. Neurosci Lett 1988; 93: 191-6.
32. Swaim MW, Pizzo SV. J Leukocyte Biol 1988; 43: 365-79.

Address for correspondence:

Dr Alexander P. Osmand,
Department of Medicine,
University of Tennessee Medical Center,
1924 Alcoa Highway, Knoxville, Tennessee 37920, USA

27 Tyrosine Phosphorylation of the Cytoplasmic Domain of Alzheimer Protein Precursors

DIRK BUNKE, URSULA MÖNNING, ROBERT M. KYPTA,
SARAH A. COURTNEIDGE, COLIN L. MASTERS
AND KONRAD T. BEYREUTHER

Alzheimer's disease (AD) is characterized by amyloid deposits principally composed of aggregates of a 42–43 residue protein, βA4. The pathogenesis of AD probably involves the abnormal proteolytic cleavage of a larger precursor protein (APP or PreA4) to yield the βA4 monomer. The predicted structure of APP indicates that it is a transmembrane cell surface receptor (1).

At least five different primary translation products can be generated by alternative splicing of the APP (PAD) gene. They give rise to a complex family of 92–135 kDa membrane-bound and soluble proteins, which are post-translationally modified by N- and O-glycosylation and tyrosine sulfation (2). The physiological functions of these different precursors are not yet understood. A functional analysis has been restricted mainly to an additional domain of the larger precursor forms APP_{751} and APP_{770}, encoding a serine protease inhibitor of the Kunitz type II family (3–5). APP_{751} has been shown to be identical with protease nexin-II (PN-II) (6,7).

There is a striking structural similarity between APP and the putative gene transcript of the ventral nervous system condensation defective (vnd) locus in *Drosophila melanogaster* (8). The vnd region is essential for the normal development of the nervous system of the fruit fly. The structural similarity suggests a related function of the APP in the mammalian nervous system, which is in agreement with earlier observations that APP may function in cell–cell or cell–matrix interaction (2,9,10).

In order to improve our understanding of the physiological functions of the Alzheimer protein precursors, we have performed a functional analysis of the cytoplasmic domain looking for post-translational modifications. Phosphorylation on tyrosine can be considered as a hallmark of proteins involved in the process of signal transduction in proliferating as well as in nonproliferating tissues: therefore we started with a tyrosine-phosphorylation assay. As the protein kinase we used $pp60^{v\text{-}src}$ and as substrates we used the synthetic APP cytoplasmic domain and in addition a control substrate which corresponds to a site which is phosphorylated on tyrosine under physiological conditions.

Alzheimer's Disease: Basic Mechanisms, Diagnosis and Therapeutic Strategies
Edited by K. Iqbal, D. R. C. McLachlan, B. Winblad and H. M. Wisniewski
© 1991 John Wiley & Sons Ltd

"Jonas"   Y T̈ S I H H G V V E   V D A A V T P E E R   H L S K M
             653

             H L S K M¦Q Q N G Y   E NP TY KFF EQ   M¦Q N
                       ¦   682   687   ¦ 695

L-22   L S K M¦Q Q N G Y E   N P T Y K F F E Q M¦   Q N
             674   ¦   682   687   ¦   695

p 6   K L I E D N E Y T   A
             409   416 418

Figure 1. Amino acid sequences of the synthetic peptides. Sequences and numbering are according to APP$_{695}$ (1) for the peptides 'Jonas' and L-22 respectively, and according to Hunter and Cooper (14) for the peptide p6. Positions of tyrosine residues are marked by numbers; cleavage sites for cyanogen bromide are indicated by dotted lines

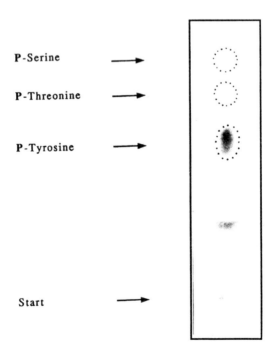

Figure 2. Phosphoamino acid analysis of the peptide 'Jonas' after phosphorylation. The phosphoamino acids were separated on a thin-layer cellulose plate by high-voltage electrophoresis in one dimension. An autoradiogram of this plate is shown. Dotted areas indicate the positions of the nonradioactive standards after ninhydrin stain

RESULTS

Choice, sequence and synthesis of the synthetic substrates

To analyse tyrosine phosphorylation of APP, we synthesized different parts of the APP (Figure 1). The peptide 'Jonas' covers the whole cytoplasmic domain of the APP. Peptide Jonas is expected to adopt the same conformation as the cytoplasmic domain of APP. Folding of this cytoplasmic domain of APP is expected to occur without interaction with other APP domains since the latter are separated from the former by the lipid bilayer. Therefore the entire synthetic cytoplasmic domain should be an ideal substrate for in-vitro phosphorylation.

Peptide L-22 corresponds to the 22 carboxy-terminal residues of peptide Jonas and of human APP transmembrane forms. Peptide L-22 includes a sequence of nine residues (Asn-Gly-Tyr-Glu-Asn-Pro-Thr-Tyr-Lys) which is identical in APP (residues 680–688 in APP_{695}) and the vnd gene transcript (residues 872–880) of *Drosophila melanogaster*.

The peptide p6 contains the major tyrosine phosphorylation site of the protein tyrosine kinase $pp60^{v\text{-}src}$, tyrosine 416. Since the apparent K_m of the peptide p6 is known and exchanges of single amino acids of p6 have shown a high specificity of this kinase for the peptide p6, we used p6 as a control substrate.

Phosphorylation of the synthetic substrates by the protein tyrosine kinase $pp60^{v\text{-}src}$

The phosphorylation of the synthetic substrates was done under conditions previously established for several synthetic substrates of the Rous sarcoma virus (RSV) transforming protein $pp60^{v\text{-}src}$ (11). We used immunoprecipated protein tyrosine kinase $pp60^{v\text{-}src}$ for the phosphorylation reaction (12). In a typical experiment, peptides were incubated with the immune complex of the enzyme in the presence of 100 μM Na_3VO_4 and 40 μM (γ^{32}P)-ATP. After removal of the excess radioactive ATP by a reverse phase–precolumn system the phosphorylated peptides were separated by reverse phase HPLC. In the presence of the immunoprecipitated kinase, each of the three peptides coelute with the radioactivity. Subsequently we ascertained by one-dimensional phosphoamino acid analysis that tyrosine is the only phosphorylated amino acid of the cytoplasmic domain that is modified under the conditions employed (Figure 2).

Determination of the site of phosphorylation

There are three tyrosine residues within the cytoplasmic domain: Y-653 is located at the amino terminal end at the border of the transmembrane domain; Y-682 and Y-687 are located in the conserved stretch of nine amino acids. By Edman degradation we determined the site of phosphorylation. The peptide L-22 was sequenced directly and the peptide Jonas after an additional cyanogen bromide cleavage step, leading to a mixture of three fragments which were sequenced in parallel. The results of the sequence analysis are summarized in Figure 3. There was a significant release

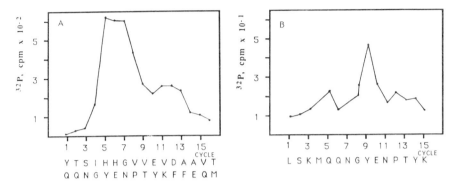

Figure 3. Sequence analysis of ^{32}P-labelled synthetic peptides. Total amounts of 35 000 cpm (A, peptide Jonas) and 14 000 cpm (B, peptide L-22) were subjected to automated Edman degradation. The figure shows the amount of radioactivity released in each degradation cycle. The sequence of the peptides is given by the one-letter code for the amino acid residues

of ^{32}P-radioactivity in the degradation steps related to tyrosine residue 682 of APP$_{695}$. There was no increase in radioactivity at positions corresponding to tyrosine 653 or tyrosine 687 of APP$_{695}$. In agreement with the results of the phosphoamino acid analysis, there was also no increase in radioactivity in the degradation steps releasing serine and threonine derivatives. Thus, sequencing clearly indicates that both peptides are specifically phosphorylated on tyrosine 682 of APP$_{695}$, and this reaction is obviously independent of the length of the two peptides.

The apparent K_m values of tyrosine phosphorylation by the kinase pp60$^{v\text{-}src}$

In order to estimate the affinity of the protein kinase pp60$^{v\text{-}src}$ to the peptides we compared the apparent Michaelis Menten K_m values (see 11) of the peptides Jonas and p6. By varying the concentration of peptide during the phosphorylation reactions, we determined the apparent K_m values for the whole cytoplasmic domain (peptide Jonas) and the phosphorylation site p6 by measurement of the radioactivity specifically incorporated into the peptides at each concentration. The results of these experiments are given in Figure 4. The linear double reciprocal plot gave an apparent K_m of 2 mM for the peptide Jonas and an apparent K_m of 1.1 mM for the peptide p6.

DISCUSSION

Until now, the phosphorylation of the cytoplasmic domain of APP has been examined using short synthetic peptides of 16 to 17 residues (13). Threonine corresponding to residue 654 and serine corresponding to residue 655 of APP$_{695}$ were phosphorylated by the Ca^{2+}/calmodulin-dependent protein kinase II; serine corresponding to position 655 of APP$_{695}$ was phosphorylated by the protein kinase C. Attempts failed

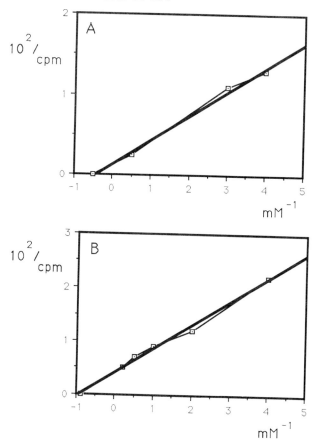

Figure 4. Apparent K_m for the phosphorylation of the peptides Jonas (A) and p6 (B). The incubation with pp60[v-src] was carried out for 5 min at 30 °C and at a total ATP concentration of 40 mM. Initial rates were determined simply as the amount of radioactivity incorporated into the peptide at each concentration

to phosphorylate any of the three tyrosine residues of the cytoplasmic domain of APP using the insulin receptor protein tyrosine kinase.

We started our experiments by synthesis of the whole cytoplasmic domain. The tyrosine residue corresponding to position 682 of the sequence of APP$_{695}$ was specifically phosphorylated by the protein tyrosine kinase pp60[v-src]. For this reaction we determined an apparent K_m of 2 mM, which is similar to the apparent K_m of 1.1 mM determined for the peptide p6, a well-characterized substrate for this kinase (11). Therefore we suggest that the tyrosine residue according to position 682 of APP$_{695}$ is a potential target site for the phosphorylation of the APP cytoplasmic domains by the protein kinase pp60[v-src] and its cellular homologue, pp60[c-src].

Protein kinase pp60[v-src] has been shown to belong to a class of tyrosine kinases that represent the transforming agent of some oncogenic viruses (14). A second class of proteins with an intrinsic tyrosine phosphorylation activity has in some cases been shown to be associated with receptors for some growth factors, such as epidermal growth factor, platelet-derived growth factor and insulin. Analysis through single amino acid substitutions and deletions have revealed that tyrosine phosphorylation is linked to the process of signal transduction and receptor regulation (15). Moreover, the affinity of receptors to their cellular ligands can be modulated by the phosphorylation/dephosphorylation of tyrosine residues (16). Therefore this enzymatic activity is not restricted to proliferating tissues (17). On the contrary, there is a high level of protein tyrosine kinase activity and a low level of growth in the adult nervous system. Synaptic vesicles and synaptosomes have been shown to have a high tyrosine kinase activity (18), and aberrant phosphorylation is thought to play a major role in the neurocytoskeletal changes which are associated with AD (19).

The protein kinase pp60^{c-src}, the cellular homologue of the kinase we have used in our assays, is evolutionarily highly conserved. Its expression in neuronal issues is developmentally regulated, starting with the differentiation of neuronal cells (20). But postmitotic neurons are also known to express high levels of this enzyme activity. Therefore this kinase and its target proteins appear to be essential for the differentiation and functional maintenance of neuronal cells. The participation of the cytoplasmic domain of the APP in these processes becomes likely since we show here that this domain is a potential target for this kinase.

The tyrosine phosphorylation site tyrosine 682 is part of a highly conserved sequence of nine amino acid residues which has also been found in the putative cytoplasmic domain of the product from the vnd region of *Drosophila melanogaster* (8). Mutations in the vnd region result in structural defects related to the organization of the nervous system during embryonic development. The structural similarity of the human APP with the product from the vnd region supports the idea of a related function for these proteins in the nervous system.

The potential tyrosine phosphorylation site described here raises the likelihood of a functional control of the APP at the post-translational level by a modification which is described for proteins involved in signal transduction. If proven, this regulation of the βA4 amyloid precursor protein may be linked to processes such as the tyrosine phosphorylation-dependent desensitization to acetylcholine of the nicotinic acetylcholine receptor (21) and provide a possible link between neuronal vulnerability and βA4 amyloid deposition in AD.

Acknowledgments

Financial support from the Deutsche Forschungs Gemeinschaft through SFB 317, the BMFT and the Fonds der chemischen Industrie is gratefully acknowledged. Dirk Bunke is a fellow of the Cusanus Werk.

REFERENCES

1. Kang J, Lemaire H-G, Unterbeck A, Salbaum JM, Masters CL, Grzeschik K-H, Multhaup G, Beyreuther K, Müller-Hill B. Nature 1987; 325: 733.

2. Weidemann A, König G, Bunke D, Fischer P, Salbaum JM, Masters CL, Beyreuther K. Cell 1989; 57: 115.
3. Kitaguchi N, Takahashi Y, Tokushima Y, Shirohiri S, Ito H. Nature 1988; 331: 385.
4. Ponte P, Gonzalez-De Whitt P, Schilling J, Miller J, Hsu D, Greenberg B, Davis K, Wallace W, Lieburg I, Fuller F, Cordell B. Nature 1988; 331: 525.
5. Tanzi RE, St George-Hyslop PH, Haines JH, Polinsky RJ, Nee L, Foncin JF, Neve RL, McClatchy AI, Coneally PM, Gusella JF. Nature 1987; 329: 156.
6. Olstersdorf T, Fritz L, Schenk DB, Lieberburg I, Jonson-Wood KL, Beatie EC, Ward PJ, Blacher RW, Dovey HF, Sinha S. Nature 1989; 341: 144.
7. Van Nostrand WE, Wagner SL, Suzuki M, Chol BH, Farrow JS, Cotman CW, Cunningham DD. Nature 1989; 341: 546.
8. Rosen DR, Martin-Morris L, Liqun L, White K. Proc Natl Acad Sci USA 1989; 86: 2478.
9. Shivers B, Hilbich C, Multhaup G, Salbaum JM, Beyreuther K, Seeburg PH. EMBO J 1988; 7: 1365.
10. Schubert D, Schroeder R, LaCorbiere M, Saitoh T, Cole G. Science 1988; 241: 223.
11. Hunter T. J Biol Chem 1982; 257: 4843.
12. Kypta RM, Hemming A, Courtneidge SA. EMBO J 1988; 7: 3837.
13. Gandy S, Czernik AJ, Greengard P. Proc Natl Acad Sci USA 1988; 85: 6218.
14. Hunter T, Cooper A. Ann Rev Biochem 1985; 54: 897.
15. Chen WS, Lazar CS. Nature 1987; 328: 820.
16. Migliaccio A, Domenico MD, Green S, de Falco A, Kajtaniak EL, Blasl F, Chambon P, Auricchio F. Mol Endocrinol 1989; 3: 1061.
17. Tuy F, Henry J, Rosenfeld C, Kahn A. Nature 1985; 305: 435.
18. Pang DT, Wang JV, Valtorta F, Benfenanil F, Greengard P. Proc Natl Acad Sci USA 1988; 85: 762.
19. Sternberger NH, Sternberger LA, Ulrich J. Proc Natl Acad Sci USA 1985; 82: 4274.
20. Sorge L, Levy BT, Manen PF. Cell 1984; 36: 249.
21. Huganir RL, Delcour AH, Greengard P, Hess GP. Nature 1986; 321: 774.

Address for correspondence:

Prof. Konrad Beyreuther,
Zentrum für Molekulare Biologie der Universität Heidelberg,
Im Neuenheimer Feld 282, D-6900 Heidelberg, Germany

28 Neuronal Expression of the Light Chain Neurofilament and Superoxide Dismutase-1 Genes in the Temporal Lobe of Alzheimer Brains

MARTIN J. SOMERVILLE, CATHERINE BERGERON,
LARRY K. K. YOONG, DONALD R. C. McLACHLAN
AND MAIRE E. PERCY

Alzheimer's disease (AD) is characterized pathologically by the presence of neuritic plaques and neurofibrillary tangles (NFT). These dramatic changes, however, overshadow less readily apparent alterations such as neuronal atrophy (1) and loss (2,3), both of which correlate closely with the dementia observed clinically (4). There are numerous models of cell death, but one that is consistent with what is already known about AD would involve cytoskeletal disruption, an event that presumably would precede the formation of the NFT that are seen in this disease. To further our understanding of the possible mechanism(s) underlying neuronal atrophy and death in AD, we studied the expression of the neurofilament light chain (NF-L) in large pyramidal neurons of layers 3 and 5 of the temporal neocortex, a cell population selectively vulnerable in AD (2). NF-L is essential to the assembly of the neurofilament protein, a major cytoskeletal element necessary for the maintenance of neuronal shape and axonal transport (5,6). Another possible mechanism of neuron death is the disruption of cellular function by free radical accumulation. Superoxide dismutase-1 (SOD-1) is the enzyme responsible for 'dismutating' oxygen free radicals to hydrogen peroxide. Any fluctuation in the expression of SOD-1 has the potential to be devastating to a cell (7).

In order to assess the contribution of these disruptive processes to the progression of AD, we have used a technique that resolves genetic activity in individual cells. In-situ hybridization to messenger RNA (mRNA) was performed in postmortem brain using labelled RNA probes to determine the relative abundance and distribution of NF-L and SOD-1 transcripts. We previously showed that the mRNA levels for NF-L and SOD-1 were not affected by the postmortem interval of 2 to 10 hours (8). Four pairs of AD and control brains were studied, matched very closely for age at death (60–65 years) and postmortem interval (2–10 hours); cases of Huntington's disease (HD) were selected as controls, because of the availability of

Alzheimer's Disease: Basic Mechanisms, Diagnosis and Therapeutic Strategies
Edited by K. Iqbal, D. R. C. McLachlan, B. Winblad and H. M. Wisniewski
© 1991 John Wiley & Sons Ltd

a large number of cases through the Canadian Brain Tissue Bank, thus allowing close matching of both sets of parameters. The use of another degenerative disorder with a lengthy debilitating course and prolonged agonal process as a control also reduced the variability of these important premortem conditions. Throughout the procedure, each AD brain and its matched HD sample were treated simultaneously, and in the same solutions, as a control for subtle variations in the experimental conditions.

HYBRIDIZATION

Portions of the middle temporal gyrus from each brain were paraffin-embedded and histological sections cut under RNase-free conditions (9). The sections were probed in situ using sense and antisense tritiated RNA, transcribed from BRL (Bethesda Research Laboratories) T3/T7 expression vectors. The cDNA used to generate NF-L and SOD-1 transcripts were obtained from Drs S. A. Lewis and Y. Groner, respectively (10,11). Hybridizations of the probes followed a previously established protocol (12). Sections were subsequently coated with a nuclear track emulsion (NTB-2; Eastman-Kodak, Rochester, New York) and exposed for several weeks in the dark, prior to staining and analysis.

ANALYSIS

All of the hybridization data was obtained with a Leco 2001 image analysis system. Individual cortical neurons were first identified by the operator in layers 3 and 5 of the cortical sections. The analyzer subsequently measured the perikaryal area of each neuron while automatically counting the number of autoradiographic grains which appeared over each of these areas. Twenty-five pyramidal cells were examined in layer 3 and in layer 5 of each case. The analyzer also recorded grain counts over defined areas that were randomly selected but did not include visible cell bodies. These counts were considered to represent the hybridization background or 'noise' and were subtracted from cell counts after adjusting for the relative cross-sectional areas.

Bielschowsky stained sections adjacent to those which were used for each hybridization allowed a determination of the extent of neurofibrillary degeneration. One hundred pyramidal cells were scored manually in layer 3 and in layer 5 of each patient and the results were tabulated as a percentage of neurons with NFT.

Statistical analysis was performed on the pooled data from patient pairs using a Student's paired t-test. Regression analysis was also used to determine the effects of autopsy interval, age at death, wet brain weight, and presence of NFT on the amount of NF-L or SOD-1 mRNA.

NEUROFILAMENT

Grain counts from each patient were tabulated against the cell sizes and percentage NFT. A consistent reduction in the amount of NF-L mRNA was seen in both layer 3

Table 1. Summary statistics, with mean values ± SEM, for brains examined. Each value represents data pooled from four patients

Source of tissue	Layer	Cell size (μm²)	NF-L count	SOD-1 count	%NFT
Huntington	3	323.23 ± 15.70	25.98 ± 1.98	20.31 ± 2.16	0
	5	335.17 ± 15.55	29.62 ± 2.07	23.71 ± 3.13	0
Alzheimer	3	260.33 ± 13.01*	13.78 ± 1.43**	12.67 ± 1.50*	21
	5	250.91 ± 10.06*	10.14 ± 0.89**	13.95 ± 1.65*	16

*P < 0.05 relative to Huntington value.
**P < 0.01 relative to Huntington value.

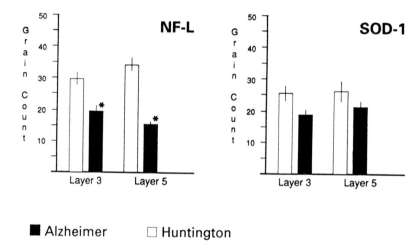

■ Alzheimer   □ Huntington

Figure 1. Histogram showing the pooled (cell size-adjusted) grain counts for NF-L and SOD-1 in the pyramidal cells of Alzheimer and Huntington middle temporal gyrus. Each bar shows the mean ± 1 SEM for four brains (100 cells). *P < 0.05

and layer 5 of each AD patient (results not shown) and pooled data indicate a greater than 45% reduction in each layer (P < 0.001) (Table 1). The AD pyramidal cells were also found to be significantly smaller than those in HD temporal lobe (P < 0.05), but when the NF-L counts were adjusted for the sizes of these cells the reduction of NF-L mRNA was still significant in AD (P < 0.05) (Figure 1). Simple regression of the relative amount of NF-L mRNA on pathology, age at death, brain weight, autopsy interval, cell cross-sectional area, and the relative number of cells with tangles indicates that the reduction of NF-L mRNA correlates only with the presence of Alzheimer's disease (P < 0.01).

SUPEROXIDE DISMUTASE-1

When the grain counts from each patient were analyzed, no consistent reduction of SOD-1 mRNA was observed in layer 3 or 5 (results not shown), but pooled data do show an approximately 40% reduction in both layers ($P < 0.05$) (Table 1). When these counts were adjusted for the size of each cell (Figure 1), however, the reductions were no longer significant. Regression analysis of the level of SOD-1 on the parameters previously listed indicated that the amount of SOD-1 mRNA is most closely associated with the cross-sectional area of the neurons ($P < 0.01$).

DISCUSSION

These results confirm and extend our previous observations in the hippocampus and cerebellum of the same cases (8) (Table 2). As in CA1 and CA2, large pyramidal neurons of the third and fifth neocortical layers show neuronal atrophy and a striking reduction in the expression of NF-L unrelated to decreased cell size. In contrast, cerebellar Purkinje cells, a neuronal population spared in AD, show no significant difference. While neurofibrillary degeneration is limited to 16–21% of large pyramidal neurons examined, the NF-L reduction is far more widespread, affecting all neurons examined. The frequency distribution of unadjusted counts in AD was uniformly shifted to a lower range of values relative to HD, with no apparent skewing or outlying values (results not shown). SOD-1 expression, however, is not significantly reduced in any of these brain regions in AD when cell size is taken into account.

The reduction in NF-L may contribute to the observed neuronal atrophy and affect several important neuronal functions such as slow axonal transport. MAP2 and tau form cross-links between neurofilaments and microtubules (13). The NF-L reduction may thus alter the interactions between these complex cytoskeletal proteins and contribute to the accumulation of abnormally phosphorylated tau that precedes the formation of neurofibrillary tangles (14). Reduced levels of NF-L expression have been reported during the period of axonal growth that follows axotomy (15). It was also shown recently that a reduction in NF-L expression coincides with chromatin condensation in the upstream regulatory region of that gene (16). Further studies are needed to determine if the decreased levels of NF-L in AD result from a change in chromatin conformation, a response to axonal damage, or the activation of a genetically determined program involved in early development.

In contrast to the AD-associated expression of NF-L, SOD-1 expression is not significantly altered in any of the brain regions (listed in Table 2) in AD when cell size is taken into account. Moreover, a very strong correlation was observed between SOD-1 expression and cell size ($P < 0.00002$), when the data from all these brain regions were pooled, but there was no significant correlation between the amount of SOD-1 mRNA and the presence or absence of AD. One interpretation of these

Table 2. Relative amounts of NF-L and SOD-1 mRNA in Alzheimer brains. All values expressed as Alzheimer/Huntington counts (adjusted for cell size)

	Cerebellum	CA1	CA2	Layer 3	Layer 5
NF-L	0.89	0.49*	0.46*	0.68*	0.46*
SOD-1	1.00	0.87	1.17	0.75	0.82

*$P < 0.05$

data is that the level of SOD-1 has nothing to do with neuron death, or perhaps only small alterations in the amount of SOD-1 have serious consequences on cellular integrity; the intriguing correlation between cell size and SOD-1 mRNA level suggests that a strong feedback system might exist for regulation of the intracellular SOD-1 concentration.

In conclusion, it would appear that neurofilament expression correlates very closely with the presence of Alzheimer's disease, whereas superoxide dismutase-1 expression correlates with the cross-sectional area of neurons. The reduction of neurofilament mRNA, which occurs in neurons that contain NFT and in adjacent neurons without Bielschowsky positive staining, may be a very sensitive indicator of the presence of Alzheimer's disease and may be part of an integrated alteration in the expression of several other growth-related genes.

Acknowledgments

This investigation would not have been possible without the tissue obtained from the Canadian Brain Tissue Bank. Partial support provided by grants to MEP from the Ontario Mental Health Foundation (934-85/87), and the Ontario Ministry of Community and Social Services Lottery Grants Programme. MJS was the recipient of a Natural Sciences and Engineering Research Council (NSERC) postgraduate scholarship, a University of Toronto Open Fellowship and an advanced student bursary from the Gerontology Research Council of Ontario. MEP was a National Health Research Scholar (NHRDP).

REFERENCES

1. Mann DMA. In Reisberg B (ed.) Alzheimer's disease: the standard reference. New York: Free Press/Macmillan 1983: 107-15.
2. Terry RD, Hansen LA. In Terry RD (ed.) Aging and the brain. New York: Raven, 1988: 109-14.
3. Mann DMA, Yates PO, Marcyniuk B. J Neurol Sci 1985: 69: 139-69.
4. Neary D, Snowden JS, Mann DMA, Bowden DM, Sims NR, Northern B, Yates PO, Davison AN. J Neurol Neurosurg Psychiat 1986; 49: 229-37.
5. Tokutake S. Int J Biochem 1990; 22: 1-6.
6. Hollenbeck PJ. J Cell Biol 1989; 108: 223-227.
7. Percy ME, Dalton AJ, Markovic VD, McLachlan DRC, Hummel JT, Rusk ACM. Am J Med Genet 1990; 35: 459-67.
8. Somerville MJ, Percy ME, Bergeron C, Yoong LKK, Grima EA, McLachlan DRC. Mol Brain Res 1991; 9: 1-8.
9. Uhl GR, Gendelman HE. In Uhl GR (ed.) In situ hybridization in brain. New York: Plenum, 1986: 264-8.
10. Lewis SA, Cowan NJ. J Cell Biol 1985; 100: 843-50.
11. Groner Y, Lieman-Hurwitz J, Dafri N, Sherman L, Levanon D, Bernstein Y, Danciger E, Elroy-Stein O. In Smith GF (ed.) Molecular structure of the number 21 chromosome and Down sydrome. Ann N Y Acad Sci New York, 1985; 450: 133-56.
12. Pardue ML. In Hames BD, Higgins SJ (eds) Nucleic acid hybridization: a practical approach. Oxford: IRL Press, 1985: 179-202.
13. Iqbal K, Grundke-Iqbal I. In Fowler CL, Carlson LA, Gottfries C-G, Winblad B (eds) Biological markers in dementia of alzheimer type. London: Smith-Gordon, 1990; 81-87.
14. Koepke-Secundo E, Grundke-Iqbal I, Iqbal K. Neurobiol Aging 1990; 11: 281.

15. Hoffman PN, Cleveland DW. Proc Natl Acad Sci USA 1988; 85: 4530-3.
16. Lukiw WJ, McLachlan DRC. Mol Brain Res 1990; 7: 227-33.

Address for correspondence:

Dr Martin J. Somerville,
Neurogenetics Laboratory,
Surrey Place Centre,
2 Surrey Place,
Toronto, Canada M5S 2C2

29 Differential Expression of Members of the Heat Shock Gene Family in Brain of Adult and Aged Rats

MARCELLE MORRISON-BOGORAD, KAREN GROSHAN, SIBILE PARDUE, BARBARA BORDER, E. KATHERINE MILLER AND JOACHIM D. RAESE

The pathological hallmark of Alzheimer's disease (AD) is the presence in specific brain regions of insoluble protein deposits, namely intracellular paired helical filaments (PHF) and extracellular senile plaques (1,2). Although the process of intracellular PHF formation is not understood, and the exact composition of PHF remains unknown, several of the proteins that comprise PHF have been identified, for example the microtubule-associated proteins (3,4). PHF could arise from abnormally modified cytoskeletal components (5). β-amyloid, a 4-kDa peptide, is the primary protein component of senile plaques and is derived from the larger amyloid precursor protein (APP) (6). The process of extracellular senile plaque formation is also not understood, but its deposition may result either from increased production and/or abnormal processing of APP (2). Neither the late onset of AD symptomatology nor the relative contributions of genetic and epidemiological factors to the etiology of this disease have been explained. We propose that the balance between the generation of abnormal proteins and their removal by different components of the heat shock system is altered in specific cell types in the aging AD brain and that this disequilibrium contributes to the gradual accumulation of the insoluble protein deposits characteristic of AD.

The synthesis of a number of heat shock proteins is induced by different stresses, most of which result in the accumulation of malfolded intracellular proteins (7,8). Among the most abundant of the heat shock proteins is a family of highly conserved proteins approximately 70 kDa in size. Members of this heat shock protein 70 (HSP-70) family share the common ability to bind ATP in a reversible manner and to bind to other proteins, preventing inappropriate protein–protein interactions (9). It has been proposed that members of the HSP-70 family may perform dual functions: a transient chaperone function that assists newly synthesized proteins in maintaining a proper conformation for intracellular transport or for multimer formation; and a stress response function that maintains malfolded proteins in a soluble state either until they can be degraded or until normal metabolism can resume (9–13). Different heat shock proteins have developed specialized roles. For example, one known

Alzheimer's Disease: Basic Mechanisms, Diagnosis and Therapeutic Strategies
Edited by K. Iqbal, D. R. C. McLachlan, B. Winblad and H. M. Wisniewski
© 1991 John Wiley & Sons Ltd

function of the major heat-inducible HSP-70 is to repair damaged nucleolar preribosomes following heat shock (14). Another specialized function of HSP-70 is to target proteins for lysosomal degradation (15). The constitutively expressed heat shock cognate protein 70 (HSC-70) member of this family is a major cytoplasmic protein that functions catalytically in the uncoating of clathrin-coated vesicles (16). A distantly related member of the HSP-70 gene family is the glucose regulated protein 78 (GRP-78). It is synthesized constitutively and is regulated by glucose deprivation and intracellular Ca^{++} flux (17). GRP-78 is localized in the endoplasmic recticulum and assists in the conformational processing of proteins destined for secretion (18,19).

Ubiquitin, another heat shock protein, is not related structurally to the HSP-70 family. However, it is under the transcriptional control of a heat shock promoter and like the members of the HSP-70 family, its synthesis is induced following heat shock and other stresses (20,21). One known function of ubiquitin is to covalently attach to intracellular proteins with high turnover rates and target them for extralysosomal degradation (10,22). Thus, different members of the heat shock family have been implicated in both lysosomal and extralysosomal pathways of protein degradation.

The initial cellular response to the presence of abnormally folded proteins may be an increase in ubiquitin synthesis, but when the ubiquitin system becomes overloaded, the HSP-70 system may be induced (10,23). As might be expected, different stressors do not uniformly induce all heat shock proteins. Ubiquitin, for example, but not HSP-70, is induced following exposure to aluminum (24) while HSP-70 related mRNAs are induced to different extents by different environmental stresses (25).

Because AD is characterized by the deposition of abnormal proteins, namely intracellular PHFs and extracellular amyloid, we suggest that synthesis of one or all heat shock proteins should be induced in compromised cells of AD brain. Indeed, ubiquitin is found in association with PHFs and with the neurites of senile plaques (26,27) and is also associated with inclusion bodies in other neurodegenerative diseases (28). In a preliminary communication, members of the HSP-70 protein family have also been reported to be present in senile plaques and PHF in AD hippocampus (29).

These results suggest the additional possibility that the balance between accumulation of abnormal proteins and their removal by different elements of the heat shock system might be altered in AD. We suggest several possible scenarios that could account for the accumulation of abnormal protein deposits in specific cell types or brain regions during aging (Figure 1). One possibility is that the stress response is decreased in AD brain. There are several ways in which this could occur (Figure 1A):

(a) The stress response could become less efficient during the process of aging. Induction of several members of the heat shock family is attenuated in aged cells in tissue culture when they are heat stressed (30–32).

(b) The stress response might vary in specific brain cell types. The cell types with the least efficient response could be those in which PHF and amyloid precursors are synthesized.

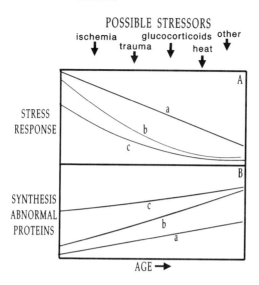

Figure 1. Possible age-related and AD-related changes in (A) the stress response and (B) the synthesis of abnormal proteins. (A) a, age-related decline in the stress response; b, accelerated age-related decline in the stress response in susceptible cells in AD; c, accelerated age-related decline in the stress response in AD caused by a mutation or polymorphisms in a heat shock gene. (B) a, age-related increase in accumulation of malfolded proteins; b, accelerated age-related increase in accumulation of malfolded proteins in AD due to a variety of stresses; c, accelerated age-related increase in accumulation of malfolded proteins in AD due to a structural mutation

(c) A subset of AD patients could have mutations or polymorphisms in genes of the heat shock system, which would further compromise the efficiency of the stress response during aging. In principle, a deficit in the stress response in AD patients could range from the complete absence of heat shock proteins to the synthesis of mutant family members less efficient than their normal counterparts. In this context, it is interesting to note that an HSP-70 gene has been localized to chromosome 21 (33). A gene on the long arm of this chromosome is linked to early onset AD (34).

The second possibility is that the synthesis of abnormal proteins is increased in AD brain (Figure 1B).

(a) Malfolded proteins could slowly accumulate during the aging process as a consequence of age-related errors in transcription or translation.
(b) Some stressors, for example ischemia, heat shock or mechanical trauma, may directly or indirectly cause the intracellular accumulation of malfolded proteins. Recent evidence shows that one form of stress directly induces synthesis of APP in glia (35). The APP promoter contains the consensus sequence for a heat shock promoter element (36), and we have preliminary evidence that APP mRNAs are induced in rat brain following amphetamine treatment (Miller, unpublished

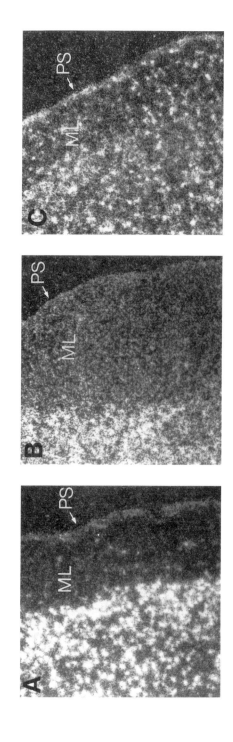

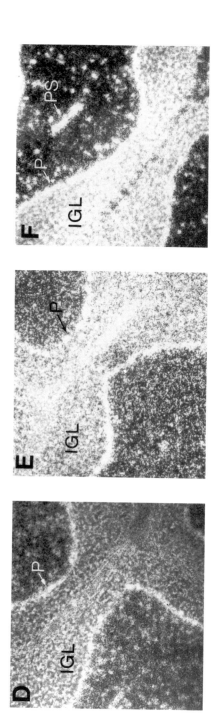

Figure 2. Dark field photomicrographs of rat brain tissue sections in situ hybridized to oligo(dT), hsc70, and hsp70 oligonucleotide probes. (A, B, C) cerebral cortex; (D, E, F) cerebellum. (A, D) oligo(dT) probe; (B, E) hsc 70 probe; (C, F) hsp70 probe. The rat was injected with 15 mg/kg amphetamine and sacrificed after 3 hours (39,40). In situ hybridization was carried out by modifications (42,48,49) of the method of Chesselet et al (50). Emulsion-coated slides were exposed for 3–7 days. PS, pial surface; ML, molecular layer; P, Purkinje cell layer; IGL, internal granular layer (×8)

observations). Overproduction of APP, as probably occurs in Down's syndrome (37), may overload the normal pathway of APP metabolism, leading to improper APP processing and ultimately to amyloid deposition.

(c) A mutation or mutations in some AD patients might result in the synthesis of abnormal proteins, overloading the stress system and eventually resulting in cell death.

We performed experiments in rat to test two of these possibilities, namely (a) that there are regional and cell-specific differences in heat shock protein 70 mRNA (hsp70 mRNA) and heat shock cognate 70 mRNA (hsc70 mRNA) expression in brain; and (b) that there is an attenuation of the heat shock response, as measured by hsp70 mRNA and hsc70 mRNA expression, in certain brain cells of the aged rat. In these studies, rats were either heat shocked or were administered amphetamine sulfate to induce hyperthermia (38-43). Inducible hsp70 mRNAs and constitutively synthesized hsc70 mRNAs were identified using oligonucleotide probes that hybridized specifically either to the hsp70 mRNA or the hsc70 mRNA (38-43). Our results showed that hsp70 mRNA was detected only in hyperthermic rats, whereas hsc70 mRNA was also present in control animals. In adult rats, both amphetamine-induced hyperthermia and heat shock robustly induced hsp70 mRNA in both cortex and cerebellum. Hsc70 mRNA was also induced to a lesser extent in hyperthermic amphetamine-treated rats and heat shocked rats (39, 40).

Quantitation of hsp70 and hsc70 mRNA levels, relative to those of 18S rRNA, in different brain regions revealed that both mRNAs were present at higher levels in cerebellum than in cerebral cortex. These results suggested that, on average, cell types in cerebellum had a more vigorous heat shock response than cells in cerebral cortex. In order to identify these cell types, we used the technique of in situ hybridization. Tissue sections from the cerebral cortex and cerebellum of adult amphetamine-treated rats were hybridized in situ to the two heat shock probes and to an oligo(dT) probe. Oligo(dT) is a probe that hybridizes to poly(A) tails of all intracellular polyadenylated mRNAs. Thus, levels of the hsp70 mRNAs and hsc70 mRNAs can be compared to the levels of total intracellular polyadenylated mRNA in specific cell types (44).

Figure 2 illustrates representative in situ hybridization experiments with the three probes to tissue sections from the cerebral cortex and cerebellum of an amphetamine-treated rat. Table 1 rates the grain densities of probe hybridization over the different cell types. In this amphetamine-treated rat, slot blot quantitation of total RNA extracted from the contralateral side of the brain showed that the relative levels of hsp70 mRNAs were approximately five times higher in cerebellum than in the cerebral cortex. Relative levels of hsc70 mRNAs were approximately three times higher in the cerebellum than in the cerebral cortex. In the cerebral cortex, the oligo(dT) probe did not hybridize to non-neuronal cells located at the pial surface or to cells located within the underlying molecular layer (Figure 2A). The oligo(dT) probe hybridized most strongly to neuronal cells just ventral to the molecular layer and showed a relatively uniform hybridization to neurons in deeper layers of the cortex. In cerebellum, Purkinje cells were intensely labelled by oligo(dT), as illustrated

Table 1. Density of grains in different cell types of rat cerebellum and cerebral cortex of amphetamine-treated rat

	Probe		
	Oligo(dT)	hsc70	hsp70
Cerebellum			
Purkinje cell	+ + + +	+ + +	+ +
Granule cell	+ +	+ +	+ + +
Glia	+	+	+ + + +
Cerebral cortex			
Pyramidal cell	+ + +	+ +	+
Glia	+	+	+ + +

+ low; + + moderate; + + + high.

by the punctate pattern of labelling in the Purkinje cell layer in Figure 2D. The most abundant cell type in the cerebellum, the granule cells of the internal granular layer (IGL), hybridized less intensely to oligo(dT). Non-neuronal cells at the pial surface, in the molecular layer, and in the white matter were sparsely labelled.

The hsc70 oligonucleotide demonstrated a similar pattern of hybridization in cerebral cortex to that of the oligo(dT) probe (Figure 2C). In cerebellum, the hsc70 probe hybridized more intensely to granule cells and to Purkinje cells, while other cell types in cerebellum were only sparsely labelled (Figure 2E).

A different overall pattern of hybridization was observed with the hsp70 oligonucleotide. In both the cerebral cortex and cerebellum (Figures 2C and 2F, respectively), the hsp70 probe hybridized most strongly to cells at the pial surface and to glia. Strong hybridization to this probe was seen in small cells within the Purkinje cell layer, most probably glia (41). As with the hsc70 probe, cerebellar granule cells hybridized much more strongly to the hsp70 probe than did neurons in the cerebral cortex (Figure 2F). These results indicated that high levels of hsp70 mRNAs and hsc70 mRNAs in cerebellar granule cells accounted for the increased levels of these mRNAs in total cerebellar RNA.

These results demonstrated that these two members of the heat shock 70 gene family were differentially localized in cells of cerebral cortex and cerebellum of hyperthermic rats. Differential localization was also present in adult rat hippocampus (results not shown). In each brain region analyzed, large neurons such as Purkinje cells and cortical or hippocampal pyramidal cells showed only a modest relative induction of hsp70 mRNA when compared to glia (41-43). Heat shock mRNAs are also strongly induced in glia of rabbit brain after LSD-induced hyperthermia (45,46). In contrast, the constitutively synthesized hsc70 mRNA was present at much higher levels in large neurons than in glia. These findings suggest that either large neurons could be at increased risk during different kinds of stress or that other members of the heat shock gene family such as hsc70 mRNA might compensate by being more highly expressed in these same neurons.

We have also examined the effect of aging on the heat shock response by comparing hsp70 mRNA and hsc70 mRNA levels in brain cells of adult and aged rats subjected to a heat stress of standardized duration and intensity. In the aged rat hippocampus, we observed a significant attentuation of hsp70 mRNA induction in neurons but not in glia (42). The relative levels of hsc70 mRNA were not significantly altered in either neurons or glia of aged rat hippocampus. These findings suggest that there was a selective attenuation in hsp70 mRNA induction in hippocampal neurons of aged rats.

These results show that (a) there are regional and cell specific differences in hsp70 and hsc70 mRNA expression in brain; large neurons, similar to those affected in AD, had an intrinsically less potent heat shock response than did small neurons or glia; and (b) there is an attenuation of the heat shock response in hippocampal cells of the aged rat; hsp70 mRNA induction was selectively decreased in hippocampal neurons. These findings are consistent with the possibility that there exists a delicate balance, in certain neuronal populations in AD, between the intracellular accumulation of abnormally folded proteins and the mediation of their removal via a member or members of the heat shock family. These results are also consistent with a shift in this balance during aging due to the diminishing ability of key neuronal populations to mount an adequate stress response.

We have focused on the hsp70 gene family in these preliminary studies. Other components of the stress response that could also be compromised include ubiquitin-mediated protein turnover (10,22), the increased synthesis of glycolytic enzymes that compensate for heat shock-induced loss of ATP (47), or the increased synthesis of GRP-78 that results from increased Ca^{++} influx (17), perhaps the result of receptor activation or of hypoxia. An analysis of mRNA levels for different members of the heat shock family between AD tissues and nondemented tissues, matched for age and for agonal variables, will be necessary to determine if there is an ongoing stress response in AD brain such as we propose here. A direct comparison of mRNA levels in stressed lymphocytes or fibroblasts from AD patients and controls would establish if there is a defect in the function of a member of the heat shock gene family that is unique to patients diagnosed with AD.

Acknowledgments

This work was supported by the following grants: NIH grants HD14886 (MM-B) and AG08013 (MM-B and JDR), the Leland Fikes Foundation (MM-B), NIH grant NS22037 (JDR); the Veterans Administration Clinical Investigation Program (JDR), and the Bio Humanics Foundation (JDR). We thank Dr Cheryl Craft for synthesizing oligonucleotides and Cheryl Beisert for word processing.

REFERENCES

1. Price DL, Koo EH, Unterbeck A. Bioessays 1989; 10: 69-74.
2. Selkoe DJ. Ann Rev Neurosci 1989; 12: 463-90.
3. Kosik KS, Joachim CL, Selkoe DJ. Proc Natl Acad Sci USA 1986; 83: 4044-8.
4. Wischik CM, Novak M, Edwards PC, Klug A, Tichelaar W, Crowther RA. Proc Natl Acad Sci USA 1988; 85: 4884-8.
5. Bancher C, Brunner C, Lassmann H, Budka H, Jellinger K, Wiche G, Seitelberger F, Grundke-Iqbal I, Iqbal K, Wisniewski HM. Brain Res 1989; 477: 90-9.
6. Lemaire HG, Salbaum JM, Multhaup G, Kang J, Bayney RM, Unterbeck A, Beyreuther K, Muller-Hill B. Nuc Acids Res 1989; 17: 517-21.

7. Lindquist S. Ann Rev Biochem 1986; 55: 1151-91.
8. Lindquist S, Craig EA. Ann Rev Genet 1988; 22: 631-77.
9. Pelham H. Nature 1988; 332: 776-7.
10. Finley D, Ozkaynak E, Varshavsky A. Cell 1987; 48: 1035-46.
11. Craig EA. CRC Crit Rev Biochem 1989; 18: 239-80.
12. Ellis JR, Hemmingsen SM. TIBS 1989; 14: 339-42.
13. Beckmann RP, Mizzen LA, Welch WJ. Science 1990; 248: 850-4.
14. Pelham HRB. Cell 1986; 46: 959-61.
15. Chiang H-L, Terlecky SR, Plant CP, Dice FJ. Science 1989; 246: 382-5.
16. Chappell TG, Konforti BB, Schmid SL, Rothman JE. J Biol Chem 1987; 262: 746-51.
17. Lee AS. Trends Biochem Sci 1987; 12: 20-3.
18. Munro S, Pelham HRB. Cell 1986; 46: 291-300.
19. Kozutsumi Y, Segal M, Normington K, Gething M-J, Sambrook J. Nature 1988; 332: 462-4.
20. Bond U, Schlesinger MJ. Mol Cell Biol 1986; 6: 4602-10.
21. Wu C, Wilson S, Walker B, Dawid I, Paisley T, Zimarino V. Ueda H. Proc Natl Acad Sci USA 1987; 84: 5991-4.
22. Rechsteiner M. Ann Rev Cell Biol 1987; 3: 1-30.
23. Munro S, Pelham HRB. EMBO J 1984; 3: 3087-93.
24. Morandi A, Los B, Osofsky L, Autilio-Gambetti L, Gambetti P. Prog Clin Biol Res 1989; 317: 819-27.
25. Tanaka K, Jay G, Isselbacher KJ. Biochim Biophys Acta 1988; 950: 138-46.
26. Mori HH, Kondo J, Ihara Y. Science 1987; 235: 1641-4.
27. Perry G, Friedman R, Shaw G, Chau V. Proc Natl Acad Sci USA 1987; 84: 3033-6.
28. Manetto V, Perry G, Tabaton M, Mulvihill P, Fried VA, Smith HT, Gambetti P, Autilio-Gambetti L. Proc Natl Acad Sci USA 1988; 85: 4501-5.
29. Hamos JE, Oblas B, Pulaski-Salo D, Apostolides PJ, Drachman DA. Neurosci Abstr 1989; 15: 1043.
30. Faassen AE, O'Leary JJ, Rodysill KJ, Bergh N, Hallgren HM. Exper Cell Res 1989; 183: 326-34.
31. Liu Ay-C, Lin Z, Choi H-S, Sorhage F, Li B. J Biol Chem 1989; 264: 12037-45.
32. Fargnoli J, Kunisada T, Fornace AJ Jr, Schneider EL, Holbrook NJ. Proc Natl Acad Sci USA 1990; 87: 846-50.
33. Harrison GS, Drabkin HA, Kao F-T, Hartz J, Hart IM, Chu EHY, Wu BJ, Morimoto RI. Som Cell Mol Genet 1987; 13: 119-30.
34. St George-Hyslop PH, Haines JL, Polinsky RJ, Tanzi RE, Farrer L, Myers RH, Gusella JF. Can J Neurol Sci 1989; 16: 465-7.
35. Siman R, Card JP, Nelson RB, Davis LG. Neuron 1989; 3: 275-85.
36. Salbaum JM, Weidemann A, Lemaire H-G, Masters CL, Beyreuther K. EMBO J 1988; 7: 2807-13.
37. Tanzi RE, Gusella JF, Watkins PC, Bruns GAP, St George-Hyslop P, Van Keuren ML, Patterson D, Pagan S, Kurnit DM, Neve RL. Science 1987; 235: 880-4.
38. Miller EK, Trulson ME, Mues GI, Munn TZ, Goggans ML, Morrison MR, Raese JD. Neurosci Abstr 1987; 13: 1709.
39. Miller EK, Raese JD, Morrison-Bogorad MR. Neurosci Abstr 1989; 15: 1127.
40. Miller EK, Raese JD, Morrison-Bogorad M. J Neurochem (in press).
41. Morrison-Bogorad M, Groshan K, Pardue S, Raese JD, Miller EK (in preparation).
42. Morrison-Bogorad M, Pardue S, Groshan K, Miller EK, Raese JD (in preparation).
43. Morrison-Bogorad MR, Groshan K, Miller EK, Raese JD. Neurosci Abstr 1989; 15: 1127.
44. Griffin WST, Alejos MA, Cox EJ, Morrison MR. J Cell Biochem 1985; 27: 205-14.
45. Sprang GK, Brown IR. Mol Brain Res 1987; 3: 89-93.

46. Masing TE, Brown IR. Neurochem Res 1989; 14: 725-31.
47. Nickells RW, Browder LW. Dev Biol 1985; 112: 391-5.
48. Willcutts M. PhD Thesis, Department of Cell and Molecular Biology, University of Texas Southwestern School of Graduate Sciences, March 1990.
49. Willcutts M, Morrison-Bogorad M. (in preparation).
50. Chesselet M-F, Weiss L, Wuenschell C, Tobin AJ, Affolter H-U. J Comp Neurol 1987; 262: 125-40.

Address for correspondence:

M. Morrison-Bogorad,
U.T. Southwestern Medical Center at Dallas,
Department of Neurology,
5323 Harry Hines Blvd,
Dallas, TX 75235-9036, USA

Part V

BRAIN AMYLOIDOSIS

30 Co-occurrence of Two Amyloid Proteins in a Patient with Familial Amyloidosis, Finnish Type

BLAS FRANGIONE, MATTI HALTIA, EFRAT LEVY,
JORGE GHISO, SARI KIURU AND FRANCES PRELLI

Familial amyloidosis, Finnish type (FAF) (1,2), also known as familial amyloid polyneuropathy type IV (3) or Meretoja's syndrome, was first described by Meretoja in 1969 (4). Although the highest incidences, up to 1:1040, are found in the Kymenlaakso and Lammi regions of southern Finland (5), cases of FAF have also been reported from Denmark (6), the Netherlands (7), and the United States (8-10). By 1978, 307 cases had been diagnosed in Finland (11). Extensive genetic studies have shown that the proportion of affected individuals in the pedigrees analyzed was 0.544, and that the sex ratio corresponded to 1:1. These features are compatible with autosomal dominant inheritance with full penetrance (5).

FAF is clinically characterized by lattice corneal dystrophy, detectable by slit-lamp examination after the age of 20 years (12). The facial skin gradually becomes loose and sagging, and resulting blepharochalasis often necessitates corrective plastic surgery. After the age of 65 years, visual acuity rapidly declines. Another hallmark of the disease is progressive cranial neuropathy, the first manifestation of which is upper facial paresis after the age of 40 years (13). Later, even the lower cranial nerves may be involved, resulting in bulbar type symptoms (4). In an early study, two out of ten patients were reported to have parkinsonism. Approximately half the patients suffer mild intermittent proteinuria. The rare homozygous cases die of a severe nephrotic syndrome by the age of 30 years (5).

Histopathological studies of kidney, skin, muscle and nerve biopsies as well as autopsy specimens have demonstrated the presence of small congophilic deposits with apple-green birefringence and red–green dichroism in polarized light in most tissues of the body. Such deposits occur particularly in blood vessel walls and in association with basement membranes, principally in the kidney glomeruli, around the epidermal appendages, in the perineurial sheaths of peripheral nerves, and in the cornea. Electron microscopy revealed that these deposits are composed of fibrils, about 7-9 nm in diameter. Earlier attempts to characterize the FAF amyloid protein have led to inconclusive or conflicting results.

Alzheimer's Disease: Basic Mechanisms, Diagnosis and Therapeutic Strategies
Edited by K. Iqbal, D. R. C. McLachlan, B. Winblad and H. M. Wisniewski
©1991 John Wiley & Sons Ltd

Our own findings (2) did not support an immunologic relationship between FAF amyloid and transthyretin or its variants (14). Moreover, we were unable to demonstrate immunocytochemical crossreactivity with any other previously identified amyloid proteins or their precursors associated with systemic or cerebral amyloidosis. Although the FAF amyloid usually is associated with basement membranes of various cell types, our immunohistochemical stainings using antibodies against a variety of basement membrane and cytoskeletal components did not disclose binding to the amyloid deposits. However, these lesions were intensely immunolabelled by an antiserum to amyloid P component, a serum and membrane associated glycoprotein found with all types of amyloid deposits tested so far (15).

The FAF amyloid deposits in tissues also reacted strongly with a rabbit antiserum raised against a purified low molecular weight subunit of amyloid fibrils, isolated from the kidney of one of our FAF patients (1,2) (Figure 1). The immunoreactivity of the anti-FAF amyloid antiserum was completely absorbed by the purified amyloid subunit, and this antiserum did not stain amyloid deposits in other types of amyloidosis or normal glomeruli. The amino-terminal sequence of this subunit was homologous to gelsolin (1), an actin-binding protein. The amyloid peptide was found to be a degradation product, starting at position 173, of the gelsolin

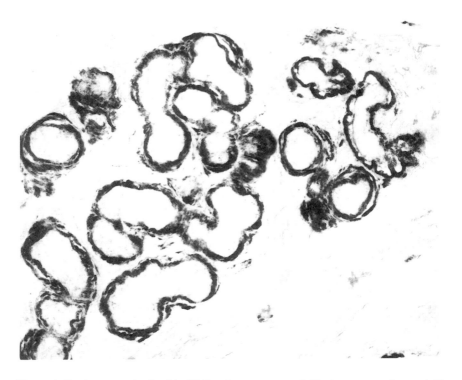

Figure 1. Eccrine sweat glands of the FAF patient are surrounded by immunoreactive amyloid deposits. Peroxidase-antiperoxidase method. Rabbit antiserum raised against purified FAF amyloid subunit 1:100 (×400)

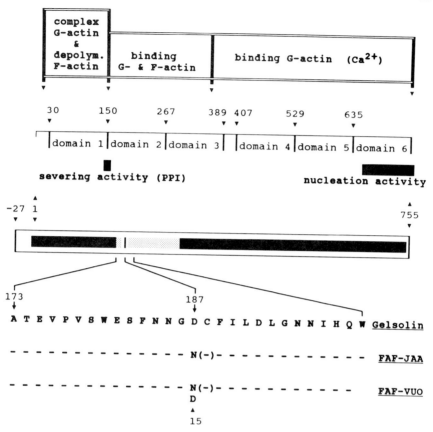

Figure 2. Schematic representation of human plasma gelsolin, as deduced from cDNA. Numbers are according to reference 20. The protein is composed of 755 residues containing six domains with internal homology. Numbers and arrowheads indicate the location of the sixfold repetitive structural motif found in gelsolin and related proteins. Top: residues 24 to 150 are related to G-actin binding as well as F-actin depolymerization activity. Domains 2 and 3 are involved in G- or F-actin binding and domains 4 to 6, in interaction with G-actin in a Ca^{2+}-dependent manner. Residues 150 to 160 mediate the PPI-regulated binding of gelsolin to the sites of actin filaments before severing. The 75-residue C-terminal peptide is related to the molecule's nucleation activity. Bottom: Amino terminal sequence of amyloid proteins VUO and JAA in comparison with human plasma gelsolin, stipple indicates location of the amyloid protein. Position 187 indicates the site of the amino acid substitution, corresponding to position 15 of the amyloid subunit. Amino acids are expressed in one-letter code; ( ), undetermined; –, homology

molecule. Other workers reported homology of tryptic peptides of FAF amyloid to gelsolin (16).

Gelsolin is a member of a class of actin-modulating proteins found in lower eukaryotes and mammals, which sever actin filaments, nucleate actin filament growth, and cap barbed filament ends (17). It is regulated by both Ca^{2+} (18) and polyphosphoinositides (19). A single gene on human chromosome 9 encodes two forms of gelsolin; one is cytoplasmic, and the other is secreted (20–22). Plasma gelsolin, originally called actin depolymerizing factor, (ADF), has a higher relative molecular mass (93 kDa) than the cytoplasmic form (90 kDa), due to an additional 25-amino acid peptide at its amino terminus. Both forms are expressed in a large variety of cell types, including neurons (17,23).

Extended amino-terminal sequence analysis of our original patient (VUO) showed heterogeneity (Asn and Asp) at position 15, while corresponding studies of a second FAF patient (JAA) showed substitution of asparagine for aspartic acid at the same position (Figure 2), corresponding to amino acid 187 of plasma gelsolin.

The presence of both amino acids at position 15 in the first patient may result from expression of normal and variant alleles in the amyloid fibril as has been shown in hereditary cerebral hemorrhage with amyloidosis, Dutch type (24,25). Alternatively, the presence of aspartic acid may be due to partial deamination of asparagine. The amino acid substitution is located in a repetitive motif (FXXXDXFIL) of unknown function, highly conserved among species (26). Position 187 is also contained in a 26-kDa fragment (positions 150–373), reported to have substantial binding capacity for both G- and F-actin, although with very low severing activity (27). It is conceivable that the replacement of an acidic residue with a neutral asparagine may result in a charge imbalance, leading to unexpected interactions with other molecules and/or triggering a particular folding responsible for abnormal degradation and fibril formation. We postulated that the variant described here may be due to a guanine to adenine transition corresponding to nucleotide 654 of the human plasma gelsolin cDNA (20). We have designated this variant of gelsolin-associated amyloidosis *Agel ASN 187*.

To test the possiblity that this mutation exists, high molecular weight genomic DNA was isolated from tissues of four autopsy cases of FAF and from fresh lymphocytes of one FAF patient. Fragments that contain nucleotide 654 were amplified with the polymerase chain reaction, using oligonucleotides that were synthesized based on the cDNA sequences encoding gelsolin. The amplified fragments were subcloned into an M13 bacteriophage vector and sequenced by dideoxy chain termination. The DNA sequences demonstrated that all five patients had one allele containing a point mutation at nucleotide 654, as well as one normal allele.

A different approach was taken to develop a diagnostic test. An oligonucleotide containing the mutation was hybridized to slot blots of amplified DNA fragments. At high stringency (65 °C), only DNA isolated from FAF patients hybridized to the probe (Figure 3).

Preliminary results with DNA isolated from affected and unaffected members of the same family suggest that the mutation (G to A) segregates with the disease, and that the slot blot analysis can be used as a diagnostic assay for prenatal evaluation for FAF in high-risk populations. These results also emphasize the importance of primary structural alterations of the precursor proteins in amyloidogenesis.

We have observed the coexistence of gelsolin variant ASN 187 with Alzheimer's β-protein and Alzheimer-type brain lesions in our original patient (VUO).

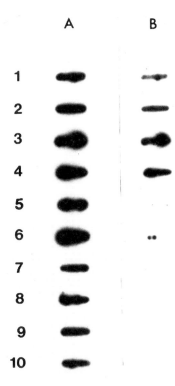

Figure 3. Slot blot analysis demonstrating the existence of a point mutation in DNA isolated from FAF patients (nos. 1-4) and its absence in DNA isolated from normal controls (nos. 5-10). Genomic DNA sequences were amplified with the polymerase chain reaction technique and blotted in duplicates. After hybridization with an oligonucleotide that contains the mutation, the blots were washed in low stringency (48 °C) (lane A) and in high stringency (65 °C) (lane B)

Furthermore, antiserum raised against FAF amyloid reacts with both classical and diffuse Lewy bodies.

CASE REPORT

Patient VUO had developed sagging facial skin and lattice corneal dystrophy over the past decades. In addition to these signs of FAF, in 1986, at the age of 69 years, he complained of loss of memory. Physical examination disclosed loss of the sense of vibration in the extremities and bilateral inguinal hernias. Psychometric tests showed extensive cognitive impairment. An electroencephalogram revealed moderate generalized changes, and computerized tomography showed widespread cerebral cortical atrophy, with parietal accentuation. Electroneuromyography gave evidence of facial nerve involvement. The results of laboratory tests were essentially within normal limits apart from evidence for mild hypothyrosis, for which substitution therapy was instituted. However, his mental condition deteriorated rapidly and he became increasingly disoriented, confused and, at times, aggressive. He died two years later, with signs of acute pneumonia.

His sister, demented at the age of 59, had died at 65, but no autopsy had been performed. She also had lattice corneal dystrophy and sagging facial skin.

Neuropathological findings

The brain weighed 1150 g and showed slight to moderate fronto-temporo-parietal gyral atrophy. Coronal sections disclosed moderate generalized ventricular dilation and mild depigmentation of the substantia nigra.

Silver stained sections showed numerous neuritic plaques throughout the cerebral cortex, many of them with congophilic cores. In addition, numerous neurofibrillary tangles were seen in the hippocampus and moderate to small amounts in most neocortical areas. Hippocampal pyramidal cells displayed granulovacuolar degeneration. In the parahippocampal and cingulate gyri and (to a lesser degree) in the temporal neocortex, slightly eosinophilic nonargyrophilic cytoplasmic inclusions with indistinct borders were seen. The substantia nigra showed moderate neuronal loss and extraneuronal pigment accumulations. The cytoplasm of many nigral neurons harbored classical spherical eosinophilic Lewy bodies with a clear halo. Occasional Lewy bodies were also seen in other brainstem nuclei, including locus ceruleus, as well as in the substantia innominata.

After pretreatment with formic acid the antiserum raised against a synthetic peptide homologous to Alzheimer's β-protein (28) reacted strongly with the neuritic plaques as well as with occasional meningeal and cortical blood vessel walls (Figure 4A). The neurofibrillary tangles were intensely stained by the antiserum raised against isolated Alzheimer neurofibrillary tangles (Figure 4B) (29). The antiserum raised against the purified low-molecular FAF amyloid subunit (2) stained the walls of occasional meningeal and cortical blood vessels. In addition, strong immunoreactivity was seen in the cytoplasm of scattered deep cortical neurons, particularly in the parahippocampal gyrus. This immunoreactivity corresponded to the intraneuronal eosinophilic inclusions (Figure 4C). The anti-FAF amyloid antiserum also stained the periphery of the classical Lewy bodies in substantia nigra and other locations (Figure 5). The same lesions were also stained by an antibody against ubiquitin. Furthermore, thread or dot-like immunoreactivity was observed diffusely in the gray matter with anti-FAF antibody as well as at the periphery of neuritic plaques, probably corresponding to dystrophic neurites. The immunoreactivity of the intraneuronal inclusions was totally absorbed by the purified low molecular weight FAF amyloid subunit but not by ubiquitin.

The immunoreactivity of the anti-FAF amyloid antiserum with classical and diffuse Lewy bodies was also tested in one case of Parkinson's disease, one case of Alzheimer's disease with nigral Lewy bodies, and one case of diffuse Lewy body disease. In all cases, both the diffuse Lewy bodies as well as the periphery of most classical Lewy bodies were intensely immunoreactive with the anti-FAF amyloid antiserum. This

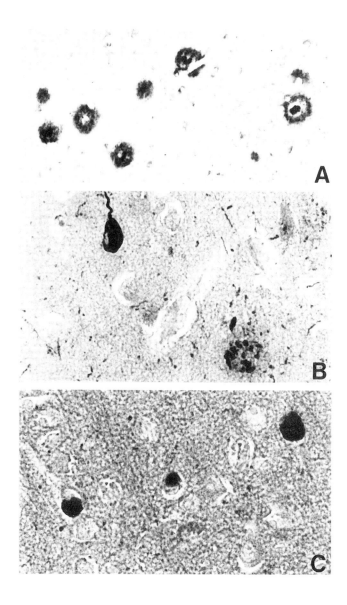

Figure 4. Temporal neocortex of FAF patient VUO. Paraffin sections stained with the peroxidase–antiperoxidase method. (A) Senile plaques immunoreactive with rabbit antiserum against a synthetic peptide homologous to Alzheimer's β-protein ($\times$100). (B) A neurofibrillary tangle and dystrophic neurites at the periphery of a neuritic plaque bind antiserum raised against Alzheimer's neurofibrillary tangles ($\times$300). (C) Scattered deep cortical neurons contain cytoplasmic bodies strongly immunoreactive with rabbit antiserum raised against purified FAF amyloid subunit ($\times$300)

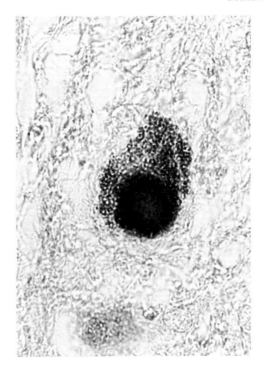

Figure 5. A classical Lewy body in a nigral neuron of FAF patient VUO. Peroxidase-antiperoxidase method. Rabbit antiserum against purified FAF amyloid subunit 1:100 (× 1000)

immunoreactivity was abolished by absorption with the purified low molecular weight FAF amyloid subunit.

DISCUSSION

Our findings document the deposition of two forms of amyloid-related proteins within the nervous system of the same patient. Little is known of the simultaneous occurrence of two chemically distinct amyloid proteins in the brain, apart from rare cases with coexistent Creutzfeldt–Jakob and Alzheimer's diseases (30). Beyond the chance coincidence of a rare with a common disease, the presence of specific tissue factors favoring the deposition of amyloid fibrils was considered in these cases. The possibility of the simultaneous occurrence of two dominantly inherited amyloidoses, FAF and familial Alzheimer-like disease, cannot be excluded in our case because the patient's sister also had developed dementia.

We also observed intraneuronal structures including classical Lewy bodies immunoreactive with the antiserum raised against the purified low molecular weight FAF amyloid subunit. These same structures were also strongly stained by an antibody against ubiquitin. However, absorption with ubiquitin did not affect the anti-FAF amyloid immunoreactivity, which was completely absorbed by the purified FAF amyloid subunit and gelsolin. These findings indicate that, in addition to ubiquitin, the intraneuronal inclusions contain an epitope crossreactive with gelsolin. Accumulation of gelsolin-related material within neuronal cells is not inconceivable in view of the expression of gelsolin in neurons (31) and its essential function in the modulation of the cytoskeleton (17,32).

CONCLUSIONS

Familial amyloidosis, Finnish type (FAF), is a form of systemic amyloidosis showing congophilic deposits in most tissues, particularly in association with blood vessel walls and basement membrane.

We have shown that:

(a) The amyloid protein is a degradation fragment of gelsolin, an actin-binding protein. It starts at position 173 of the gelsolin molecule and has an amino acid substitution (Asn for Asp) at position 187.

(b) Nucleotide 654 of the gelsolin gene, located in chromosome 9, is mutated (A for G).

(c) Gelsolin-associated lesions coexist with Alzheimer's β-protein and Alzheimer-type lesions in the brain of a patient with FAF.

(d) Antiserum raised against FAF amyloid reacts with classical and diffuse Lewy bodies, suggesting a role of gelsolin in the pathogenesis of diffuse Lewy body disease and Parkinson's disease.

This variant of gelsolin-associated amyloidosis is designated Agel ASN 187.

REFERENCES

1. Haltia M, Prelli F, Ghiso J et al. Biochem Biophys Res Comm 1990; 167: 927-32.
2. Haltia M, Ghiso J, Prelli F et al. Am J Pathol 1990; 136: 1223-8.
3. Cohen AS, Rubinow A. In Dyck PJ, Thomas PK, Lambert EH, Bunge R (eds) Peripheral neuropathy, Vol. II, Philadelphia: W. B. Saunders, 1866.
4. Meretoja J. Ann Clin Res 1969; 1: 314-24.
5. Meretoja J. Clin Genet 1973; 4: 173-85.
6. Boysen G, Galassi G, Kamieniecka Z, Schlaeer J, Trojaborg W. J Neurol Neurosurg Psychiat 1979; 42: 1020-30.
7. Winkelman JE, Delleman JW, Ansink BJJ. Klin Monatsbl Augenheilkd 1971; 159: 618-23.
8. Purcell JJ Jr, Rodrigues M, Chishti MI, Riner RN, Dooley JM. Ophthalmology 1983; 90: 1512-17.
9. Sack GH, Dumars KW, Gummerson KS, Law A, McKusick VA. Johns Hopkins Med J 1981; 149: 239-47.
10. Darras BT, Adelman LS, Mora JS, Bodziner RA, Munsat TL. Neurology 1986; 36: 432-5.
11. Meretoja J, Hollmén T, Meretoja T, Penttinen R. Med Biol 1978; 56: 17-22.
12. Meretoja J. Ophthalmologica 1972; 165: 15-37.
13. Meretoja J, Teppo L. APMIS Section A, 1971; 79: 432-40.
14. Maury CPJ, Teppo A-M, Kariniemi A-L, Koeppen AH. Am J Clin Pathol 1988; 89: 359-64.
15. Castaño EM, Frangione B. Lab Invest 1988; 58: 122-32.

16. Maury CPJ, Alli K, Baumann M. FEBS Lett 1990; 260: 85-7.
17. Stossel T, Chaponnier C, Ezzel R et al. Ann Rev Cell Biol 1985; 1: 353-402.
18. Chaponnier C, Yin H, Stossel T. J Exp Med 1987; 165: 97-106.
19. Janmey P, Stossel T. Nature (London) 1987; 325: 362-64.
20. Kwiatkowski DJ, Stossel TP, Orkin SH et al. Nature 1986; 323: 455-8.
21. Kwiatkowski DJ, Westbrook CA, Bruns GAP et al. Am J Hum Genet 1988; 42: 565-72.
22. Kwiatkowski DJ, Mehl R, Yin HL. J Cell Biol 1988; 106: 375-84.
23. Yin HL, Kwiatkowski DJ, Mole JE et al. J Biol Chem 1984; 259: 5271-6.
24. Levy E, Carman MD, Fernandez-Madrid I et al. Science 1990; 248: 1124-6.
25. Prelli F, Levy E, Van Duinen SG et al. Biochem Biophys Res Comm 1990; 170: 301-7.
26. Way M, Weeds A. J Mol Biol 1988; 203: 1127-33.
27. Bryan J. J Cell Biol 1988; 106: 1553-62.
28. Castaño EM, Ghiso J, Prelli F et al. Biochem Biophys Res Comm 1986; 141: 782-9.
29. Gorevic PD, Goñi F, Pons-Estel B et al. J Neuropath Exp Neurol 1986; 45: 647-69.
30. Brown P, Jannotta F, Gibbs CJ et al. Neurology 1990; 40: 226-8.
31. Petrucci TC, Thomas C, Bray D. J Neurochem 1983; 40: 1507-16.
32. Forscher P. Trends Neurol Sci 1989; 12: 468-74.

Address for correspondence:

Blas Frangione,
Department of Pathology,
New York University Medical Center,
550 First Avenue,
New York, NY 10016, USA

31 Proteolysis in the Formation of Amyloid Fibrils in Alzheimer's Disease

GEORGE G. GLENNER, PAIGE M. MEHLHAFF AND HIROO KAWANO

The selective localization of β-protein amyloid fibers (1) to the brain and more selectively to vessels in the leptomeninges and the grey matter has been explained by compartmentalization of 'amyloidogenic' enzymes involved in cleavage of the 695 amino acid β-protein gene product (βGP) (2) to release a circulating β-protein precursor (βPP) and subsequently to form the 28–39 amino acid β-protein amyloid fibril (3).

Recent progress in the investigation of the post-translational modification of the βGP by proteolysis to form the β-protein which composes the amyloid fibrils of the senile plaque core and cerebrovasculature in Alzheimer's disease may provide insight into the course of amyloid fibril deposition as well as a therapeutic approach to Alzheimer's disease. It has been shown in vitro that some segments of the β-protein have an intrinsic β-pleated sheet structure and form nonbranching fibrils. These have been designated the 'amyloidogenic regions'. As in other proteins, the presence of β-pleated sheet segments in the β-protein strongly suggests that these regions contribute to the insolubility and resistance to proteolysis of the β-protein in vitro (4). However, other segments under in-vivo conditions may also contribute to these characteristics.

Earlier suggestions (3,5) have been presented that the site(s) of proteolytic cleavage of the βGP and βPP might predicate whether amyloid fibrils composed of the β-protein will be formed. These suggestions appear to have some experimental basis. The βGP has been proposed as a ubiquitous, glycosylated membrane protein with intracytoplasmic, transmembranal and extracellular domains. Release or secretion of the βPP from the βGP at the plasmalemma would occur by cleavage of about two-thirds of the β-protein segment incorporated extracellularly near the C-terminal region of the βGP from the remaining intramembranal one-third. This would leave approximately 28 residues of the β-protein at the C-terminus of the released βPP. If further proteolytic cleavage approximately halves this 28-residue segment, further cleavage of βPP just prior to residue 1 of the β protein might not in the absence of the intact 1–28 amyloidogenic segment result in amyloid fibril formation.

Such an intra-β protein cleavage site may well be the cleavage site common to normal individuals, i.e. those not having Alzheimer's disease. In fact the gene coding for the enzyme catalyzing this cleavage may well be absent in familial Alzheimer's

Alzheimer's Disease: Basic Mechanisms, Diagnosis and Therapeutic Strategies
Edited by K. Iqbal, D. R. C. McLachlan, B. Winblad and H. M. Wisniewski
© 1991 John Wiley & Sons Ltd

disease (FAD), i.e. the FAD marker gene, thus predisposing these families to amyloid fibril formation as the result of further proteolytic cleavage of βPP prior to residue 1 of the β protein and release of intact 1-28 β-protein to form amyloid fibrils. As noted above, a variety of in-vitro studies have shown that certain segments of the β-protein have 'amyloidogenic' capabilities.

Nonetheless, if the 1-28 β-protein domain (occupying the C-terminus of βPP) fails to be internally cleaved as the result of an absent or defective FAD gene coding for the specific proteolytic enzyme or as the result of an acquired inhibitor of this enzyme, e.g. in sporadic Alzheimer's disease, then a subsequent cleavage prior to residue 1 would release the intact 1-28 β-protein to form amyloid fibrils. Inhibition of this latter proteolytic step, which would produce the N-terminus of the amyloid β-protein, might completely prevent amyloid fibril formation from βPP. Such inhibition would, therefore, provide a therapeutic approach to the treatment of Alzheimer's disease, if, as we have suggested, Alzheimer's disease is the result of cerebral amyloid fibril formation.

A hypothetical example of β-protein amyloid formation is the following. The 1-41 β-protein domain with an N-terminal tripeptide of the βPP is:

-2 1   5   16

Val-Lys-Met-Asp-Ala-Glu-Phe-Arg-His-Asp-Ser-Gly-Tyr-Glu-Val-His-His-Gln-Lys-

28

Leu-Val-Phe-Phe-Ala-Glu-Asp-Val-Gly-Ser-Asn-Lys-Gly-Ala-Ile-Gly-Leu-Met-Val-

40

Gly-Gly-Val-Val-Ile

An assumption is made that all proteolytic cleavages of the β-protein gene product (βGP) are the result of trypsin-like serine proteases. If enzyme 1 cleaves the Lys[28]-Gly[29] bond of the βGP at the membrane surface, it will release (secrete) the βPP. If normally enzyme 2 cleaves the Lys[16]-Leu[17] intra-β protein bond, it will release the C-terminal segment (approximately one-half) of the β-protein. If enzyme 3 cleaves the Lys[-2]-Met[-1] bond it will release the remaining segment of the β-protein having a Met N-terminus. Aminopeptidase activity would further cleave the Met[-1] residue to yield the consistently reported Asp N-terminal segment of the β-protein (1,2,4,7,8). Because of their predilection for lysyl residues, it is postulated that cleavage by enzyme 1, 2 or 3 at the Arg[5]-His[6] bond does not occur. Because of factors related to the formation of the β-pleated sheet, fibrillogenesis (6) would be prevented by the prior cleavage of the β-protein region of βPP by enzyme 2 into two nonamyloidogenic segments and consequently amyloid fibrils would not form.

However, if enzyme 2 is absent (e.g. in FAD) or inhibited (e.g. in acquired Alzheimer's disease), the whole β-protein domain would be released by enzyme 3 (in association with an aminopeptidase cleavage of the N-terminal Met) to provide the intact 1-28 β-protein. This would result in amyloid fibril formation. It is of interest that the consistent presence of the N-terminal Asp of β-protein may be the result of the reduced activity of some aminopeptidases on N-terminal Asp residues (15 times less than on N-terminal Asn residues). Though this scheme of proteolytic formation of β-protein amyloid fibrils is strictly theoretical, e.g. we do not know if enzymes 1, 2 and 3 are a single or different enzymes, the strong likelihood is proposed that enzyme 2 differs markedly from 1 and 3 and all differ from each other in V_{max} and K_m values in their activity at the various cleavage sites. Abnormal processing of the βPP consistent with that presented here has recently been implicated in amyloid formation in Alzheimer's disease (7). In addition evidence that a βPP 'secretase' cleaves at or near Lys[16] has recently been presented (8) (the term 'secretase' would appear to be more appropriate for an enzyme cleaving at Lys[28], the N-terminus of the trasmembrane region of βGP). Therefore, the result of the above hypothetical process would be that a synthetic inhibitor of enzyme 3 would most probably prevent amyloid formation and would, as postulated, abort the progress of Alzheimer's disease.

Partial purification and characterization has been achieved of an enzyme from leptomeningeal vessels in normal and Alzheimer's disease patients having the characteristic of enzyme 3, i.e. completely cleaving the Lys^{-2}-Met^{-1} bond of the synthetic substrate VKMDA, i.e. the predicted tryptic cleavage site leading to β-amyloid fibril formation by subsequent aminopeptidase release of Met^{-1}. This enzyme cleaves on the carboxyl side of 11 different peptides containing an internal lysyl residue, but has no activity on internal arginyl residues. The enzyme has been purified by ammonium sulfate fractionation (30–60% saturation) and the use of Prozorb, a serine protease affinity column matrix. Serine protease inhibitor TLCK significantly inhibited enzyme activity. If amyloid fibril formation in Alzheimer's disease is to be prevented, this enzyme appears to be the postulated candidate for inhibition. Further studies are in progress to purify and define further the affinity of this enzyme for the βPP.

Acknowledgments

This work was supported by the Metropolitan Life Foundation and by grants from the National Institute on Aging (AG05683), the American Health Assistance Foundation and the National Alzheimer's Association.

REFERENCES

1. Glenner GG, Wong CW. Alzheimer's disease: initial report of the purification and characterization of a novel cerebrovascular amyloid protein. Biochem Biophys Res Comm 1984; 120: 885–90.
2. Kang J, Lemaire HG, Unterbeck A, Salbaum JM, Masters CL, Gryeschik KH, Multhaup G, Beyreuther K, Muller-Hill B. The precursor of Alzheimer's disease amyloid A4 protein resembles a cell-surface receptor. Nature 1987; 234: 733–6.
3. Glenner GG, Ein D, Eanes ED, Bladen HA, Terry W, Page D. The creation of 'amyloid' fibrils from Bence Jones proteins in vitro. Science 1971; 174: 712–14.
4. Gorevic PD, Castaño EM, Sarma R, Frangione B. Ten to fourteen residue peptides of Alzheimer's disease protein are sufficient for amyloid fibril formation and its characteristic X-ray diffraction pattern. Biochem Biophys Res Comm 1987; 147: 854–62.
5. Glenner GG. Alzheimer's disease: its proteins and genes. Cell 1988; 52: 307–8.

6. Glenner GG. Amyloid deposits and amyloidosis: the β-fibrilloses (Medical Progress Report). N Engl J Med 1980; 302: 1283-92.
7. Sisodia SS, Koo EH, Beyreuther K, Unterbeck A, Price DL. Evidence that β-amyloid protein Alzheimer's disease is not derived by normal processing. Science 1990; 248: 492-5.
8. Esch FS, Keim PS, Beattie EC, Blacher RW, Culwell AR, Oltersdorf T, McClure D, Ward PJ. Cleavage of amyloid β-peptide during constitutive processing of its precursor. Science 1990; 248: 1122-4.

Address for correspondence:

Dr George G. Glenner,
University of California, San Diego,
School of Medicine,
Pathology Department 0612,
La Jolla, CA 92093, USA

32 The Alzheimer's β-Amyloid Peptide is Cleaved During Constitutive Processing of the Amyloid Precursor Protein

F. S. ESCH, P. S. KEIM, E. C. BEATTIE, R. W. BLACHER,
A. R. CULWELL, T. OLTERSDORF, D. McCLURE AND
P. J. WARD

The beta-amyloid peptide (β-AP) which forms the central core of senile plaques in the Alzheimer's disease (AD) brain is a small fragment of the much larger amyloid precursor protein (APP). The nearly ubiquitous distribution of APP throughout the body and the relative absence of β-AP deposition in normal brain suggests that altered processing of APP occurs in AD and may represent a key pathogenic event in the disease. Constitutive processing of APP results in the secretion of a large, soluble NH_2-terminal fragment and the generation of a membrane-bound 9-kDa COOH-terminal fragment. We have purified both APP fragments from human embryonic kidney 293 cells transfected with cDNAs encoding the 695 and 751 amino acid forms of the APP; direct protein microsequencing, mass spectrometry and amino acid analyses of these NH_2- and COOH-terminal APP fragments have established that they are generated by *proteolytic cleavage within the β-AP sequence*. Thus, the *formation and deposition of β-AP is precluded by normal constitutive processing in 293 cells*. These observations suggest that β-AP deposition and the pathological formation of amyloid-bearing senile plaques in Alzheimer's disease could result from a deficiency in this processing event.

INTRODUCTION

The central core of senile plaques in Alzheimer's disease is composed of the insoluble 4-kDa β-AP, a small fragment of the 90–130 kDa glycosylated, membrane-bound amyloid precursor protein (APP) (1–6). Alternative mRNA splicing gives rise to three forms of APP which contain the β-AP sequence and may give rise to β-AP deposition. These putative β-AP precursors contain 770 (APP_{770}), 751 (APP_{751}) and 695 (APP_{695}) amino acids, respectively, and differ from one another primarily by the presence (APP_{770} and APP_{751}) or absence (APP_{695}) of a Kunitz-type protease inhibitor insert (7–9). Proteolytic processing of APP results in the secretion of a

Alzheimer's Disease: Basic Mechanisms, Diagnosis and Therapeutic Strategies
Edited by K. Iqbal, D. R. C. McLachlan, B. Winblad and H. M. Wisniewski
Published 1991 by John Wiley & Sons Ltd

large (> 100 kDa), soluble NH_2-terminal APP fragment (10,11), recently identified as protease nexin II (12,13) and the generation of a low molecular mass, membrane-associated COOH-terminal APP fragment (5). Although immunochemical studies (5,14–16) have provided some important insights into APP processing events, the exact site of the proteolytic cleavage within APP which gives rise to the NH_2- and COOH-terminal APP fragments remains unidentified. To rigorously answer this question we have purified these fragments from human embryonic 293 cells stably transfected with cDNA constructs encoding full-length forms of APP_{751} and APP_{695} and have structurally characterized the amino acid sequence around this processing site.

9-kDa COOH-TERMINAL APP FRAGMENT PURIFICATION AND CHARACTERIZATION

The 9-kDa COOH-terminal APP fragment (this fragment migrates aberrantly on SDS-PAGE with an apparent molecular mass of 10–14 kDa) was identified throughout the purification by western blotting employing an antibody directed against the COOH-terminal sequence of APP: anti-APP_{695}(590–695) (17). The purification protocol (18) took advantage of the strong tendency of the 9-kDa COOH-terminal APP fragment to aggregate in the absence of strong detergent. Briefly, the crude cell pellet was solubilized in formic acid and chromatographed over a Sephacryl HR S-100 column equilibrated in 10% formic acid. The high molecular weight aggregate containing the 9-kDa fragment was then dissociated in 1% SDS and rechromatographed over a similar column equilibrated in 0.1% SDS; this effectively resolved the 9-kDa fragment from the bulk of the protein and achieved a high degree of purification. Final purification steps employed reverse phase HPLC in 0.1% SDS and preparative SDS-PAGE electroblotting. Microsequencing of the electroblotted 9-kDa fragment yielded two major sequences for both the APP_{751}- and APP_{695}-derived samples: the NH_2-terminal sequence of ubiquinol cytochrome C reductase (a contaminating protein), and the sequence of β-AP beginning at β-AP (Leu[17]) (Table 1).

CHARACTERIZATION OF THE COOH-TERMINI OF THE SECRETED NH_2-TERMINAL APP_{695} AND APP_{751} FRAGMENTS

That cleavage occurred within the β-AP sequence itself was confirmed through identification of the COOH-terminus of the secreted, soluble fragments of APP_{695}

Table 1. Microsequence analyses of the 9-kDa COOH-terminal APP fragments

Protein	Sequence*
9 kDa APP_{751} fragment	XVFFA XdVXS X. . .
Ubiquinol cyt. C reductase	XREFG NLTRM RHVIX YX. . .
9 kDa APP_{695} fragment	XVFFA EDVGX X. . .
Ubiquitol cyt. C reductase	XREFG XLTXX RHXIX X. . .

*PTH-amino acid identifications were made in the 1–10 pmol range. Unidentifiable residues are shown as 'X' and tentative identifications are denoted with the lower case one-letter amino acid code. From Esch et al (18) with permission; copyright 1990 by the AAAS.

Table 2. Structural analyses of the COOH-terminal cyanogen bromide digestion fragments of the secreted forms of APP_{695} and APP_{751}

	Amino acid compositions				Microsequence analyses		
	Amino acid ratios					Yields (pmol)	
Amino acid	APP_{695}	APP_{751}	β-AP(1–15)	Cycle	PTH-AA	APP_{695}	APP_{751}
Asp	2.19	1.98	2	1	Asp	47.5	73.7
Glu	3.42	3.35	3	2	Ala	76.5	130.6
Ser	0.85	0.91	1	3	Glu	55.4	64.7
Gly	1.12	1.19	1	4	Phe	57.1	87.6
His	2.97	2.92	3	5	Arg	73.2	156.5
Arg	1.12	1.06	1	6	His	26.1	46.5
Thr	0	0	0	7	Asp	37.2	67.3
Ala	0.98	1.05	1	8	Ser	11.5	18.6
Pro	0	0	0	9	Gly	31.1	48.0
Tyr	0.69	0.74	1	10	Tyr	29.7	46.2
Val	0.79	0.89	1	11	Glu	22.7	38.3
Met	0	0	0	12	Val	18.3	35.1
Cys	0	0	0	13	His	10.3	20.7
Ile	0	0	0	14	His	12.3	23.9
Phe	0.88	0.93	1	15	Gln	5.0	11.0
Lys	0	0	0				

FAB mass spectrometry of each COOH-terminal cyanogen bromide digestion fragment yielded protonated molecular mass ions of 1826.72 which are identical with the calculated mass of the predicted COOH-terminal β-AP(1–15) peptide. From Esch et al (18) with permission; copyright 1990 by the AAAS.

and APP_{751}. This was accomplished by structurally characterizing the COOH-terminal cyanogen bromide digestion fragments of these secreted proteins by amino acid analyses, microsequencing and mass spectrometry as indicated in Table 2. The resulting data unequivocally show that the secreted forms of both APP_{695} and APP_{751} terminate at β-AP(Gln[15]) in the interior of the β-AP sequence.

DISCUSSION

These data demonstrate that the proteolytic event which results in secretion of the ~ 100 kDa soluble NH_2-terminal APP fragment, terminating at β-AP(Gln[15]), and concomitant generation of a 9-kDa membrane-bound COOH-terminal APP fragment, whose NH_2-terminal sequence begins at β-AP(Leu[17]) (Figure 1), is mediated by a protease which we have termed the APP secretase. Removal of β-AP(Lys[16]) is most probably effected by a basic exopeptidase (19–22). Since the APP secretase constitutively cleaves APP in the interior of the amyloid peptide sequence, β-AP formation and deposition by this pathway is precluded in 293 cells.

Previous hypothetical pathogenic mechanisms linking aberrant APP processing to amyloid deposition have tended to emphasize the importance of anomalous extracellular or intracellular APP cleavage at the NH_2-terminus of β-AP. However, one can now speculate that such inappropriate cleavage leads to β-AP deposition only in the absence of efficient constitutive APP processing. Thus, the key etiological event in AD may be inefficient secretase cleavage within the β-AP sequence.

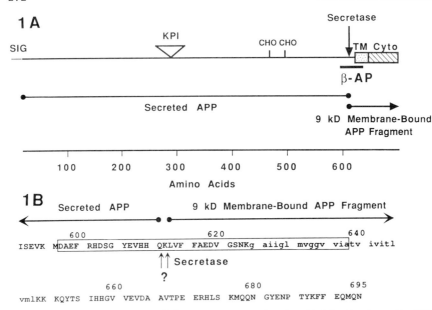

Figure 1. Diagram showing the APP secretase processing site. (A) The signal peptide (SIG), Kunitz protease inhibitor domain (KPI), N-linked glycosylation sites (CHO), transmembrane (TM) and cytoplasmic (Cyto) domains of the APP are shown. The sequences of the secreted APP fragments begin at APP(Leu[18]) and extend to β-AP(Gln[15]). The sequences of the residual membrane-bound 9-kDa APP fragments begin at β-AP(Leu[17]) and may extend to or near the C-terminus of the APP. (B) The β-AP sequence is boxed, the transmembrane segment appears in lower case single-letter amino acid code and the putative APP secretase processing sites at β-AP(Gln[15]-Lys[16]) and β-AP(Lys[16]-Leu[17]) are indicated with arrows (from Esch et al (18) with permission; copyright 1990 by the AAAS)

The resulting pathogenic accumulation of membrane-bound forms of APP which cannot be effectively cleared from the cell may then be the source of amyloid plaque formation in the brain. Recent evidence for β-AP deposition in AD peripheral tissues suggests that aberrant APP processing may occur throughout the body (23), and yet AD symptomatology is primarily limited to the brain. This may simply reflect the unique vulnerability of nonregenerating CNS neurons to the irreversible accumulation of β-AP in AD.

Note added in proof: Sisodia et al (Science 1990; 248: 492) have recently confirmed that normal APP metabolism results in the proteolysis of β-AP in African green monkey Cos-1 cells, mouse Ltk-cells, Chinese hamster ovary cells and human embryonic kidney 293 cells.

Note: Large portions of text are excerpted from Esch et al (18) with permission; copyright 1990 by the AAAS.

REFERENCES

1. Kang J, Lemaire H-G, Unterbeck A, Salbaum JM, Masters CL, Grzeschik KH, Multhaup G, Beyreuther K, Muller-Hill B. Nature 1987; 325: 733-6.

2. Goldgaber D, Lerman MI, Mcbride OW, Saffiotti U, Gajdusek DC. Science 1987; 235: 877-80.
3. Tanzi RE, Gusella JF, Watkins PC, Bruns GAP, St George-Hyslop P, van Keuren ML, Patterson D, Pagan S, Kurnit DM, Neve RL. Science 1987; 235: 880-3.
4. Robakis NK, Ramakrishna N, Wolfe G, Wisniewski HM. Proc Natl Acad Sci USA 1987; 84: 4190-4.
5. Selkoe DJ, Podlisny MB, Joachim CL, Vickers EA, Lee G, Fritz LC, Oltersdorf T. Proc Natl Acad Sci USA 1988; 85: 7341-5.
6. Weidemann A, Konig G, Bunke D, Fischer P, Salbaum JM, Masters CL, Beyreuther K. Cell 1989; 57: 115-26.
7. Ponte P, Gonzalez-DeWhitt P, Schilling J, Miller J, Hsu D, Greenberg B, Davis K, Wallace W, Lieberburg I, Fuller F, Cordell B. Nature 1988; 311: 525-7.
8. Tanzi RE, McClatchey AI, Lamperti EE, Villa-Komaroff L, Gusella JF, Neve RL. Nature 1988; 311: 528-30.
9. Kitaguchi N, Takahashi Y, Tokushima Y, Shiojiri S, Ito H. Nature 1988; 311: 530-2.
10. Weidemann A, Konig G, Bunke D, Fischer P, Salbaum JM, Masters CL, Beyreuther K. Cell 1989; 57: 115-26.
11. Schubert D, LaCorbiere M, Saitoh T, Cole G. Proc Natl Acad Sci USA 1989; 86: 2066-9.
12. Oltersdorf T, Fritz LC, Schenk DB, Lieberburg I, Johnson-Wood KL, Beattie EC, Ward PJ, Blacher RW, Dovey HF, Sinha S. Nature 1989; 341: 144-7.
13. Van Nostrand WE, Wagner SL, Suzuki M, Choi BH, Farrow JS, Geddes JW, Cotman CW, Cunningham DD. Nature 1989; 341; 546-9.
14. Palmert MR, Podlisny MB, Witker DS, Oltersdorf T, Younkin LH, Selkoe DJ, Younkin SG. Proc Natl Acad Sci USA 1989; 86: 6338-42.
15. Ghiso J, Tagliavini F, Timmers WF, Frangione B. Biochem Biophys Res Comm 1989; 163: 430-7.
16. Palmert MR, Siedlak SL, Podlisny MB, Greenberg B, Shelton ER, Chan HW, Usiak M, Selkoe DJ, Perry G, Younkin SG. Biochem Biophys Res Comm 1989; 165: 182-8.
17. Oltersdorf TO, Ward PJ, Henriksson T, Beattie EC, Neve R, Lieberburg I, Fritz L. J Biol Chem 1990; 265: 4492-7.
18. Esch FS, Keim PS, Beattie EC, Blacher RW, Culwell AR, Oltersdorf T, McClure D, Ward PJ. Science 1990; 248: 1122-4.
19. Ito Y, Mizutani S, Kurauchi O, Kasugai M, Narita O, Tomoda Y. Enzyme (Switz) 1989; 42: 8-14.
20. Skidgel RA, Davis RM, Tan F. J Biol Chem 1989; 264: 2236-41.
21. Rautenberg W, Tschesche H. Hoppe Seylers Z Physiol Chem 1984; 365: 49-58.
22. Gainer H, Russell JT, Loh YP. FEBS Lett 1984; 175: 135-9.
23. Joachim CL, Mori H, Selkoe DJ. Nature 1989; 341: 226-30.

Address for correspondence:

Dr F. S. Esch,
Athena Neurosciences Inc.,
800F Gateway Blvd,
South San Francisco, CA 94080, USA

33 The Alzheimer Amyloid Components α_1-Antichymotrypsin and β-Protein Form a Stable Complex In Vitro

HUNTINGTON POTTER, CARMELA R. ABRAHAM AND
DAVID DRESSLER

The protease inhibitor α_1-antichymotrypsin (ACT) and the 42-amino acid β-protein are integral components of the brain amyloid deposits of Alzheimer's disease, Down's syndrome, and normal aging. This indicates that there is a special affinity between ACT and the β-protein, perhaps essential to amyloid formation. A basis for this association is suggested by the similarity of the N-terminus of β-protein to the active site of serine proteases. In vitro experiments demonstrate that ACT and β-protein form a complex that reflects the specificity and stability of a protease–inhibitor interaction. These results suggest a model for the amyloid filament and a physiological function for the β-protein.

An analysis of a number of amyloidoses has shown that ACT and β-protein always occur together in the amyloid filaments — even in a newly discovered Dutch variant of hereditary cerebral hemorrhage with amyloidosis that shows little clinical or neuropathological similarity to Alzheimer's disease (1–3). The biochemical characteristics of ACT and the β-protein suggest a basis for this special association. First, ACT is a serine protease inhibitor that functions by acting as a pseudosubstrate and binding covalently to its target protease to form a long-lived complex (4). Second, an inspection of the sequence of the β-protein reveals a striking similarity to one segment of the active site of serine proteases, including the key serine amino acid (Table 1). Thus, it seemed possible that ACT and β-protein might be able to form a complex by virtue of a protease–inhibitor type of interaction and that this complex contributes to the stability of Alzheimer amyloid filaments. We have tested this hypothesis and found that, in fact, the β-protein is able to bind specifically and stably to the inhibitory active site of ACT (5; Potter et al, in preparation).

Figure 1 shows the results of pre-incubating ACT with an approximately fourfold molar excess of synthetic peptides corresponding to amino acids 1–12 or 1–28 of the β-peptide prior to the addition of chymotrypsin and the assay of protease activity through cleavage of a chromogenic substrate. We found that when the ACT/chymotrypsin molar ratio was approximately 1:1, the ACT inhibited over 90% of the chymotrypsin activity. However, in the presence of either the 1–12 or 1–28

Alzheimer's Disease: Basic Mechanisms, Diagnosis and Therapeutic Strategies
Edited by K. Iqbal, D. R. C. McLachlan, B. Winblad and H. M. Wisniewski
© 1991 John Wiley & Sons Ltd

Table 1. Homology between β-protein and the active site of serine proteases

β-protein	¹Asp Ala Glu Phe Arg His Asp Ser Gly Tyr Glu Val . . .⁴²
β-protein	[1]Asp Ala Glu Phe Arg His Asp Ser Gly Tyr Glu Val . . .[42]
T cell protease	Ala Ser Phe Arg Gly Asp Ser Gly Gly
Trypsin	Asp Ser Cys Gln Gly Asp Ser Gly Gly
Chymotrypsin	Ser Ser Cys Met Gly Asp Ser Gly Gly

amino acid β-protein peptide, the inhibitory activity of ACT was substantially reduced and the chymotrypsin reaction rate increased two- to fivefold. In contrast, pre-incubation with even a tenfold molar excess of a peptide corresponding to amino acids 258–277 of the β-protein precursor (which shows no similarity to the active site of serine proteases) failed to interfere with ACT. These data indicate that peptides showing similarity to the region around the key serine in the active site of serine proteases, and in particular the Alzheimer amyloid β-protein, are able to interfere with the inhibitory function of a serine protease inhibitor, ACT. The specificity of the interaction indicates that it is occurring at the inhibitory active site of ACT.

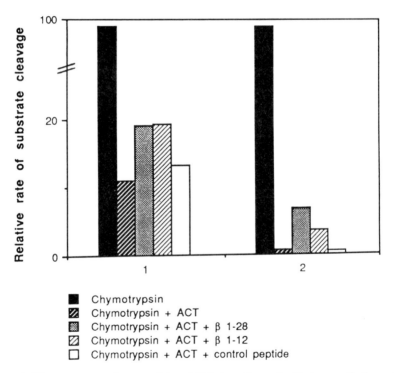

■ Chymotrypsin
▨ Chymotrypsin + ACT
▨ Chymotrypsin + ACT + β 1-28
▨ Chymotrypsin + ACT + β 1-12
☐ Chymotrypsin + ACT + control peptide

Figure 1. The protease regulatory activity of Alzheimer β-protein. Various synthetic peptides were tested for their effect on the inhibition of chymotrypsin by ACT in vitro. The activity of chymotrypsin was measured by cleavage of the chromogenic substrate succinyl-Ala-Ala-Pro-Phe-nitroanilide. The graphs compare the relative slopes of the reaction curves (all straight lines) normalized to the reaction rate of chymotrypsin alone. The data shown represent the average of four independent assays in which 0.5 (left) or 0.6 (right) μg of ACT were incubated with 0.3 μg of chymotrypsin ± peptide

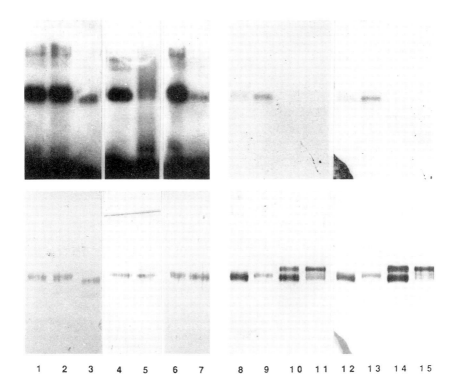

1 2 3 4 5 6 7 8 9 10 11 12 13 14 15

Figure 2. Stable interaction between α_1-antichymotrypsin and β-protein. The ability of synthetic fragments of β-protein to inhibit ACT (Figure 1) indicates that at least a transient complex can form between the two proteins. The stability of such complexes can be demonstrated by incubating ACT with radiolabeled β-protein fragments under various conditions, and then analyzing the complex formation by polyacrylamide gel electrophoresis. In some experiments, a protein cross-linking agent (DSS) was used to stabilize the complex prior to gel electrophoresis (lanes 1-6, 8-11). However, even in the absence of cross-linking, a complex is formed which is stable to boiling in SDS and β-mercaptoethanol (lanes 7, 12 and 13). The addition of an equal molar amount of chymotrypsin to ACT blocks the active site and prevents the complex formation (lanes 5, 10, 11, 14, 15). Denaturing the ACT protein by heat (lane 3) also prevents the complex formation. Immunostaining of the blotted protein with antibodies to α_1-antichymotrypsin (lower panel) indicated that neither the heat nor the chymotrypsin treatment destroyed the ACT. Thin layer chromatography (not shown) confirmed that the amount of chymotrypsin added to the ACT was not sufficient to digest the peptide

The data in Figure 2 showing that the ACT-β-protein interaction occurs at the protease inhibitory site of ACT was confirmed by the fact that the addition of chymotrypsin to ACT prior to the radioactive peptide prevented the formation of the ACT-peptide complex. TLC and gel analysis confirmed that the chymotrypsin added was not, however, sufficient to damage either the ACT protein or the peptide (not shown).

The fact that serine protease inhibitors form stable complexes with their target proteases and that a serine protease inhibitor, ACT, is an integral component of the insoluble Alzheimer amyloid deposits, suggested that this protein might be incorporated into the filaments through a stable inhibitor–protease interaction. We therefore investigated the stability of the interaction between α_1-antichymotrypsin and the β-protein. As shown in Figure 2, radio-iodinated peptides corresponding to amino acids 1–12 and 1–28 of the β-protein were prepared, incubated in the presence of ACT under various conditions, and the mixture electrophoresed on SDS-polyacrylamide gels. The formation of a β-protein–ACT complex was indicated by a new radioactive band generated at a position corresponding to a molecular weight a few thousand daltons larger than the ACT protein.

These results suggest a model for the structure of the Alzheimer amyloid filaments, shown in Figure 3. The hydrophobic C-terminal portion of β-protein molecules making up the filament would be tucked into the interior, while the hydrophilic central segment (amino acids 12–28) would form the surface of the filament. Finally, the protease-active-site-related amino acids at the N-terminus would form an arm projecting from the surface of the filament and available for binding by ACT.

The experiments do not address the questions as to whether ACT binds to β-protein before, during, or after filament formation. However, the latter seems at least possible, inasmuch as the β-protein alone can form filaments in vitro having a β-pleated sheet conformation (6,7). However, these filaments can easily be solubilized and therefore must lack a key component or structural conformation characteristic of true Alzheimer amyloid filaments. It is possible that the binding of a β-protein core filament to the relatively protease-resistant ACT provides the required extra stability.

These results also suggest a potential biological function for the β-protein. Since the β-protein can competitively interact with the active site of a serine protease inhibitor in vitro, it might be expected to be able to play a similar role in vivo. By decoying protease inhibitors (including the Kunitz-type inhibitor in the β-protein precursor), the β-protein, though not itself a protease, would serve as a protease enhancer — effectively increasing proteolytic activity in its vicinity. Overproduction

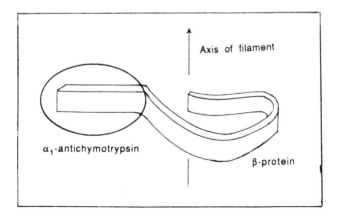

Figure 3. A model structure of the Alzheimer amyloid filaments, based on the interaction between ACT and β-protein. Filaments accumulate as amyloid deposits in Alzheimer's disease

of the β-protein, as would result for instance from increased proteolytic degradation of the β-protein precursor, could thus lead to a further increase in protease activity, with progressively adverse consequences.

Acknowledgments

The work of the laboratory was supported by NIH grants GM35967 and AG08084, a grant to H. P. from the ADRDA and support to C. R. A. from the Freudenberger family. We are grateful to Stefan Cooke for excellent assistance in the experiments and the preparation of the manuscript.

REFERENCES

1. Abraham CR, Selkoe DJ, Potter H. Immunochemical identification of the serine protease inhibitor α_1-antichymotrypsin in the brain amyloid deposits of Alzheimer's disease. Cell 1988; 52: 487-501.
2. Picken MM, Coria F, Larrondo-Lillo M, Gallow GR, Shelanski ML, Frangione B. Distribution of the protease inhibitor α_1-antichymotrypsin in cerebral and systematic amyloid. Am J Pathol 1989; 134: 749.
3. Abraham CR, Shirahama T, Potter H. The protease inhibitor α_1-antichymotrypsin is associated solely with amyloid deposits containing the β-protein and is localized in specific cells of both normal and diseased brain. Neurobiol Aging 1990; 11: 123-9.
4. Travis J, Salvesen GS. Human plasma proteinase inhibitors. Ann Rev Biochem 1983; 52: 655-709.
5. Dressler D, Abraham CR, Amsterdam P, Potter H. In vitro studies of the interaction between the Alzheimer components α_1-antichymotrypsin and β-protein. Soc Neurosci Abstr. 1989; 414.20.
6. Kirschner DA, Abraham CR, Selkoe DJ. X-ray diffraction from intraneuronal paired helical filaments and extraneuronal amyloid fibers in Alzheimer disease indicates cross-β conformation. Proc Natl Acad Sci USA 1986; 83: 503-7.
7. Kirschner DA, Inouye H, Duffy LK, Sinclair A, Lind M, Selkoe DJ. Synthetic peptide homologous to β protein from Alzheimer disease forms amyloid-like fibrils in vitro. Proc Natl Acad Sci USA 1987; 84: 6953-7.

Address for correspondence:

Dr Huntington Potter,
Department of Neurobiology,
Harvard Medical School,
Boston, MA 02115, USA

34 Membrane Insertion Prevents Aggregation of Precursor Fragments Containing the β/A4 Sequence of Alzheimer's Disease

THOMAS DYRKS, ELKE MACK, COLIN L. MASTERS AND KONRAD BEYREUTHER

Amyloid β/A4 protein is the biological marker for Alzheimer's disease (1–3). Its sequence is included in that of at least four membrane-bound amyloid precursor proteins (APP_{mem}) (APP_{695}, APP_{714}, APP_{751} and APP_{770}) (4–8). These amyloid precursor proteins arise through alternative splicing. The two longest APP forms (APP_{751}, APP_{770}) carry an additional domain with a protease inhibitor function and homology to the Kunitz type II serine protease inhibitors (KPI-domain), which is absent in APP_{695} and APP_{714} (7,9). APP_{714} and APP_{770} have an additional 19-residue domain with homology to MRC OX-2 proteins.

We have previously shown that the major APP forms (APP_{695}, APP_{751} and APP_{770}) are synthesized as N- and O-glycosylated integral transmembrane proteins. These proteins are built up from three to five extracellular domains, a transmembrane domain and a 47-residue cytoplasmic domain (10–12). In cell cultures, 30% of these transmembrane proteins are converted by proteolytic processing to secretory forms which comprise the extracellular part (12). The thus produced secretory forms of APP, APP_{751sec} and APP_{770sec}, are identical to protease nexin II (9,13). The proteolytic cleavage generating the APP_{sec} forms occurs within the amyloid β/A4 sequence, N-terminal of Val 17 in the β/A4 sequence (14,15). This suggests that the N-terminus of the amyloid β/A4 protein is not produced by the normal cleavage which leads to secretory APPs.

We have proposed that the initial step of the abnormal proteolytic processing of full-length APP in Alzheimer's disease that leads to the amyloid β/A4 protein may generate the N-terminus of the β/A4 sequence and produce a C-terminal fragment which includes the amyloid β/A4 sequence, the transmembrane and cytoplasmic domain of all known APP_{mem} forms (11). To study the properties of this hypothetical 'preamyloid' protein, we expressed the C-terminal 100 residues of APP_{mem} with and without a signal sequence at the N-terminus, termed by us SPA4CT and A4CT, respectively.

Alzheimer's Disease: Basic Mechanisms, Diagnosis and Therapeutic Strategies
Edited by K. Iqbal, D. R. C. McLachlan, B. Winblad and H. M. Wisniewski

Here we report expression of this hypothetical 'preamyloid' A4CT in a eukaryotic cell-free system, in *E. coli* and in HeLa cells. Synthesized in the first two systems, A4CT is shown to aggregate. We provide evidence that membrane insertion of A4CT prevents this aggregation, and that post-translational removal of the membranes restores the high tendency of A4CT for self-aggregation. In contrast, expression of A4CT in HeLa cells results in monomeric forms with the SDS-PAGE assay which cannot be transformed into aggregates, suggesting the presence of so far unknown mechanisms that prevent A4CT aggregation in eukaryotic cells. We suggest that these mechanisms are disturbed in Alzheimer's disease.

RESULTS

Expression of A4CT in vitro

For expression in a cell-free system we used plasmid SP65/A4CT. It encodes A4CT (Figure 1) that has the methionine codon 596 of APP_{695} in front of codons 597–695 of APP_{695}. A4CT includes the β/A4 sequence, the transmembrane domain and the cytoplasmic domain. In contrast to full-length APP forms, this protein is not inserted into membranes through the signal sequence pathway, and its proposed aggregation should not be sterically hindered by additional N-terminal sequences. Expression of SP65/A4CT was done in rabbit reticulocyte lysates and aggregation of A4CT was analysed by SDS-polyacrylamide gel electrophoresis (SDS-PAGE) (10,11).

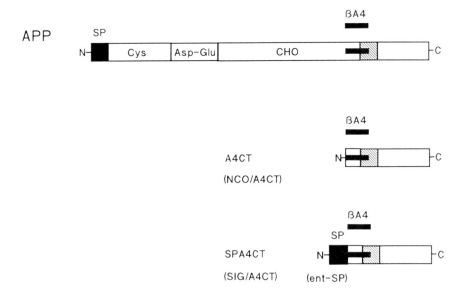

Figure 1. Schematic representation of APP695 and A4CT. SP, APP-signal peptide; ent-SP, enterotoxin-signal peptide; shaded bar, transmembrane sequence; black bar, β/A4 sequence; Cys, cysteine domain; CHO, *N*-glycosylation domain; Asp-Glu, domain rich in Asp and Glu

Translation of A4CT in rabbit reticulocyte lysates in the presence and absence of membranes did not result in a single band in the SDS-PAGE, but gave rise to a broad smear between 10 and 18 kDa and additional bands at approximately 20, 30, 40 kDa and higher molecular masses.

To study the behavior of A4CT when inserted into membranes, we expressed plasmid SP65/SPA4CT which encodes the APP signal sequence (codon 1-17) and two additional residues (codon 18-19) from APP together with the A4CT sequence (Figure 1). The two additional codons were included to ensure correct signal peptidase cleavage. Expression of this protein in the reticulocyte system in the absence of membranes resulted in an aggregation pattern comparable to that found for A4CT. In the presence of microsomal membranes, expression of SPA4CT gives rise to a prominent broad band between 12 and 18 kDa. No additional bands at higher molecular masses were detected.

Evidence for the insertion of SPA4CT into membranes was obtained with the sedimentation assay for integral membrane proteins (16). The translation product obtained in the presence of microsomes could be selectively sedimentated with the sodium carbonate technique. This strongly suggests that membrane insertion of A4CT prevents its aggregation.

To study the effect of membrane damage as experimentally realized by membrane removal, we extracted the microsomal vesicles with chloroform/methanol prior to the addition of SDS sample buffer. Subsequent protein analysis by SDS-PAGE revealed that SPA4CT aggregates now formed. Heating the extracted APP fragment for 10 min at 100 °C enhances the aggregation process. We assume that the lipid removal allows the necessary conformation change to take place that leads to aggregation. The amyloid β/A4 sequence, which has a predicted tendency to adopt a β-sheet conformation in aqueous solutions, is probably responsible for this aggregation (10,11).

Expression of A4CT in *E. coli*

For expression of A4CT in *E. coli* we used plasmid NCO/A4CT. The *E. coli* expression product is soluble in 70% formic acid and SDS-sample buffer but not in non-ionic detergents such as Triton X-100 or NP-40. Western blot analysis of the NCO/A4CT expression product revealed a dominant band at 17 kDa and an aggregation pattern similar to that of in-vitro expressed A4CT. The primary polyclonal rabbit antibody used (anti-A4) was raised against synthetic amyloid β/A4 protein in an aggregated form. This antibody stains amyloid plaques, vascular amyloid and extracellular tangles, but not APP in brain sections of patients with Alzheimer's disease.

To express membrane-inserted A4CT in *E. coli*, we used the construct SIG/A4CT, which has the enterotoxin signal sequence in front of the A4CT sequence (Figure 1). Western blot analysis of SIG/A4CT, done as specified for NCO/A4CT, revealed a weakly stained monomeric band at 17 kDa. In contrast to what was found for NCO/A4CT expression, there was no indication of higher aggregates.

In western blot analysis using another polyclonal rabbit antibody (anti CT-II) which was raised against a peptide corresponding to residues 665–677 of APP_{695}, both expression products (NCO/A4CT and SIG/A4CT) showed a comparable band intensity at 17 kDa, but only NCO/A4CT showed the presence of higher aggregates. This suggests that also in the prokaryotic expression system, membrane insertion of A4CT prevents its aggregation. The difference in reaction of NCO/A4CT and SIG/A4CT expression products with the antiamyloid β/A4 antibody (anti-A4) could be due to a different conformation for the epitopes of NCO/A4CT and SIG/A4CT. The former may adopt the β-sheet structure of the antigen and then be recognized. SIG/A4CT inserted into the membrane may adopt an α-helical conformation and therefore not react with the antibody. Such an interpretation is in agreement with the finding that membrane insertion of SPA4CT prevents aggregation, and the finding that transmembrane domains are in an α-helical conformation if inserted into the membrane.

Expression of A4CT in HeLa cells

HeLa cells transfected with constructs CMV/SPA4CT or CMV/A4CT, coding for SPA4CT and A4CT respectively, were metabolically labeled with ^{35}S-methionine. The immunoprecipitates of cell lysates obtained with anti-A4CT, a polyclonal rabbit antibody raised against A4CT expressed in *E. coli*, were subsequently separated on SDS-PAGE. Cell lysates from CMV/SPA4CT-transfected HeLa cells revealed a prominent band at 17 kDa in addition to the precursor bands present in the control experiment. The same analysis if performed with lysates from CMV/A4CT-transfected HeLa cells revealed a band at 17 kDa. The difference in molecular mass in SDS-PAGE is due to the two additional amino acids present in mature SPA4CT which were introduced together with the signal peptide sequence.

We were also unable to detect aggregates of A4CT and SPA4CT expressed in HeLa cells after chloroform/methanol extraction. This shows that eukaryotic cells are able to handle these precursor fragments in a way which prevents their aggregation.

DISCUSSION

The findings that an aggregating APP fragment (A4CT) can be synthesized in vitro in a eukaryotic cell-free system as well as in *E. coli* provides further experimental evidence in favour of a crucial role of A4CT-like proteins as potential intermediates in the process of amyloid β/A4 protein formation.

Expression of A4CT in *E. coli* allowed the identification of the protein and the determination of its relative molecular mass of 17 kDa. This protein has aggregational properties similar to that of A4CT synthesized in a eukaryotic cell-free system. The solubility properties of bacterial A4CT resemble that of amyloid β/A4 protein (2). Strong acids such as 70% formic acid and strong denaturants such as 9 M urea, which are known to dissolve amyloid β/A4 protein, are also required to dissolve A4CT aggregates. Membrane insertion of A4CT in a cell-free system and in *E. coli* brought about by the addition of a signal sequence interferes with aggregation of this molecule.

We suggest that the β/A4-sequence with the high β-pleated sheet potential adopts an α-helical conformation when inserted into membranes leading to an A4CT molecule unable to aggregate (17,18). Without membranes, the β-sheet conformation required for amyloid formation is expected to be adopted and to dominate, and therefore to promote aggregation (Figure 2).

Expression of SPA4CT and A4CT in HeLa cells resulted only in the monomeric forms. Neither SPA4CT nor A4CT show aggregation, not even after membrane removal, which was shown to promote aggregation of the same molecules when expressed in a eukaryotic cell-free system. The fate of the precursor fragments in HeLa cells is therefore altered by mechanisms which are not present in the cell-free system. One explanation for the altered properties could be that post-translational modifications such as O-glycosylation occur and interfere with the aggregation process.

Expression of A4CT *in vitro*

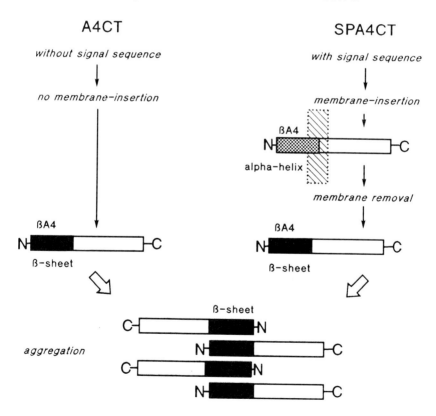

Figure 2. Predicted conformational changes leading to aggregation of membrane-inserted SPA4CT. Black bar, β/A4 sequence

286

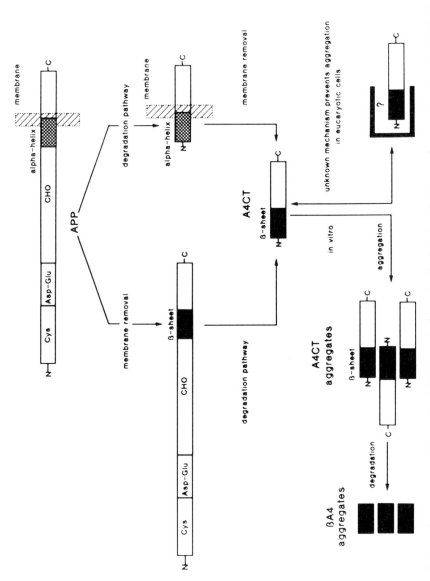

Figure 3. Hypothetic pathway suggested for amyloid β/A4 protein formation in Alzheimer's disease. Cys, cysteine domain; CHO, *N*-glycosylation domain; Asp-Glu, domain rich in Asp and Glu

We predict proteolytic cleavage of APP_{mem} which generates the N-terminus of amyloid $\beta/A4$ protein to be a crucial step for amyloid $\beta/A4$ formation if these protective mechanisms are disturbed (Figure 3). This may be the case in Alzheimer's disease. The cleavage produces A4CT. The latter is shown to have a high tendency to aggregate if it is released from the membrane by, for instance, membrane damage. This would lead to A4CT aggregates which upon further processing yield amyloid.

Acknowledgments

We thank Caroline Hilbich and Gerd Multhaup for anti-A4 and anti-CT-II serum. Financial support from the Deutsche Forschungsgemeinschaft through SFB 317, the BMFT of Germany, the Thyssen Stiftung and the Fonds der chemischen Industrie is gratefully acknowledged. Colin L. Masters is supported by the National Health and Medical Research Council of Australia and by a grant from the Alzheimer's Disease and Related Disorders Association.

REFERENCES

1. Glenner GG, Wong CW. Biochem Biophys Res Comm 1984; 122: 1131-5.
2. Masters CL, Simms G, Weinmann NA, Multhaup G, McDonald BL, Beyreuther K. Proc Natl Acad Sci USA 1985; 82: 4245-9.
3. Masters CL, Multhaup G, Simms G, Pottgiesser J, Martins RN, Beyreuther K. EMBO J 1985; 4: 2757-63.
4. Kang J, Lemaire H-G, Unterbeck A, Salbaum JM, Masters CL, Grzeschik K-H, Multhaup G, Beyreuther K, Müller-Hill B. Nature 1987; 325: 733-6.
5. Ponte P, Gonzalez-DeWhitt P, Schilling J, Miller J, Hsu D, Greenberg B, Davis K, Wallace W, Lieberburg I, Fuller F, Cordell B. Nature 1988; 331: 525-7.
6. Tanzi RE, McClatchey AI, Lamerti ED, Villa-Komaroff L, Gusella JF, Neve RL. Nature 1988; 311: 528-30.
7. Kitaguchi N, Takahashi Y, Tokushima Y, Shiogiri S, Ito H. Nature 1988; 331: 530-2.
8. Kang J, Müller-Hill B. Biochem Biophys Res Comm 1990; 166: 1192-200.
9. Oltersdorf T, Fritz LC, Schenk DB, Lieberburg I, Johnson-Wood KL, Beattie EC, Ward PJ, Blacher RW, Dovey HJ, Sinha S. Nature 1989; 341: 144-7.
10. Dyrks T, Weidemann A, Multhaup G, Salbaum JM, Lemaire HG, Kang J, Müller-Hill B, Masters CL, Beyreuther K. EMBO J 1988; 7: 949-57.
11. Dyrks T, König G, Hilbich C, Masters CL, Beyreuther K. Prog Clin Biol Res 1989; 317: 877-91.
12. Weidemann A, König G, Bunke D, Fischer P, Salbaum J-M, Masters CL, Beyreuther K. Cell 1989; 57: 115-26.
13. Knauer DJ, Cunningham DD. Proc Natl Acad Sci USA 1982; 79: 2310-14.
14. Sisodia SS, Koo EH, Beyreuther K, Unterbeck A, Price DL. Science 1990; 248: 492-5.
15. Esch FS, Keim PL, Beattie EC, Blacher RW, Culwell AR, Oltersdorf T, McClure D, Ward PJ. Science 1990; 248: 1122-4.
16. Fujiki Y, Hubbard AL, Fowler S, Lazarow PB. J Cell Biol 1982; 93: 97-102.
17. Rao JKM, Argos P. Biochim Biophys Acta 1986; 869: 197-214.
18. Kyte J, Dolittle RF. J Mol Biol 1982; 157: 105-32.

Address for correspondence:

Dr T. Dyrks,
Center for Molecular Biology,
University of Heidelberg,
Im Neuenheimer Feld 282,
D-6900 Heidelberg 1, Germany

35 Basement Membrane Heparan Sulphate Proteoglycan is Part of Isolated Alzheimer's Amyloid Plaques

S. NARINDRASORASAK, I. YOUNG, S. AUBIN,
S. K. LUDWIN AND R. KISILEVSKY

Highly sulphated glycosaminoglycans (GAGs) have been identified as part of all amyloid deposits examined to date (1). Where it has been possible to identify the proteoglycan, it has been shown to be the heparan sulphate proteoglycan (HSPG), which has now been identified in at least five diverse forms of amyloid. These include AA amyloid in inflammation (2,3) the β-amyloid associated with Alzheimer's disease (4), the prealbumin amyloid seen in familial amyloidotic polyneuropathy (5), the IAPP form of amyloid seen in diabetes (6), and prion amyloid seen in the Gerstmann-Sträussler-Scheinker syndrome (7). In amyloid associated with inflammation, the HSPG is deposited coincidentally with the amyloid peptide, regardless of the induction procedure used, or tissue site of deposition (8). In addition, sulphate ions probably as part of HSPG have been shown to play a role in maintaining AA amyloid fibril structure (9). Previous light and electron microscopic studies have shown the GAG to be part of the plaque amyloid fibril (10,11), and in plaque-like lesions which do not contain an amyloid core.

The above findings prompted us to isolate neuritic plaques to determine whether the isolated plaques contain the proteoglycan of interest.

MATERIALS AND METHODS

Neuritic plaque isolation

Plaques were isolated by the procedure of Selkoe et al (12). Briefly, frozen brains which were previously assessed by histological criteria to show that they contained significant numbers of plaques were dissected free of white matter and visible blood vessels. The grey matter was homogenized in 2% SDS, 0.1 M β-mercaptoethanol buffer, heated to 100 °C for 10 minutes, sieved through 110-μm nylon mesh (Nitrex) and subjected to centrifugation at $300\,g$ for 30 min. The pelleted material was

Alzheimer's Disease: Basic Mechanisms, Diagnosis and Therapeutic Strategies
Edited by K. Iqbal, D. R. C. McLachlan, B. Winblad and H. M. Wisniewski
© 1991 John Wiley & Sons Ltd

washed three times in 0.1% SDS, 150 mM NaCl and 0.02% NaN$_3$, rehomogenized and sieved through 35-μm Nitrex. The sieved material was loaded on a step gradient of 1.2, 1.4, 1.6 and 1.8 M sucrose in 1% SDS, 50 mM Tris, pH 7.5 and centrifuged in an SW 28 rotor at 72 000 g for 60 min. The 1.4/1.6 M and 1.6/1.8 M interfaces provided the greatest enrichment. The yield of plaque core material was approximately 1–7 μg/g of grey matter.

Histological assessment

A drop of the preparation from the sucrose gradients was placed on a glass slide, allowed to dry, and stained either with the sulphated Alcian blue technique (SAB) (13), or the alkaline Congo red technique (14).

Heparan sulphate proteoglycan isolation and antibody preparation

Mouse EHS tumours (a kind gift of Hynda Kleinman, National Institutes of Health, Bethesda, Maryland) were grown in C57B1/J mice and used as a source of heparan sulphate proteoglycan. The isolation procedure followed was that of Ledbetter et al (15). The purified protein was used for immunization purposes in rabbits. The protein which had previously been purified to homogeneity was coupled to a cyanogen bromide Sepharose column, and used to purify the HSPG antibodies. The antibodies were characterized and shown not to have any crossreactivity to any other basement membrane components.

Solubilization of plaque core proteins

Attempts to solubilize the plaque cores with formic acid led to complete loss of Alcian blue staining of these cores, indicating the destruction of any sulphated glycosaminoglycans. The cores were therefore first solubilized in 6.8 M guanidine thiocyanate for 4 hours at 37 °C, dialysed extensively against distilled water, and lyophilized. The lyophilized material was either then left untreated, or treated with nitrous acid (16) or papain, 3 units in 50 mM sodium acetate, pH 4.5, overnight at 37 °C. Each preparation was then dialysed, lyophilized, and subjected to electrophoresis in 2% agarose 40 mM Tris, pH 8.0, 20 mM sodium acetate, and 2 mM EDTA. Western blotting with the affinity purified antibody to HSPG was performed according to the method of Burnette (17), using a goat anti-rabbit IgG conjugated alkaline phosphatase.

RESULTS

Table 1 is a partial listing of the various forms of amyloid which we have examined for highly sulphated GAGs. All amyloids examined to date possess such highly sulphated glycosaminoglycans. Table 2 is a listing of amyloid which has been examined with antisera to the HSPG and which indicates that five diverse forms of amyloid possess the HSPG.

Table 1. A comparison of the diverse forms of amyloid proteins and the presence of highly sulphated glycosaminoglycans

Amyloid protein	Presence of sulphated GAGs
AA	+
AL	+
Prealbumin	+
Procalcitonin	+
Beta-2 microglobulin	+
IAPP	+
Beta amyloid	+
Prion protein	+

Table 2. A comparison of diverse forms of amyloid proteins and presence of the basement membrane form of heparan sulphate proteoglycan

Amyloid protein	Basement membrane form of heparan proteoglycan
AA	+
Beta amyloid	+
IAPP	+
Prealbumin	+
Prion (GSS)	+

A representative section from a brain containing significant numbers of neuritic plaques stained with the SAB technique to show sulphated carbohydrates is demonstrated in Figure 1. Material such as this was used for plaque isolation. A representative preparation of such isolated plaques is demonstrated in Figure 2. This preparation has been stained with the SAB technique, and demonstrates that sulphated carbohydrates are present in the plaque cores. Evidence that these cores really represent the amyloid cores is confirmed in Figure 3 where the preparation has been stained with Congo red and viewed under crossed-polars. These cores show the typical Maltese-cross appearance and red–green birefringence, characteristic of these cores in situ.

Electrophoresis and western blotting of the guanidine thiocyanate solubilized material is demonstrated in Figure 4. Intact cores fail to penetrate the gel to any significant degree (lane c). Solubilizing the material in guanidine thiocyanate allows the protein to penetrate the gel (lane b). The material appears as a relatively broad smear, which is not surprising. The brains used to prepare the plaque cores are usually gathered from individuals who have died sometime prior to necropsy. Treatment of the guanidine thiocyanate solubilized material with nitrous acid (a technique specific for fragmentation of the heparan sulphated side-chains) leads to a significant decrease in the molecular weight of the material detectable with the HSPG antibodies (lane a). The treatment of the thiocyanate solubilized material with papain leads to its complete destruction (lane d).

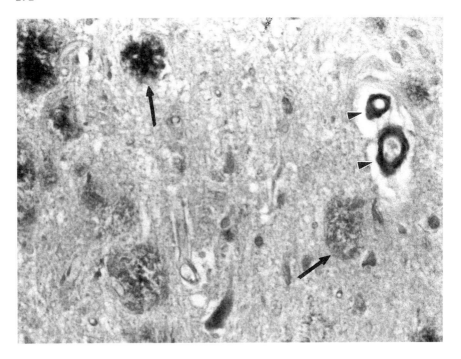

Figure 1. A section of cerebral cortex stained with sulphated Alcian blue demonstrating neuritic plaques with and without amyloid cores (arrows). Congophilic angiopathy is also seen (arrowheads) (×505)

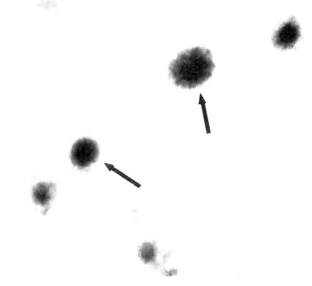

Figure 2. Isolated neuritic plaques (arrows), following sucrose gradient density purification stained with sulphated Alcian blue (×810)

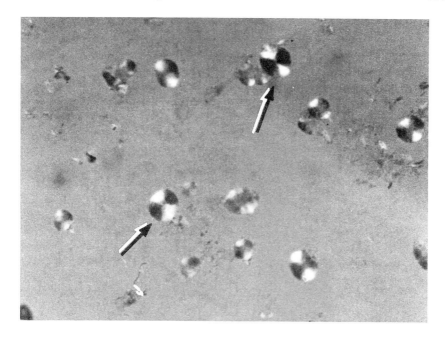

Figure 3. Isolated neuritic plaques (arrows), following sucrose gradient density purification, stained with Congo red and viewed under crossed-polars (×810)

DISCUSSION

This work corroborates previous observations made in our own laboratory (1,2), and in the hands of others (3). Using histochemical techniques, we have shown previously that highly sulphated GAGs are part of the amyloid deposits seen in association with the senile plaques, the neurofibrillary tangles, and the congophilic angiopathy (18). Ultrastructural analysis has shown that the GAGs are closely linked to the fibril structure (10,11). Immunohistochemical studies by Snow et al (4), using an antibody to the basement membrane form of HSPG, suggested that the HSPG protein core was also part of plaque structure.

In the present work we wished to examine whether the HSPG is present in isolated plaques when using existing procedures to purify senile plaques. The results indicated that following purification of the plaque cores, they continued to stain positively with the sulphated Alcian blue technique, showing the presence of a sulphated carbohydrate. Attempts to solubilize these isolated senile plaques in formic acid, for subsequent electrophoresis, led to the loss of their Alcian blue staining properties. Using an alternative technique for solubilizing the isolated plaques, guanidine thiocyanate, we were able to preserve their Alcian blue staining properties which indicated the preservation of the carbohydrate side-chains. We then employed western blotting and specific antisera to test for the presence of the HSPG protein core. Treatment of the isolated plaques with guanidine thiocyanate solubilized them

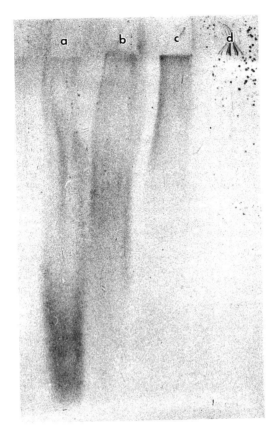

Figure 4. Agarose electrophoresis, western blotting of guanidine thiocyanate solubilized plaque cores using affinity purified anti-basement membrane HSPG antibodies. Lane (a) guanidine thiocyanate, and nitrous acid treated plaque cores; lane (b) guanidine thiocyanate treated plaque cores; lane (c) intact plaque cores, untreated; and (d) guanidine thiocyanate, and papain-treated plaque cores

sufficiently so that they penetrated the agarose gel adequately for subsequent western blotting. This solubilized material was clearly sensitive to papain which destroyed all immunoreactive material. Treatment with nitrous acid, which destroys GAGs containing nitrogen sulphur linkages, reduced the molecular weight of the HSPG protein core as anticipated.

The aesthetic quality of the western blots leaves a great deal to be desired. However, it should be remembered that the neuritic plaques have been isolated from the brains of patients who have died many hours prior to necropsy. This gives ample time for the plaques to be subjected to proteolytic attack within the brain following death. In addition, these neuritic plaques have existed within these patients for many years and presumably have undergone significant modifications during this period. Attack by local cellular or extracellular enzymes is highly likely. It is therefore not surprising that the HSPG protein cores do not exist as a single protein species, but rather fragments of many sizes.

Our working hypothesis is that the HSPG plays an important role in the genesis of these lesions. The size of the HSPG molecule probably precludes significant diffusion of HSPG from areas distant to sites of neuritic plaque generation. The HSPG protein core has a molecular weight greater than 400 000 and with its carbohydrate side-chains is of the order of 600 000-700 000 (15). Such a molecule is too large to diffuse to any significant degree. Further it has never been demonstrated that this molecule is present in the circulation. It is therefore our feeling that this molecule is produced and has its effects locally. A variety of neural cell types are known to be capable of producing basement membranes. These include not only neuronal cells, but glial cells as well. Preliminary evidence in our laboratory indicates that astrocytes possess the potential to produce HSPG, as do neurons. Both these cell types have also been shown to produce the β-amyloid precursor protein (19-22). It is therefore not far-fetched to conclude that one or other, or perhaps both, of these cells may be directly involved in the synthesis and genesis of the components seen in the Alzheimer's neuritic plaques.

Acknowledgments

This work was supported by grants MT-3153, MA-10477 and the Upjohn Company of Canada. We thank Mrs B. Latimer and Ms K. Wowk for their able secretarial assistance.

REFERENCES

1. Snow AD, Willmer J, Kisilevsky R. Lab Invest 1987; 56: 120-3.
2. Snow AD, Kisilevsky R, Wight TN. In Isobe T, Araki S, Uchino F, Kito S, Tsuburu E (eds) Amyloid and amyloidosis. New York: Plenum, 1988; 87-93.
3. Norling B, Westermark GT, Westermark P. Clin Exp Immunol 1988; 73: 333-7.
4. Snow AD, Mar H, Nochlin D, Kimata K, Kato M, Suzuki S, Hassell J, Wight TN. Am J Pathol 1988; 133: 456-63.
5. Saraiva M, Snow AD (personal communication).
6. Young I, Ailles L, Narindrasorasak S, Kisilevsky, R. Hum Pathol (submitted for publication).
7. Snow AD (personal communication).
8. Snow AD, Kisilevsky R. Lab Invest 1985; 53: 37-44.
9. Wong S, Kisilevsky R. Scand J Immunol 1990; 32: 225-32.
10. Snow AD, Lara S, Nochlin D, Wight TN. Acta Neuropathol 1989; 78: 113-23.
11. Young ID, Willmer JP, Kisilevsky R. Acta Neuropathol 1989; 78: 202-9.
12. Selkoe DS, Abraham CR, Podlisny MB, Duffy LK. Neurochem 1986; 46: 1820-33.
13. Lendrum AC, Sidders W, Fraser S. J Clin Pathol 1972; 25: 373-96.
14. Puchtler H, Sweat F, Levine M. J Histochem Cytochem 1962; 10: 355-64.
15. Ledbetter SR, Fisher LW, Hassell JR. Biochemistry 1987; 26: 988-95.
16. Shively JE, Conrad HE. Biochemistry 1976; 15: 3932-42.
17. Burnette WN. Anal Biochem 1981; 112: 195-203.
18. Snow AD, Willmer J, Kisilevsky R. Hum Pathol 1987; 18: 506-10.
19. Siman R, Card JP, Nelson RB, Davis LG. Neuron 1989; 3: 275-85.
20. Quon D, Catalano R, Cordell B. Biochem Biophys Res Comm 1990; 167: 96-102.

21. Berkenbosch F, Refolo LM, Friedrich VL, Casper D, Blum M, Robakis NK. J Neurosci Res 1990; 25: 431–40.
22. Selkoe DJ. Neurobiol Aging 1989; 10: 387–95.

Address for correspondence:

Dr R. Kisilevsky,
Department of Pathology,
Queen's University,
Kingston, Ontario K7L 3N6, Canada

36 Release of a Putative 60-kDa Amyloidogenic Alzheimer Amyloid Precursor Protein from PC-12 Cells, and the Isolation of AD-Fibroblast Hybrids

FRED BASKIN, ROGER N. ROSENBERG, STUART A. STEIN
AND BARRY D. GREENBERG

Amyloidotic plaque cores of Alzheimer's disease (AD) and Down's syndrome (DS) brain, composed of a 41–43 amino acid peptide (A4), are derived from a transmembrane amyloid precursor protein (APP). As this protein is cleaved in transfected cells *within* A4, increased extracellular A4 peptides in AD and DS require the release of abnormally cleaved APP, containing intact A4. We report the increased release of a 60-kDa protein from stressed PC-12 cultures into serum-free media, which is detected with nine antisera elicited by four peptides within the carboxyl half of APP, including the carboxyl-terminus and A4 domains. Whereas many of these antisera crossreact with bovine serum albumin producing a broad band at 68 kDa, a 60-kDa band either distinct from, or partially overlapping, the stained BSA band is resolved on autoradiograms of conditioned media immunoblots. Antisera elicited by six peptides within the amino-terminal half of APP detect the normal 120-kDa APP_{751} cleavage product but not a 60-kDa species. These and partial sequencing data indicate that this 60-kDa APP-like fragment corresponds to amino acids 436–751 of PC-12 APP_{751}. Further 2-D gel, metabolic labeling and sequencing experiments may confirm this structure and establish PC-12 cells as the source of this protein. Increased amounts of this potentially amyloidogenic APP are released from PC-12 cultures maintained with membrane damaging and lysosomal inhibiting but not from those maintained with cytoskeletal disrupting agents or one APP inducer, phorbol ester. These data suggest the possible importance of specific pre-existing neural injuries in AD and DS amyloidogenesis.

We also report the induction of APP_{751} mRNA in PC-12 cells by 7S NGF, interleukin-1 and phorbol ester, and the cloning of control and AD fibroblast-neuroblastoma cell hybrids. In future work we will examine the fibroblast–neural hybrids for the possible expression of altered APP cleavage or other AD markers, the relative importance of APP induction and neural damage on the release of

Alzheimer's Disease: Basic Mechanisms, Diagnosis and Therapeutic Strategies
Edited by K. Iqbal, D. R. C. McLachlan, B. Winblad and H. M. Wisniewski
©1991 John Wiley & Sons Ltd

amyloidogenic APP fragments in this cell culture model, and the relevance of these studies to amyloidogenesis in human brain.

INTRODUCTION

APP, the precursor of the extracellular A4 plaque peptide seen in early Alzheimer's disease (AD) and Down's syndrome (DS) brain, is a glycosylated transmembrane protein (1,2). As it is cleaved in transfected cells within the A4 domain (3,4) releasing 120-kDa nexin-II (5), accumulation of A4 peptides requires that some APP escape this cleavage and be released from neural (2) or peripheral (6) tissues with an intact A4 domain. Mechanisms as to how this may occur include (a) overproduction (7) of one or more APP forms and (b) pre-existing physical (8,9) or metabolic (10) cell injury. As 3T3 cells release a similar transmembrane protein, EGF-receptor precursor (11), into *serum-free* media, we analyzed proteins released by PC-12 cells stressfully maintained in serum-free media alone or with the addition of APP inducers (13,14) or injurious agents. Because of possible nonspecific immunochemical identification (12), we have used 35 APP peptide-elicited polyclonal antisera, representing 10 distinct APP peptides, to examine both cell conditioned media and serum proteins. We have also selected and cloned familial AD (FAD) and control fibroblast-neuroblastoma hybrids in which the FAD gene may be differentially expressed.

METHODS AND RESULTS

Induction of APP mRNA

Total RNAs were gel fractionated and hybridized with an APP cDNA probe (15) binding all APP mRNAs (Figure 1). PC-12 (ATTC) cultures, grown with either 7S NGF (100 ng/ml), phorbol ester (250 ng/nl) or interleukin-1A or B (10 units/ml) for 8 hours, generally produced 2-, 3- or 4-fold inductions of APP_{751}, respectively. Growth with phorbol ester for 4 or 24 hours produced smaller 1.5–2.0 fold increases. Only traces of APP_{695} mRNA were detected with a junction probe (16) which at 58 °C and $1 \times SSC$ binds only APP_{695} mRNA.

Immunoprecipitation, microsequencing and immunoblot analyses of A4-containing APP in PC-12 conditioned media

Semiconfluent PC-12 cultures were rinsed (three times, for 20 min) and placed in serum-free media (17) containing 10% of the normal transferrin and 5 μl/ml leupeptin (32). In some cases, a membrane-damaging agent—SDS (0.003% or 0.005%); an APP inducer—phorbol ester (250 ng/ml); lysosomal inhibitors—chloroquine (60 μM) or NH_4Cl (25 mM); or other injurious agents were added. Cells remained viable by intact mRNA and dye-exclusion criteria. After 18 hours 1 mM PMSF was added, and media were concentrated (Centriprep tubes) and either iodinated for immunoprecipitation with Pansorbin and PAGE fractionated, or directly fractionated on 10% polyacrylamide gels (32) and transferred to Immobilon filters. Western blots were exposed to characterized (6,18–23) antisera (Table 1) overnight and to ^{125}I-protein A for 2 hours. Filters were subjected to enhanced autoradiography, and quantitated by densitometry.

AGENT:

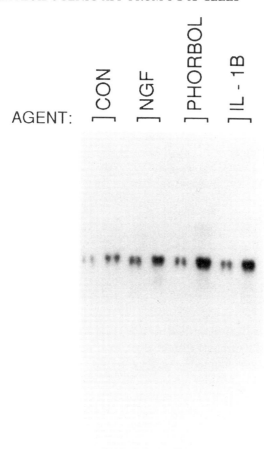

LANE: 1 2 3 4 5 6 7 8

Figure 1. Autoradiogram of PC-12 RNA, fractionated on agarose gels, and hybridized with an APP cDNA probe (15). Successive lanes contain 6 μg or 12 μg total RNA, respectively, from control, NGF, phorbol ester and IL-1B induced cells

Immunoprecipitation with Ab-12 (anti-A4) of PC-12 conditioned media containing 0.005% SDS revealed a 60-kDa band not present in preabsorbed Ab-12 or anti-IgG controls (32). Microsequencing of similarly purified 60-kDa protein revealed an N-terminus of E-T-H-M-A, identical to amino acids 436–440 of APP_{751} (16). Two- to fivefold reduced amounts of this protein were released in the absence of SDS.

Western analysis of these media with antisera elicited by peptides within the amino-terminal portion of APP revealed strong 120-kDa bands and weaker 100-kDa bands (32). Two Kunitz-type protease inhibitor (KPI) domain antisera revealed only

Table 1.

	Antisera	Eliciting peptide AA*	Ref.	60 kDa	120 kDa
1.	Mab22C11	60-80	(18)	–	+
2.	Anti-3	20-304		–	+
3.	IAF2	95-110	(20)	–	+
4.	Alz-4	190-208	(20)	–	+
5.	Alz-13	281-294	(21)	–	+
6.	Anti-F4:2	319-334		–	+
7.	Anti-KPI	319-334	(22)	–	+
8.	Alz-6	357-375	(21)	–	+
9.	IAF5	475-491	(20)	+	+
10.	Anti-5	500-648		+	+
11.	Alz-10	A4 1-17	(23)	+	+
12.	Angela	Amyloid	(24)	+	–
13.	Corina	Amyloid	(24)	+	–
14A.	Anti-B1	A4 1-43		+	–
14B.	Yoshiko	A4 1-38	(6)	+	–
15A.	Anti-Cl	732-751	(6)	+	–
15B.	IAF-8	704-751	(20)	+	–

*Based on the APP_{751} sequence

120-kDa bands consistent with its derivation from APP_{751}. Immunoblot analyses
with five A4, two APP carboxyl-terminus, or two other APP peptide-elicited antisera
(see Table 1), corresponding to the carboxyl-terminal portion of APP, all revealed
60-kDa bands (Figure 2). Although broad bands centered at 68 kDa were seen on
bovine serum albumin (BSA) immunoblots with several of these antisera,
experimental lanes containing 125 μg cell-conditioned media protein revealed 60-kDa
band 5 with these nine antisera distinct from or partially overlapping stained BSA
bands in these lanes. Similar analyses of conditioned media containing injurious
or APP-inducing agents suggest increased release with SDS or two lysosomal

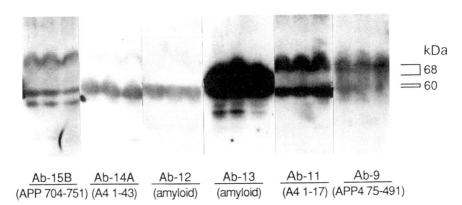

Ab-15B	Ab-14A	Ab-12	Ab-13	Ab-11	Ab-9
(APP 704-751)	(A4 1-43)	(amyloid)	(amyloid)	(A4 1-17)	(APP4 75-491)

Figure 2. Autoradiogram of triplicate isolates of PC-12 conditioned serum-free media proteins,
fractionated by PAGE, transferred to Immobilon filters and immunoblotted with Abs 15b,
14a, 12, 11, 13 and 9, respectively (see Table 1 for characterization of these antisera)

Table 2. Effect of various injurious agents on APP cleavage products in PC-12 media

Agent	60-kDa APP	120-kDa APP
Control — no serum	0	0
0.003% SDS	+	−
Chloroquine	+	0
NH_4Cl	+	0
Vincristine	−	−
Cytochalasin B	−	−
NaF	−	−
Phorbol ester	0	0

inhibitors, but not cytoskeletal disrupters or one APP inducer (Table 2). Together with the immunoprecipitation and sequencing data (above), these data suggest a stress-mediated release of a 60-kDa APP-like protein corresponding to amino acids 436–751 of APP_{751} (16) which includes the intact A4 domain. Whereas a protein of 315 amino acids would have a mass of 32 kDa, hydrophobic domains or O-glycosyl side-chains could cause migration on SDS-PAGE gels at 60 kDa.

Similar immunoblot analyses of fetal, newborn, calf and bovine sera with Abs 11–14b (see Table 1) also reveal a 60-kDa protein. However, this protein, unlike the 60-kDa protein released from PC-12 cells, is not seen in immunoblots with Abs 15a or b. This serum protein may therefore be derived from the normally cleaved 120-kDa APP seen in CSF (23).

Selection and cloning of FAD and control fibroblast–neuroblastoma hybrids

An HGPRT⁻ mutant of human neuroblastoma N-GP, NGP-1A-TRI, donated by Dr E. J. Stanbridge, was rendered Geneticin-resistant by electrophoresis of a Gen-R-plasmid construct. This clone was fused with one of four control or four FAD-fibroblast clones with polyethylene glycol. After selection with Geneticin (400 μg/ml) and HAT, surviving cells formed colonies which were grown in conditioned media containing both selective agents (Figure 3). Although FAD fibroblasts grew more vigorously than age and passage-matched controls, the opposite is observed for their neural hybrids.

DISCUSSION

Whereas a 90-kDa protein in human sera (26) and a 58-kDa (27) protein in brain (27) were detected with APP antisera elicited by peptides in or near A4, their correspondence to APP is unclear (12). A 72-kDa protein, detected in normal and AD brain with both A4 and APP carboxyl-terminus elicited antisera (28,29), may represent an amyloidogenic APP fragment (12). This is the first report, however, of a potentially amyloidogenic putative APP product specifically released from stressed neural cells. Whereas some APP peptide-elicited antisera capriciously bind

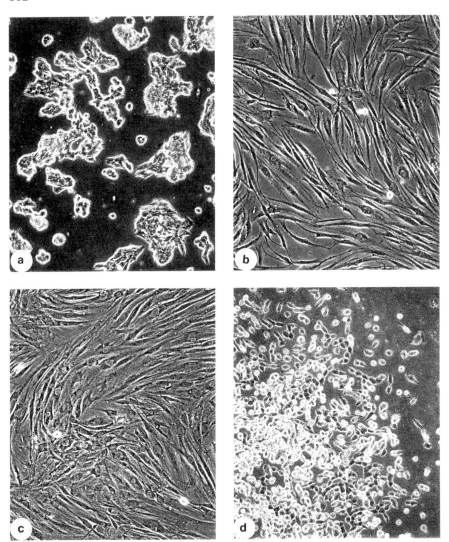

Figure 3. Microphotographs of (a) NGP-IA-TRI-GEN[R] (neuroblastoma), (b) GM 00967C (control fibroblast), (c) AG 04402A (FAD fibroblast) cells and representative NGP-fibroblast, (d) control, and (e,f) AD hybrids (×250)

BSA and other non-APP proteins (12), our detection of an apparently distinct 60-kDa protein with nine antisera elicited by four distinct APP peptides including the carboxyl-terminus and A4 domains supports this conclusion. Crossreactions of several APP antisera with bovine serum albumin (BSA) and the proximity of stained BSA to 60-kDa immunoreactivity on some blots, suggest additional experiments with metabolically labeled cell-conditioned media analyzed by 2D-PAGE to confirm our conclusion that the 60-kDa protein is derived from PC-12 APP. Purification and

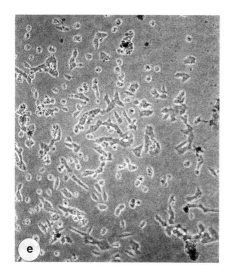
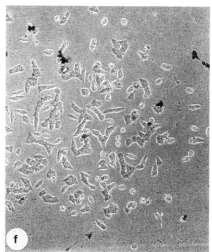

Figure 3 (e) and (f). *(caption opposite)*

sequencing of this 60-kDa protein will prove that it contains an intact A4 domain and is therefore potentially amyloidogenic.

The fact that increased release of a 60-kDa putative APP product was seen when PC-12 cells were subjected to serum-free media or the additional stress of SDS or lysosomal inhibitors but not other injurious agents or one APP inducer, suggests a role for specific pre-existing neuronal injuries in AD amyloidogenesis. Longer APP inductions with additional agents and additional experiments with more specific membrane or lysosomally active agents are needed to confirm these conclusions. The effect of lysosomal inhibitors is consistent with reports of increased APP fragments in AD brain lysosomes (10). We will determine whether the abnormal cleavage and release of this putative amyloidogenic APP fragment from PC-12 cells, which principally express APP_{751} (containing the KPI (16) protease inhibitor), might not occur in cell lines principally expressing APP_{695}. This would support the importance of specific APP forms in AD amyloidogenesis (30,31).

Future analyses of the immortal AD-neural hybrid clones in which the FAD gene may be expressed in a unique neural milieu may establish their use in future research on both AD mechanisms and therapies.

Acknowledgments

We thank Dr E. J. Stanbridge for the NGP-1A-TRI neuroblastoma mutant; and Dr I. Lieberburg, Athena Neurosciences Corp, The Upjohn Co. and Drs D. Selkoe, S. Younkin and K. Beyreuther for antisera, peptides and many helpful comments. We especially acknowledge the careful and dedicated assistance of Richard Davis and Sumedha Bhaghat. This work was supported in part by the ADRDA; NIH, NIA (AG-00813-02) and the Zale Medical Foundation.

REFERENCES

1. Dyrks T et al. EMBO J 1988; 7: 949-57.
2. Weidemann A et al. Cell 1989; 57: 115-26.
3. Sisodia SS et al. Science 1990; 248: 492-5.
4. Esch FS et al. Science 1990; 248: 1122-4.
5. Oltersdorf T et al. Nature 1989; 341: 144-7
6. Joachim CL, Mori H, Selkoe DJ. Nature 1989; 341: 226-30.
7. Neve RL. Neurobiol Aging 1989; 10: 400-2.
8. Koo EH et al. Proc Natl Acad Sci USA 1990; 87: 1561-5.
9. Siman R et al. Soc Neurosci 1989; 541: 15.
10. Benowitz LI et al. Exp Neurol 1989; 106: 237-50.
11. Mroczkowski B et al. Molec Cell Biol 1989; 9: 2771-8.
12. Stern RA, Trojanowski J, Lee VM-Y. FEBS Lett 1990; 264: 43-8.
13. Refolo LM et al. Biochem Biophys Res Comm 1989; 164: 664-70.
14. Goldgaber D et al. Proc Natl Acad Sci USA 1989; 86: 7606-10.
15. Goldgaber D et al. Science 1987; 237: 77-80.
16. Ponte P et al. Nature 1988; 331: 525-7.
17. Schubert D et al. Proc Natl Acad Sci USA 1989; 86: 2066-9.
18. Kang J et al. Nature 1987; 325: 733-4.
19. Bottenstein JE, Sato GH. Proc Natl Acad Sci USA 1979; 76: 514-17.
20. Greenberg BD et al (in preparation).
21. Arai H et al. Proc Natl Acad Sci USA 1990; 87: 2249-58.
22. Palmert MR et al. Proc Natl Acad Sci USA 1989; 86: 6338-42.
23. Palmert MR et al. Biochem Biophys Res Comm 1989; 165: 182-8.
24. Selkoe DJ, Abraham CR, Podlisny MB, Duffy LK. J Neurochem 1986; 46: 1820-34.
25. Selkoe DJ et al. Proc Natl Acad Sci USA 1988; 85: 7341-5.
26. Rumble B et al. New Engl J Med 1989; 320: 1446-52.
27. Landon M et al. Prog Clin Biol Res 1989; 317: 902-17.
28. Simpson J et al. FEBS Lett 1988; 237: 196-8.
29. Kametani F et al. Biomed Res 1989; 10: 179-83.
30. Johnson SA et al. Science 1990; 248: 854-7.
31. Anderson JP et al. EMBO J 1989; 8: 3627-32.
32. Baskin F et al (in preparation).

Address for correspondence:

Dr Fred Baskin,
Department of Neurology,
University of Texas Southwestern Medical Center,
5323 Harry Hines Boulevard,
Dallas, Texas 75235, USA

37 A Neurotrophic Role for Basic Fibroblast Growth Factor in Alzheimer's Disease

EDWARD G. STOPA, ANA-MARIA GONZALEZ,
REGINA CHORSKY, ROBERT J. CORONA, JAIME ALVAREZ,
EDWARD D. BIRD AND ANDREW BAIRD

Although nerve growth factor has been considered for therapeutic use in the treatment of Alzheimer's disease (1), basic fibroblast growth factor (FGF) is also effective in supporting the growth of basal forebrain cholinergic neurons (2). Furthermore, because of its ability to support noncholinergic neurons in vitro (3–6), its relatively high concentration in brain (7), and its widespread localization within the central nervous system (8–10), basic FGF is a prime candidate for neurotrophic activity in brain.

Various biological and biochemical properties of basic FGF favor the involvement of this neurotrophic factor in the pathogenesis of Alzheimer's disease. The amyloid β/A4 protein has recently been found in tissues other than brain in Alzheimer patients, suggesting that Alzheimer's disease may result from a widespread systemic disorder (11). Expression of the β-amyloid protein precursor mRNA by nonneuronal cells in the adult human brain and meninges also supports this hypothesis (12). Basic FGF is present in many body tissues (8), and has been shown to induce the synthesis of the amyloid β/A4 protein precursor mRNA in cultured glial cells (13) and increase the secretion of the amyloid β/A4 protein precursor more effectively than nerve growth factor in PC-12 cells (14). In addition, heparan sulfate-like proteoglycans (HSPG), normally associated with basic FGF within the basement membrane and extracellular matrix of different tissues (14–17), have been identified in both the neuritic plaques and vascular amyloid deposits present in the brains of Alzheimer patients (19). In view of these observations, it seems quite likely that the interactions of the amyloid β/A4 protein with both basic FGF and the heparan sulfate-like proteoglycans of the extracellular matrix may be important in the pathogenesis of Alzheimer's disease. This association may also relate to the appearance of the amyloid β/A4 protein in peripheral tissues, many of which contain high concentrations of both basic FGF and heparan sulfate-like proteoglycans.

Alzheimer's Disease: Basic Mechanisms, Diagnosis and Therapeutic Strategies
Edited by K. Iqbal, D. R. C. McLachlan, B. Winblad and H. M. Wisniewski
© 1991 John Wiley & Sons Ltd

IMMUNOCYTOCHEMICAL LOCALIZATION OF BASIC FGF

Control

To define the distribution of basic FGF in the normal human brain, immuno-cytochemical localization was performed using a modification of the avidin-biotin complex technique and a specific polyclonal anti-FGF (1-24) antibody (773) raised against the amino-terminus of synthetic basic FGF (16,20). In normal controls ($n = 5$), this growth factor was found to be widely distributed throughout the three brain regions examined (prefrontal cortex, hippocampus, and hypothalamus). Unlike in peripheral tissues, where basic FGF is often associated with the heparan sulfate-like proteoglycans of the extracellular matrix and basement membrane (14–17), immunoreactivity was observed within astrocytes in both the grey and white matter, as well as within neuronal perikarya (Figure 1). In general, the staining was more uniform and intense within the astrocytic population. Neuronal staining was less robust and varied considerably in different brain regions. Scattered pyramidal-shaped immunoreactive neurons were evident within both the prefrontal cortex and hippocampus. Light staining was also seen in the media and adventitia of cerebral blood vessels.

Alzheimer's disease

In comparison with the control brains, basic FGF in the brains of Alzheimer patients was not distributed in the normal fashion, but was found in association with the lesions that characterize this disease. Brain tissues that were obtained from Alzheimer patients ($n = 4$) showed a substantial increase in the overall specific staining of astrocytes and neurons, particularly in areas of reactive gliosis (Figure 2A). In contrast to normal control brain specimens, focal concentration of immunoreactive basic FGF was evident within the neuritic plaques, and could be clearly seen in association with the neurofibrillary tangles present within neuronal perikarya (Figure 2B). Control experiments performed using the basic FGF affinity column 'flow through' of antibody 773 (16), as well as the omission of primary antibody from the protocol, failed to yield any specific staining.

BASIC FGF mRNA IN-SITU HYBRIDIZATION STUDIES

To further examine the role of basic FGF in Alzheimer's disease, in-situ hybridization with a specific probe for basic FGF mRNA was performed on samples of prefrontal cortex and hippocampus obtained from the brains used for immunocytochemical analyses. The in-situ hybridization procedures were performed as described by Emoto et al (9). A riboprobe containing the sequence of human basic FGF was constructed by inserting the coding region of a synthetic human basic FGF gene into bluescript (Stratagene, La Jolla, CA). The probes were labeled with alpha ^{35}S-UTP in a transcriptional run-off reaction using the T3 or T7 promoters as described by the manufacturer. The hybridizing solution consisted of 50% formamide, 0.3 M NaCl, 10 mM TRIS (pH 8.0), 1 mM EDTA, 10 mM dithiothreiotol, 1× Denhardt's solution

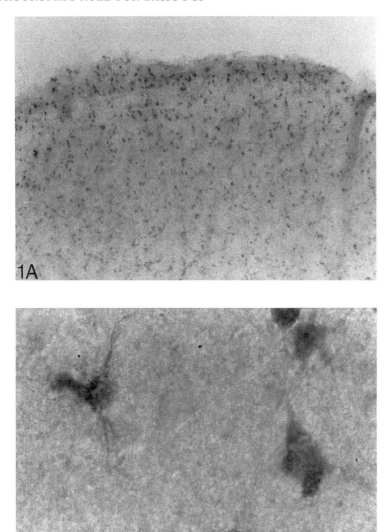

Figure 1. Immunocytochemical detection of basic FGF in normal human prefrontal cortex. (A) Low magnification (×20) photomicrograph showing the widespread distribution of immunoreactive basic FGF in a 55-year-old female patient who died of a myocardial infarction. (B) High magnification (×1000) view demonstrating the presence of basic FGF immunoreactivity in both an astrocyte (left) and a pyramidal-shaped neuron (right). Both control and Alzheimer brain tissues were obtained within 6–18 hours postmortem and fixed by immersion for 15–24 hours in 4% paraformaldehyde in 0.1 M phosphate buffer (pH 7.4), sunk in 30% sucrose in 0.1 M phosphate buffer (pH 7.4) and then serially sectioned at 60 μm on a freezing microtome. The immunocytochemical procedures used were identical to those previously described (16)

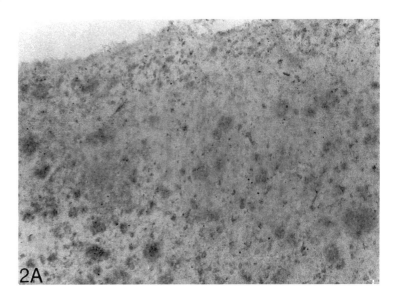

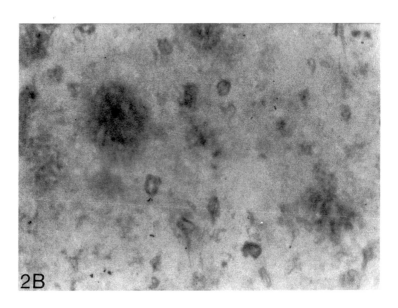

Figure 2. Immunoreactive basic FGF in Alzheimer's disease. (A) Low magnification (×20) photomicrograph showing the increase in immunoreactive basic FGF observed in the prefrontal cortex of a 78-year-old female patient with Alzheimer's disease (compare to Figure 1A). (B) High magnification (×400) image illustrating the intimate association of basic FGF immunoreactivity with neuritic plaques and neurofibrillary tangles

and 10% dextran sulfate (W/V). Unless otherwise indicated, total yeast RNA and tRNA (0.5 µg/ml) was used as blocking RNA. The 15-µm sections were washed with 4× SSC (0.6 M NaCl/0.06 M Na citrate, pH 7.0) at room temperature and treated with ribonuclease A (20 µg/ml) for 30 min at 37 °C. The sections were then thoroughly washed in 0.2× SSC, 1 mM DTT at 65 °C dehydrated with ethanol; dried and coated with Kodak NTB2 liquid autoradiographic emulsion. After a 2-3 week exposure at 4 °C, the slides were developed in Kodak D19, rinsed and the silver grains were examined by light and dark field microscopy.

The intensity of the hybridization reaction varied among specimens within each experimental group, possibly as a result of differences in both postmortem degradation and premortem agonal events. Despite this limitation, the autoradiographic grain density signal overlying both neurons and astrocytes was consistently more robust in brain samples from Alzheimer patients (not shown). This observation suggests that synthesis of basic FGF mRNA may be increased as a consequence of Alzheimer's disease.

BASIC FGF PROTEIN ANALYSES

The increase in basic FGF was also confirmed by protein analyses. Molecular (Western blotting) and quantitative (radioimmunoassay with antibody 773) analyses for basic FGF were performed as previously described (20,22) on fresh frozen samples of prefrontal and temporal cortex obtained from control ($n = 5$) and Alzheimer ($n = 5$) patients that were matched for age (8th decade), sex, Brodmann area, and postmortem interval (range 4-17 h). Consistent with both the immunocytochemical and in-situ hybridization data, the amounts of immunoreactive basic FGF in extracts from both prefrontal and temporal cortex were greater in tissues from Alzheimer patients than their control counterparts. Brodmann areas 10 and 11 contained 10.8 ± 1.1 ng/mg basic FGF in control specimens vs 23.2 ± 1.6 ng/mg in Alzheimer tissue ($P < 0.01$). Brodmann areas 21 and 22 contained 10.1 ± 0.9 ng/mg in control specimens vs 18.6 ± 4.4 ng/mg in Alzheimer tissue ($P < 0.01$). All of the samples were also shown to contain a biologically active basic FGF, which upon analysis by western blotting revealed the presence of the 18 000 dalton form of basic FGF and its 20-25 kDa variants (21).

CONCLUSIONS

Our results clearly demonstrate that basic FGF is widely present in the adult human brain. They further establish that basic FGF is increased as a consequence of the pathological alterations occurring in Alzheimer's disease. These observations have a number of important implications. First, they provide evidence in support of the hypothesis that basic FGF may function as a neurotrophic factor in the human brain, as previously suggested by the ability of basic FGF to both enhance neuronal survival in vitro (3-6) and prevent neuronal degeneration in vivo (2). Second, in view of the ability of basic FGF to stimulate the synthesis of the amyloid β/A4 protein precursor mRNA in cultured glial cells (13), and increase the secretion of the amyloid

β/A4 protein precursor in PC-12 cells (14), our data support the hypothesis that basic FGF may be a stimulus for the increased production of the amyloid β/A4 protein seen in Alzheimer's disease. Finally, the presence of basic FGF within the neuritic plaques and neurofibrillary tangles suggests that the heparan sulfate-like proteoglycans integrated within the amyloidotic lesions of Alzheimer's disease (19) may serve to sequester basic FGF and decrease its bioavailability to surrounding cells. This process is normally seen in peripheral tissues and would be consistent with the role that heparan sulfate-like proteoglycans are thought to play in the regulation of basic FGF activity (8,17,18,23). Thus, the appearance of heparan sulfate-containing structures (i.e. neuritic plaques, neurofibrillary tangles and amyloid angiopathy) may negate the increased synthesis of basic FGF by sequestering the mitogen. The ensuing decrease in bioavailable FGF would predictably lead to decreased maintenance of functional synapses and failure of surrounding neurons to survive. Accordingly, further elucidation of the influence of basic FGF and its antagonists (20,24) could have important implications in the treatment of Alzheimer's disease.

Acknowledgments

The authors wish to acknowledge Ms Dorothy Stechyshyn, Ms Dawn Chapman, Ms Lisa A. Kanaley, Dr George Collins, Mr James Ferris and Mr Michael Ong for their helpful suggestions and assistance.

REFERENCES

1. Phelps CH, Gage FH, Growdon JH, Hefti F, Harbaugh R, Johnston MV, Khachaturian ZS, Mobley WC, Price DL, Raskino M, Simpkins J, Thal LJ, Woodstock J. Neurobiol Aging 1989; 10: 205-207.
2. Anderson KJ, Dam D, Lee S, Cotman CW. Nature 1988; 332: 306-61.
3. Walicke P, Cowan WM, Ueno N, Baird A, Guillemin R. Proc Natl Acad Sci USA 1986; 83: 3012-15.
4. Walicke PA, Baird A. Prog Brain Res 1988; 78: 333-8.
5. Walicke PA. J Neurosci 1988; 8: 2618-27.
6. Morrison RS, Sharma A, DeVellis J, Bradshaw RA. Proc Natl Acad Sci USA 1986; 83: 7537-41.
7. Bohlen P, Esch F, Baird A, Jones KL, Gospodarowicz D. FEBS Lett 1985; 185: 177-81.
8. Baird A, Walicke PA. Br Med Bull 1989; 45: 438-52.
9. Emoto N, Gonzalez AM, Walicke PA, Wada E, Simmons DM, Shimasaki S, Baird A. Growth Factors 1989; 2: 21-9.
10. Pettman B, Labourdette G, Weihel M, Sensenbrenner M. Neurosci Lett 1986; 68: 175-80.
11. Joachim CL, Mori H, Selkoe DJ. Nature 1989; 341: 226-30.
12. Golde TE, Estus S, Usiak M, Younkin LH, Younkin SG. Neuron 1990; 4: 253-67.
13. Quon D, Catalano R, Cordell B. Biochem Biophys Res Comm 1990; 163: 96-102.
14. Schubert D, Jin LW, Saitoh T, Cole E. Neuron 1989; 3: 689-94.
15. Baird A, Ling N. Biochem Biophys Res Comm 1987; 142: 428-35.
16. Gonzalez AM, Buscaglia M, Ong M, Baird A. J Cell Biol 1990; 110: 347-58.
17. Folkman J, Klagsbrun M, Sasse J, Wadzinski MG, Inger D, Vlodavsky I. Am J Pathol 1988; 230: 393-400.
18. Vlodavsky I, Folkman J, Sullivan R, Fridman R, Ishai-Michaeli R, Sasse J, Klagsbrun M. Proc Natl. Acad Sci USA 1987; 84: 2292-6.

19. Snow AD, Mar H, Nochlin D, Kimata K, Kato M, Suzuki S, Hassell J, Wright TN. Am J Pathol 1988; 113: 456-63.
20. Lappi DA, Martineau D, Baird A. Biochem Biophys Res Comm 1989; 160: 917-23.
21. Florkiewicz RZ, Sommer A. Proc Natl Acad Sci USA 1989; 86: 3678-981.
22. Baird A, Bohlen P, Ling N, Gullemin R. Reg Peptides 1985; 10: 309-17.
23. Baird A, Bohlen P. Handbook of Experimental Pharmacology 1990; 95: 369-418.
24. Baird A, Schubert D, Ling N, Guillemin R. Proc Natl Acad Sci USA 1988; 85: 2324-8.

Address for correspondence:

Dr Edward G. Stopa,
Department of Pathology (Neuropathology Division),
State University of New York,
Health Science Center, 750 East Adams Street,
Syracuse, NY 13210, USA

38 Differential Expression of Three Types of Amyloid β-Protein Precursor mRNA in the Brain and Nonneural Tissues

S. TANAKA, S. SHIOJIRI, Y. TAKAHASHI, N. KITAGUCHI,
J. KIMURA, S. NAKAMURA AND K. UEDA

Three types of amyloid β-protein precursor (APP) mRNA are produced by alternative splicing; they are APP_{770} and APP_{751} harboring a protease inhibitor (APPI), and APP_{695} lacking the APPI. We examined, using the RNase protection assay, the ratio of the three types of APP mRNA, and obtained the following results: (1) the expression of APP_{695} mRNA was specific for the brain; (2) the ratio of APP_{770} and APP_{751} mRNAs was tissue-specific; (3) the ratio of $APP_{770}/APP_{751}/APP_{695}$ mRNAs was approximately 1:10:20 in normal cerebral cortices; (4) the ratio of APP_{751} plus APP_{770} mRNAs increased 1.05 ~ 1.41-fold in the brain of Alzheimer's disease (AD) relative to control. Furthermore, an enzyme-linked immunosorbent assay (ELISA) of the cerebrospinal fluid (CSF) showed that the concentration of APPI increased in AD patients compared with control. These results support the idea that an increase in APPI may disturb the normal processing of APPs and thus lead to amyloid deposition.

Deposition of amyloid β-protein, i.e. ~ 40-amino acid peptide, in the brain as senile plaque cores and amyloid angiopathy is characteristic of AD. Amyloid β-protein is derived from larger precursors that have structural features characteristic of cell surface receptors (1). Three types of APP mRNA are produced from a single gene transcript by alternative splicing of exons 7 and 8 (2,3). APP_{770} and APP_{751} harbor an identical 56-amino acid sequence (APPI) encoded by exon 7, that is highly homologous to the Kunitz-type basic protease inhibitors, while APP_{695} lacks this APPI segment (Figure 1). In fact, transfection and expression of APP_{770} cDNA in COS-1 cells induced a higher inhibitory activity against trypsin than those of APP_{695} cDNA (2).

The role of APPI in amyloid deposition, i.e. the effect of APPI on the processing of APPs, has not been elucidated. In order to clarify this point, we analyzed expression of three types of APP mRNA in various tissues, including the brain, with reference to AD versus control. The concentration of APPI in CSF was also measured.

Alzheimer's Disease: Basic Mechanisms, Diagnosis and Therapeutic Strategies
Edited by K. Iqbal, D. R. C. McLachlan, B. Winblad and H. M. Wisniewski
© 1991 John Wiley & Sons Ltd

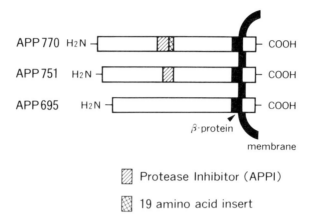

Figure 1. Structure of three types of APP

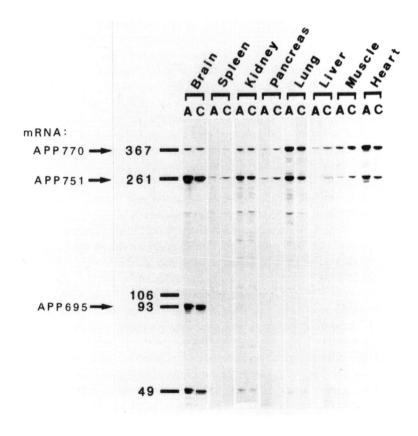

Figure 2(a). *(Caption opposite)*

EXPRESSION OF THREE TYPES OF APP mRNA IN HUMAN BRAIN AND OTHER TISSUES

The RNase protection assay was carried out using an antisense RNA fragment which spans over the APPI sequence (4). Three types of APP mRNA were detected in the brain, and the ratio of $APP_{770}/APP_{751}/APP_{695}$ mRNAs was approximately 1:10:20 in the frontal cortex of control brain. APP_{770} and APP_{751} mRNAs, but not APP_{695}, were also found in other nonneural tissues (Figure 2); thus, the expression of APP_{695} mRNA was specific for the brain. The ratio of APP_{770}/APP_{751} mRNAs varied markedly among tissues, indicating a tissue-specific splicing of the APP gene transcript; APP_{770} was predominant in the heart and muscle; APP_{751} was predominant in the spleen, kidney and pancreas; the two types were comparable in the lung and liver. This ratio did not differ significantly among individuals, irrespective of control (five cases) or AD (one case). More cases would need to be analyzed before making the conclusion that APP mRNAs are not expressed differentially in nonneural tissues of AD.

Accumulation of β-protein was reportedly found in other nonneural tissues (skin and colon) of AD (5). Investigation of nonneural tissues in more detail might lead to development of a useful method for diagnosis of AD.

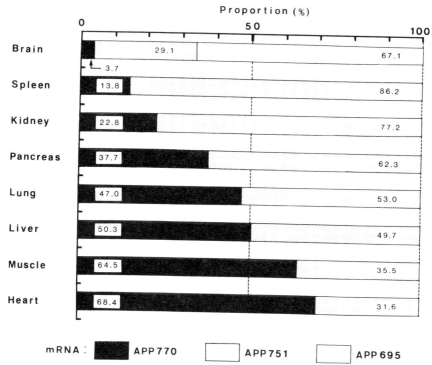

Figure 2. Analysis of APP mRNAs expression in various tissues by RNase protection assay (ref. 4). (a) Autoradiogram of AD (A) and one case of control (C). (b) Proportion of three types of APP mRNA in controls ($n = 5$)

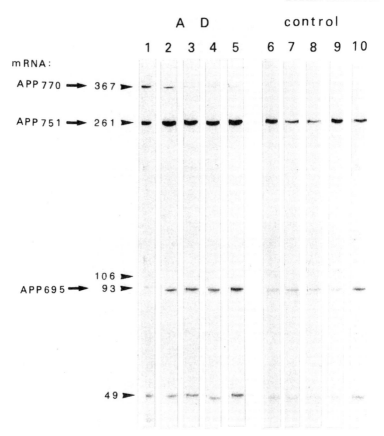

Figure 3(a). *(Caption opposite)*

DIFFERENTIAL EXPRESSION OF THREE TYPES OF APP mRNA IN THE BRAIN OF AD

Our previous study using oligonucleotide probes in Northern blot analysis showed that the expression of APP_{770} mRNA increased significantly in the brain (frontal cortex) of AD compared with nondemented control (6). In the present study using the RNase protection assay, we analyzed the ratio of three types of APP mRNA in various brain regions of AD and nondemented control (4). The mean ratio of $APP_{770}/APP_{751}/APP_{695}$ mRNAs was approximately 1:10:20 in various brain regions (except cerebellum) of control. The ratio of APP_{770} plus APP_{751} mRNAs increased $1.07 \sim 1.41$-fold in the cerebral cortex and 1.28-fold in the hippocampus of AD relative to control (Figure 3).

As for the expression of APP mRNAs, there have been contradictory reports; our results indicate an enhanced expression of APP_{770} and APP_{751} mRNAs. Johnson et al (7) also showed a twofold increase in the ratio of APP_{751}/APP_{695} mRNAs. On the contrary, Palmert et al, using an in-situ hybridization technique, reported an

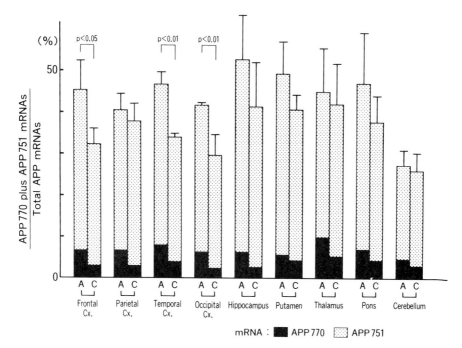

Figure 3. Analysis of APP mRNAs expression in various brain regions by RNase protection assay (ref. 4). (a) Autoradiogram of AD (1–5) and control (6–10) in the frontal cortex. (b) Ratios of APP_{770} plus APP_{751} mRNAs in nine brain regions of AD and control groups (mean value ± SD). Significance of the difference between the groups was analyzed by Student's t-test

increased expression of APP_{695} mRNA in specific regions of the brain (locus ceruleus and nucleus basalis) of AD compared with control (8). Johnson's and our results support the view that the increase in the proportion of APPI-harboring types to an APPI-lacking type may disturb the balance between the protease and its inhibitor in the processing of APPs, and eventually lead to accumulation of β-protein as amyloid (Figure 4). Recent reports (9,10) suggest that the initial cleavage of APPs occurs in the interior of β-protein. Although the protease engaged in this cleavage of β-protein has not been identified, APPI might inhibit this initial cleavage and possibly subsequent cleavages. Whether the change in APP mRNAs proportion in the brain of AD results from a differential splicing of APP gene transcript or the change in the proportion of APPI-producing cells, such as gliosis, is currently under investigation.

CONCENTRATION OF APPI IN CSF

There have been several reports on detection of soluble (secreted) form of APPs in CSF by immunoblot analysis (11,12). These reports suggested that the ratios of APPs or the concentration of APPI in CSF might change in AD patients. We developed a new sandwich ELISA with a trypsin-coated plate for detection of APPI (13).

Hypothesis

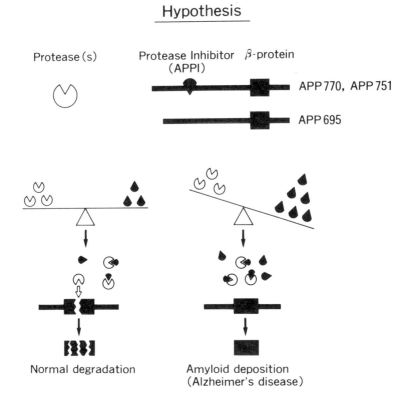

Figure 4. A possible mechanism of amyloid deposition in the brain of AD

Our preliminary study indicated that the concentration of APPI in CSF was significantly elevated in AD patients compared with multi-infarct dementia or nondemented controls. This finding is consistent with the results of APP mRNA analyses. Our new ELISA of APPI in CSF may provide a most promising avenue to the early diagnosis of AD.

REFERENCES

1. Kang J, Lemaire H-G, Unterbeck A, Salbaum JM, Masters CL, Grzeschik K-H, Multhaup G, Beyreuther K, Müller-Hill B. Nature 1987; 325: 733-6.
2. Kitaguchi N, Takahashi Y, Tokushima Y, Shiojiri S, Ito H. Nature 1988; 331: 530-2.
3. Lemaire HG, Salbaum JM, Multhaup G, Kang J, Bayney RM, Unterbeck A, Beyreuther K, Müller-Hill B. Nuc Acids Res 1989; 17: 517-22.
4. Tanaka S, Shiojiri S, Takahashi Y, Kitaguchi N, Ito H, Kameyama M, Kimura J, Nakamura S, Ueda K. Biochem Biophys Res Comm 1989; 165: 1406-14.
5. Joachim CL, Mori H, Selkoe DJ. Nature 1989; 341: 226-30.
6. Tanaka S, Nakamura S, Ueda K, Kameyama M, Shiojiri S, Takahashi Y, Kitaguchi N, Ito H. Biochem Biophys Res Comm 1988; 157: 472-9.
7. Johnson SA, McNeill T, Cordell B, Finch CE. Science 1990; 248: 854-7.

8. Palmert MR, Golde TE, Cohen ML, Kovacs DM, Tanzi RE, Gusella JF, Usiak MF, Younkin LH, Younkin SG. Science 1988; 241: 1080-4.
9. Sisodia SS, Koo KH, Beyreuther K, Unterbeck A, Price DL. Science 1990; 248: 492-5.
10. Esch FS, Keim PS, Beattie EC, Blacher RW, Culwell AR, Oltersdorf T, McClure D, Ward PJ. Science 1990; 248: 1122-4.
11. Weidemann A, Koenig G, Bunke D, Fisher P, Salbaum JM, Masters CL, Beyreuther K. Cell 1989; 57: 115-26.
12. Palmert MR, Podlisny MB, Witker DS, Oltersdorf T, Younkin LH, Selkoe DJ, Younkin SG. Proc Natl Acad Sci USA 1989; 86: 6338-42.
13. Kitaguchi N, Tokushima Y, Oishi K, Takahashi Y, Shiojiri S, Nakamura S, Tanaka S, Ito H. Biochem Biophys Res Comm 1990; 166: 1453-9.

Address for correspondence:

Dr Seigo Tanaka,
Department of Neurology,
Kyoto University Faculty of Medicine,
Sakyo-ku, Kyoto 606, Japan

39 Amyloid β-Protein Precursor Accumulates in Dystrophic Neurites of Senile Plaques in Alzheimer-Type Dementia

MIKIO SHOJI, YASUO HARIGAYA, TAKESHI KAWARABAYASHI,
KOJI ISHIGURO, ETSURO MATSUBARA,
HARUYASU YAMAGUCHI, KOICHI OKAMOTO,
SHUNSAKU HIRAI AND MASAMITSU TAKATAMA

We raised two rabbit antisera against synthetic peptides corresponding to the carboxyl- and amino-terminal regions of the predicted amyloid β-protein precursor (APP). Both antisera recognized the same 106–135 kDa proteins of human brain extract by immunoblot analysis. Immunocytochemical studies showed that these antisera both reacted with the same dystrophic neurites within the senile plaques of Alzheimer brains. These results indicated that APP accumulated in the dystrophic neurites of the senile plaques.

INTRODUCTION

Alzheimer-type dementia (ATD) is a frequent cause of mental deterioration in the elderly. Alzheimer's neurofibrillary tangles and senile plaques are characteristic changes seen in Alzheimer brains. The major component of senile plaque amyloid — β-protein (1) or A4 protein (2) — is suspected to be derived from larger precursor protein, i.e. amyloid β-protein precursor (APP) (3). In-situ hybridization studies have shown that the mRNA encoding APP is expressed in the neurons and some glial cells of the cerebral cortex (4,5). However, the localization of APP at the protein level is still unclear. In this study, we prepared antisera to both terminal ends of APP, and investigated the histological localization of APP in Alzheimer-type dementia brains.

MATERIALS AND METHODS

We examined tissues of four brains from patients with ATD aged between 80 and 87 years. Tissue blocks were taken from the frontal cortex, the temporal cortex,

Alzheimer's Disease: Basic Mechanisms, Diagnosis and Therapeutic Strategies
Edited by K. Iqbal, D. R. C. McLachlan, B. Winblad and H. M. Wisniewski
© 1991 John Wiley & Sons Ltd

and the hippocampus. They were fixed with 0.1 M phosphate buffer saline containing 4% paraformaldehyde and 0.3% picric acid (pH 7.6, 4 °C), and embedded in paraffin. Serial 3-μm sections were then prepared. The two rabbit antisera to APP_{18-38} (amino-terminus of APP; W63N, 1:200) and $APP_{666-695}$ (carboxyl-terminus of APP; W61C, 1:500) were used. The characteristics and specificity have been reported elsewhere (6). Antiserum to β-protein (28K1, 1:500) (7) was used to detect senile plaque amyloids, and antiserum to tau protein (generously provided by Dr Y. Ihara, Tokyo Metropolitan Institute of Gerontology, Tokyo, Japan; 1:500) (8) was used to detect the dystrophic neurites of senile plaques. Each section was stained using the Elite avidin-biotin peroxidase complex (ABC) method (Vector Lab. Burlingame, CA). Intrinsic peroxidase activity was blocked by incubation for 10 min with 0.5% periodic acid solution. For β-protein immunostaining, sections were pretreated for 5 min with 99% formic acid.

Samples of membrane-associated proteins were prepared from the 2% Triton X-100 extract of frontal lobe homogenates of four normal human brains, as

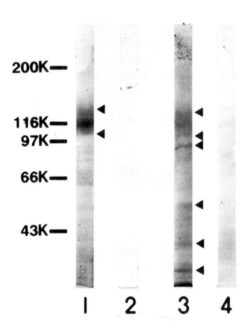

Figure 1. Immunoblots of the Triton X-100 extract from normal brain homogenates. Lane 1, W61C (antiserum against a synthetic peptide corresponding to the APP_{695} C-terminus: $APP_{666-695}$; 1:500); lane 2, W61C after absorption; lane 3, W63N (antiserum against a synthetic peptide corresponding to the N-terminus of APP_{695}: APP_{18-38}; 1:200); lane 4, W63N after absorption. Molecular weight markers are 200, 116, 97, 66, and 43 kDa. W61C labeled the 106–135 kDa proteins (arrowed). W63N labeled the same bands detected by W61C, as well as additional 93, 52, 30 and 17 kDa bands (arrowed). These immunoreactive bands were abolished by preabsorption

described by Selkoe et al (9). Blots of a 4-12% gradient of SDS-polyacrylamide gels on polyvinylidinene difluoride membranes (Millipore, Bedford, MA) were immunostained by the Elite-ABC method.

RESULTS AND DISCUSSION

The W61C antibody labeled 106-135 kDa proteins in the Western blot analysis. W63N labeled the same bands detected by W61C, as well as additional 93, 52, 30 and 17 kDa bands (Figure 1). These 106-135 kDa proteins have already been identified in the Triton X-100 extract from human brains by immunoblots using antiserum to the C-terminus (residues 675-695) of APP_{695} (9). Antiserum to the N-terminus (residues 45-62) of APP_{695} has also been shown to label a set of 106-135 kDa and 55 kDa proteins (10). In addition, the antibody to a recombinant bacterial APP_{695} fusion protein detected 103-130 kDa proteins, which were suspected to be the N- and O-glycosylated forms of APP_{695}, APP_{751}, and APP_{770} (11). We showed that these 106-135 kDa proteins were actually almost the full length of native APP, because these proteins had both terminal epitopes. Kunitz-type protease inhibitor-like inserts (12) and glycosylation could explain the differences in molecular weight of the labeled bands. The bands detected with W63N below the 106-135 kDa proteins were suspected to be proteolytic fragments of APP.

In the immunocytochemical study, W61C showed many patches of immuno-reactivity, consisting of small clusters of swollen and bulbous profiles in the frontal and temporal cortices and the hippocampal regions of the four ATD brains. Their distribution corresponded to the primitive and classical plaques on the adjacent sections stained with 28K1 (Figure 2a, b). Amyloid cores were not stained by W61C. These immunoreactive cluster-like structures were seen in the crowns of classic plaques, and collected in primitive plaques (Figure 2c). Diffuse plaques (7), which consist of amorphous β-protein deposits, and compact plaques (7) were not stained. These immunoreactive cluster-like structures were widely distributed in the frontal and temporal cerebral cortex, and many were also seen in the subiculum of the hippocampus.

W63N showed cluster-like immunoreactive structures in the crowns of classical plaques and in primitive plaques similarly to W61C. Compared with W61C, W63N stained the cluster-like immunoreactive structures in a more granular and intense manner.

A few neurons and glial cells showed dot-like immunoreactivity for both W61C and W63N in their cell bodies (Figure 2d). Neither amyloid components of the senile plaques, nor subpial amyloid deposits (7), nor cerebrovascular amyloid, were stained with these antisera. The 28K1 antiserum labeled only amyloid deposits. Anti-tau antiserum immunostained many Alzheimer's neuro-fibrillary tangles, and the dystrophic neurites in classical and primitive plaques, as well as neurons and curly fibers (8).

We carefully examined serial sections stained with W61C, W63N, 28K1, and anti-tau protein serum, and evaluated the staining of the same regions of the

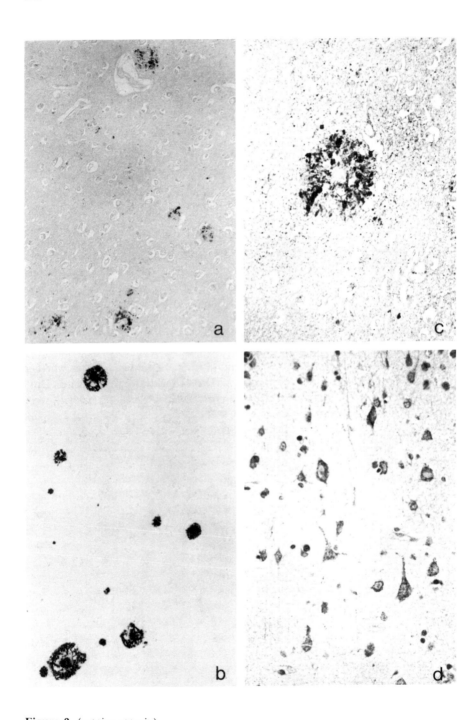

Figure 2. (*caption opposite*)

senile plaques. Each cluster-like profile labeled by W61C was also immuno-stained by W63N (Figure 3a, b). Tau protein immunoreactivity was detected in many of the same structures demonstrated by W61C and W63N (Figure 3c, d). However, 28K1 selectively labeled the amyloid component of senile plaques, and did not stain these cluster-like regions (Figure 3e, f). These findings indicated that the structures stained by W61C and W63N were dystrophic neurites, and not the amyloid component of senile plaques. Moreover, these results showed that native APP is accumulated in the dystrophic neurites of senile plaques.

By in-situ hybridization, the messenger RNA encoding APP has been found to be expressed in cortical neurons and some glial cells (4,5). Immunocytochemical study of APP in the rat brain has also shown that it is widely distributed in the neurons and some glial cells of the central nervous system (13,14). These data suggest that specific alterations of neuronal APP result in the formation of senile plaque amyloid. However, immunocytochemical analysis of Alzheimer brains using antisera against the different portions of APP has unexpectedly shown that APP was present in the senile plaques. Selkoe et al have reported that only some amyloid-bearing plaques, not the dystrophic neurites of senile plaques, were labeled by antiserum to the carboxyl-terminus of APP_{695} ($APP_{675-695}$) (9). The same result was shown by Palmert et al using antiserum to the amino-terminus of APP_{695} (APP_{45-62}) (10). Tate-Ostroff et al used antiserum to residues 413–429 (APP_{695}), and found that APP was present in the neurons, astrocytes, and blood vessels of normal brains (15). They also noted immunoreactivity of senile plaques, but it was unclear whether the reaction was located in the amyloid component or the dystrophic neurites. Only Ishii's group has demonstrated dystrophic neurites in senile plaques which were labeled with antiserum to synthetic carboxyl-terminus peptides ($APP_{681-695}$) (16). We consider that this discrepancy was caused by the nature of the antiserum used against different portions of APP and by variations in immunostaining techniques. In order to clarify this discrepancy, we used two antisera that recognized different portions of APP, and performed the immunostaining procedures with meticulous care. Furthermore, we compared the findings using β-protein and tau protein immunostaining on thin serial sections to clarify the exact localization of APP. Our findings are that native APP was accumulated in the dystrophic neurites of senile plaques, and not in senile plaque amyloid deposits.

Figure 2. Adjacent sections (a, b) of the entorhinal cortex of the hippocampus from an ATD brain (×100). (a) Immunostaining with W61C; 1:500. (b) β-protein immunostaining; 1:500. The distribution of cluster-like structures labeled with W61C corresponded to the primitive and classical plaques detected by 28K1. (c) Classical plaque stained by W61C antiserum (×200). Amyloid core was not stained. Immunoreactive cluster-like structures were seen in the crown. (d) The pyramidal cells and astrocytes showed dot-like immunoreactivity for W61C antiserum in their cell bodies. Temporal lobe cortex from a normal control brain (×200).

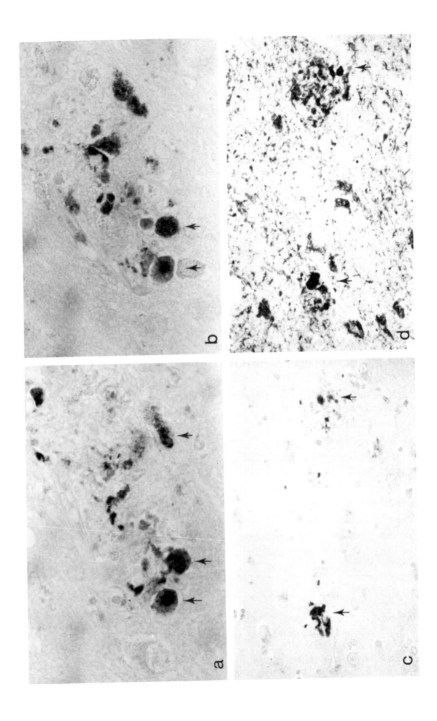

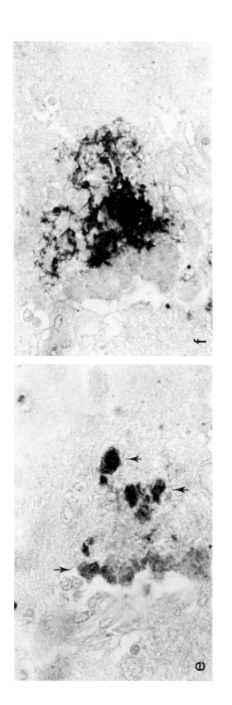

Figure 3. (a) and (b), (c) and (d), (e) and (f) are adjacent sections of the subiculum of the hippocampus from an SDAT brain (×400). (a) W61C, 1:500; (b) W63N, 1:200. The cluster-like structures labeled with W61C are also stained with W63N (arrow). (c) W61C, 1:500 and (d) anti-tau protein serum, 1:500. These structures are stained with anti-tau protein serum (arrow). (e) W63N, 1:200; (f) 28K1, 1:500. W63N labeled the dystrophic neurites (arrow); 28K1 immunostained only amyloid components, and not dystrophic neurites in the senile plaques

REFERENCES

1. Glenner GG, Wong CW. Biochem Biophys Res Comm 1984; 120: 885-90.
2. Masters CL, Simms G, Weinman NA, Multhaup G, McDonard BL, Beyreuther K. Proc Natl Acad Sci USA 1985; 82: 4245-9.
3. Kang J, Lemaire HG, Unterbeck A, Salbaum JM, Masters CL, Grzeshik KH, Multhaup G, Beyreuther K, Muller-Hill B. Nature 1987; 325: 733-6.
4. Bahmanyar S, Higgins GA, Goldgaber D, Lewis DA, Morrison JH, Wilson MC, Shankar SK, Gajdusek DC. Science 1987; 237: 77-80.
5. Neve RL, Finch EA, Dawes LR. Neuron 1988; 1: 669-77.
6. Shoji M, Hirai S, Yamaguchi H, Harigaya Y, Kawarabayashi T. Brain Res 1990; 512: 164-8.
7. Yamaguchi H, Hirai S, Morimatsu M, Shoji M, Harigaya Y. Acta Neuropathol 1988; 77: 113-19.
8. Ihara Y. Brain Res 1988; 459: 138-148.
9. Selkoe DJ, Podlisny MB, Joachim CL, Vickers EA, Lee G, Fritz LC, Oltersdorf T. Proc Natl Acad Sci USA 1988; 85: 7341-5.
10. Palmert MR, Podlisny MB, Witker DS, Oltersdorf T, Younkin LH, Selkoe DJ, Younkin SG. Biochem Biophys Res Comm 1988; 156: 432-7.
11. Weidemann A, Konig G, Bunke D, Fisher P, Saubaum JM, Masters CL, Beyreuther K. Cell 1989; 57: 115-26.
12. Kitaguchi N, Takahashi Y, Tokushima Y, Shiojiri S, Ito H. Nature 1988; 331: 530-2.
13. Shivers BD, Hilbich C, Multhaup G, Salbaum M, Beyreuther K, Seeburg P. EMBO J 1988; 7: 1365-70.
14. Card JP, Meade RP, Davis LG. Neuron 1988; 1: 835-46.
15. Tate-Ostroff B, Majocha R, Marotta CA. Proc Natl Acad Sci USA 1989; 86: 745-9.
16. Ishii T, Kametani F, Haga S, Sato M. Neuropath Appl Neurobiol 1989; 15: 135-47.

Address for correspondence:

Mikio Shoji,
Department of Neurology
Gunma University School of Medicine,
Maebashi,
Gunma 371, Japan

40 Synaptic Alterations in Preamyloid Deposits

ORSO BUGIANI, LAURA VERGA, FABRIZIO TAGLIAVINI,
BIANCA POLLO, BERNARDINO GHETTI, BLAS FRANGIONE
AND GIORGIO GIACCONE

In Alzheimer's disease and related disorders, the neuropil contains nonbirefringent, nonfluorescent deposits of nonfibrillary electrodense material recognized by antibodies to the amyloid β-protein (1–4). It is likely that these preamyloid deposits are made up of intermediate cleavage products of the amyloid precursor protein (APP) with the β-protein fragment and represent the earliest morphological change that one can relate to the aging process and/or age-related diseases of the brain. No neuritic changes detectable by means of antibodies against paired helical filaments (PHF), putative PHF precursors or related cytoskeleton abnormalities were ever observed within preamyloid deposits. The present study showed that in Alzheimer's disease and Down's syndrome a relationship exists between preamyloid deposits, whatever their site in the brain, and presynaptic terminal swellings immunoreactive with antibodies to synaptophysin and ubiquitin.

This study was carried out on brain samples from two Alzheimer patients and two Down patients. Serial sections were alternately stained with thioflavine S for tissue changes with amyloid fibrils and cell changes with PHFs, anti-SP28 (a rabbit polyclonal antibody to the 28-residue synthetic peptide homologous to the NH_2-terminal region of amyloid β-protein) (5) immunoperoxidase (IP) for preamyloid and amyloid deposits, antisynaptophysin antibody IP for the vesicle-associated protein localized in presynaptic terminals (6), antiubiquitin antibody IP for altered and/or abnormal proteins (7), and Alz-50 IP for PHFs and PHF putative precursors (8). As a result, it was found that neuritic swellings immunolabeled by antisynaptophysin, antiubiquitin and Alz-50 antibodies were present in senile plaques. At variance with plaques, no Alz-50 immunoreactive structures were associated with any preamyloid deposits, while neuritic swellings recognized by antisynaptophysin antibody were related with two preamyloid deposits out of three and neuritic swellings immunoreactive with antiubiquitin antibody were present in one preamyloid deposit out of three (Figure 1). Finally, one preamyloid deposit out of three was found to be devoid of any neuritic changes.

These findings suggest that neuritic swellings filled with antisynaptophysin immunoreactive material represent a peculiar neuronal reaction that involves presynaptic terminals and is associated with the extracellular deposition of APP

Alzheimer's Disease: Basic Mechanisms, Diagnosis and Therapeutic Strategies
Edited by K. Iqbal, D. R. C. McLachlan, B. Winblad and H. M. Wisniewski
© 1991 John Wiley & Sons Ltd

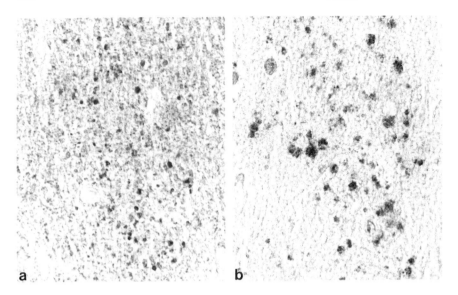

Figure 1. Molecular layer of the cerebellum, Alzheimer's disease, immunocytochemical staining with (a) antisynaptophysin antibody (Dako, 1:10 at 4 °C overnight, 7-μm thick section, Paraplast-embedded block, × 1100) and (b) antiubiquitin antibody (Chemicon, 1:200 at 4 °C overnight, 7-μm thick section, Paraplast-embedded block, × 1100) immunoperoxidase. The area corresponding to the preamyloid deposit contains several round bodies immunoreactive with antisynaptophysin and antiubiquitin antibodies. Bodies evidenced by anti-synaptophysin antibody are up to 6 μm in size, while those evidenced by antiubiquitin antibody are up to 20 μm in size

intermediate cleavage products including the amyloid β-protein fragment. Such a neuritic reaction might be due to the APP itself and/or its intermediate cleavage products that when present in large amounts in the neuropil may act as a growth factor (9) on neuritic terminals. Accordingly, antiubiquitin immunoreactive swellings within preamyloid deposits might have to do with altered and/or abnormal proteins resulting from overproduction of APP, synaptophysin or proteins necessary to neuritic sprouting. Whether the presynaptic terminal changes that are present within preamyloid deposits may in certain regions of the brain evolve toward the neuritic degeneration characterized by cytoskeleton abnormalities with straight filaments or PHFs remains to be established.

Acknowledgments

Supported in part by the Italian Ministry of Health, Department of Social Services, the US National Institutes of Health (Grants AG05891 and AG08721 to B. F.) and gifts from relatives of Alzheimer patients (to O. B. and B. G.). Dr P. Davies kindly provided Alz-50.

REFERENCES

1. Tagliavini F, Giaccone G, Frangione B, Bugiani O. Neurosci Lett 1988; 93: 191-6.
2. Giaccone G, Tagliavini F, Linoli G, Bouras C, Frigerio L, Frangione B, Bugiani O. Neurosci Lett 1989; 97: 232-8.

3. Bugiani O, Giaccone G, Frangione B, Ghetti B, Tagliavini F. Neurosci Lett 1989; 103: 263-8.
4. Verga L, Frangione B, Tagliavini F, Giaccone G, Migheli A, Bugiani O. Neurosci Lett 1989; 106: 294-9.
5. Castaño EN, Ghiso J, Prelli F, Gorevic PD, Migheli A, Frangione B. Biochem Biophys Res Comm 1986; 141: 782-9.
6. Wiedenmann B, Franke WW. Cell 1985; 41: 1017-28.
7. Parag HA, Raboy B, Kulka RG. EMBO J 1987; 6: 55-61.
8. Wolozin B, Pruchnicki A, Dickson DW, Davies P. Science 1986; 232: 648-50.
9. Saito T, Sundsmo M, Roch JM, Kimura N, Cole G, Shubert D, Oltersdorf T, Schenk DB. Cell 1989; 58: 615-22.

Address for correspondence:

Dr Orso Bugiani,
Istituto neurologico Carlo Besta, via Celoria 11,
20133 Milano MI, Italy

41 The Cellular Basis for β-Amyloid Fibril Formation and Removal

H. M. WISNIEWSKI, J. WEGIEL, A. W. VORBRODT,
M. BARCIKOWSKA AND T. G. BURRAGE

Amyloid is a collective term for pathological fibrils that are derived from any one of a number of host proteins. The deposition of amyloid fibrils occurs during normal aging, in Down's sydrome and Alzheimer's disease (AD) as well as in unconventional viral diseases. In AD, the β-amyloid plaque constitutes the major lesion. The plaque is composed of the amyloid fibrils (β-amyloid fibrils in varying stages of orientation and compaction), microglial cells, abnormal neuritic processes and reactive astrocytes (1-3). In-situ hybridization and immunohistochemical studies have shown that many cell types both within and outside of the central nervous system could generate the β-protein precursor. Recent morphological studies have shown a primarily manufacturing relationship between the cytoplasmic and plasma membranes of microglial cells and amyloid fibrils (3-5). In addition, we have recently shown that macrophages are directly involved in the removal of β-amyloid deposits in individuals with stroke (Wisniewski et al, submitted for publication).

This chapter reviews the evidence for the cellular basis of amyloid deposition and degradation using transmission electron microscopy, three-dimensional reconstruction techniques, and immunohistochemistry and cytochemistry at the light and electron microscope levels.

SITE OF FORMATION OF β-AMYLOID FIBRILS

The cellular basis of amyloid fibril formation is most clearly seen by the three-dimensional reconstruction of the classical plaque (5). The general features of ultrathin sections of plaques include the irregular surface of the amyloid star, the spatial arrangement of the four or five associated microglial cells and the presence of abnormal neurites and proliferating astrocytic processes (Figure 1).

Three morphological forms of microglial cells can be distinguished by their topological relationship to the plaque, extent of contact with the amyloid star, overall size and shape. The most numerous morphological type was a cap-like microglial cell which also had the greatest contact with the amyloid star (25-40% of cell surface). The cytoplasm contained a well-developed system of rough and smooth endoplasmic reticulum (RER and SER), numerous mitochondria and polymorphic dense bodies.

Alzheimer's Disease: Basic Mechanisms, Diagnosis and Therapeutic Strategies
Edited by K. Iqbal, D. R. C. McLachlan, B. Winblad and H. M. Wisniewski
© 1991 John Wiley & Sons Ltd

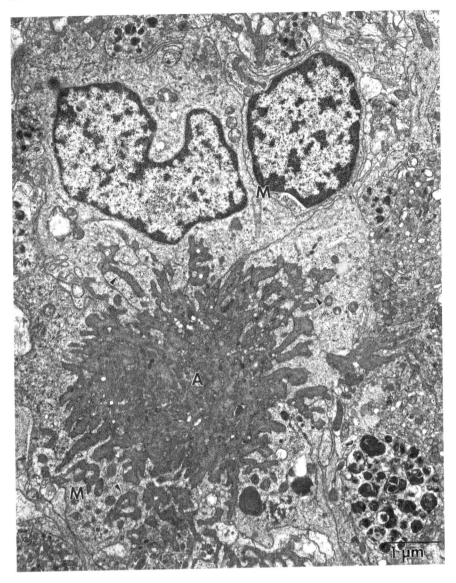

Figure 1. A classical plaque with cap-like microglial cells (M) surrounding the amyloid core (A). The cell membrane forms a labyrinth of channels filled with amyloid (arrows)

Some segments of the RER were in continuity with distended SER membranes and deep infoldings of the plasma membrane. The plasma membrane facing the star consisted of a labyrinth of channels filled with newly formed amyloid fibrils. Each of the classical plaques had at least one or two macrophage-like cells associated with it. These macrophage cells were large and extended from the amyloid star to the plaque periphery, but the area of contact was less (13–25% of cell surface) than the cap-like microglial cell. Numerous polymorphic, osmiophilic bodies were found in this cell type as well as phagocytic vacuoles containing degenerating cytoplasmic organelles. A third type of microglial cell, called an octopus microglial cell because of its radiating arms and position at the periphery of the plaque, had the smallest contact zone with the amyloid star.

The first amyloid fibrils appear in the distended cisterns of the SER. With increasing accumulations of amyloid, the altered ER forms a complex labyrinth of channels whose membranes appear to fuse with the cell membrane. Frequently, smooth and coated vesicles will appear to fuse with the membranes of the amyloid-containing channels. There are three zones in the amyloid star. The peripheral zone is composed of finger-like aggregates of amyloid channels and outpocketing of microglial cytoplasm. The second zone, called the transient zone, is composed of aggregates of amyloid and degenerating cytoplasm trapped between the aggregates. The core of the amyloid star is made up of compacted clusters of amyloid fibrils which still retain their parallel array. The amyloid core is free of cytoplasmic debris and dense bodies. The occurrence of fibrillar material in the endoplasmic reticulum and adjacent to the plasma membrane and a gradient of organization and density in the amyloid star gives distinct morphological evidence of the fibril-forming role of the microglial cells. The constructive role for these cells is also borne out by evidence from NDPase cytochemistry.

CO-LOCALIZATION OF NUCLEOSIDE DIPHOSPHATASE ACTIVITY AND β-AMYLOID FIBRILS

Nucleoside diphosphatase (NDPase) has been used to distinguish between cells of ectodermal origin (neurons, astroglia, and oligodendrocytes) and cells of mesodermal origin (endothelial cells, pericytes, and microglial cells). In the ectodermal cells, the NDPase is intracellular, whereas in the mesodermal cells the NDPase is associated primarily with the cell surface (6) and to a much lesser extent the SER. Plasmalemma-bound NDPase is a cytochemical marker for microglial cells in normal and pathological brains (7). In experimental murine scrapie, microglial cells appear directly associated with the amyloid fibrils in the neuritic plaques (8). In addition, NDPase activity is present on both the surface of these cells and in the distended cisternae of the ER filled with amyloid fibrils (4). These observations suggest that microglial cells are engaged in the production or final elaboration of amyloid in scrapie plaques and that the NDPase molecules are engaged in glycosylation of amyloid fibrils (3,4,8).

Studies were undertaken to determine if similar events take place with microglial cells in neuritic plaques in human and animal brain (9). The cytochemical reaction for NDPase was more evident at the periphery of the amyloid star than at the center (Figure 2). In addition to classical plaques with stars, there were numerous primitive plaques with disperse deposits of amyloid fibrils; the fibrils were frequently packaged in elongated channels (Figure 2). They were interconnected and often formed a labyrinth. These channels showed a strong reaction for NDPase. The

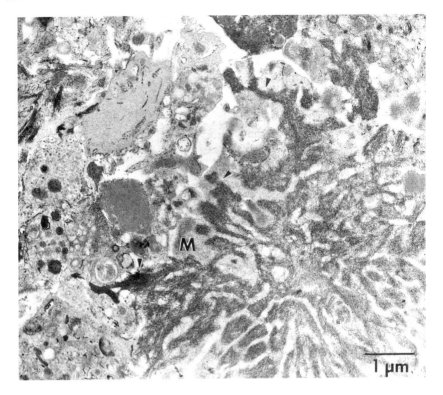

Figure 2. A section of human cerebral cortex incubated for NDPase activity. The most intense cytochemical reaction occurs at the plasma membrane of the microglia cell and with the bundles of the amyloid fibrils in the channels at the periphery of the plaque (arrows)

presence of NDPase activity on the surface of the microglial cells and especially within the ER cisternae that are filled with amyloid fibrils and that are in apparent continuity with extracellular amyloid deposits in plaques suggests that in AD, as in scrapie, these cells are engaged in glycosylation of the amyloid fibril protein.

CELLS INVOLVED IN DEGRADATION OF β-AMYLOID FIBRILS

In order to further distinguish between microglial/macrophage cells involved in fibril formation and those involved in removal of amyloid deposits, we have recently examined the cells involved in β-amyloid fibril removal (phagocytosis) after a stroke (Wisniewski et al, submitted for publication). The individuals who died because of stroke and had numerous (more than 40 in 1 mm^2) neuritic and amyloid plaques in their cortex were studied. Macrophages showing β-amyloid immunoreactivity (specifically demonstrated by immunostaining with mAb 4G8, 10) were found in areas of amyloid deposits. Immunoelectron microscopy of these macrophages (using protein A gold) revealed presence of intact amyloid fibrils and fuzzy, disintegrating fibrillar material in secondary lysosomes (Wisniewski et al, submitted for publication).

Another cell participating in the degradation of amyloid deposits in the plaque is the fibrous astrocyte. The astrocytes increase in number in plaque-rich regions in AD and senile dementia of Alzheimer's type (SDAT) (11,12). Astrocytes accumulate in the periphery of the plaque and their processes penetrate into the plaque. Three-dimensional reconstruction of astrocytes and their processes (Wisniewski and Wegiel, submitted for publication) has revealed close association between the numerous astrocytic processes and the amyloid fibrils. Morphological observations suggest that astrocytes participate in fragmentation and disintegration of amyloid deposits probably through membranous contact with the amyloid.

SPECTRUM OF APPEARANCE OF DEPOSITS CONTAINING β-AMYLOID

The amyloid deposits in the form of classical and primitive plaques are well described and can be easily detected with a variety of histological techniques (e.g. silver stain, Congo red, thioflavine S) as well as monoclonal and polyclonal antibodies. The increased specificity and sensitivity of the immunocytochemical procedures have revealed diffuse and ribbon-like infiltrations, granular deposits in the white matter, dispersed deposits in the molecular layer of the cerebellar cortex and the basal ganglia, star-shaped deposits in the Purkinje cell layer and amyloid angiopathy (10,13). All these lesions, however, are characterized by the presence of extracellular fibrils which are ultrastructurally similar (14), confirming the biochemical evidence of the similarity between vascular amyloid and amyloid of plaque cores (15,16).

As indicated above, various morphological forms have been described in the brains of AD and Down's patients (10,17,18). These observations were made using immunocytochemical methods highly sensitive and specific for the β-protein. This type of plaque is variously called 'diffuse', 'pale', 'very primitive' or 'preamyloid'. These lesions remain negative or are difficult to visualize with other histological techniques which usually detect amyloid (e.g. Congo red, thioflavine S) and do not have a neuritic component. These properties led investigators to suggest that the diffuse deposits were an early stage of plaque formation and that these deposits appear in the absence of reactive microglial cells or neurites (18–21). It has been our recent experience with the three-dimensional reconstruction studies that even diffuse deposits in the brain cortex are associated with microglial cells and the presence of a few dystrophic neurites (22). Like Yamaguchi et al (18) and Giaccone et al (19) in these areas, we see both wisps of fibrillar amyloid deposits as well as accumulations of indistinct floccular and granular material. In our electron microscope experience, the granular–floccular material, in contrast to the fibrillar deposits, labels poorly with the anti-β antibody. In our opinion, therefore, on the basis of morphological studies only, it is impossible to determine whether the granular–floccular material represents degradation product of the fibrils or a nonpolymerized form of amyloid.

SUMMARY

The stimulus for the initiation of deposition of amyloid fibrils is still unknown. However, the cells involved with the formation of the fibrils have been clearly identified as the microglial cells. It remains to be determined precisely if the microglial cells themselves or other cells serve as the source of the amyloid precursor protein (APP) which is then processed, or more probably, improperly processed into the amyloid fibrils. Of similar interest is the determination of the role of the other proteins (α_1-antichymotrypsin, amyloid P component, proteoglycans) which accompany the deposits of β-amyloid fibrils.

We conclusively demonstrated that the amyloid fibrils can be readily degraded by the lysosomal enzymes of the macrophages. Astrocytes also appear to be engaged in the removal of the amyloid fibrils. The astrocytes accomplish this by isolation and dispersal of the amyloid fibrils. We hypothesize that the fibrils are being degraded by ectoenzymes present on the surface of the astrocytes.

Acknowledgments

Supported in part by funds from the New York State Institute for Basic Research in Developmental Disabilities and a grant from the National Institute on Aging NIH AGO-4220-6.

REFERENCES

1. Wisniewski HM, Terry RD. Prog Neuropathol 1973; 11: 1-26.
2. Wisniewski HM, Moretz RC, Lossinsky AC. Ann Neurol 1981; 10: 517-22.
3. Wisniewski HM, Wegiel J, Wang KC, Kujawa M, Lach B. Can J Neurol Sci 1989; 16: 535-42.
4. Wisniewski HM, Vorbrodt AW, Wegiel J, Morys J, Lossinsky AS. Am J Med Gen 1990; 37 (in press).
5. Wegiel J, Wisniewski HM. Acta Neuropathol 1990 (in press).
6. Vorbrodt AW, Wisniewski HM. J Histochem Cytochem 1982; 30: 418-24.
7. Merz GS, Schwenk J, Schuller-Levis G, Gruca S, Wisniewski HM. Acta Neuropathol 1987; 72: 240-7.
8. Burrage TG, Lossinsky AS, Kascsak R, Carp R, Wisniewski HM. J Cell Biol 1990 (abstr. 0917).
9. Wisniewski HM, Johnson AB, Raine CS, Kay WJ, Terry RD. Lab Invest 1970; 23: 287-96.
10. Wisniewski HM, Bancher C, Barcikowska M, Wen GY, Currie J. Acta Neuropathol 1989; 78: 337-47.
11. Dickson DW, Farlo J, Davies P, Crystal H, Fuld P, Yen SC. Am J Pathol 1988; 132: 86-101.
12. Duffy PE, Rapport M, Graft L. Neurology 1980; 30: 778-82.
13. Selkoe DJ. Neurobiol Aging 1989; 10: 387-95.
14. Okamoto K, Yamaguchi H, Hirai S, Shoji M, Harigaya Y, Takatama M. Alz Dis Assoc Disord 1988; 2: 269 (abstr.).
15. Miller DL, Currie JR, Iqbal K, Potempska A, Styles J. Alz Dis Assoc Disord 1988; 2: 253 (abstr.).
16. Ikeda S-I, Wong CW, Allsop D, Landon M, Kidd M, Glenner GG. Lab Invest 1987; 57: 446-9.
17. Probst A, Brunnschweiler H, Lautenschlager C, Ulrich J. Acta Neuropathol 1988; 74: 133-41.

18. Yamaguchi H, Nakazato Y, Hirai S, Shoji S, Harigaya Y. Am J Pathol 1989; 135: 593-7.
19. Giaccone G, Tagliavini F, Linoli G, Bouras C, Fregeres L, Frangione B, Bugiani O. Neurosci Lett 1989; 97: 232-8.
20. Tagliavini F, Giaccone G, Frangione B, Bugiani O. Neurosci Lett 1988; 93: 191-6.
21. Joachim CL, Morris JH, Selkoe DJ. Am J Pathol 1989; 135: 309-19.
22. Wegiel J, Wisniewski HM. J Neuropath Exp Neurol 1990; 49: 268 (abstr.).

Address for correspondence:

Dr H. M. Wisniewski,
Department of Pathological Neurobiology,
Institute for Basic Research in Developmental Disabilities,
1050 Forest Hill Road, Staten Island, New York 10314, USA

Part VI

RISK FACTORS AND EPIDEMIOLOGY

42 Epidemiologic Studies of Dementia in Rochester, Minnesota

EMRE KOKMEN AND C. MARY BEARD

Epidemiologic studies of Alzheimer's disease are necessary for accurate descriptions of the clinical course, for planning of health care resources, and for development of theories of pathogenesis. Many population-based studies of prevalence of dementing illness have been carried out (1,2). The only population-based studies of incidence of dementing illness in North America have been published based on data obtained from Rochester, Minnesota (3,4). Other population-based studies include those from Gothenburg, Sweden (5), two western islands in Sweden (6), Lundby, Sweden (7,8), Turku, Finland (9) and Israel (10).

MATERIALS AND METHODS

Rochester is a town of approximately 62 000 population (1980) in southeastern Minnesota. The closest large urban centers are the twin cities of Minneapolis and St Paul some 90 miles away. Most medical care to the community is provided by the Mayo Clinic, a multispecialty group practice and its affiliated hospitals. A record linkage system provides access to all medical records from all health care delivery resources in the community. Medical diagnosis for all inhabitants of Olmsted County (Rochester is the county seat) are coded and entered into a computer-based data bank. The only resource for autopsies in the county is the Mayo Clinic and the only emergency trauma center is located in one of its affiliated hospitals.

We identified all incidence cases with a diagnosis that might be construed as dementia (Table 1) between 1 January 1959 and 31 December 1986. An investigator (E.K.) then reviewed each medical record looking for preselected diagnostic criteria (Table 2). The medical record then was reviewed in greater detail to ascertain the year of onset of symptoms of dementia. A specialist clerk determined whether the patient was a resident of Rochester, Minnesota, during the year of onset (index year). The residency criteria were as follows:

1. The patient should have continuously resided in the city limits of Rochester, Minnesota, during the index year and the year immediately preceding it. The city directory and city maps of the particular index year were utilized.

Alzheimer's Disease: Basic Mechanisms, Diagnosis and Therapeutic Strategies
Edited by K. Iqbal, D. R. C. McLachlan, B. Winblad and H. M. Wisniewski
© 1991 John Wiley & Sons Ltd

Table 1. Diagnostic rubrics utilized in medical record reviews for dementing illnesses

Alzheimer's disease	Cortical atrophy/cortical degeneration
Atherosclerosis or arteriosclerosis	Dementia/delirium/encephalopathy
Acute brain syndrome	Encephalitis
Brain atrophy	Encephalomalacia
Brain degeneration	Generalized brain atrophy
Brain syndrome	Huntington's disease
Brain damage	Lesions of the central nervous system
Brain sclerosis	Inflammation of brain
Brain softening	Depression
Brain disease	Pick's disease
Chronic brain syndrome	Personality disorder
Cerebral arteriosclerosis	Mental changes
Cerebrovascular disease	Senility/senile brain disease/senescence
Creutzfeldt-Jakob disease	

Table 2. Diagnostic criteria utilized for dementia and Alzheimer's disease

Diagnostic criteria for dementia

Documented evidence of:

previously normal intellectual and social function
progressive decline of intellectual/cognitive/social function which is irreversible with medical or psychiatric treatment
evidence of memory impairment
dementia sufficiently important to impair age/education/occupation — appropriate lifestyle adjustment

In addition to this, documented evidence for at least two of the following:

disorientation
personality/behavioral problems
dyscalculia
aphasia or apraxia or agnosia
impairment of judgment/abstract thinking

Diagnostic criteria for Alzheimer's disease

Clinical diagnosis (probable Alzheimer's disease):

presence of dementia as defined above
insidious onset of symptoms of dementia
gradual progression and irreversible course
other potential causes of dementia are either not present or occurred definitely after the onset of symptoms of dementia

Neuropathological diagnosis (definite Alzheimer's disease):

presence of clinical Alzheimer's disease as defined above
presence of abundant neuritic (senile) plaques and/or neurofibrillary tangles in neocortical regions excluding hippocampus and subiculum

2. The patient should not have moved to Rochester for purposes of treatment and management of dementing illness.

A trained nurse abstractor then reviewed the medical record and collected information utilizing a predetermined protocol. Death certificates and autopsy protocols (if autopsy was done) were uniformly available. Only cases whose dementia lasted for six months or longer were accepted.

After the cases were identified, the investigator reviewed the history once more, and, based on all available clinical and postmortem data, made a diagnosis of the cause of dementia.

To establish the incidence cohort, medical records with a diagnosis relatable to dementia up to seven years beyond the last incidence year were reviewed. We thus feel confident that we have included all cases whose dementia may have started many years before their diagnosis was recorded. To establish the prevalence cohort, we included all cases that were known to be residing in the community with dementia on the prevalence date.

For each case of dementia, five potential controls from a list of registrations for care—matched for age (±3 years) and of same sex—who did not have a diagnostic rubric relatable to dementia were identified. The investigator reviewed each of these individuals' medical records and accepted the first one who had a medical evaluation of sufficient depth within one year of the index year and who did not have evidence of dementia as a potential control. The residency specialist then reviewed the potential controls to determine residency status utilizing the criteria mentioned above. The control medical record was abstracted using the same protocol as the cases.

Age-specific and sex-specific incidence rates for each of the four quinquennial periods from 1960 were then calculated. Prevalence rates for 1 January 1975 were also calculated. Matched-pair odds ratios using the conditional logistic regression techniques of Breslow and Day were estimated for a series of medical and neurological conditions.

To study the relationship between Hashimoto's thyroiditis and Alzheimer's disease, we performed a cohort study by following a group of individuals with surgically proven Hashimoto's disease for the occurrence of Alzheimer's disease (16).

RESULTS

Age-specific and sex-specific incidence rates for dementia (Figure 1) and Alzheimer's disease (Figure 2) show remarkable stability over the twenty years. A sharp rise of incidence rates occurs with each advancing decade of life. Tables 3 and 4 indicate age-adjusted incidence rates (US white 1980 population) for the four quinquennial periods, again showing a remarkable stability of the incidence rates.

Relative survival is depicted for dementia in Figure 3 and for Alzheimer's disease in Figure 4. Relative survival at five and ten years after onset was significantly longer ($P < 0.05$) for females only in the 1960-64 period. The survivorship trend has not changed over time in the four quinquennial periods.

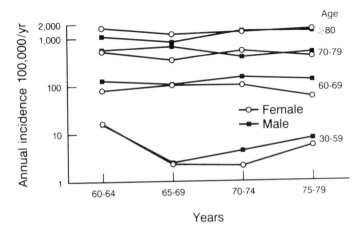

Figure 1. Age-specific and sex-specific incidence rates (/100 000 per year total population) for dementia due to all causes in four quinquennial periods 1960–1979 in Rochester, Minnesota

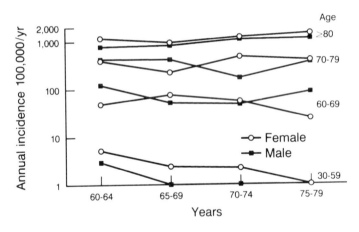

Figure 2. Age-specific and sex-specific incidence rates (/100 000 per year per total population) for Alzheimer's disease in four quinquennial periods 1960–1979 in Rochester, Minnesota

Prevalence on 1 January 1975 in Rochester, Minnesota, shows a marked increase of rates with age (Figure 5) (11).

In the study of selected risk factors for previously occurring severe head trauma with loss of consciousness, the odds ratio was 1.25 with a 95% confidence interval of 0.34 to 4.66 (12). Ongoing studies of a cohort of Olmsted County residents who had suffered head trauma with presumed brain injury also suggest that the standardized morbidity ratio (ratio of observed to expected cases) was not significantly elevated for dementia or Alzheimer's disease (13).

Table 3. Adjusted annual incidence per 100 000* for dementia in Rochester, Minnesota, in four quinquennial periods 1960-1979

	1960-64		1965-69		1970-74		1975-79	
	PY†	n	PY	n	PY	n	PY	n
		rate		rate		rate		rate
		(95% CI)		(95% CI)		(95% CI)		(95% CI)
Age-adjusted:								
females	114.9	117	133.5	108	149.0	170	155.5	194
		116.6		82.7		103.6		96.8
		(95.5-137.7)		(67.1-98.4)		(87.8-119.4)		(82.6-110.4)
males	94.3	61	110.7	64	123.7	79	129.6	91
		105.2		94.7		101.9		108.3
		(78.3-132.2)		(71.4-118.0)		(79.4-124.3)		(86.0-130.6)
Age- and sex-	209.2	178	244.2	172	272.7	249	285.2	285
adjusted		113.9		88.7		103.1		102.2
total		(97.1-130.8)		(75.4-102.0)		(90.1-116.0)		(90.1-114.4)

*Using age groups 0-29, 30-59, 60-69, 70-79, 80+ years and the US white 1980 population as the adjusting population.
†Person years of observation in thousands.
Reprinted by permission from Neurology 1989; 39: 773-6.

Table 4. Adjusted annual incidence per 100 000* for Alzheimer's disease in Rochester, Minnesota, in four quinquennial periods 1960-1979

	1960-64		1965-69		1970-74		1975-79	
	PY†	n	PY	n	PY	n	PY	n
		rate		rate		rate		rate
		(95% CI)		(95% CI)		(95% CI)		(95% CI)
Age-adjusted:								
females	114.9	76	133.5	78	149.0	140	155.5	168
		75.7		57.3		84.0		81.6
		(58.7-92.7)		(44.3-70.3)		(69.9-98.0)		(69.1-94.2)
males	94.3	41	110.7	42	123.7	42	129.6	63
		72.0		63.6		54.6		76.0
		(49.6-94.4)		(44.3-82.90)		(38.1-71.1)		(57.2-94.8)
Age- and sex-	209.2	117	244.2	117	272.7	182	285.2	231
adjusted		75.7		60.6		72.4		80.5
total		(61.9-89.4)		(49.1-70.9)		(61.8-83.0)		(69.9-91.1)

*Using age groups 0-29, 30-59, 60-69, 70-79, 80+ years and the US white 1980 population as the adjusting population.
†Person years of observation in thousands.
Reprinted by permission from Neurology 1989; 39: 773-6.

For the multiplicity of medical, neurologic, and psychiatric disorders, we found elevated odds ratio for only episodic depression. None of the other variables reached statistical significance (14).

We identified a subgroup of our cases and controls who had been exposed to therapeutic radiation. Odds ratios for any prior exposure to therapeutic radiation as well as direct exposure limited to the head were calculated and were found to be not significantly elevated (15).

In the cohort study of the influence of pre-existing Hashimoto's disease on subsequent development of Alzheimer's disease, we did not find an association with previously diagnosed (by biopsy) Hashimoto's thyroiditis and subsequent

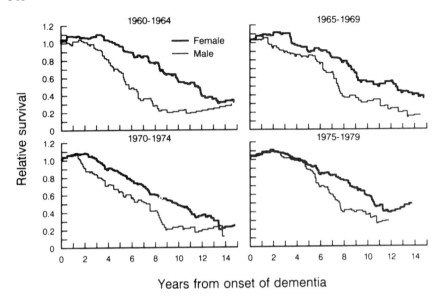

Years from onset of dementia

Figure 3. Relative survival (observed/expected) in four quinquennial periods 1960–1979, females and males separate, all dementia

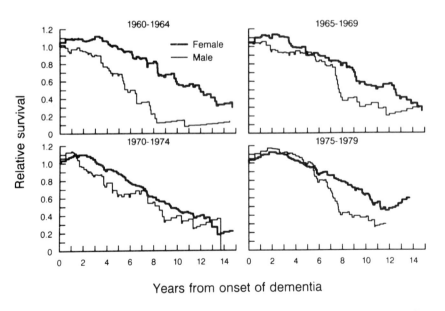

Years from onset of dementia

Figure 4. Relative survival (observed/expected), females and males separate, in four quinquennial periods 1960–1979, Alzheimer's disease only

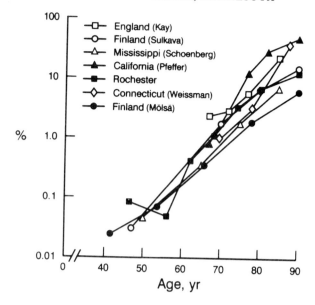

Figure 5. Age-specific prevalence rates (%) of primary progressive degenerative dementia from seven separate studies (on an arithmetic scale). Reprinted by permission from Neurology 1989; 39: 773-776

development of Alzheimer's disease. In the case-control study of previous thyroid disease and Alzheimer's, there was a positive association of Alzheimer's disease and myxedema (matched-pair odds ratio 2.0 with a 95% confidence interval of 0.75-5.33), but this failed to reach significance (16).

DISCUSSION

There have been no other population-based reports on the incidence of dementing illness from North American communities. Our incidence figures show considerable concordance with age-specific incidence reports from other parts of the world (2,3). The Rochester population contains only a very small percentage of minorities such as Hispanics and blacks; therefore, it would not be possible to make any comments about the incidence of dementia in diverse ethnic cultural backgrounds based on the Rochester, Minnesota, data. Our prevalence figures are quite similar to many prevalence figures reported from elsewhere in the world (Figure 5) (11). Two recent studies reported from North American communities (17,18) indicate higher prevalence rates than other estimates in the literature. The main reason for this discrepancy would appear to be case definition: those two studies relied heavily on standardized psychometric tests. Most other investigators used clinical definitions of cases.

Our methods of measuring incidence and prevalence rely exclusively on review of medical records. It can be argued that patients who do not come to medical attention might be missed by our method of case ascertainment. This, indeed, is a serious consideration. However, we feel that we capture most, if not all, dementing illness since our population at risk (i.e. 65 years and older) are estimated to come to medical attention at least once every three years, and we have access to all medical records, which often cover the lifetime of a patient. A comparison of our incidence figures to those presented from other parts of the world utilizing community survey methods suggest that our case ascertainment is quite adequate (1).

To establish incidence rates by utilizing a prospective community survey in the US would require longitudinal follow-up of an entire population. This may take many years and may be very expensive.

Analysis of risk factors for dementing illness in general and Alzheimer's disease in particular has relied heavily on case-control studies (2,20). Of the putative risk factors (19) that have been proposed for dementing illness, cigarette smoking (21) and previously experienced thyroid disease (22) remain unconfirmed (23,24). Our data, at present, do not support the head trauma hypothesis. Frequency of family history of dementing illness or other degenerative diseases such as parkinsonism has been recently reported to be increased in Alzheimer's disease (25). Because of the nature of the medical record information, we were unable to address cigarette smoking, potential exposure to toxic materials and drugs, and family history of dementia in our studies.

Acknowledgments

The authors are grateful to Mrs Lavonne Gates and Mrs Virginia Hanson for assistance in data abstraction and to many collaborators who, over the years, assisted in certain phases of these projects: Bruce S. Schoenberg MD, Vijay Chandra MD, L. T. Kurland MD, David Ballard PhD, F. Yoshimasu MD, J. P. Whisnant MD, H. Okazaki MD, K. P. Offord MS and D. B. Williams MD.

REFERENCES

1. Rocca WA, Amaducci LA, Schoenberg BS. Epidemiology of clinically diagnosed Alzheimer's disease. Ann Neurol 1986; 19: 415-24.
2. Rocca WA, Amaducci LA. Epidemiology of Alzheimer's disease. In Schoenberg BS, Anderson DW (eds) Neuroepidemiology. Boca Raton, FL: CRC Press (in press).
3. Schoenberg BS, Kokmen E, Okazaki H. Alzheimer's disease and other dementing illnesses in a defined United States population: incidence rates and clinical features. Ann Neurol 1987, 22: 724-9.
4. Kokmen E, Chandra V, Schoenberg BS. Trends in incidence of dementing illness in Rochester, Minnesota, in three quinquennial periods, 1960-1974. Neurology 1988; 38: 975-80.
5. Nilsson LV. Incidence of severe dementia in an urban sample followed from 70 to 79 years of age. Acta Psychiatr Scand 1984; 70: 478-86.
6. Akesson HO. A population study of senile and arteriosclerotic psychoses. Human Heredity 1969; 19: 546-66.
7. Hagnell O, Lanke J, Rorsman B et al. Current trends in the incidence of senile and multi-infarct dementia. Arch Psychiatr Nervenkr 1983; 233: 423-38.
8. Rorsman B, Hagnell O. Prevalence and incidence of senile dementia and multi-infarct dementia in Lundby. Neuropsychobiol 1986; 15: 122-9.
9. Molsa. Epidemiology of dementia in Finland. Acta Neurol Scand 1982; 65: 541-52.

10. Treves T, Korczyn AD, Zilber N et al. Presenile dementia in Israel. Arch Neurol 1986; 43: 26-9.
11. Kokmen E, Beard CM, Offord KP, Kurland LT. Prevalence of medically diagnosed dementia in a defined United States population: Rochester, Minnesota, January 1, 1975. Neurology 1989; 39: 773-6.
12. Chandra V, Kokmen E, Schoenberg BS, Beard CM. Head trauma with loss of consciousness as a risk factor for Alzheimer's disease. Neurology 1989; 39: 1576-8.
13. Williams DB, Annegers JF, Kokmen E, Kurland LT. Brain injury and its neurological sequelae: a prospective study of dementia, parkinsonism, and amyotrophic lateral sclerosis. Neurology 1990; 40: 419 (abstr.).
14. Kokmen E, Beard CM, Chandra V et al. Case-control study of Alzheimer's disease in Rochester, Minnesota (1960-1974). Neurology 1989; 39: 179 (abstr.).
15. Kokmen E, Beard CM, Offord KP, Anderson JA. Therapeutic radiation exposure in Alzheimer's disease: a case-control study. Neurology 1989; 39: 1980 (abstr.).
16. Yoshimasu F, Kokmen E, Hay ID et al. An association between Alzheimer's disease and thyroid diseases in Rochester, Minnesota. Neurology 1990; 40: 347 (abstr.).
17. Pfeffer RI, Afifi AA, Chance JM. Prevalence of Alzheimer's disease in a retirement community. Am J Epidemiol 1987; 125: 420-36.
18. Evans DA, Funkenstein HH, Albert MS et al. Prevalence of Alzheimer's disease in a community population of older persons. JAMA 1989; 262: 2551-6.
19. Henderson AS. The risk factors for Alzheimer's disease: a review and a hypothesis. Acta Psychiatr Scand 1988; 78: 257-75.
20. Shalat SL, Seltzer B, Pidcock C, Baker EL Jr. Risk factors for Alzheimer's disease: a case-control study. Neurology 1987; 37: 1630-3.
21. Heyman A, Wilkinson WE, Stafford JA et al. Alzheimer's disease: a study of epidemiological aspects. Ann Neurol 1984; 15: 335-41.
22. Amaducci LA, Fratiglioni L, Rocca WA et al. Risk factors for clinically diagnosed Alzheimer's disease: a case-control study of an Italian population. Neurology 1986; 36: 922-31.
23. Chandra V, Philipose V, Bell PA et al. Case-control study of late onset 'probable Alzheimer's disease'. Neurology 1987; 37: 1295-1300.
24. Hofman A, Schulte W, Tanja TA et al. History of dementia and Parkinson's disease in 1st-degree relatives of patients with Alzheimer's disease. Neurology 1989; 39: 1589-92.

Address for correspondence:

Dr Emre Kokmen,
Mayo Clinic,
Rochester, Minnesota, USA

43 Age-Associated Cognitive Decline is Related to Biological Life Events

PETER J. HOUX, FRED W. VREELING AND JELLEMER JOLLES

Several studies consistently show a decline of cognitive abilities that is associated with aging. Most of this research was directed towards the deterioration of memory functions (1). Up to now, studies have typically been concerned with a group of elderly subjects of about 70 years or older, whose performance was compared with that of younger adults, mostly students. In addition, hardly any attention has been paid to the possibility of brain dysfunction in supposedly normal and healthy volunteers. This approach can have a serious drawback, as old people are more likely to have been exposed to some agent that hampers the optimal functioning of the brain. For these agents the term 'biological life events' (BLE) is proposed here. BLE are factors that are known to damage optimal brain functioning, other than severely impairing conditions such as trauma, psychiatric disease with cognitive disorders, or dementia. As yet, no consensus exists about these factors. Examples of BLE are mild, closed head injuries (2), repeated anaesthesia, or intoxication (3).

The present study investigates the possibility that BLE might interact with aging in its effect on memory. The hypothesis was tested that there is little or no memory decline in successive age groups from 20 to 80 years when no demonstrable BLE has been sustained by any of the volunteers. In addition, it was hypothesized that when one or more BLE can be identified in individuals, their average performance is inferior, and this gap widens between older age groups. This contradicts the prevailing notion that memory impairment is a normal, inevitable concomitant of advancing age (see for instance reference 4).

METHOD
Subjects

Data are presented of 112 subjects, who were assigned to seven distinct age groups with mean ages of 20 to 80 years, centered around whole tens of years (20 ± 2 years, 30 ± 2 years, etc.). Within each group subjects were balanced for sex and level of education. Prior to, as well as during, the actual testing, a very thorough health screening for BLE took place. Subjects had subjectively rated their health by filling in a questionnaire concerning general health and in particular brain functioning (e.g. dementia, severe trauma, closed head injury, intoxication, hypoxia, ischemia).

Alzheimer's Disease: Basic Mechanisms, Diagnosis and Therapeutic Strategies
Edited by K. Iqbal, D. R. C. McLachlan, B. Winblad and H. M. Wisniewski
©1991 John Wiley & Sons Ltd

Applicants who had sustained anything that is known to hamper optimal brain functioning were excluded. Thus, none of the subjects had an a priori likelihood of brain dysfunctioning. During the examination the subjects were interviewed about BLE by an experienced neurologist who, when in doubt, consulted their medical files. The following BLE were regarded as criteria to assign subjects to a separate BLE group, as opposed to a group of subjects of equal size:

1. present or past treatment by a neurologist for epilepsy, migraine, meningitis, encephalitis, etc.
2. present or past treatment for diseases with possible brain impact (e.g. renal dysfunction or hypertension)
3. more than three closed head injuries, or one with amnesia of more than 1 hour
4. undergoing general anaesthesia more than three times, or one time lasting for more than 3 hours
5. medication affecting driving ability or consciousness
6. heavy drinking—i.e. more than 35 glasses per week (for men) or 21 glasses per week (for women)
7. other neurotoxic factors (e.g. chronic exposure to organic solvents)
8. treatment for psychiatric problems within the last 5 years
9. perinatal complications or developmental problems of early childhood.

Having sustained any of these factors sufficed for the subjects to be assigned to the BLE group. Thus, in each age group there were eight subjects who had sustained BLE, and eight subjects who had not. All subjects were paid for their participation in the experiment.

Neuropsychological tests

Experimental evidence presented here concerns several aspects of memory functioning, along with another well-known test (5):

1. visual and auditory short-term memory: block span and digit span
2. speed of memory scanning and sensomotoric processing: a paper-and-pencil information processing task
3. verbal memory consolidation and retrieval: free-recall verbal learning test with testing of delayed recall and recognition
4. speeded reading, color naming and perceptual interference susceptibility: Stroop test.

Procedure

Health screening and testing were part of a standardized procedure which took about two hours. An extensive neurological examination with special focus on pathological and primitive reflexes took place (6). Apart from the tests mentioned above, several other areas of cognitive functioning were studied (7).

RESULTS

Figure 1 depicts the performance on the memory scanning task. Subjects were requested to memorize a set of 1–4 characters. The time needed to cross out 24 target characters on a test sheet with 120 distractor letters is plotted against the number of different targets that have to be memorized. In this vein, speed of cognitive processing relative to the memory load can be assessed. When the target character is the salient '%' sign, the memory load is negligible. Digits still place little load on the memory, as they can easily be discerned from the distractor letters (8).

Every successive age group needed more time to cross out all '%' signs ($F[6,96] = 10.03$, $P < 0.001$), indicating that perceptual and motor processes were slower in all older subjects. Subdivision based on BLE was not statistically significant ($F[1,96] = 2.79$, $P < 0.1$). Crossing out digits was also slower in all elderly subjects ($F[6,96] = 13.68$, $P < 0.001$). Moreover, BLE-affected subjects needed even more time ($F[1,96] = 8.33$, $P < 0.01$). In addition, the effect of memory load was larger in the elderly ($F[6,96] = 3.06$, $P < 0.001$), and in the BLE group ($F[1,96] = 5.10$, $P < 0.01$). When target characters were letters, and therefore the memory load was greatest, this pattern of results was repeated, only more clearly so. The occurrence of BLE and age even appeared to interact significantly with memory load: with increasing memory set and group age the performance was slower, and slower still if BLE had been sustained.

Test performance on the verbal learning test is graphically summarized in Figure 2. A list of 15 monosyllabic words was administered for five successive learning trials

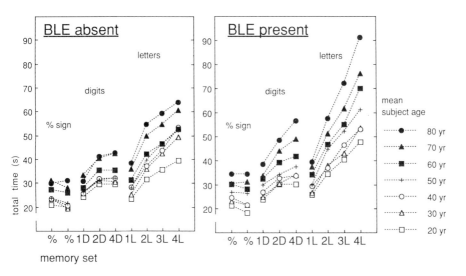

Figure 1. Memory scanning speed. Performance on paper-and-pencil memory scanning task in seven age groups, and in subjects who have (right) or have not (left) sustained biological life events (BLE). The x-axis represents the number and nature of different target items to be remembered and subsequently crossed out: % sign (2 trials), 1/2/4 digits, and 1/2/3/4 letters. Each sheet contains 24 targets among 120 distractors

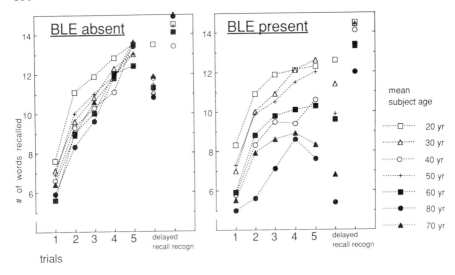

Figure 2. Immediate and delayed repeated free recall of verbal material. Repeated free recall of 15 monosyllabic words, after five repeated presentations in seven age groups, with or without BLE. Not connected by lines are delayed recall and recognition after 20 minutes

at which immediate free recall was tested. Delayed free recall was examined after some 20 minutes, followed by a recognition trial in which the words had to be identified among 15 others.

Subject age significantly affected the performance over all five learning trials ($F[6,98] = 9.87$, $P < 0.001$), as did BLE ($F[1,98] = 24.21$, $P < 0.001$). These effects also interacted ($F[6,98] = 3.16$, $P < 0.01$), indicating that age-related decline of memory performance is further aggravated by BLE. Subjects in the BLE group appeared to profit less from repeated presentation of the words ($F[4,392] = 16.40$, $P < 0.001$). The BLE-unaffected group showed very little age-related decline of the maximal trial score, whereas the elderly BLE subjects did ($F[1,98] = 130.73$, $P < 0.001$), and this effect interacted with age ($F[6,98] = 10.10$, $P < 0.001$), which means that elderly BLE subjects have much less memory capacity than the corresponding BLE-free age groups. Their ability to recall items after 20 minutes was also sharply reduced: $F[1,98] = 155.57$, $P < 0.001$ (main effect); $F[6,98] = 17.93$, $P < 0.001$ (interaction). Delayed recognition was only affected by age if BLE had been sustained: $F[1,98] = 7.13$, $P < 0.01$ (main effect); $F[6,98] = 4.25$, $P < 0.001$ (interaction).

Figure 3 (left) depicts the auditory and visual memory span performance. Analysis showed effects of age group ($F[6,97] = 2.97$, $P < 0.05$) and BLE ($F[1,98] = 4.46$, $P < 0.05$). There was no interaction between these main effects.

Not only memory-related tests showed effects of age or BLE. All factors yielded large and significant main and interaction effects in Stroop performance. Moreover, the susceptibility to perceptual interference proved showed effects of age ($F[6,97] = 11.52$, $P < 0.001$), BLE ($F[1,97] = 22.58$, $P < 0.001$), and a large

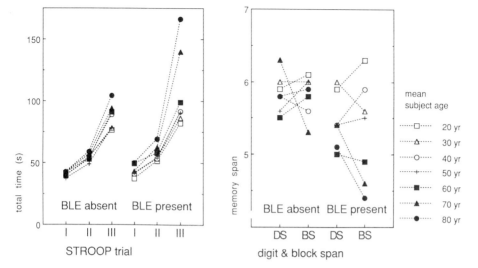

Figure 3. Stroop performance and memory span. Left: performance on three consecutive trials of the Stroop test, involving speeded word reading (I), color naming (II), and colored word reading with language interference. Right: immediate span of auditory and visual memory, as measured by digit span and block span. Both graphs depict seven age groups with either BLE present or absent

interaction effect ($F[6,97] = 4.12$, $P < 0.001$). This suggests that the occurrence of BLE severely aggravates the age-related increase of interference susceptibility.

DISCUSSION

The results show a very small but systematic cross-sectional effect of advancing age in nearly all aspects of memory that were studied in the subjects who were free of biological life events (BLE). The immediate memory span is slightly reduced, the speed and ease of memory search processes (including perceptual and motor processes), verbal memory performance during repeated item presentation, delayed retrieval of newly learned information, and consolidation into memory. An important exception is the maximal performance after repeated presentation. When given time and opportunity to rehearse, healthy elderly people performed almost as well as young subjects. These data are inconsistent with a homogeneous decline in the whole aging population (4). All age-related performance decrements were substantially larger in the BLE age groups. However, this group effect of BLE was already apparent in younger subjects (sometimes as young as 20 or 30 years). The interaction between the effects of age and BLE was not confined to memory functions. Interference susceptibility showed a similar pattern of outcomes, as did several other aspects of cognitive functioning (7). This also implies that health screening is obligatory in experimental research with normal (and therefore supposedly healthy) elderly volunteers.

In elderly BLE-affected subjects, the global cognitive decrement in performance was compatible with the dysfunctions found in incipient dementia. This is best illustrated with the finding of an incomplete memory consolidation, exclusively in the older BLE groups: some of the previously learned items were not even recognized, which is a common finding in dementing patients (1). It is thus proposed that BLE can contribute to the appearance of dementia in the later stages of life. As was stated above, none of the subjects had an a priori likelihood of cognitive dysfunctions due to major brain damage or dementia. The observed group differences are therefore attributable to BLE, instead of any disorder or biological aging. BLE may well be one of the risk factors for incipient dementia. This is consistent with the findings of Amaducci et al (9) who identified a number of risk factors for clinically diagnosed Alzheimer's disease. Presently, a follow-up study is planned with the same subjects. It is hypothesized that the BLE-affected subjects will show more cognitive deterioration and that the incidence of dementia will be highest in the BLE groups.

REFERENCES

1. Jolles J. Prog Brain Res 1986; 70: 15-39.
2. Binder LM. J Clin Exp Neuropsychol 1986; 8: 323-46.
3. Hartman DE. Neuropsychological toxicology: identification and assessment of human neurotoxic syndromes. New York: Pergamon, 1988.
4. Craik FIM. In Birren JE, Schaie KW (eds) Handbook of the psychology of aging. New York: Van Nostrand Reinhold, 1977: 384-420.
5. Lezak MD. Neuropsychological assessment, 2nd edn. New York: Oxford University Press, 1983.
6. Vreeling FW, Houx PJ, Jolles J. In Verhofstad AAJ, Van Bezooijen CFA, Ravid R (eds) From gene to man: gerontological research in The Netherlands. The Hague: Pasmans (in press).
7. Houx PJ, Vreeling FW, Jolles J. In Wurtman MD, Corkin SH, Growdon JH, Ritter-Walker E (eds) Alzheimer's Disease: Advances in Basic Research and Therapies. Proceedings of the Fifth Meeting of the International Study Group on the Pharmacology of Memory Disorders Associated with Aging. Cambridge, MA: Center for Brain Sciences and Metabolism Charitable Trust, 1989: 413-17.
8. Brand AN, Jolles J. Psychol Med 1986; 17: 145-54.
9. Amaducci LA, Fratiglioni L, Rocca WA et al. Neurol 1986; 36: 923-31.

Address for correspondence:

Dr Peter J. Houx,
Department of Neuropsychology and Psychobiology,
University of Limburg, PO Box 616,
NL-6200 MD Maastricht, The Netherlands.
Tel. 31-43888430

44 Prevalence of Dementia in Advanced Age: Preliminary Results from the Kungsholmen Project

L. FRATIGLIONI, M. GRUT, Y. FORSELL, M. GRAFSTRÖM, K. HOLMEN, K. ERIKSSON, P. SANDMAN, P. JOHNSON, L. FORSELL, M. VIITANEN AND B. WINBLAD

Alzheimer's disease (AD) and other dementias are age-related disorders (1). Many studies have been performed on the natural history of AD (occurrence, prognosis, risk factors). Most of them included subjects aged no more than 75–80 years, or a low number of subjects in the oldest age groups.

For this reason a longitudinal study, called the Kungsholmen Project, is being carried out in Stockholm, Sweden. This study includes a population of 2368 individuals aged 75 years and over. The project concerns aging and the related medical and social problems with particular emphasis on dementia.

The preliminary results on the prevalence of dementia from the cross-sectional phase are reported here.

SUBJECTS AND METHODS

The study population consists of all the inhabitants living in a parish of Stockholm in October 1987, born in 1912 or earlier: 2368 subjects, 76% female. People living in institutions were included.

The ascertainment of the cases was done by means of a two-phase study design. During phase I, all subjects were administered mini-mental state examination (MMSE) (2) in order to discriminate between subjects with and without cognitive impairment (screening test). A score of 23/24 was used as cut-off. In phase II, subjects who screened positive (i.e. suspected to be affected by dementia, $MMSE \leq 23$) were extensively evaluated to reach a clinical diagnosis of AD or other dementias. The same procedure was used for a sample of subjects screened negative (suspected not to be affected by dementia, $MMSE \geq 24$). The sample was randomly selected from all the negatives, matched by age and sex with the positives.

The phase II procedure included a complete clinical examination, a social interview, a structured family interview, laboratory tests and neuropsychological tests.

Alzheimer's Disease: Basic Mechanisms, Diagnosis and Therapeutic Strategies
Edited by K. Iqbal, D. R. C. McLachlan, B. Winblad and H. M. Wisniewski
© 1991 John Wiley & Sons Ltd

DSMIII-R (3) diagnostic criteria for dementia and AD were used. The diagnostic process included three steps:

1. A first preliminary diagnosis was put after a common discussion among the physicians (M. G., Y. F., M. V.) who had examined the patient and the nurse who had performed the social and family interview.
2. A second preliminary diagnosis was put independently by an extraneous physician (extraneous regarding the data collection; L. F.).
3. A comparison between preliminary and second diagnoses was performed. The diagnoses in agreement were accepted in the study as final diagnoses. In case of disagreement, the data were re-examined and the final diagnosis was put by a supervisor (B. W.).

Prevalence ratios were calculated at December 1987. The numerator included all the ascertained plus the estimated cases. The estimate was based on two types of inference:

—the number of false negatives in the whole population was estimated from the sample of screened negatives after stratification by age, sex and MMSE;
—the number of missed cases among the drop-outs of the screened positives was estimated from the examined screened positives after stratification by age, sex and MMSE.

The denominator included the whole screened population. Ninety-five percent confidence intervals were calculated based on the normal distribution (4).

PRELIMINARY RESULTS

The distribution by age and sex of the screened population is shown in Table 1 together with the same figures from the drop-outs in phase I. The drop-outs were 22.8% of the study population and were caused by death in 33.5%, refusal in 53.8%, and moving from the parish in 12.7%.

Among the 1827 screened subjects, 380 screened positive (MMSE ≤ 23). Out of them, 314 subjects underwent phase II. A sample of 393 screened negatives was selected and 354 subjects examined. In total the drop-outs in phase II were 105 (13.6%); 73.3% due to refusal, 19.1% to moving and 7.6% to death.

The estimated prevalence of dementia at December 1987 is reported in Table 2. The age-specific ratios presented no difference between sexes and an exponential increase with age.

As regards to the dementia types, 54% was due to AD, 23% to vascular dementia, 11% to other secondary dementias. Uncertain dementias and uncertain types of dementia represented the remaining 12%. The secondary dementias included 13 cases classified as alcoholic dementia because of the positive history of heavy intake of alcohol, 7 as dementia in Parkinson's disease, 3 as mixed vascular and degenerative dementia and 1 as dementia due to chronic subdural hematoma.

Table 1. Distribution by age and sex of the screened population and the drop-outs of phase I

Age at Dec. 1987 (years)	Screened population M	F	Drop-outs of phase I M	F
75-79	195	530	50	132
80-84	157	464	43	136
85-89	59	264	26	101
90-94	24	111	12	36
95+	3	20	0	5
Total	438	1389	131	410

Table 2. Estimated prevalence (P) for dementia at December 1987

Age (years)	Male P (%)	Female P (%)	Total P (%)
75-79	7.2 (3.6-10.8)*	7.7 (5.5-10.0)	7.6 (5.7-9.5)
80-84	19.8 (13.5-26.0)	12.7 (9.7-15.7)	14.5 (11.7-17.3)
85-89	23.7 (12.9-34.6)	26.9 (21.5-32.2)	26.3 (21.5-31.1)
90+	29.6 (12.4-46.8)	38.9 (30.6-47.3)	37.3 (29.8-37.3)
All	15.3 (11.9-18.7)	16.0 (14.1-17.9)	15.8 (14.1-17.5)

*In parentheses 95% confidence interval.

DISCUSSION

Our study has the following main advantages:

1. It is a population-based study, including all the subjects both living at home and in institution.
2. The ascertainment of the cases was done by means of a clinical examination of all the positive subjects in MMSE used as screening test.
3. A sample of screened negatives was clinically examined in order to estimate the number of false negatives at the screening test.
4. The response rate of the population was very high: only 12% of the study population refused to participate in phase I and 10% in phase II.
5. The size of the study population was sufficiently large to give stable prevalence estimates in the age- and sex-specific strata.

The present results are preliminary as studies still are ongoing of the subjects who have migrated in and out the study area in the last five years preceding the onset of the research. Moreover the drop-outs of phase I caused by death and moving need to be evaluated by means of death certificates and/or clinical records in order to ascertain the number of dementia cases. It seems likely that demented subjects have a higher proportion in these two groups when compared with the proportion in the screened population. For this reason we think that our preliminary results are slightly underestimated.

Our results on dementia have the same magnitude of some previously reported data. In particular, Jorm (5) estimated age- and sex-specific prevalence ratios from all the cross-sectional studies performed up to 1985, very close to our data. Recent original data from Italy (6) show similar age-specific prevalence ratios for dementia and AD, but the data are very different as regards to sex distribution and vascular dementia. A possible explanation is that the Italian study has a very low number of cases when sex is added to age in the stratification or different causes of dementia are taken into account. A study from Rochester, USA (7), reported no difference between sexes in dementia and AD prevalence as well as our study.

Our data are in disagreement with the results from the Baltimore longitudinal study (8): it is interesting to note that their figures for AD are completely overlapping our figures for dementia as a whole. Finally our estimated prevalence for dementia seems even lower than the reported data on AD only from East Boston (9).

In conclusion the main results from our study are:

1. The prevalence of dementia is high but not over 12% in the age group 75-84 years and 34% in people aged 85 years and over.
2. There is no difference between male and female as regards the prevalence of dementia and types of dementia.
3. The prevalence of dementia increases exponentially with age, also in advanced ages.
4. AD accounts for 50% and vascular dementia for 25% of the cases.

REFERENCES

1. Henderson AS. Acta Psychiatr Scan 1988; 78: 257-75.
2. Folstein MF, Folstein SE, McHugh PR. J Psychiatr Res 1975; 12: 189-98.
3. American Psychiatric Association. Diagnostic and statistical manual of mental disorders, 3rd edn. Washington, DC: APA, 1987: 97-163.
4. Ahlbom A. Biostatistik för epidemiologer. Lund: Studentlitteratur, 1990: 59-60.
5. Jorm AF, Korten AE, Henderson AS. Acta Psychiatr Scan 1987; 76: 465-79.
6. Rocca WA, Bonaiuto S, Lippi A, Luciani P, Turtu F, Caverzeran F, Amaducci L. Neurology 1990; 40: 626-31.
7. Kokmen E, Beard M, Offord KP, Kurland LT. Neurology 1989; 39: 773-6.
8. Sayetta RB. J Chron Dis 1986; 39: 271-86.
9. Evans AD, Funkenstein HH, Albert MS, Scherr PA, Cook NR, Chown MJ, Hebert LE, Hennekens CH, Taylor JO. JAMA 1989; 262: 2551-6.

Address for correspondence:

Dr L. Fratiglioni,
Stockholm Gerontology Research Center
and Department of Geriatric Medicine,
Karolinksa Institute, S-14186 Huddinge, Sweden

45 Risk Factors in Clinically Diagnosed Alzheimer's Disease: A Case-Control Study in Colombia (South America)

CLAUDIA J. JOYA-PARDO, JUAN L. LONDOÑO, AND
CARLOS A. PARDO

INTRODUCTION

Alzheimer's disease (AD) is the major cause of dementia in elderly individuals (1), and its prevalence has an epidemic proportion in developed countries (2,3). However, the magnitude of dementia and AD in developing countries is unknown due to the absence of descriptive and analytical epidemiological studies. In some Latin American countries, the elderly population has increased significantly due to improvements in life expectancy, which is now greater than 65 years of age (4). In Colombia, life expectancy has increased from 58.5 years (between 1965 and 1970) to 65.4 years (1985), and it is projected to increase to 70.8 years between 1995 and 2000 (5). In addition, projections show that the percentage of the population >60 years of age will grow from 6.0% in 1985 to 6.8% between 1995 and 2000 (5). These demographic trends translate into an increase in the number of patients with neurological diseases associated with aging and AD. As part of an investigation of the characteristics of AD in the Colombian population, a case-control study was conducted to determine the roles of various hypothetical, causative, or contributing factors to AD. We examined whether risk factors studied previously in developed countries (for review, see Rocca et al (3) and Henderson (6) influenced the presence of AD in developing countries or whether additional factors contributed to AD in those countries.

MATERIALS AND METHODS

The present study was conducted on 43 patients with clinical diagnoses of AD and 86 control subjects from an urban population of Medellin, Antioquia, in northwest Colombia. All AD patients (14 male, 29 female) were enrolled in comprehensive, clinical, and epidemiological studies at Facultad Nacional de Salud Pública Universidad de Antioquia and the Neurology Service of the Facultad de Medicina. Patients were identified in nursing homes and in the three major university hospitals: Hospital Universitario 'San Vicente de Paul'; Instituto de Seguros Sociales; and Hospital 'Pablo Tobón Uribe'.

Alzheimer's Disease: Basic Mechanisms, Diagnosis and Therapeutic Strategies
Edited by K. Iqbal, D. R. C. McLachlan, B. Winblad and H. M. Wisniewski
© 1991 John Wiley & Sons Ltd

Each AD patient had a complete clinical and neurological examination as well as laboratory tests and computerized tomographic scans to exclude causes of dementia other than AD (e.g. multi-infarct dementia and dementia secondary to alcoholism, depression, or metabolic disorders). All patients fulfilled criteria for the clinical diagnosis of probable AD (7).

For each AD patient involved in the study, two control subjects were matched for age (± 3 years), sex, and socioeconomic status. Control subjects for cases from university hospitals were randomly selected from nonneurological outpatients and neighbors of the patient. For patients from nursing homes, control subjects were randomly selected from the same institutions. When information was not adequate or complete, patients or controls were excluded. All control subjects had clinical and neurological examinations to exclude cognitive changes or dementia. Information was obtained uniformly from a close family member, with priority to spouses and first-degree relatives. Structured questionnaires and interviews were used to obtain information concerning possible risk factors including: previous history of infectious diseases, including those with high incidence in Colombia (e.g. malaria and tuberculosis); surgical procedures; anesthesia; exposure to toxins and drugs; and familial histories of lymphoproliferative and neurodegenerative disorders. Emphasis was placed on questions referring to: parental age at subject birth; parental siblings; birth order; woman's parity; history of head trauma; chronic ingestion of aluminum-containing antacids; previous thyroid diseases; cigarette smoking; and familial histories of Down's syndrome, mental retardation, or dementia. Personal interviews were conducted by one of the researchers. A matched-paired method and conditional logistical regression model were used for the analysis of data. As a first step, the Mantel-Haenszel procedure was applied for assessing possible confounding variables (8). As a second step, a conditional logistical regression analysis was used for the analysis of data (9). The odds ratio, as an estimate of the relative risk, was calculated, and 95% confidence intervals were obtained for the adjusted relative risk.

RESULTS

The age range in the case group was 52–89 years of age, and the mean age at onset of dementia was 72.5 years. Of the 43 patients, 20 were under the care of geriatric institutions, and 23 were outpatients from university hospitals, living at home. Surrogate respondents interviewed to collect information from the case group included: spouses (6 cases = 14.0%); offspring (19 cases = 44.2%); siblings (9 cases = 20.9%); and kin (9 cases = 20.9%). Demographic characteristics of cases and control subjects under study are shown in Table 1.

At the beginning of the investigation, we conducted an unmatched analysis for all factors included in the questionnaire, and, subsequently, we selected the most relevant risk factors found for the matched analysis. Head trauma, aluminum-containing antacids, and histories of thyroid disease were not significant. Although a significant difference was not observed for a history of Down's syndrome in unmatched analysis (odds ratio = 4.30; $p = 0.183$), this factor was considered for the matched-pair analysis due to its higher frequency among cases (four) than controls (two). A positive

Table 1. Demographic characteristics of subjects

Characteristics	Cases		Controls	
Number	43		86	
Mean age (years)	76.9		76.8	
Men	14		28	
Women	29		58	
Marital status				
single	15	(34.9%)	17	(19.8%)
married	12	(27.9%)	27	(31.4%)
widowed or other	16	(37.2%)	32	(48.8%)
Mean formal education (years)	6.7		7.1	
MMSE score*	12.6		28.0	

*Eight patients were excluded for aphasia and severe demential stage

association for AD, but not significant (odds ratio = 1.5), was achieved for marital status after grouping the 'single' category vs others, and marital status was also considered for the subsequent analysis. The analysis of cigarette smoking showed an increased association (odds ratio = 2.13; $p = 0.10$) when a person smoked > 20 cigarettes per day and was used for the matched analysis.

Family histories of dementia were significantly higher in the AD group than in the control population (odds ratio = 3.46; $p = 0.007$) in the unmatched analysis. Individuals with AD had a total of 15 first-degree relatives and 4 second-degree relatives affected with the disease, and controls reported 6 first-degree relatives, and 9 second-degree relatives. Other selected factors studied for association with AD are listed in Table 2, but statistically significant differences were not observed. The results of the analysis regarding the initial matching on some of the factors are presented in Table 3 and show that only the familial history of dementia and excessive cigarette smoking appeared to be associated with AD.

The final model of conditional logistic regression included variables of familial history of dementia and excessive use of tobacco showing a significant association

Table 2. Means and statistical tests on selected variables

Variables	Cases	Controls	F^a	p^b
Number	43.00	86.00		
Parental siblings	8.23	9.23	1.356	0.123
Birth order	4.67	5.60	1.369	0.122
Mother age/subject birth	27.05	29.00[c]	2.023	0.078
Father age/subject birth	33.32[c]	35.06[c]	0.979	0.169
Parity[d]	3.65	4.62	0.647	0.212
Tobacco use duration (years)	41.66[e]	43.20[f]	0.103	0.377
Suspension tobacco use (years)	2.50[e]	2.41[f]	0.089	0.388

[a]Snedecor's F statistic.
[b]Significance.
[c]In two cases, data not available.
[d]For all women.
[e]Obtained from 26 tobacco users.
[f]Obtained from 44 tobacco users.

Table 3. Results on matched analysis in selected variables

Variables	Odds ratio	95% CL*	Chi^2	Significance (p)
Marital status, single/other	2.00	0.95-4.56	2.65	0.052
Down's syndrome, familial history	4.00	0.83-19.2	1.19	0.096
Aluminum-containing antacids, use of	0.56	0.20-1.60	0.72	0.198
Thyroid disease, history	0.25	0.04-1.71	1.13	0.144
Excessive tobacco use	2.25	0.89-5.68	2.13	0.072
Dementia, family history	3.30	1.52-7.16	7.97	0.002

*Confidence limits.

with AD ($p = 0.004$ and 0.07, respectively). Thus, the regression of these variables accounts for 11.98% of log likelihood. The relative risks in the logistical regression analysis are shown in Table 4.

DISCUSSION

This study, performed on a mestizo population in Colombia, showed a significant association of AD with the presence of a familial history of dementia. This risk factor has been found to be significant in other case-control studies previously performed in developed countries (10–12), suggesting a possible role for genetic factors in the pathogenesis of AD. A family history of Down's syndrome was more frequent in AD cases than controls, but this difference was not significant. This study found that the relative risk of AD increased when the number of cigarettes smoked per day was > 20 and when the familial history of dementia was considered concomitantly in the conditional logistical regression analysis. A similar association was also found by Shalat (13) in a veterans hospital population in the United States. The significance of this possible risk factor in this mestizo population is interesting; until recent years, Colombians smoked dark, nonfiltered cigarettes or 'black' tobacco that contained more nicotine than other refined light cigarettes (14). It is possible that nicotine contained in this type of 'black' tobacco may affect the brain nicotinic receptors, producing neurochemical changes in the cholinergic system. Previously, it has been suggested that chronic and excessive consumption of nicotine may cause desensitizing of nicotinic receptors in the brain (13). This study, as well as previous ones, suggests that risk factors (e.g. head trauma, ingestion of aluminum-containing antacids, or history of thyroid disease) are not associated with AD. Hypothesized risk factors (e.g. parental age at the subject birth, birth order, fertility, and woman's parity)

Table 4. Results on the logistical regression analysis

Independent variable	Coefficient	Relative risk	95% CL*
Dementia, family history	1.0781	2.939	1.319-6.546
Tobacco use excess	0.9324	2.540	0.900-7.171

*Confidence limits.

were not significant. In Colombia, and in many developing countries, one of the characteristics of the family is its large size (mean of parental siblings is 8.23 in AD subjects in this study); this family characteristic does not appear to affect the presence of AD. Typical regional health problems (e.g. malaria and tuberculosis) or other infectious conditions do not appear to be related to AD.

Although considerable effort was made in obtaining precise data, recall bias cannot be excluded in this study, whereas information was obtained from close relatives. However, previous studies have shown this source to be reliable (15). The relatively small size of the sample group might have affected the number of significant associations and may have included some type-II errors.

In conclusion, this study, conducted in a mestizo population in Colombia, showed that a familial history of dementia as well as excessive use of tobacco appear to be the most significant risk factors in the presence of AD, and these risk factors are probably similar in developed as well as developing countries.

Acknowledgments

This work was supported by grants from the Comité Departamental de Cafeteros de Antioquia, Hospital San Vicente de Paul-Universidad de Antioquia and Servicio Seccional de Salud de Antioquia.

REFERENCES

1. Katzman R. Arch Neurol 1976; 33: 217-8.
2. Evans DA, Funkenstein HH, Albert MS, Scherr PA, Cook NR, Chown MJ, Hebert LE, Hennekens CH, Taylor JO. J Am Med Associ 1989; 262: 2551-6.
3. Rocca WA, Amaducci LA, Schoenberg BS. Ann Neurol 1986; 19: 415-24.
4. 1987 Demographic Yearbook (Annuaire démographique). New York, United Nations: 1989.
5. Departmento Administrativo Nacionale de Estadistica, Colombia. Avance de resultados preliminares del censo 1985. Bogota: 1986.
6. Henderson AS. Acta Psychiatr Scand 1988; 78: 257-75.
7. McKhann G, Drachman D, Folstein M, Katzman R, Price D, Stadlan EM. Neurology 1984; 34: 939-44.
8. Mantel N, Haenszel W. J Natl Cancer Inst 1959; 22: 719-48.
9. Breslow NE, Day NE. The analysis of case-control studies, vol. 1. Statistical methods in cancer. Lyon, International Agency for Research on Cancer: 1980.
10. Amaducci LA, Fratiglioni L, Rocca WA, Fieschi C, Livrea P, Pedone D, Bracco L, Lippi A, Gandolfo C, Bino G, Prencipe M, Bonatti ML, Girotti F, Carella F, Tavolato B, Ferla S, Lenzi GL, Carolei A, Gambi A, Grigoletto F, Schoenberg BS. Neurology 1986; 36: 922-31.
11. De Braekeleer M, Cholette A, Mathieu J, Boily C, Robitalle Y, Gauvreau D. Eur Neurol 1989; 29 (suppl): 2-8.
12. Heyman A, Wilkinson WE, Stafford JA, Helms MJ, Sigmon AH, Weinberg T. Ann Neurol 1984; 15: 335-41.
13. Shalat SL, Seltzer B, Pidcock C, Baker EL Jr. Neurology 1987; 37: 1630-3.

14. Restrepo HE, Correa P, Haenszel W, Brinton LA, Franco A. Bull PAHO 1989; 23: 405-13.
15. Kolonel LN, Hirohata T, Nomura AMY. Am J Epidemiol 1977; 106: 476-84.

Address for correspondence:

Dr Carlos A. Pardo,
The Johns Hopkins University School of Medicine,
Neuropathology Laboratory,
600 North Wolfe Street, 509 Pathology Building,
Baltimore, Maryland 21205-2181, USA

46 Risk Factors for Alzheimer's Disease Projected into the 21st Century

ELAINE NEWMAN ROGAN AND
THOMAS M. SULLIVAN

This paper addressed to the risk factors in Alzheimer's disease, concerns: (1) projected population longevity rates in varying societies; (2) availability of mental health facilities within these societies; and (3) the inter-relationship between these two. Our first priority is to identify populations at risk based on age for Alzheimer's disease worldwide as reported by United Nations population projections.

According to the United Nations World Population Prospects—1988 (1), 432 million people in 1985 were over age 60 comprising 9% of the total world population. However, by the year 2000, this number will be 612 million comprising 10% of the world population. Even more significant than these facts by 2025 the elderly population will be about 15% of the total world population.

Table 1. Percentage increase in population age 60 and over by world region* between 1990 and 2025

	1990	2025	% increase
West, Central & East Africa	4.63	7.69	66.1
Southern Africa	5.30	9.30	75.4
Central America	5.61	10.25	82.7
Central Asia	6.00	11.20	86.6
North Africa/Middle East	6.03	10.67	76.9
Southeast Asia/South Pacific	6.12	13.54	121.2
South Asia	6.15	11.47	86.5
Western South America	6.34	11.14	75.7
Eastern South America	7.82	12.60	61.1
Caribbean	9.30	16.88	81.5
East Asia	11.45	23.75	107.3
Australia/New Zealand	15.20	23.65	55.6
Southern Europe	15.80	24.56	55.4
North America	16.30	27.20	66.9
Eastern Europe	16.65	22.80	36.9
United Kingdom	17.30	22.95	32.7
Western Europe	19.26	29.66	53.9
Northern Europe	19.84	29.60	49.4

*World regions named above as defined by Rogan, Dunham and Sullivan in 1973 which closely approximates the current definition of world regions as defined by the United Nations.

Alzheimer's Disease: Basic Mechanisms, Diagnosis and Therapeutic Strategies
Edited by K. Iqbal, D. R. C. McLachlan, B. Winblad and H. M. Wisniewski
© 1991 John Wiley & Sons Ltd

The trends of growth among the elderly population differ significantly among world regions as described in Table 1 (3). The greater percentage increase in those age 60 and over is projected to occur in those world regions defined by the UN as 'less developed'. Using 'fertility level' criteria (2), the regions defined by the United Nations as 'less developed' include all regions of Africa, Asia (excluding Japan), Latin America, and Oceania (excluding Australia and New Zealand). The 'more developed' regions of the world include Europe, USSR, North America, Japan, Australia and New Zealand.

Data describing the population over 60 emphasize the increasing risk of becoming an Alzheimer's disease patient. A recent study shows 10% of the population worldwide over 65 have Alzheimer's disease (4). Statistics increase to 50% for those over 85 which identify a tremendous health problem among the aging. Moreover, Alzheimer's disease not only attacks the person but also their families suffer as well because of the everyday stress of providing physical and financial care which demand support systems for the caretakers.

The need for services for Alzheimer's disease patients and their families is overwhelming. To assess the current state and projected adequacies of facilities, a recent survey by world region was conducted. In this survey 685 psychiatrists practicing in 100 countries responded to two questions in a mailed questionnaire: (A) 'In your opinion, do your present psychiatric facilities meet the mental health needs of your country?' (B) 'In your country, do the plans for future expansion include any of the following: (1) Expansion of custodial mental hospitals, (2) Incorporation of psychiatric units in general hospitals, (3) Outpatient services . . . Adults, (4) Outpatient services . . . Children, (5) Rehabilitation services, (6) Day hospitals, (7) Night hospitals, (8) Aftercare service, (9) Development of community mental health centers with designated catchment areas and (10) Social clubs for ex-mental patients.'

Table 2. Do your present psychiatric facilities meet the mental health needs of your country?

Region	Yes	No	Uncertain	% positive response
Eastern Europe	20	14	2	58
East Asia	9	24	5	27
North Africa/Middle East	7	19	3	26
United Kingdom	12	38	4	24
Northern Europe	15	48	9	23
Western Europe	9	32	3	21
Caribbean	3	10	2	21
Central Asia	2	10	2	16
North America	24	124	10	16
Australia/New Zealand	5	28	7	15
Southeast Asia/South Pacific	2	17	3	10
Southern Europe	3	28	1	9
West, Central and East Africa	2	22	0	8
Western South America	1	13	1	6
Eastern South America	1	23	2	4
Central America	1	23	0	4
South Asia	1	38	0	2
Southern Africa	0	11	0	0
Total	117	522	54	18

Table 3. Regional ranking of plans for future expansion

	REGIONS																		Rank
	1	2	3	4	5	6	7	8	9	10	11	12	13	14	15	16	17	18	
Custodial mental hospitals	6	8	7	5	7	9	8	10	7	8	7	7	10	10	10	10	10	8	9
Psychiatric units in general hospitals	3	5	1	4	2	1	2	8	4	1	1	5	7	3	7	9	6	6	4
Outpatient services — adult	1	1	2	1	1	2	1	1	1	3	3	1	1	6	1	5	3	1	1
Outpatient services — children	2	2	3	2	3	2	5	4	3	4	6	2	3	2	4	3	4	2	2
Rehabilitation services	5	4	5	3	4	4	3	3	6	7	5	6	4	1	2	4	2	5	3
Day hospitals	9	7	8	6	6	5	7	5	2	5	2	8	5	4	6	2	1	3	6
Night hospitals	10	10	10	9	9	7	9	9	8	2	9	9	9	9	5	6	8	9	8
Aftercare services	4	3	4	7	5	6	4	2	9	9	4	3	2	5	3	1	5	3	5
Community mental health centers	8	6	6	8	8	8	6	7	5	6	8	4	6	8	9	8	7	7	7
Social clubs for ex-mental patients	7	9	9	10	10	10	10	6	10	10	10	10	8	7	8	7	9	10	10

REGION

1 – Southern Africa
2 – West, Central and East Africa
3 – North Africa/Middle East
4 – Central Asia
5 – South Asia
6 – East Asia
7 – Southeast Asia/South Pacific
8 – Australia/New Zealand
9 – Eastern South America

10 – Western South America
11 – Caribbean
12 – Central America
13 – North America
14 – United Kingdom
15 – Western Europe
16 – Northern Europe
17 – Eastern Europe
18 – Southern Europe

NOTE: 1 = highest rank

Responses were rather evenly distributed between the 'less developed' and the 'more developed' world regions. Referring to question (A) concerning the adequacy of psychiatric facilities; 117 said 'yes', 522 answered 'no', 44 were 'uncertain' and 2 did not respond (Table 2). To question (B), plans for future mental health services (Table 3), the 'less developed' world regions are more likely to plan for hospital services while the 'more developed' world regions gave first priority to outpatient services.

In summary, we are concerned with three risk factors: (1) the increased risk of becoming an Alzheimer's disease patient with the rapid aging of the world population, (2) the risk of not having available facilities for treatment as indicated in a worldwide survey and (3) the risk of not having available support services for the caretakers as is well documented in the literature. In addressing these risks it is crucial that we note that those countries who are most likely to have the greatest percentage increase in persons age 60 or older with enhanced vulnerability to the risk of Alzheimer's disease, are the least likely to have the necessary psychiatric facilities.

This information should shed light in planning for the needs for Alzheimer's disease facilities into the 21st century worldwide, particularly in developing countries.

REFERENCES

1. World Population Prospects 1988 (United Nations publication, Sales No 88. XIII.7).
2. World Population Prospects as Assessed in 1963 (United Nations publication, Sales No. 66. XIII.2).
3. Rogan EN, Dunham HW, Sullivan TM. A worldwide transcultural survey of diagnostic, treatment and etiological approaches in schizophrenia, Transcultural Psychiatric Research Review 1973; 10: 107–110.
4. Alzheimer's Medicines in Development. Presented by the Pharmaceutical Manufacturers Association and the Alzheimer's Association, 16 Medicine in Testing, 11/89.

Address for correspondence:

Dr Elaine Newman Rogan,
Department of Psychiatry,
Wayne State University School of Medicine,
Detroit, Michigan 48210, USA

Part VII

ENVIRONMENTAL FACTORS

47 Amyotrophic Lateral Sclerosis-Parkinsonism Dementia Complex of Guam as a Model of Alzheimer's Disease

DANIEL P. PERL, JOHN C. STEELE, ARTHUR LOERZEL
AND LEONARD T. KURLAND

The Marianas are a chain of fifteen islands of volcanic origin, eight of which are inhabited. Guam lies at the southernmost end of this chain and is the largest island in the North Pacific Ocean between Hawaii and the Philippines and between Japan and New Guinea. Guam, with an area of approximately 225 square miles, has a total civilian population of 100 000 (approximately 50 000 indigenous 'Chamorros', 30 000 Filipinos, and 20 000 other ethnicities). In the decade following the end of World War II, an extremely high prevalence of amyotrophic lateral sclerosis (ALS) and a form of parkinsonism associated with dementia (parkinsonism dementia complex or PDC) was identified among the Chamorro indigenes of the island of Guam and the adjacent island of Rota (1-3). This tragic epidemic continues to plague the island and has stimulated, over the past 35 years, extensive research studies into the source and nature of this unusual geographic isolate of neurodegenerative disease.

In the initial years, the classic studies of Hirano and colleagues characterized most of the neuropathologic features encountered in the brains and spinal cords of affected Guamanians (2-4). Because of the way Guamanian ALS and parkinsonism dementia complex were originally described they have come to be considered by many as two distinct and separate entities. The cases of amyotrophic lateral sclerosis have been considered to show all of the typical clinical features of the disease as seen elsewhere in the world (1,5). Accordingly, much of the research effort involved a search for etiologic factors which might have relevance to ALS, as seen elsewhere in the world. However, clinical and neuropathologic studies have repeatedly shown that pure cases of amyotrophic lateral sclerosis or parkinsonism dementia complex are relatively rare (6-8). The majority of cases encountered on the island represent a mixture of both entitites with either amyotrophic or parkinsonian features predominating.

Initially, research approaches continued to emphasize the use of the Guam epidemic as a model of amyotrophic lateral sclerosis and generally failed to consider other features of what is a complex spectrum of clinical and neuropathologic involvement

Alzheimer's Disease: Basic Mechanisms, Diagnosis and Therapeutic Strategies
Edited by K. Iqbal, D. R. C. McLachlan, B. Winblad and H. M. Wisniewski

demonstrating many features in common with other forms of neurodegenerative disease. Specifically, as reviewed here, most of the characteristic neuropathologic features of ALS/PDC of Guam are also encountered in cases of Alzheimer's disease seen elsewhere in the world.

The following represents a list of the principal neuropathologic features of Alzheimer's disease:

1. neurofibrillary tangles
2. senile or neuritic plaques
3. granulovacuolar degeneration (of Simchowitz)
4. Hirano bodies
5. cell loss in the basal forebrain
6. congophilic angiopathy.

As we will discuss, with the exception of extracellular amyloid deposition, all of these neuropathologic features are encountered in cases of Guam ALS/parkinsonism dementia complex. Indeed, in this setting they are generally present in a more severe degree than is usually observed in cases of Alzheimer's disease elsewhere in the world. It is our belief that the neurodegenerative diseases encountered among the natives of Guam can serve as an important opportunity for the study of many aspects of Alzheimer's disease.

NEUROPATHOLOGIC FEATURES ENCOUNTERED IN BOTH ALZHEIMER'S DISEASE *AND* ALS/PDC OF GUAM

Neurofibrillary tangle

The neurofibrillary tangle and the senile or neuritic plaque represent the two cardinal neuropathologic features of Alzheimer's disease. Neurofibrillary tangles were originally noted by Malamud in cases of Guam parkinsonism dementia complex (3). Subsequently, neurofibrillary tangles were also identified in Guamanian patients with predominantly ALS symptomatology (4,9,10). Ultrastructurally and immunohisto-chemically, the neurofibrillary tangles of Guam ALS/PDC are identical to those of Alzheimer's disease (11,12). The extent of involvement by neurofibrillary tangles in the Guam cases is particularly severe in the H1 region of the hippocampus, inferior aspects of the temporal lobes and the amygdala. Hirano and co-workers (9) mapped out the distribution of neurofibrillary tangles in cases of Guam ALS and noted that although the degree of involvement was more severe, there was a significant overlap in the distribution of neurofibrillary tangles in cases of Alzheimer's disease seen in the continental United States. It is of interest to note that cases of Guam ALS may have extensive involvement with neurofibrillary tangles in several limbic structures and yet be apparently free of overt cognitive impairment (13).

Granulovacuolar degeneration

In 1911, granulovacuolar degeneration was first described by Simchowitz in cases of Alzheimer's disease (14). This neuronal alteration consists of multiple cytoplasmic vacuoles each containing a dense basophilic granule. Granulovacuolar degeneration occurs almost exclusively in the border zone between the H1 and H2 regions of the Ammon's horn of the hippocampus. Although classically described in the brains of Alzheimer's disease patients, a lesser extent of granulovacuolar degeneration is also encountered in nondemented elderly controls (15,16). Studies have shown a high correlation of the presence of prominent granulovacuolar degeneration in the posterior portion of the hippocampus and the diagnosis of Alzheimer's disease (15,16). Cases of Guam ALS/PDC also show a severe degree of posterior hippocampal granulovacuolar degeneration (17). In the Guam-derived cases the number of neurons involved by granulovacuolar degeneration is much greater than is typically seen in US mainland Alzheimer's disease cases and the degree of involvement of individual affected neurons is also greater.

Hirano body

The discovery of the Hirano body represents a particularly illustrative example of the concept that Guam ALS/PDC represents an important opportunity to explore aspects of Alzheimer's disease. Beginning in 1961, Hirano conducted his pioneering clinico-pathologic studies on Guam. While evaluating the brains of a number of autopsied cases of Guam Chamorro ALS/PDC, Hirano noticed the presence of large numbers of eosinophilic rod-shaped bodies immediately adjacent to the pyramidal neurons of the hippocampus. In 1966, he published the first morphologic description of these eosinophilic bodies which have now come to be referred to as Hirano bodies (18). The eosinophilic inclusion bodies were initially considered to be specific for the Guam disorders. However, following his return to the mainland United States, Hirano recognized that identical eosinophilic inclusion bodies were also encountered in the hippocampus of some cases of Alzheimer's disease and Pick's disease (17). When present, their numbers were much smaller than he had become accustomed to seeing in the brains of ALS/PDC patients on Guam.

It is clear that several generations of neuropathologists had failed to recognize these rather large inclusion bodies in cases of Alzheimer's disease until they were first identified in such large numbers in ALS/PDC. Ultimately, rare examples of Hirano bodies were identified in the hippocampus of elderly nondemented controls in the continental United States and in middle-aged adults on Guam (17). The exaggerated form of this neuropathologic lesion was obvious in the Guam-derived specimens which led to the recognition of the more subtle form in cases of Alzheimer's disease and finally in association with normal aging.

Cell loss in nucleus basalis of Meynert

Cell loss in the nucleus basalis of Meynert of the basal forebrain represents an important finding in Alzheimer's disease patients (19). It has been proposed that the neocortical deficits encountered in association with Alzheimer's disease are the result of loss of cholinergic input arising from this nucleus (20). The specificity of this loss for Alzheimer's disease has been questioned with identification of comparable cell losses in cases of idiopathic Parkinson's disease (21). Cell loss in the basal forebrain is seen in cases of Guam ALS/PDC and typically this nucleus is much more severely affected than one commonly finds in cases of Alzheimer's disease (22,23). Unfortunately, no systematic studies of neurotransmitter biochemistry have been reported on Guam. This is of particular interest since cases with predominantly an ALS clinical pattern appear to retain cognitive function.

NEUROPATHOLOGIC FEATURES ENCOUNTERED IN ALZHEIMER'S DISEASE AND CHARACTERISTICALLY *ABSENT* IN ALS/PDC OF GUAM

The two principal features associated with Alzheimer's disease which have remained conspicuously absent in cases of ALS/PDC of Guam relate to the deposition of extracellular amyloid. These are senile plaque formation and congophilic angiopathy. Indeed, as will be pointed out, the Chamorros of Guam appear particularly resistant to the development of extracellular amyloid accumulations in the brain, both in the setting of ALS/PDC and in neurologically intact, normal, elderly Chamorros.

Senile plaques

Acceptance of the diseases on Guam as a model of age-related dementing disorders has met with resistance since, as originally described, the cases of Guam ALS and parkinsonism dementia complex were free of evidence of senile and neuritic plaques, despite the presence of large number of neurofibrillary tangles. Indeed, in the early classic neuropathologic descriptions, mention was repeatedly made of the absence of senile plaques in the Guam cases (3,9,10). The brain specimens from Guam have represented an important example that patients may have large numbers of neurofibrillary tangles, presumably acquired over a relatively long disease course, in the absence of any accompanying senile or neuritic plaques.

More recently, we have identified two Chamorro cases with typical Guamanian ALS/PDC (one with predominantly amyotrophic symptoms, the other manifesting parkinsonian features) who, at autopsy, demonstrated extensive widespread amyloid plaques in the neocortex and hippocampus. The vast majority of these plaques had the appearance of 'primitive' plaques but a small number were encountered with well-formed amyloid cores. Neuritic pathology was rarely encountered in the periphery of the plaques of these cases. The plaques stained with a monoclonal antibody raised to a synthetic peptide within the β-peptide sequence. The two patients at death were aged 64 and 67 years. We feel that it is highly unlikely that they represent either age-related changes or superimposed Alzheimer's disease.

The uniqueness of these two individuals is further emphasized by reviewing a neuropathologic study conducted on the brains of neurologically intact (and presumably nondemented) Guamanian subjects, dying of unrelated causes, who were examined as medical examiner's cases. This study reported neuropathologic findings on Guamanians who died at a wide range of ages, including several who were in their 70s and 80s. Surprisingly, the elderly subjects failed to show the presence of neuritic plaques in most elderly Chamorros (24). This observation, embedded in a long article regarding neurofibrillary tangle formation, is worth considering by itself. Based on experience in mainland US derived autopsy series, one would expect most patients of this age to display some degree of senile plaque formation on the basis of 'normal aging' alone. Surveys of the prevalence of senile plaques among normal non-Guamanian elderly individuals repeatedly show a significant percentage with some degree of plaque formation (25,26).

Is it possible that the Guamanian Chamorro is not only extremely prone to neurofibrillary tangle formation and accompanying neurodegenerative disease but is also somehow protected from the development of neuritic plaques? The nature of this apparent lack of extracellular amyloid deposition or neuritic pathology in the face of extensive neuronal pathology remains an important issue requiring further exploration. Furthermore, observations of the aging native Guamanian suggest that such changes are *not* necessarily inherent in the aging process.

Congophilic angiopathy

Little attention has been paid to the incidence and distribution of amyloid deposits in the cerebral cortical and leptomeningeal blood vessels of Guam brains. To date, most of the cases described in the literature have been of a relatively young age, although a few older patients have been examined. More recently, the age of onset and age at death of affected Guamanians has been rising and currently it is not uncommon to see ALS/PDC patients dying in their 60s and even 70s (a very rare occurrence in previous decades). We are not aware of any description or discussion of vascular amyloid involvement in any of the previous literature on the disease. It has been our observation that Guam ALS/PDC patients typically are free of vascular amyloid deposits, even at advanced age. The few cases with senile plaque formation do show mild congophilic angiopathy but most cases are free of any vascular involvement, despite relatively advanced age.

We recently had an opportunity to examine at autopsy two PDC patients who died at age 75 years. Despite extensive cerebral cortical sectioning and staining with thioflavine S, Congo red and β-peptide immunohistochemistry, no evidence of vascular amyloid deposits were identified. In our experience in a mainland US derived autopsy population, this is most unusual at this age, even in individuals without accompanying age-related neurofibrillary tangles and senile plaques. Obviously further investigation will be needed to substantiate our impression that the degree of vascular amyloid deposition is strikingly less than one normally encounters among elderly subjects (whether normal elderly or certainly those with Alzheimer's disease).

SUMMARY

As we have pointed out, although Guam ALS/PDC has long served as a model for the study of etiologic and pathogenetic factors involved in amyotrophic lateral sclerosis, the neurodegenerative disorder of the native Guamanian also shares much in common with Alzheimer's disease (see Table 1). In particular, the cellular pathology associated with Alzheimer's disease is well represented in the Guam cases

Table 1. Extent of neuropathologic involvement of various features of Alzheimer's disease in AD and Guam ALS/PDC

Neuropathologic feature	Alzheimer's disease	Guam ALS/PDC
Cortical atrophy and ventriculomegaly	1+ to 4+	3+ to 4+
Neurofibrillary tangles	1+ to 3+	3+ to 4+
Granulovacuolar degeneration	1+ to 2+	3+ to 4+
Hirano bodies	1+ to 2+	3+ to 4+
Cell loss in basal forebrain	1+ to 3+	3+ to 4+
Senile plaques	1+ to 4+	0 (1+ to 2+ rarely)
Congophilic angiopathy	2+ to 4+	0 (1+ rarely)

0, none; 1+, mild involvement; 2+, moderate involvement; 3+, severe involvement; 4+, very severe involvement.

and even appears to show an exaggerated degree of involvement. Accordingly, alterations which are obvious in the central nervous system of Guamanian patients may be of a subtler quality in cases of Alzheimer's disease or in normal elderly subjects.

The major difference between Guam ALS/PDC and Alzheimer's disease regards the lack of evidence of extracellular deposition of β-amyloid in Chamorros, an observation which needs further confirmation. If this condition remains true then we believe that it has important implications for our understanding of the role of amyloid in the dementing disorders and in normal aging.

Finally, one must consider the implications of the overlaps (and disparities) in the neuropathologic features of Guam ALS/PDC and Alzheimer's disease to our understanding of etiologic mechanisms. Extensive epidemiologic studies have repeatedly pointed to the importance of local environmental factors rather than genetic predisposition as the underlying cause(s) of this remarkable constellation of clinical and pathologic neurodegenerative phenomena seen on Guam (27,28). Gajdusek has written with regard to Guam ALS, 'Discovery of its cause and pathogenesis in these intensely affected populations will surely contribute to a better understanding of the disease [ALS] elsewhere' (29). We would extend that approach and suggest that the remarkable tendency of the Chamorros living on Guam to develop large numbers of neurofibrillary tangles, Hirano bodies, granulovacuolar degeneration and cell loss in the nucleus basalis of Meynert represents a similar opportunity for Alzheimer's disease. If the local environment on Guam can induce so many aspects of the neuropathologic lesions of Alzheimer's disease, then we argue that clues regarding similar potential environmental factors related to Alzheimer's disease pathogenesis might be actively pursued in the context of the Chamorros of Guam. In the same way that the high-risk pedigrees of familial Alzheimer's disease are particularly informative on relevant genetic factors, we consider the high-risk villages of southern Guam to represent unique opportunities to identify environmental factors of relevance not only to Guam ALS/PDC but also to Alzheimer's disease as well.

Acknowledgments

The authors wish to thank Dr Douglas Hanks, US Naval Hospital, Agana, Guam for providing postmortem material. We also thank Gina Georgescu, Isadora Quarles and Essie Smith for technical and secretarial assistance. Supported, in part, by grants AG-05138, AG-08802 and ES-00928 from the National Institutes of Health.

REFERENCES

1. Kurland LT, Mulder DW. Neurology 1954; 4: 355-78.
2. Hirano A, Kurland LT et al. Brain 1961; 84: 717-24.
3. Hirano A, Malamud N et al. Brain 1961; 84: 642-79.
4. Malamud N, Hirano H et al. Neurology 1961; 5: 401-14.
5. Bobowick AR, Brody JA. N Engl J Med 1973; 288: 1047-55.
6. Elizan TS, Hirano A et al. Arch Neurol 1966; 14: 356-68.
7. Hirano A, Malamud N et al. Arch Neurol 1966; 15: 35-51.
8. Rogers-Johnson P, Garruto RM et al. Neurology 1985; 36: 7-13.
9. Hirano A, Arumugasamy N et al. Neurology 1967; 16: 357-63.
10. Hirano A, Malamud N et al. Arch Neurol 1966; 15: 35-51.
11. Shankar SK, Yanagihara R et al. Ann Neurol 1989; 25: 146-51.
12. Wisniewski H, Terry RD et al. J Neuropath Exp Neurol 1970; 29: 163-76.
13. Personal observation (DPP, JCS); unfortunately this observation has not been confirmed by formal cognitive testing. Although in the late stages of the disease these patients are semiparalyzed, we continue to be amazed, despite extensive neurofibrillary tangle formation, how well they are able to communicate with their families and are able to follow complex commands.
14. Simchowitz T. Histol Histopath Arb Grosshirn 1911; 4: 267-444.
15. Tomlinson BE, Kitchener DJ. J Pathol 1972; 106: 165-85.
16. Ball MJ, Juttall K. Neuropath Appl Neurobiol 1981; 7: 13-20.
17. Hirano A, Dembitzer HM et al. J Neuropath Exp Neurol 1968; 27: 167-82.
18. Hirano A. Amytrophic lateral sclerosis: a reappraisal. In Gajdusek DC, Gibbs CJ Jr, Alpers M (eds) Slow latent and temperate virus infections, NINDB Monograph No. 2. Washington, DC: US Gov Printing Office, 1965: 13-22.
19. Whitehouse PJ, Price DL et al. Science 1982; 215: 1237-9.
20. Coyle JT, Price DL et al. Science 1983; 219: 1184-90.
21. Whitehouse PJ, Hedreen JC et al. Ann Neurol 1983; 13: 243-8.
22. Nakano I, Hirano A. Ann Neurol 1982; 13: 87-91.
23. Masullo C, Pocchiari M et al. Neuropath Appl Neurobiol 1989; 15: 193-206.
24. Anderson FH, Richardson EP et al. Brain 1979; 102: 65-77.
25. Tomlinson BE, Blessed G et al. J Neurol Sci 1968; 7: 331-56.
26. Ogomori K, Kitamoto T et al. Am J Pathol 1989; 134: 243-53.
27. Garruto RM, Yase Y. Trends Neurosci 1986; 9: 368-374.
28. Kurland LT. Trends Neurosci 1988; 11: 51-4.
29. Gajdusek DC. Adv Neurol 1982; 36: 363-93.

Address for correspondence:

Dr Daniel P. Perl,
Neuropathology Division,
Mount Sinai Medical Center,
New York, NY 10029, USA

48 Aluminium in the Causation of Alzheimer's Disease: Population-Based Studies in England and Wales

C. N. MARTYN AND J. CANDY

Aluminium has been detected in the cores of senile plaques and in neurofibrillary tangle-bearing neurones in the brains of patients with Alzheimer's disease (1,2). These observations suggest that exposure to aluminium may be important in the causation of Alzheimer's disease. Epidemiological methods provide a way of testing this hypothesis. This chapter outlines two population-based studies that were designed to investigate the relation between exposure to environmental sources of aluminium and risk of developing Alzheimer's disease. The first of these has already been described in detail elsewhere (3).

GEOGRAPHICAL RELATION BETWEEN ALZHEIMER'S DISEASE AND ALUMINIUM IN DRINKING WATER

Aluminium is found widely in the environment and it is estimated that British adults ingest several mg each day from food and water. Little is known about absorption of different aluminium-containing compounds from the gastrointestinal tract but much of the aluminium present in the diet is in highly insoluble form and is probably largely unabsorbed. In many parts of England and Wales aluminium sulphate is used as a coagulant in the treatment of water before it goes into supply. Aluminium coagulation effectively removes suspended particulate matter and humic acids rendering the water colourless and reducing the dose of chlorine required to achieve satisfactory microbiological standards. Low concentrations of aluminium, up to 200–300 μg/l, may pass into supply following such treatment. As a proportion of total daily intake, the contribution of aluminium from this source is small. However, aluminium in drinking water is largely uncomplexed and it is possible that it makes a disproportionate contribution to the total amount of aluminium absorbed.

A survey was conducted in 88 county districts within England and Wales. Details of residual aluminium concentrations in all important water sources supplying these districts over the previous decade were made available to us by the local water authorities. From these data mean aluminium concentrations were calculated. The incidence of Alzheimer's disease, other causes of dementia and epilepsy in people

Alzheimer's Disease: Basic Mechanisms, Diagnosis and Therapeutic Strategies
Edited by K. Iqbal, D. R. C. McLachlan, B. Winblad and H. M. Wisniewski
©1991 John Wiley & Sons Ltd

Table 1. Relative risks (95% CI) of Alzheimer's disease, dementia from other causes, and epilepsy in patients aged 40-69 years in county districts grouped according to water aluminium concentration (risks adjusted for distance from CT scanning unit and CT scanning rate). Reproduced by kind permission of The Lancet

Aluminium concentration (mg/l)	Probable Alzheimer's disease $n=445$	Possible Alzheimer's disease $n=221$	Other causes of dementia $n=519$	Epilepsy $n=2920$
0-0.01	1	1	1	1
0.02-0.04	1.5 (1.0-2.2)	1.1 (0.7-1.8)	1.2 (0.9-1.7)	0.9 (0.8-1.1)
0.05-0.07	1.4 (1.0-1.9)	1.1 (0.7-1.7)	1.1 (0.8-1.4)	0.9 (0.8-1.0)
0.08-0.11	1.3 (0.9-2.0)	0.8 (0.5-1.4)	1.0 (0.7-1.4)	0.9 (0.8-1.1)
>0.11	1.5 (1.1-2.2)	1.2 (0.7-1.9)	1.2 (0.8-1.6)	0.9 (0.8-1.1)

aged 40-69 years was estimated from the records of neurological centres serving the local population of these districts. Rates of disease for each diagnosis were directly age-standardised to the 40-69-year-old population of England and Wales of 1983.

Concentrations of aluminium in the water supply in these districts varied between 0 and 200 µg/l. For the purposes of analysis estimates of mean aluminium concentration were divided into five groups. The first group contained county districts with concentrations of 10 µg/l or less. None of these districts had used aluminium coagulation in treatment processes during the previous 10 years and aluminium in their waters was usually undetectable. The other four groups were divided so that they contained approximately equal numbers of people at risk.

The relation between aluminium and rates of disease in the different diagnostic categories is summarised in Tables 1 and 2. Rates of each disease in districts where concentrations of aluminium in water were less than 10 µg/l have been taken as a baseline. Rates of disease in the other four groupings of districts have been expressed as a risk relative to this baseline.

A positive association between diagnostic rates of Alzheimer's disease and the average residual aluminium concentrations present in drinking water supplies was present. The relationship stands out more clearly when only those under the age of 65 years are considered (Table 2). This probably reflects a more aggressive policy

Table 2. Relative risks (95% CI) of Alzheimer's disease, dementia from other causes, and epilepsy in patients aged 40-64 years (risks adjusted for distance from CT scanning unit and CT scanning rate). Reproduced by kind permission of The Lancet

Aluminium concentration (mg/l)	Probable Alzheimer's disease $n=307$	Possible Alzheimer's disease $n=153$	Other causes of dementia $n=372$	Epilepsy $n=2461$
0-0.01	1	1	1	1
0.02-0.04	1.4 (1.0-2.2)	0.9 (0.5-1.5)	1.2 (0.8-1.7)	1.0 (0.8-1.1)
0.05-0.07	1.4 (1.0-2.2)	1.1 (0.7-1.8)	1.1 (0.8-1.6)	0.9 (0.8-1.1)
0.08-0.11	1.6 (1.0-2.5)	0.6 (0.3-1.2)	1.2 (0.8-1.8)	1.0 (0.9-1.2)
>0.11	1.7 (1.1-2.7)	0.9 (0.5-1.6)	1.2 (0.8-1.8)	1.0 (0.8-1.1)

Table 3. Numbers of subjects ($n = 149$, age range 70-98 years) with senile plaques present in the temporal cortex. Subjects are grouped according to bone aluminium concentration

Bone aluminium group	Plaques	
	None	Any
1 (lowest)	15	18
2	9	20
3	10	16
4	13	18
5 (highest)	11	19
Total	58	91

in the investigation of younger demented patients, a greater likelihood of younger patients receiving a CT scan and therefore more complete case ascertainment by the methods used in this study. No relation between diagnostic rates of non-Alzheimer dementia or late-onset epilepsy and water aluminium concentrations was found.

Although the results of this study suggest a causal relation between aluminium and Alzheimer's disease, they should be interpreted with care. All epidemiological surveys are vulnerable to confounding and it is possible that the relation observed here is due to the operation of some unknown confounding variable. Confirmation will require replication of these results using a different methodological approach in a different population. We are currently carrying out a case-control study in which exposure to aluminium is assessed retrospectively in cases of presenile Alzheimer's disease and in controls in order to address this need.

BONE CONTENT OF ALUMINIUM AND PREVALENCE OF PATHOLOGICAL FEATURES OF ALZHEIMER'S DISEASE

A straightforward prediction from the hypothesis linking aluminium to Alzheimer's disease is that individuals exposed to larger amounts of aluminium will be at higher risk of developing the disease. We carried out a study to examine the relation between

Table 4. Numbers of subjects ($n = 157$, age range 70-98 years) with neurofibrillary tangles present in the temporal cortex. Subjects are grouped according to bone aluminium concentration

Bone aluminium group	Tangles	
	None	Any
1 (lowest)	28	8
2	28	3
3	21	6
4	26	6
5 (highest)	27	4
Total	130	27

bone aluminium concentration (as an indicator of long-term exposure to aluminium) and the presence of histopathological features of Alzheimer's disease.

Consecutive autopsies of patients over the age of 70 years from five general hospitals within England and Wales provided specimens of bone and cerebral cortex. Bone was taken from the iliac crest and its aluminium content measured by flameless atomic absorption spectrometry. Histopathological features of Alzheimer's disease were identified and quantified in silver-stained sections from blocks of temporal cortex. The results of this work are summarised in Tables 3 and 4. No relation between the presence of senile plaques or neurofibrillary tangle-bearing neurones and concentration of aluminium in bone is apparent. A systematic analysis of these data, including the use of multivariate techniques, failed to identify subgroups of patients in whom such a relation was present. No tendency for aluminium concentration of bone to increase with increasing age was found, although, at any age, bone aluminium concentration was higher in women than it was in men. Nor was there a clear relation between the prevalence of senile plaques or neurofibrillary tangles and the age of the patient at death.

Although estimates of bone aluminium concentrations have been used extensively in the investigation of bone disease in patients undergoing renal dialysis, their validity as a marker for exposure to aluminium at the lower concentrations encountered in subjects with normal renal function is less clearly established. Further, the range of bone aluminium concentrations in this series of patients was limited. The lack of a relation between aluminium in bone and the presence of pathological features of Alzheimer's disease in this data is hard to interpret. While these results provide no support for the hypothesis linking aluminium and Alzheimer's disease, they cannot be thought of as strong evidence against it.

REFERENCES

1. Candy JM, Oakley AE, Klinowski J et al. Lancet 1986; i: 354-7.
2. Perl D, Brody AR. Science 1980; 208: 297-9.
3. Martyn CN, Barker DJP, Osmond C et al. Lancet 1989; i: 59-62.

Address for correspondence:

Dr C. N. Martyn,
MRC Environmental Epidemiology Unit,
Southampton General Hospital,
Southampton SO9 4XY, UK

49 Study of the Relationship Between Aluminium Concentration in Drinking Water and Risk of Alzheimer's Disease

P. MICHEL, D. COMMENGES, J. F. DARTIGUES, M. GAGNON,
P. BARBERGER-GATEAU, L. LETENNEUR
AND THE PAQUID RESEARCH GROUP

Among several hypotheses, chronic exposure to aluminium has been proposed to be a possible risk factor of Alzheimer's disease (1). This hypothesis was suggested by the presence of aluminium in both senile plaques (2) and neurofibrillary tangle-bearing neurons (3) in brains of patients with Alzheimer's disease. This hypothesis has been further supported by the existence of encephalopathies due to aluminium poisoning both in animals (4) and in patients submitted to recurrent haemodialysis (5).

In the four previously published epidemiological studies which have been conducted to investigate this relationship, aluminium content in drinking water was found to be significantly related to Alzheimer's disease (6-9).

The results of these studies, however, are not completely convincing because of methodological limitations. Among many possible drawbacks, major problems were the use of death certificates to make the diagnosis of senile or presenile dementia (6,7), the indirect measurement of aluminium intake (8), and the selection and diagnosis of the cases based on the computerized tomographic (CT) scan records (9).

The goal of this study, which was part of the Paquid research program, was to investigate the relationship between aluminium concentration in drinking water and the risk of Alzheimer's disease, while avoiding the biases of the previous studies.

METHOD

Study population and design

The target population was that of the community residents aged 65 years and older living in the department of Gironde, an area of 41 308 km^2 around its main town, Bordeaux. A random sample of 4050 subjects was drawn according to a three-stage sampling design, using the French administrative divisions, cantons (districts) and

Alzheimer's Disease: Basic Mechanisms, Diagnosis and Therapeutic Strategies
Edited by K. Iqbal, D. R. C. McLachlan, B. Winblad and H. M. Wisniewski
© 1991 John Wiley & Sons Ltd

commutes (parishes). The first two stages resulted in the selection of 37 communes distributed in all areas of the department; the subjects were then randomly chosen from electoral lists after stratification by age and sex.

Among the 4050 subjects drawn, 1258 refused to participate in the study, and 2792 subjects were visited. The distribution of age and sex of this final sample was the same as in the target population (10).

The questionnaire included age, sex, educational level and a battery of pyschometric tests including Folstein, Folstein and McHugh's mini-mental state examination.

Diagnosis of Alzheimer's disease

The diagnosis of Alzheimer's disease was made by a two-stage process. The screening stage was done by psychologists, based on the DSM-III criteria for dementia and documented by psychometric tests. The final diagnosis was done in a second stage by two senior neurologists (S. A. and B. R.), after an interview and a clinical examination, according to the NINCDS-ADRDA criteria for Alzheimer's disease. Biological tests and CT scan were performed when accepted. Both the psychologists and the neurologists were not aware of the aluminium concentration values at the time of diagnostic investigation.

Aluminium concentration in drinking water

For each of the 37 communes, the number of wells, their depth, their relative contribution to water supply and the aluminium concentration were obtained from the sanitary authorities and the water distribution companies. When several wells contributed to the water supply in a commune, a weighted mean was computed to evaluate the exposure in this commune.

Statistical analysis

In the first analysis, the Spearman rank correlation coefficient was used for testing whether there was an association between aluminium concentration and Alzheimer's disease prevalence in the communes. This was done on both crude prevalence and prevalence standardized on age and educational level, which was found to be related to Alzheimer's disease in some studies (10): two classes of age—65-74 years and > 74 years—and two classes of educational level—no education and grade school, versus high school and university—were defined; the reference population for standardization was that of the total sample.

In a second analysis, the subjects were considered as independent; the data were analysed by a chi-squared test and for adjusting on possible confounding factors by a Cox's proportional hazard model.

RESULTS

Of the 2792 subjects who accepted to participate in the study, 101 (3.62%) were considered to meet the DSM-III criteria for dementia by the pyschologists. Of those

Table 1. Results of the two-stage diagnosis process according to aluminium concentration (Paquid, 1989)

	Aluminium concentration (mg/l)			
	≤0.01	0.02-0.04	0.05-0.07	≥0.08
Probable Alzheimer's disease*	0	23	8	9
	(0%)	(1.2%)	(1.6%)	(5.8%)
Possible Alzheimer's disease*	0	6	3	2
	(0%)	(0.3%)	(0.6%)	(1.3%)
Other dementia	0	7	7	1
	(0%)	(0.4%)	(1.4%)	(0.6%)
False positive cases*	0	8	7	3
Refusals	1	3	6	5
Dead	0	2	0	0
DSM-III negative cases of the screening stage	146	1935	475	135
Total	147	1984	506	155
	(100%)	(100%)	(100%)	(100%)

*See definitions in method section.

subjects, 17 could not be submitted to the neurological examination: 2 had died between the two stages and 15 refused. Eighteen subjects (21.4% of those examined) were considered as nondemented by the neurologists. The 66 demented subjects were classified as having probably Alzheimer's disease in 40 cases (60%), possible Alzheimer's disease in 11 cases (17%) and another type of dementia in 15 cases (23%). The aluminium concentration in water ranged from 0.01 to 0.16 mg/l.

The possible effect of aluminium was first studied by examining the correlation between aluminium concentration and the estimated prevalence of Alzheimer's disease in the communes. The Spearman rank correlation coefficient was significantly different from zero for both crude ($r = 0.44$, $P = 0.004$) and standardized ($r = 0.40$, $P = 0.01$) prevalences.

Table 1 synthesizes the data by classifying the subjects according to categories of aluminium concentration in water—the same as in Martyn et al (9), except that the last two classes are grouped. There is an association between probable Alzheimer's disease and class of aluminium concentration ($x^2 = 26.3$ with 3 d.f. $P < 0.001$).

We performed an analysis adjusted for educational level and rural or urban residence. Educational level was classified into three categories (no education, grade school, high school or university level); rural residence was defined as living in a commune of fewer than 2000 inhabitants. Age was automatically taken into account into the Cox's model that was used. Aluminium was entered as a continuous explanatory variable. The analysis was performed on a sample including the 40 probable Alzheimer's disease cases and the 2691 nondemented subjects.

The relative risk was estimated to be 1.16 for an increase of 0.01 mg/l of aluminium concentration, and was significantly different from 1 ($P = 0.0014$). For an increase of 0.1 mg/l the relative risk is 4.53 (95% confidence interval: [3.36-6.10]).

DISCUSSION

We have found a significant relationship between the aluminium concentration in drinking water and the risk of Alzheimer's disease which persists after adjustment for age, educational level and place of residence. This result is in general agreement with the previous studies (6-9). Our study, however, is free from some of the biases which hampered those studies. The importance of the measurement error on aluminium concentration is not known; also there may be a large variability of the true aluminium concentrations at different moments.

However, possible errors in aluminium concentrations or in the diagnosis of Alzheimer's disease should only tend to weaken the relationship.

It is difficult to explain this relationship by a confounding factor which would have to be related to both Alzheimer's disease and aluminium concentration. The strength of the relative risk (4.53 for an increase of 0.10 mg/l of aluminium) is an argument in favour of a direct effect of aluminium in Alzheimer's disease.

Acknowledgments

This research was supported by grants from the Fondation de France, Sandoz laboratories, AXA Insurance Group, French Ministry for Research and Technology, French Social Security (CNAMTS and MSA), Institut du Cerveau, Conseil Régional d'Aquitaine, Conseil Général de Gironde et de Dordogne, DRASS d'Aquitaine, Caisse de Retraite Interentreprises and CAPIMMEC.

We thank Mr Roche from the 'Lyonnaise des eaux' water company, and Mr Cazaux from the DDASS, for their help in collecting the aluminium concentration values.

REFERENCES

1. Crapper DR, Krishnan SS, Dalton AJ. Brain aluminium distribution in Alzheimer's disease and experimental neurofibrillary degeneration. Science 1973; 180: 511.
2. Candy JM, Oakley AE, Klinowski J et al. Aluminosilicates and senile plaque formation in AD. Lancet 1986; i: 354-6.
3. Perl DP, Brody AR. Alzheimer's disease: X-ray spectometric evidence of aluminium accumulation in neurofibrillary tangle-bearing neurones. Science 1980; 208: 297-9.
4. Terry RD, Pena C. Experimental production of neurofibrillary degeneration: I: light microscopic observation. J Neuropath Exp Neurol 1965; 24: 187-99.
5. Alfrey AC. Dialysis encephalopathy syndrome. Ann Rev Med 1978; 29: 93.
6. Vogt T. Water quality and health study for a possible relationship between aluminium in drinking water and dementia. Sosiale og okonom stud 1986; 61: 1-99.
7. Flaten TP. Geographical associations between aluminium in drinking water and registered death rates with dementia (including Alzheimer's disease) in Norway. Proceedings of the Second International Symposium on Geochemistry and Health, London (in press).
8. Still CN, Kelley P. On the incidence of primary degenerative dementia vs. water fluoride content in South Carolina. Neurotoxicology 1980; 1: 125-31.
9. Martyn CN, Barker DPJ, Osmond C, Harris EC, Edwardson JA, Lacey RF. Geographical relation between Alzheimer's disease and aluminium in drinking water. Lancet 1989; i: 59-62.

10. Dartiques JF, Gagnon M, Michel P et al. Le programme de recherche Paquid sur l'épidémiologie de la démence. Méthode et résultats initiaux. Rev Neurol (in press).

Address for correspondence:

Dr P. Michel,
Unité INSERM 330,
Université de Bordeaux II,
146 rue Léo Saignat,
33076 Bordeaux, France

50 The Effect of Aluminum(III) on the Integrity of Plasmatic Membranes: Relevance to Alzheimer's Disease

B. CORAIN, M. PERAZZOLO, L. FONTANA, A. TAPPARO,
M. FAVARATO, G. G. BOMBI, C. CORVAJA, M. NICOLINI
AND P. ZATTA

The unique polypeptide A4, identified as an important building block of the amyloid deposits typical of senile plaques (SP) of Alzheimer's disease (AD) (1), might possibly represent a piece of 'chemical memory' related to an initial degenerative process involving the gradual loss of integrity of the neuronal plasmatic membrane (2). Thus, investigation on the effects of neurotoxins on plasmatic membranes, or on relevant chemical models, are likely to be pertinent to the yet mysterious etiology of AD.

Aluminum(III) is an established neurotoxin (3) and an extensive literature illustrates its ability to induce alterations in the function of plasmatic membranes (4), although the molecular bases of these observations are still obscure.

Recent biochemical and biophysical work (5,6) has shown that aluminum(III) at μM concentrations induces phase separation, aggregation, dye release and membrane rigidification in phosphatidylserine- and phosphatidylethanolamine-containing lipid vesicles.

In 1978, aluminum(III) was recognized as a chemical aggressor to biological membranes (7), on the basis of physicochemical evidence. Thus, $[Al(OH_2)_6^{3+}]$ was found to induce a significant reduction of membrane fluidity in *Thermoplasma acidophilum* at pH 3, as revealed by ESR measurements on the ghosts of bacterial cells exposed to aluminum(III) after labelling with 5-NSA (2-(3-carboxypropyl)-2-tridecyl-4,4-dimethyl-3-oxazolyndinyloxyl).

In 1988, we reported (8,9) that rabbit erythrocytes suspended in aqueous solution of the hydrolytically stable lipophilic (10) complex $Al(acac)_3$ (acac = 2,4-pentanedionate) undergo a prominent morphological effect (echinoacanthocytosis) accompanied by a significant increase of osmotic fragility at physiological pH values. $Al(malt)_3$ (malt = 3-hydroxy-2-methyl-4-pyronate) (hydrolytically stable, hydrophilic) (10) and $Al(lact)_3$ (hydrolytically metastable, hydrophilic) (10) were found to be ineffective in terms of morphological modifications and slightly effective in terms of osmotic fragility. Equally inactive were found to be both the ligand Hacac and the complex $Fe(acac)_3$, which is quite related to $Al(acac)_3$ in terms of basic

Alzheimer's Disease: Basic Mechanisms, Diagnosis and Therapeutic Strategies
Edited by K. Iqbal, D. R. C. McLachlan, B. Winblad and H. M. Wisniewski
© 1991 John Wiley & Sons Ltd

physico-chemical properties. These results appeared to be particularly interesting in that they offered a clear example of a prominent aggression of aluminum(III) to biological membranes at physiological pH values.

CHEMICAL ASPECTS OF Al(acac)$_3$ ACTION

Echinoacanthocytosis is produced at Al(III) concentrations in the range of 0.34–8 mM on 2 ml of washed packed rabbit erythrocytes in 8 ml of physiological buffered solution (2 hours). The same effect is observed for rat and human erythrocytes, although in this latter case the morphological modification becomes apparent only at 8 mM Al(acac)$_3$.

SDS-PAGE analysis of the ghosts of rabbit echinoacanthocytes (11) has revealed so far that exposure to Al(acac)$_3$ produces no significant change in the structure of membrane proteins. Repeated washing–centrifuging (3×5 ml phosphate buffer solution 3.4 mM, pH 7.4) of the echinoanthocytes did not reverse the dramatic morphological effect caused by aluminum(III), thus demonstrating that the Al(acac)$_3$-induced echinoacanthocytosis is irreversible.

The metal-induced pathological effect is accompanied, in fact, by a large increase of aluminum concentration inside the ghosts of treated erythrocytes (from 11 p.p.m. to 5700 p.p.m. dry weight). The data, depicted in Figure 1, show a marked correlation between aluminum concentration in the membranes and in the solutions to which they were exposed.

All these data demonstrate that (a) exposure of the erythrocytes to Al(acac)$_3$ is accompanied by the formation of relatively strong (i.e. covalent) bonds between Al(III) and the membrane (possibly at the membrane surface); (b) such bonds do not seem to involve the proteic component of the plasmatic membrane; and (c) echinoacanthocytosis is speciation dependent, i.e. it is induced only by a lipophilic form of aluminum(III).

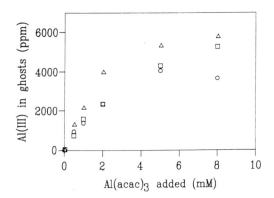

Figure 1. Al concentrations in ghosts from rabbit (△), rat (○) and human (□) erythrocytes (w/w in dry samples) observed after exposition to aqueous Al(acac)$_3$ in the 0.34–8 mM concentration range

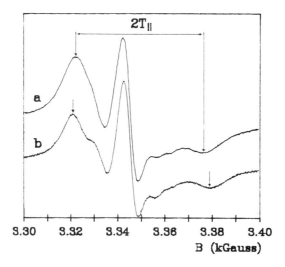

Figure 2. ESR spectrum of rabbit erythrocyte ghosts labelled with 5-NSA; (a) untreated; (b) treated with 2 mM Al(acac)$_3$

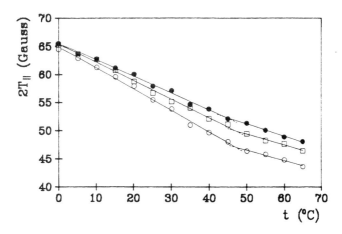

Figure 3. Temperature effect on 2T$\|$, observed for rabbit erythrocyte ghosts (controls, ○) after treatment with Al(acac)$_3$ (●), Al(lact)$_3$ (□), and labelling with 5-NSA (9). Al(malt)$_3$ behaves as Al(lact)$_3$. Estimated error: ordinate ± 0.2 gauss; abscissa ± 0.2 °C. Notice the crystalline–fluid crystalline phase transition temperature around 45 °C

PHYSICOCHEMICAL ASPECTS OF Al(acac)$_3$ ACTION

In order to shed light on the physicochemical aspects of the essentially biophysical effects caused by Al(acac)$_3$ on erythrocytes (i.e. echinoacanthocytosis and osmotic fragility), we considered potential changes of a fundamental property of biological membranes, i.e. the effect of Al(III) on their fluidity (7). It is well known that a proper degree of fluidity is a crucial feature of 'healthy' membranes and this biophysical parameter can be evaluated, inter alia, by ESR measurements after labelling with paramagnetic probes (e.g. 5-NSA) which, when inserted into the biological bilayers, can provide rather subtle and well-rationalized information on membrane fluidity (12,13). Our relevant data are collected in Figures 2 and 3.

It is seen that the exposure of rabbit erythrocytes to Al(acac)₃ causes a consistent increase of $2T\|$ (Figure 2). This parameter is related to the spin label mobility and its increase indicates a significant lowering of membrane fluidity (12,13). This observation is confirmed by the dependence of $2T\|$ on the temperature (Figure 3); from the same figure it appears that also Al(malt)₃ and Al(lact)₃ do affect membrane fluidity, albeit to a lesser extent.

Similar results were obtained for rat erythrocytes, while no significant reduction of membrane fluidity was observed for human samples.

MOLECULAR HYPOTHESIS FOR Al(III) MEMBRANE TOXICITY

In rather general terms, it can be stated that Al(III) is likely to bind both to carboxylate and phosphate groups present in biomolecules, with a preference for phosphate oxoanions (14). The phosphate hydrophilic head groups of membrane phospholipids appear to be a plausible 'anchoring' site, able to react with Al(III) toxins sufficiently lipophilic in character to diffuse *at* the bilayer surface or *just below it*. The definitely hydrophilic species Al(malt)₃ and Al(lact)₃ are expected to reside in the water phase, while the prevalently lipophilic Al(acac)₃ may be expected to reach the membrane bilayer surface and to form true covalent bonds with the phosphate head groups present in the lipid fraction of rabbit and human erythrocytes (15) (Figure 4). The remarkable affinity of Al(III), at neutral pH, for phosphatidylcholine artificial vesicles has been recently documented on the basis of equilibrium dialysis and electrophoresis experiments (16).

The consequences of the formation of phospholipid–Al(acac)₂ molecular species in terms of biophysical effects appear rather predictable. Thus, the diffuse

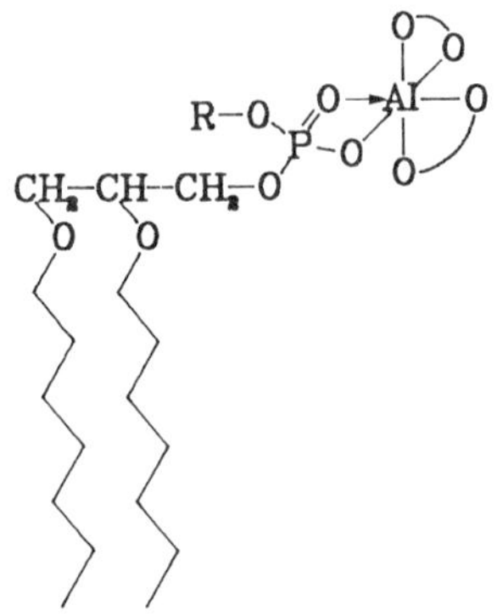

Figure 4. Tentative proposal for the formation of covalent adducts between lipophilic Al(acac)₃ and membrane phospholipids of rabbit and rat erythrocytes

perturbation of the bilayer architecture will imply both structural effects (osmotic fragility and morphological alterations) and dynamic effects (reduction of membrane fluidity). As to the morphological alteration, it is worthwhile to point out that an effect similar to that produced by Al(acac)$_3$ is also observed when erythrocytes are exposed to a variety of amphipathic drugs (17). This effect was interpreted as due to 'simple' insertion (intercalation) of these molecules in the external half of the membrane bilayer, with a consequent expansion of the exterior surface area of the membrane, able to give rise to the overall observed crenation effect (17). In the model presented here the irreversible nature of the morphological effect is a strong support to the formation of covalent bonds between aluminum and the membrane phospholipids.

CONCLUSIONS

The lipophilic, hydrolytically stable, artificial aluminum(III) toxin, Al(acac)$_3$, is a chemical aggressor of the membrane of rabbit and rat erythrocytes. Its action is accompanied by prominent irreversible morphological changes (echinoacanthocytosis), with concomitant incorporation of large amounts of Al(III) inside (or at the surface of) the ghosts preparation and significant decrease of membrane fluidity. Echinoacanthocytosis is observed also for human erythrocytes, but only at higher doses; moreover, the incorporation of aluminum(III) in the corresponding ghosts is not accompanied by a significant decrease of membrane fluidity. The reason for these important differences will be a matter of further investigation by biophysical measurements, e.g. ESR, by employing other properly chosen spin labels.

Acknowledgments

We are grateful to Parke Davis and to Shering Plough for research fellowships to M. P. and L. F.

REFERENCES

1. Price DL, Koo EH, Muma NA, Applegate MD, Wagster MU, Walker LC, Struble RG, Troncoso JC, Cark LC. In Henderson AS, Henderson JH (eds) Etiology of dementia of Alzheimer's type. Chichester: John Wiley, 1988: 65-81.
2. Masters CL, Beyreuther K. In Terry ED (ed.) Aging and the brain. New York: Raven Press, 1988: 183-204.
3. Sturman JA, Wisniewski HM. In Boudy SC, Prasad KN (eds) Metal neurotoxicity. Boca Raton: CRC Press, 1988: 61-85.
4. Banks WA, Kastin AJ. Neurosci Behav Sci 1989; 13: 47-53.
5. Deleers M, Servais J-P, Wülfer E. Biochim Biophys Acta 1985; 813: 195-200.
6. Deleers M, Servais J-P, Wülfer E. Biochim Biophys Acta 1986; 855: 271-6.
7. Vierstra R, Haug A. Biochem Biophys Res Comm 1988; 84: 138-43.
8. Zatta P, Perazzolo M, Corain B. Toxicol Lett 1989; 45: 15-21.
9. Zatta P, Perazzolo M, Bombi GG, Corain B, Nicolini M. In Iqbal K, Wisniewski HM, Winblad B (eds) Alzheimer's disease and related disorders. New York: Alan R. Liss, 1989: 1087-94.

10. Tapparo A, Perazzolo M. Int J Anal Chem 1989; 36: 13-16.
11. Montecucco C. In Azzi A, Masotti L, Vecli A (eds) Membrane proteins isolation and characterisation. Berlin: Springer, 1986: 119-23.
12. Berliner LE. Spin labelling. Theory and applications vol. I, II. New York: 1976, 1979.
13. Markesbery WR, Leung PK, Butterfield A. J Neurol Sci 1980; 45: 323-30.
14. Martin B. Clin Chem 1986; 32: 1797-1806.
15. Brewer G. In The red cell (7th Ann Arbor Conference). New York: Alan R. Liss, 1989: 162-9.
16. Akeson MA, Munns DN, Buran RG. Biochim Biophys Acta 1989; 986: 33-40.
17. Shutz MP, Singer SJ. Proc Natl Acad Sci USA 1974; 71: 4457-61.

Address for correspondence:

Dr B. Corain,
University of Padova,
Dipartimento di Chimica Inorganica, Metallorganica ed Analitica,
via Marzolo 1, I-35131 Padova, Italy

51 Chromatographic Resolution of Aluminum Binding Components in Human Serum

MOSÈ FAVARATO, CRAIG A. MIZZEN,
THEODORE P. A. KRUCK, BHUMA KRISHNAN,
PAOLO F. ZATTA AND DONALD R. McLACHLAN

The toxic properties of aluminum in dialysis dementia are well established (1) even though the specific biochemical mechanisms by which aluminum toxicity is expressed in this disease are not known. Aluminum has been proposed to be a risk factor in the etiology of Alzheimer's disease and other neuropathies (2-6). Abundant evidence from epidemiological and neuropathological studies presented at this conference clearly indicates that further investigation of the role of environmental exposure to aluminum in the pathogenesis of neurodegenerative disease is warranted.

Since aluminum in blood is bound to several serum proteins (7-16,18), identification and characterization of plasma constituents that bind aluminum and may facilitate transfer of aluminum from the blood stream to the central nervous system (CNS) are fundamental to understanding the mechanisms of aluminum accumulation and toxicity in disease states.

Aluminum binding to serum proteins has been studied by several authors employing gel filtration chromatography (GFC) (8-15). They concluded that albumin and transferrin are the major aluminum carriers (8-10,12,13). Recently, Khalil and co-workers (15) suggested that a low molecular weight protein is the major aluminum carrier in sera of hemodialysis patients.

Utilizing GFC (16), we have studied serum aluminum distribution in renal dialysis and Alzheimer patients and demonstrated the presence of a proteinaceous component with high affinity for aluminum that has not been described previously.

MATERIAL AND METHODS

Blood samples were collected from five hemodialysis and five Alzheimer patients. Sera were prepared by centrifugation at $1500\,g$ for 10 min and samples stored at $-80\,°C$ until processed.

Aluminum concentrations in sera and GFC fractions were determined by electrothermal atomic absorption spectrometry (EAAS).

Alzheimer's Disease: Basic Mechanisms, Diagnosis and Therapeutic Strategies
Edited by K. Iqbal, D. R. C. McLachlan, B. Winblad and H. M. Wisniewski
©1991 John Wiley & Sons Ltd

Serum samples were fractionated by GFC on a 1.6 cm × 100 cm column packed with Toyopearl TSK-GEL HW-55S gel as described (16).

Sodium dodecylsulfate polyacrylamide gel electrophoresis (SDS-PAGE) was performed according to the method of Laemmli (17). Samples were heated at 100 °C for 5 minutes prior to application on 9% polyacrylamide gels. Proteins were visualized with Coomassie Brilliant Blue.

RESULTS

Representative elution profiles for patients on renal dialysis, patients with Alzheimer's disease and healthy volunteers are shown in Figures 1, 2 and 3 respectively.

Differences between the protein profiles in Figures 1, 2 and 3 are found in the high molecular weight regions of the chromatograms. Peak ii (Figure 1) contains a heterogeneous collection of proteins of high molecular weight, the predominant species being α_2-macroglobulin, immunoglobulins, hepatoglobin and several proteins that were not identified. These components were better resolved in chromatograms of Alzheimer or control sera samples (Figures 2 and 3) where SDS-PAGE analysis revealed that peak 1 contains α_2-macroglobulin and peak ii contains immunoglobulins and hepatoglobin.

In all three patient groups, the major fraction of aluminum, peak b, coelutes with transferrin and albumin, peak 3 (Figures 1–3). Aluminum also elutes with a group of proteins in a volume consistent with a molecular weight of 18 000 daltons,

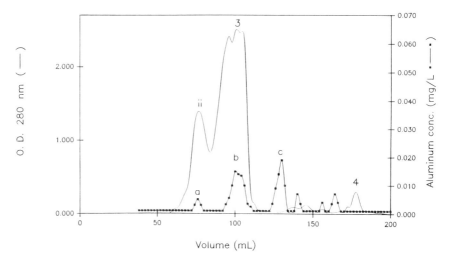

Figure 1. Gel filtration chromatography analysis of hemodialysis sera. One ml of serum obtained from a chronic hemodialysis patient was loaded on a TSK-GEL HW-55S column and eluted at 12 ml/h with 50 mM Tris pH 7.4, 50 mM NaCl, 3 mM NaN₃. Fractions (2 ml) were collected and protein elution (solid line) determined by measuring optical density of fractions at 280 nm (left axis). Aluminum elution (■) was determined by EAAS measurement of aluminum concentration in fractions (right axis)

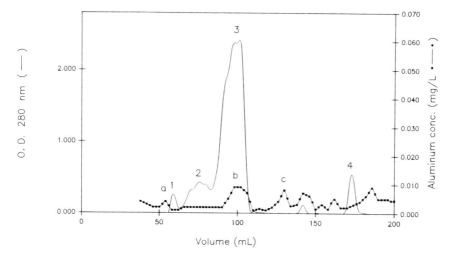

Figure 2. Gel filtration chromatography analysis of Alzheimer sera. One ml of serum obtained from an Alzheimer patient was chromatographed as described in Figure 1

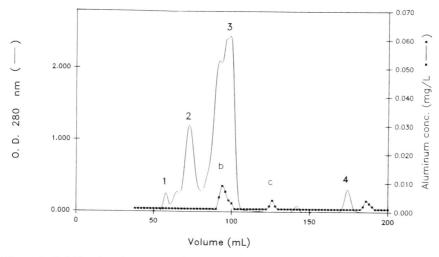

Figure 3. Gel filtration chromatography analysis of normal sera. One ml of serum obtained from a healthy volunteer was chromatographed as described in Figure 1

peak c (Figures 1-3). The amount of aluminum eluting in peak c is significantly greater in samples from hemodialysis patients (Figure 1) compared to those from Alzheimer or normal subjects (Figures 2 and 3). It is of interest to note that relatively little absorbancy at 280 nm is associated with fractions in this region.

In addition to peaks b and c (Figures 1-3), aluminum elutes as a high molecular weight component (peak a of Figures 1 and 2) and several low molecular weight components in hemodialysis and Alzheimer disease samples (Figures 1 and 2) in contrast to normal sera (Figure 3).

ENVIRONMENTAL FACTORS

DISCUSSION

The differences in the protein profiles between the three subject groups are possibly a consequence of the disease state or perhaps are due to protein aggregation. The protein elution profile in Alzheimer patients is similar to the pattern obtained in normal subjects. Serum proteins of hemodialysis patients are less well resolved. Reasons for the reduced resolution are not apparent. The chromatogram shown in Figure 1 is similar to that obtained upon the addition of aluminum chloride to normal serum in vitro (16), suggesting that aluminum concentrations in hemodialysis sera are sufficient to induce protein aggregation.

Our observations confirm that in Alzheimer and nonhyperaluminemic dialysis patients, aluminum in serum is bound primarily to transferrin and albumin (8-10,12,13).

However, as serum aluminum concentrations exceed normal levels, other serum proteins become involved in aluminum binding. Serum aluminum levels are generally considered normal if the aluminum concentration is less than 400 nmol/l. The chromatogram presented in Figure 1 was obtained from a hemodialysis patient whose total serum aluminum was 7925 nmol/l. We suggest that as transferrin and albumin binding of aluminum approaches saturation, serum proteins with lesser affinity (i.e. immunoglobulins) can compete for aluminum binding.

Even though the existence of these aluminum-protein complexes has been demonstrated, their role in aluminum transport has not been established. It is not known whether any of these aluminum complexes can cross the blood-brain barrier (BBB). Indeed, these aluminum binding proteins may protect against aluminum intoxication by preventing the formation of low molecular weight aluminum complexes (i.e. Al-citrate) that may be capable of crossing the BBB and mediate aluminum entry into the brain.

The newly identified aluminum binding serum component (peak c of Figures 1, 2, 3) has an affinity for aluminum equal to or greater than that of transferrin. GFC analysis of patient samples before and after Desferal® (trivalent metal chelator) treatment reveals that this high-affinity chelator reduces the amount of aluminum eluting in peak a and other components (18). Yet, the amount of aluminum associated with peak b (transferrin and albumin) does not change significantly while the quantity in peak c increases markedly. Control experiments demonstrate that peak c is not an aluminum-Desferal® complex. Analysis of peak c by SDS-PAGE electrophoresis invariably shows the presence of proteins with molecular weight ranging from 20 000 to 150 000 daltons. The aluminum binding properties of each of these proteins are currently under investigation.

Acknowledgments

The authors would like to acknowledge the assistance of the Clinical Investigation Unit of Toronto General Hospital and thank the Peterborough chapter of the Alzheimer's Society and Parke-Davis (Italy) for financial support. We acknowledge Dr M. K. Sutherland and Dr S. Zanoni for their help in manuscript preparation.

REFERENCES

1. Alfrey AC, Mishell JM, Burks J. Trans Am Soc Artif Inter Organs 1972; 18: 257-61.
2. Crapper DR, Krishnan SS, Dalton AJ. Science 1973; 180: 511-13.
3. Crapper DR, Krishnan SS, Quittkat S. Brain 1976; 99: 67-79.
4. Crapper DR, Quittkat S, Krishnan SS, Dalton AJ, DeBoni U. Acta Neuropathol (Berl) 1980; 50: 19-24.
5. Perl DP, Gajdusek DC, Garruto RM, Yanagihara RT, Gibbs CJ. Science 1982; 217: 1053-5.
6. Martyn CN, Osmond C, Edwardson JA, Barker DJP, Harris EC, Lacey RF. Lancet 1989; i: 59-62.
7. Lundin AP, Caruso C, Sass M, Berlyne GM. Clin Res 1978; 26: 636A.
8. King SW, Wills MR, Savory J. Res Comm Chem Pathol Pharmacol 1979; 26: 161-9.
9. King SW, Savory J, Wills MR. Ann Clin Lab Sci 1982; 12: 143-9.
10. Trapp GA. Life Sci 1983; 33: 311-16.
11. Bertholf RL, Wills MR, Savory J. Clin Physiol Biochem 1985; 3: 271-6.
12. Leung FY, Hodsman AB, Muirhead N, Henderson AR. Clin Chem 1985; 31: 20-3.
13. Cochran M, Patterson D, Neoh S, Stevens B, Mazzachi R. Clin Chem 1985; 31: 1314-16.
14. Bertholf RL, Savory J, Wills MR. Trace Elem Med 986; 3: 157-60.
15. Khalil-Manesh F, Agness C, Gonick HC. Nephron 1989; 52: 323-8.
16. Favarato M, Mizzen C, Kruck TPA, McLachlan DR (in preparation).
17. Laemmli UK. Nature 1970; 227: 680.
18. Favarato M, Mizzen C, Kruck TPA, McLachlan DR (in preparation).

Address for correspondence:

Dr Mosè Favarato,
Department of Physiology and
Centre for Research in Neurodegenerative Diseases,
Faculty of Medicine, University of Toronto,
Toronto M5S 1A8, Ontario, Canada

Part VIII

GENETIC MECHANISMS

52 RNA Metabolism in Alzheimer's Disease: Selective Increase in GFAP RNA

DAVID G. MORGAN, CALEB E. FINCH AND
STEVEN A. JOHNSON

RNA was isolated from over 300 Alzheimer's disease (AD) and age-matched control (CTL) brain samples obtained post mortem. Total RNA yields and poly(A+)RNA yields were generally similar for AD and CTL tissue specimens, except for a slight reduction (15%) in total RNA yield in temporal cortex. Ethidium bromide stained agarose gels indicated that the RNA from AD samples was on average more degraded than CTL RNA; however, considerable overlap between the two groups was present. No difference was found in [^{35}S]methionine incorporation into in-vitro translation products using AD and CTL RNA, and most translation products resolved on two-dimensional polyacrylamide gels were of similar intensities. One exception was an AD-related increase in bands which migrated in the region where glial fibrillary acidic protein (GFAP) is expected to migrate. Northern blot and solution hybridization studies confirmed a threefold to fourfold increase in GFAP RNA prevalence in AD. This study shows that the prevalence of most abundant RNA sequences is similar in AD and CTL brain samples, and that normal yields of reasonably intact RNA can be obtained. These results encourage further examination of RNA from AD samples using molecular genetic technologies.

INTRODUCTION

Over the last five years we have performed a series of studies to evaluate RNA metabolism in AD, directed toward identifying sequences with altered abundance which may be causally linked to disease etiology or symptomatology. The present report summarizes our data on RNA yields in AD, and some of our characterization data concerning RNA obtained from AD cases. While the utilization of post-mortem human tissue presents methodological difficulties, our data suggest that the RNA from some AD and age-matched control (CTL) patients is of sufficient quality to quantify prevalence of specific RNA sequences, and for molecular cloning studies.

Alzheimer's Disease: Basic Mechanisms, Diagnosis and Therapeutic Strategies
Edited by K. Iqbal, D. R. C. McLachlan, B. Winblad and H. M. Wisniewski
©1991 John Wiley & Sons Ltd

MATERIALS AND METHODS

Materials

Human postmortem brain samples were obtained from the Alzheimer Disease Research Consortium of Southern California (Los Angeles County General Hospital), Rancho Los Amigos Medical Center, Downey, CA, and the Biogerontology Research Institute, Sun City, AZ. Samples of frontal, temporal and occipital cortex, hippocampus and cerebellum were obtained at autopsy. Alzheimer cases were diagnosed using neuropathologic and clinical criteria; cases with multi-infarct dementia or parkinsonian dementia are not included in the analyses presented here. Age-matched control (CTL) cases were identified by similar criteria to be free of psychiatric and neurologic dysfunction, and failed to exhibit neuritic plaque and neurofibrillary tangle pathology consistent with Alzheimer-type dementia.

RNA preparation

Frozen tissue samples (0.5–2 g) were broken into smaller fragments in a dry-ice cooled mortar, and added directly to freshly prepared 5M guanidinium isothiocyanate, 50 mM Tris (pH 8.0), 50 mM EDTA and 4% 2-mercaptoethanol and extensively disrupted with a Dounce homogenizer. After homogenization, sodium lauryl sarcosine was added to 3% final concentration and the homogenate was centrifuged (12 000 g for 10 min) to remove insoluble material. CsCl was added to 0.15 g/ml, the homogenates were underlayered with 2 ml of 5.7 M CsCl, and centrifuged overnight (112 000 g at 20 °C). The resulting RNA pellet was resuspended in diethylpyrocarbonate (DEP) treated water, extracted with phenol, chloroform/isoamyl alcohol (Sevag), and ether, ethanol precipitated (using 250 mM potassium acetate), resuspended in DEP treated water, and RNA content was estimated at A_{260} (1.0 o.d. = 43 μg/ml). Control studies used radiolabeled RNA (1.1 kb, GFAP) and DNA (nick-translated 1.4 kb beta-tubulin) probes to evaluate the degree of separation afforded by this technique. The pellet contained 93% of the added radioactivity when an RNA probe was added to the homogenate, while only 2% of the added radioactivity was found in the pellet when a DNA probe was added to the homogenate, indicating that RNA recovery was high, and DNA contamination was low in this procedure.

Poly(A+)RNA was selected by two or three binding elution cycles over oligo(dT)cellulose, using either a column (1) or batch procedure, depending upon the brain region, and measured by A_{260}. Because no attempt was made to isolate polysomal RNA, the sequences detected in this fraction may be nuclear or cytoplasmic untranslated RNA in addition to true mRNA loaded onto polysomes.

In-vitro translation

Five μg of total RNA were added to a rabbit reticulocyte translation mix (BRL Laboratories, Bethesda, MD) using [^{35}S] methionine to label translation products. Incorporation was measured by TCA precipitation after hydrolysis of aminoacyl tRNA. Translation products from samples with similar incorporation were resolved on two-dimensional gels using a modification of the O'Farrell method with isoelectric focusing in the first dimension followed by 12.5% acrylamide-SDS gel electrophoresis in the second dimension. Gels were dehydrated in DMSO, impregnated with 2,5-diphenyloxazole (PPO), dried and exposed to X-ray film. The autoradiograms were analyzed by computer-based video densitometry, and the data for each spot expressed as the ratio of the integrated optical density in the AD gel divided by the integrated optical density in the matched CTL gel. Five pairs of samples were analyzed in this manner.

RNA gel blot hybridization

Five μg of AD and CTL total RNA samples were electrophoresed on denaturing 1% agarose/2.2 M formaldehyde gels and blotted onto nylon membranes. The membranes were baked at 80 °C for 2 hours, and hybridized overnight with [^{32}P]antisense RNA probes prepared from recombinant transcription vectors (Bluescript; Stratagene, San Diego, CA) in $5 \times$ SSC, 0.1% SDS, 10% dextran sulfate, 25 μg/μl poly(A)- and poly(C)RNA, 100 μg/ml sheared, denatured salmon sperm DNA, and 0.5% nonfat dry milk at 75 °C. Hybridized blots were washed in successively decreasing salt concentrations down to $0.5 \times$ SSC at 75 °C. Blots were then exposed to X-ray film and the resulting autoradiograms quantified by computer-based video densitometry calibrated with a photographic density wedge.

Solution hybridization; nuclease protection/titration analysis

For each RNA sample, five concentrations of total RNA (0–2 μg) in triplicate were hybridized overnight with 1 ng of [^{32}P]GFAP antisense RNA (20 μl volume with 0.4 M NaCl, 50% formamide, sample RNA with yeast tRNA to give 10 μg RNA, 50 °C). Single-stranded cRNA probe was digested with RNase A and RNase T1, and probe-target hybrids were precipitated with 1 M HCl, 0.1 M $Na_4P_2O_7$ and collected by filtration. The amount of target RNA in the sample was calculated from the specific activity of the cRNA probe, the probe length as a fraction of the target RNA, and the slope of the line relating added total RNA with precipitated c.p.m. Additional details are presented in Goss et al (2).

RESULTS

RNA yields in Alzheimer's disease cerebral cortex

When analyzed together, RNA isolated from over 200 AD and CTL tissue samples from frontal, temporal and occipital cortices showed no significant differences in total RNA yield per gram tissue (Figure 1). The AD samples' mean value is 7% lower than the CTL value, but this is due to a larger number of AD samples with very low yield values (less than 200 μg RNA per gram tissue). Yields this low were invariably associated with extreme degradation, with very little 28S or 18S rRNA

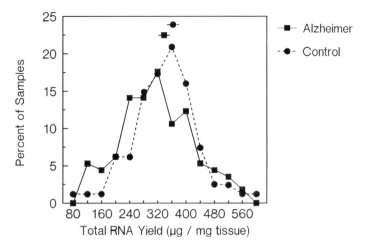

Figure 1. Total RNA recovery from cerebral cortical samples of Alzheimer and control cases. Total RNA was isolated from 113 AD and 81 control specimens as described in Methods. The histogram represents the percentage of the total data set falling into each group of 40 μg/mg tissue. The two datapoints above the histograms represent the mean and SEM for each group. There is no statistically significant difference between the two distributions (*t*-test, *P* > 0.1)

visible on ethidium bromide stained gels. However, when the cortical samples are grouped into subregions, a significant 17% loss of total RNA is detected in AD temporal cortex samples. RNA recovery from frontal and occipital cortices was unaltered in AD cases, as were the recoveries from hippocampal and cerebellar samples (Table 1).

Poly(A+)RNA was prepared by multiple binding–elution cycles over oligo(DT)-cellulose. The yield of poly(A+)RNA per μg total RNA added to the column was

Table 1. Total RNA yields in Alzheimer's disease

	μg RNA/mg tissue				
	Fntl CX	Temp CX	Occ CX	HPC	CER
CTL					
Mean	360	359	371	332	378
SD	76	93	116	88	84
SEM	13	17	28	18	19
n	33	29	17	25	19
AD					
Mean	347	298★	391	357	369
SD	90	88	76	82	81
SEM	13	14	13	14	17
n	49	42	33	35	22

★Significantly different from CTL, *P* < 0.01, *t*-test.
Fntl CX, frontal cortex; Temp CX, temporal cortex; Occ CX, occipital cortex; HPC, hippocampus; CER, cerebellum; SD, standard deviation; SEM, standard error of the mean; *n*, number of samples analyzed per group.

POLY(A+)RNA YIELDS IN ALZHEIMER DISEASE

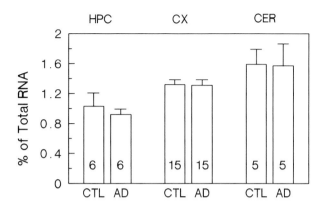

Figure 2. Poly(A+)RNA recovery from RNA samples isolated from Alzheimer and control cases. Poly(A+)RNA was isolated from total RNA using oligo(dT)cellulose chromatography as described in Methods. Data are presented as the percentage of the total RNA recovered in the poly(A+)RNA fraction after two or three cycles of binding and elution. HPC, hippocampus; CX, cerebral cortex; CER, cerebellum. The number of samples analyzed is indicated within each bar. Error bars represent standard errors of the means

the same for AD and CTL RNA samples in cortical, hippocampal and cerebellar samples, although some regional differences in poly(A+)RNA yield were observed, resulting at least partially from minor procedural differences (number of binding-elution cycles; column versus batch procedures; Figure 2).

While yields were normal in AD, the RNA recovered was, on the average, slightly less intact as evaluated by ethidium bromide gel staining patterns (Table 2). There was considerable overlap, however, between the AD and CTL populations. For further studies with these RNA samples, attempts were made to use CTL and AD pairs with equivalent integrity.

Table 2. RNA integrity in Alzeimer's disease

	Temporal cortex		Frontal cortex		Occipital cortex	
	CTL	AD	CTL	AD	CTL	AD
Mean	2.9	2.0*	3.3	2.2**	3.1	2.0*
SEM	0.3	0.3	0.2	0.2	0.3	0.4
n	7	11	17	21	10	8

Integrity was estimated from ethidium-bromide stained denaturing agarose gels of total RNA. A four-point rating scale was established by comparison of the staining intensity of the 28S and 18S rRNA bands: 4, 28S twice 18S; 3, 28S greater than 18S; 2, 28S equivalent to 18S; 1, 28S less than 18S. Photographs of ethidium-bromide stained gels were rated by three different investigators who were unaware of the identity of each sample. The average of these three ratings was used in the present analysis. *$P < 0.05$; **$P < 0.01$.

In-vitro translation of AD RNA

AD and CTL total RNA samples were translated in vitro in a reticulocyte lysate system, and the translation products were labeled with [³⁵S]methionine. No difference in TCA-precipitable incorporation was observed in the AD and CTL samples (AD, 10 700 ± 1800 c.p.m./μg RNA; CTL, 12 900 ± 1700 c.p.m./μg RNA; $n = 10$ per group). Translation products were resolved on two-dimensional gels for five pairs of AD and CTL samples. The gels were fluorographed and the autoradiograms were analyzed by computer-based video densitometry. At least 200 bands could be recognized on each autoradiogram, and very few of these changed consistently in AD. Figure 3 shows the optical density ratios for four bands which appear elevated in AD samples, four bands representative of the many bands which were the same in AD and CTL samples, and four bands which were reduced in the AD cases. The bands H, I and J (M_r 50 000, pI 5.6, 5.5, and 5.4 respectively) are in the region of the two-dimensional gel where others have reported that GFAP bands migrate (3). A second band of specific interest is band A (M_r 20 000, pI 6.7), which was consistently repressed in AD samples. The most striking feature of the two-dimensional gel analyses is the similarity in the patterns between AD and CTL samples for these abundant RNA sequences detected by in-vitro translation of total RNA.

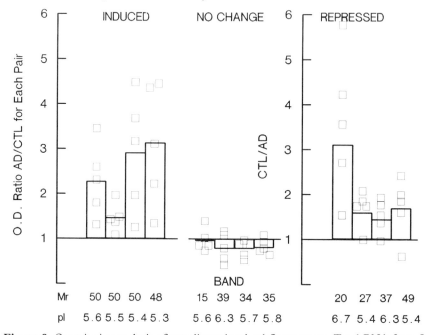

Figure 3. Quantitative analysis of two-dimensional gel fluorograms. Total RNA from five pairs of AD and CTL samples was translated in vitro and the [³⁵S]-labeled polypeptide products were resolved on two-dimensional acrylamide gels. Fluorograms were analyzed by video densitometry, and the total optical density for each of the spots was measured. The ratios of the AD to CTL samples were calculated for each spot, and are shown on the graph. The bar represents the mean of the AD/CTL ratios. Note that the y-axis for the right one-third of the figure is inverted (CTL/AD) so that repressions are on the same scale as inductions

RNA hybridization analyses

We assayed total RNA from AD and CTL cortex for the prevalence of several specific RNA sequences. One of these, GFAP, was elevated threefold in AD samples by northern blot hybridization (Figure 4). In contrast, signals for beta-tubulin or thy-1 RNA were not different between the AD and CTL samples (Figure 4). However, because of inherent problems in northern blot quantitation, especially with RNA samples that are partially degraded, the AD-related change in GFAP RNA was quantified by the more rigorously quantitative solution hybridization nuclease protection assay. Using a different series of AD and CTL samples from those used for the northern blot studies, this analysis revealed a fourfold elevation of GFAP RNA in AD temporal cortex, but no change in cerebellum relative to CTL samples (Figure 5).

DISCUSSION

The most prominent finding of this report is a threefold to fourfold elevation of GFAP RNA in AD cerebral cortex samples. The results of the solution hybridization and northern blot hybridization analyses are consistent with the results of two-dimensional gel fluorography of in-vitro translation products, where several bands in the region of the GFAP cluster described by others (4) are elevated in the AD samples. Surprisingly, another study of AD RNA prevalence using dot blot analysis detected only a 40% elevation of GFAP RNA in AD (5).

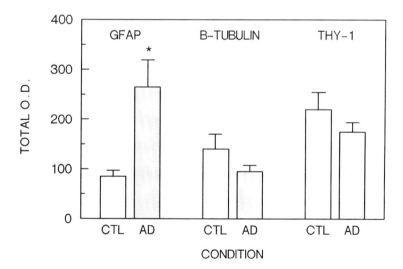

Figure 4. Quantitation of northern blot hybridizations. Hybridization and quantification are as described in Methods. The increase in GFAP RNA in AD samples was significant at $P < 0.001$. No significant differences were apparent when [^{32}P]beta-tubulin or [^{32}P]thy-1 antigen antisense RNAs were used in the hybridization reactions of sister blots. Error bars represent standard errors of the means

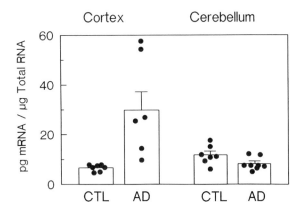

Figure 5. Quantitation of solution hybridization for GFAP. Solution hybridization analysis (nuclease protection/titration analysis) was performed on AD and CTL RNA samples for cerebral cortex (cortex) and cerebellum. Each marker represents the results from a single case. The error bars represent standard errors of the means. There was a significant increase in GFAP RNA in AD samples from the cerebral cortex ($P < 0.001$), but not in samples from the cerebellum

Two phenomena may contribute to this elevation in GFAP RNA in AD. The first is a reaction to neuronal degeneration occurring in AD. Acute brain lesions produce reactive astrocytosis, which involves a change in gray matter astrocytes from protoplasmic to primarily a reactive, more fibrous form (6), which develops over weeks and fades over several months (7). This increase in fibrous character is due to increased abundance of intermediate filaments constructed of GFAP (8). The chronic neurodegeneration occurring in AD may produce a persistent but somewhat smaller increase in the synthesis of this protein. A second factor contributing to the enhanced GFAP RNA abundance may be secondary to the prolonged terminal phase of many AD patients characterized by gradual wasting. In a mouse wasting model, we observed a twofold to threefold elevation of GFAP RNA, similar to that found in AD (9). We consider it plausible that the terminal phase and neurodegeneration may combine to cause the elevation of GFAP RNA found in AD samples. This increase in GFAP RNA is also consistent with the increased number of GFAP-positive astrocytes found in AD cortex (10,11), and the elevation of GFAP protein (12).

The extensive analysis of RNA yield from AD cerebral cortex conducted in this study showed no major change in total RNA recovery (Table 1), although the average yield is slightly reduced in temporal cortical samples. This is consistent with most published reports of RNA yield from AD tissue measured chemically (13-17). One group reported a 50% reduction in total RNA yields from AD cerebral cortex (4). However, these authors reported low yields compared to most groups, even in their control samples, had a small number of samples (four CTL and six AD), and remarked that the AD RNA they isolated was degraded. It is possible that the results obtained in this study derive from an unfortunate use of AD samples which happened to have highly degraded RNA. As mentioned in Results (Table 2), lower RNA integrity is observed in some AD samples, but this is not a uniform characteristic of the disorder. It is probable that uncontrolled premorbid and postmortem variables account for the RNA degradation, although we and others have demonstrated that postmortem interval per se does not lead to RNA degradation (1,18). Tissue handling may also be a critical variable, as Morrison et al (19) report that RNA from AD tissue is more sensitive to degradation if the tissue is thawed slightly prior to homogenization. It is important to recognize that the guanidinium isothiocyanate/cesium cushion method of RNA isolation is poor at recovering RNAs less than 400 nt (20). Thus, highly degraded RNA with a majority of the sequences less than 400 nt in length would be expected to give low yields by this method.

The data concerning poly(A+)RNA yield are more equivocal than total yields. While in the three regions we examined (cerebral cortex, hippocampus and cerebellum) we found no change per μg total RNA, as did Sajdel-Sulkowska and Marotta (4), others found 30–50% declines in poly(A+)RNA yield (16,17), while a third study group reported a twofold increase in poly(A+)RNA in AD brain samples (14). Wallace and Winblad (15) and Långström et al (21) report a decreased polysome yield and polysomal translation in AD tissues which is consistent with a loss of poly(A+)RNA. As we have only measured poly(A+)RNA yields from a small number of AD and CTL cortical samples, the issue of poly(A+)RNA yield in AD remains unresolved.

Anatomical evidence concerning the RNA content of neurons measured microspectrophotometrically (usually after azure blue staining) consistently finds 30–50% reductions in neuronal RNA in AD (22–25). On the surface, these anatomical measures seem contradictory to the chemical measures reporting no change in total RNA in AD. However, if one considers that the anatomically measured neurons are generally smaller in AD, and that glial RNA may increase as a percentage of total brain RNA, it is possible that both findings are correct.

In conclusion, our data suggest that the total amount of RNA in AD cortex does not change substantially per g weight, and those changes which are observed may result more from RNA degradation than reduced quantities in vivo. Moreover, major changes in the abundance of most prevalent class proteins do not occur in AD, as evaluated by in-vitro translation of CTL and AD RNAs. However, moderate shifts in the ratio of neuronal versus glial RNA sequences are probable, and changes in protein reflecting cell damage are likely, as evidenced by the large increase in RNA coding for GFAP.

Acknowledgments

D. G. M. was supported by the Anna Greenwall Award from the American Federation for Aging Research, grant AG-07892 from NIA, and an Established Investigator Award from the American Heart Association; S. A. J. was supported by the Samuel A. Blank Research Grant from the Alzheimer's Disease and Related Disorders Association; C. E. F. received support from the Alzheimer's Research Consortium of Southern California, and LEAD Award AG-7909 from NIA.

REFERENCES

1. Johnson SA, Morgan DG, Finch CE. J Neurosci Res 1986; 16: 267–80.
2. Goss JR, Finch CE, Morgan DG. Neurobiol Aging 1990 (in press).
3. Sajdel-Sulkowska EM, Majocha RE, Salim M, Fulwiler CE, Manz HJ, Zain SB, Marotta CA. Neurosci Soc Abstr 1986; 12: 1400.
4. Sajdel-Sulkowska EM, Marotta CA. Science 1984; 225: 947–9.
5. McLachlan DRC, Lukiw WJ, Wong L, Bergeron C, Bech-Hansen NT. Mol Brain Res 1988; 3: 255–62.
6. Matyja E. Exp Neurol 1986; 92: 609–23.
7. Brock TO, O'Callaghan JP. J Neurosci 1987; 7: 931–42.
8. Issacson O, Fischer W, Wictorin K, Dawbarn D, Bjorklund A. Neurosci 1987; 20: 1043–56.
9. Goss JR, Finch CE, Morgan DG. Exp Neurol 1990; 108: 266–8.
10. Schechter R, Yen SHC, Terry RD. J Neuropath Exp Neurol 1981; 40: 95–101.
11. Mancardi GL, Liwnicz BH, Mandybur TI. Acta Neuropathol (Berl) 1983; 61: 76–80.
12. Panter SS, McSwigan JD, Sheppard JR, Emory CR, Frey III WH. Neurochem Res 1985; 10: 1567–76.
13. DeKosky ST, Bass NH. Neurology 1982; 32: 1227–33.
14. Morrison MR, Griffin WST, White III CL. In Guiditta A (ed.) The role of DNA in brain activity. Boston: Martinus Nijhoff.
15. Wallace W, Winblad B. Neuropsychopharmacol Biol Psychiat 1986; 10: 657–63.
16. Taylor GR, Carter GR, Crow TJ, Johnson JA, Fairbairn AF, Perry EK, Perry RH. Exp Mol Pathol 1986; 44: 111–16.
17. Guillemette JG, Wong L, McLachlan DRC, Lewis PN. J Neurochem 1986; 47: 987–97.
18. Barton AJL, Hardy JA. Biochem Soc Trans 1985; 15: 558–9.
19. Morrison MR, Pardue S, Maschoff K, Griffin WST, White CL, Gilbert J, Roses A. Biochem Soc Transact 1986; 15: 133–4.
20. Bird RC. Biotechniques 1986; 4: 202–4.
21. Långström NS, Anderson JP, Lindroos HG, Winblad B, Wallace WC. Mol Brain Res 1989; 5: 259–69.
22. Doebler JA, Markesbery WR, Anthony A, Rhoads RE. J Neuropath Exp Neurol 1987; 46: 28–39.
23. Mann DMA. Mech Ageing Dev 1985; 31: 213–55.
24. Neary D, Snowden JS, Mann DMA, Bowen DM, Sims NR, Northen B, Yates PO, Davison AN. J Neurol Neurosurg Psychiatr 1986; 49: 229–37.
25. Uemura E, Hartmann HA. J Neuropath Exp Neurol 1978; 38: 487–96.

Address for correspondence:

Dr David G. Morgan,
School of Gerontology,
University of Southern California,
Los Angeles, CA 90089-0191, USA

53 Developing a Coherent Strategy for Locating the Gene(s) Predisposing to Alzheimer's Disease

JOHN HARDY

The isolation of the genetic locus causing systic fibrosis represents a triumph for the application of reverse genetics (1). In contrast, the controversy and uncertainty surrounding the localizing of the 'predisposing genes' for schizophrenia and affective disorder indicate that the use of the simple reverse genetic approach (as presently practised) is unlikely to solve more complex disorders (reviewed in reference 2). However, the application of molecular genetics to coronary artery disease has been successful largely because molecular biology had generated probes for useful candidate genes.

The application of reverse genetics to the problem of Alzheimer's disease has been moderately successful in that the original report of linkage to chromosome 21 (3) has been independently replicated (reviewed in reference 4). However, precise localization of the causative mutation has been disappointingly slow.

In this chapter, I briefly discuss the application of molecular genetics to cystic fibrosis, depression and schizophrenia, and coronary artery disease, and discuss what lessons can be drawn for the application of molecular genetics to Alzheimer's disease.

Localization of the mutation leading to cystic fibrosis: successful application of the reverse genetic approach to a simple genetic disorder

Cystic fibrosis is a relatively common, easily diagnosed, autosomal recessive disorder. Reverse genetics has allowed the identification of the causative mutations by the following route:

(a) Identification of genetic linkage. The inheritance of polymorphic loci of known chromosomal localization throughout the genome was followed in families multiply affected by the disorder. Eventually, markers were identified which usually cosegregated with the disease (outlined in reference 1).

Alzheimer's Disease: Basic Mechanisms, Diagnosis and Therapeutic Strategies
Edited by K. Iqbal, D. R. C. McLachlan, B. Winblad and H. M. Wisniewski
© 1991 John Wiley & Sons Ltd

(b) Identification of closer and flanking markers. The inheritance of other markers from the same chromosomal region was followed in the same families. The segregation of these latter markers was compared. In this way, flanking markers were identified (5).

(c) The genetic homogeneity of the disease was tested. Recombinants for a close flanking marker were tested to see whether these individuals were also recombinant at the flanking marker on the other side of the disease locus. If individuals had been found who were apparently recombinant at both flanking markers, it would have suggested that these cases of the disease were encoded at a different locus. Since they were not, this indicated that the disease was encoded at a single locus.

(d) The chromosomal region between the flanking markers was rigorously characterized and genes identified. The flanking markers were about 500 kb apart: in this region there were only a limited number of genes.

The important lesson to be drawn from this success story is that it was the unequivocal interpretation of recombinant individuals which allowed the disease locus to be localized and genetic homogeneity to be established. Recombination between marker loci and disease gave clear directional and positional information: even so, there were at least two genes in the region defined by genetic analysis and this led to premature hopes that the gene had been cloned two years before it was.

Localizing mutations leading to schizophrenia and affective disorder: pitfalls in the application of the reverse genetic approach to complex disorders

Schizophrenia and affective disorders are familial: most workers agree that this familiality in part reflects a genetic predisposition. However, the mode of inheritance of the disorders is not known and may be heterogeneous. While impressive pedigrees have been collected which purport to illustrate particular modes of inheritance, these large pedigrees are rare and their significance is difficult to assess because of ascertainment bias. If disorders are common and familial, families multiply affected by disease are relatively easy to find. It is dangerous to impose particular modes of inheritance upon these families, especially if the diagnosis is uncertain and the phenotype variable and common. Thus, whereas linkage analysis in cystic fibrosis had a single goal (to localize the gene), in these disorders there are two goals: determination of the mode of inheritance, and localization of the disease-causing gene(s). Since linkage analysis requires estimates of the mode of inheritance to be entered into the calculation, this is akin to trying to solve a single equation for two variables.

With this background, it is unsurprising that reports of linkage to these disorders have not been repeated (2). More sophisticated analyses, which are robust to the mode of inheritance, are needed and are being developed (reference 6). However, it is likely that programmes which co-analyse genetic information from all chromosomal linkage groups are most likely to be successful at localizing genes for such complex disorders. This is a formidable exercise which is becoming possible from a molecular point of view but is, as yet, beyond the capabilities of genetic analysis programmes. Furthermore, more complex and robust analyses require a very large amount of genetic information (i.e. very large numbers of families and thus much intergroup coordination).

The important lesson to be drawn from the debacle of the application of molecular genetics to these psychiatric disorders is that simple analyses of small numbers of families with complex inheritance of disease are unlikely to yield reproducible results. Large collaborative programmes are, despite their drawbacks, likely to be the only successful route forward.

Coronary artery disease: candidate genes help the progress towards complete understanding

Coronary artery disease is often familial. In a few rare families it segregates as an early-onset, biochemically defined dominant disorder. Cholesterol is an established risk factor for heart disease. Identification and cloning of genes related to cholesterol metabolism, identification of genetic variants within these genes and segregation analysis revealed that the rare early-onset families were caused directly by mutations within these genes. Most, however, of the familial clustering is caused by polygenic effects. The task for molecular biologists and molecular geneticists now is to identify other candidate genes and mutations and for geneticists and epidemiologists it is to ascribe the overall risk factors for coronary artery disease within the general population, recognizing that the disease may have different causes in different families (7).

Two lessons may be drawn from this story: first, that pathology-derived candidate genes offer a route forward to developing an understanding of complex disorders. Second, families with rare, severe and clearly genetic forms of the disorder offer a vital substrate to test these candidate genes upon.

Alzheimer's disease

The epidemiological genetics of Alzheimer's disease, like schizophrenia, affective disorder and coronary artery disease, are complex. However, it is considerably easier to work on the genetics of Alzheimer's disease than on the other psychiatric disorders for two reasons. First, while clinical diagnosis is difficult and uncertain, pathological confirmation is available. Second, while the disease is common in the elderly, it is very rare before the age of 60 years: within this latter group, there are many well-documented families where the disease appears to segregate as an autosomal dominant disorder. Because the disease in this age group is so rare, we can be fairly confident that the disease is actually autosomal dominant and not an artefact caused by ascertainment bias (see reference 4 et seq). In this, there are clear parallels with some biochemical subgroups of early-onset, familial coronary artery disease.

Together, these observations suggest that the early onset familial disorder is a good model for conventional linkage analysis. In contrast, they suggest that it will be much less easy to apply linkage analysis to the late-onset disorder since in this group we do not know the mode of inheritance, and the diagnosis of individuals as 'unaffected' is difficult (in an elderly population, most people will have the disease pathology). Here too, there are clear parallels with coronary artery disease.

Genetic linkage analysis by three groups using early-onset families have demonstrated linkage to chromosome 21 markers (4). This suggests that a high proportion of such cases must be caused at this locus. However, a fourth group has not observed linkage in early-onset families (8). Furthermore, a combined analysis of data from many groups, while confirming linkage, has shown that there are many apparent recombinants between the disease locus and presently available chromosome 21 markers. These latter two pieces of information suggest that the early-onset disease may be genetically heterogeneous (9). If this is the case, it will make precise genetic localization of the defects very difficult because it will not be possible to interpret recombinants in the way it was for cystic fibrosis. Precise localization of the causative gene is already hampered by the small numbers of families, their poor pedigree structure, diagnostic uncertainty, the late age of onset of the disorder and the possible occurrence of 'nongenetic' cases or genetic heterogeneity. All these factors make the observation and clear interpretation of recombination between the disease locus and close genetic markers hazardous. Because of this, it is likely that reverse genetics will only allow the identification of a region of several megabases as containing the Alzheimer gene. This means that the region known to contain the Alzheimer's disease gene on chromosome 21 will be between one and two orders of magnitude greater than the region which was known to contain the gene for cystic fibrosis.

In a disease as complex and little understood at Alzheimer's disease, it is difficult to derive with certainty a clear understanding of the pathogenesis from the pathology. There are many candidate genes suggested by the pathology. The observation that a mutation in the β-amyloid gene co-segregates with Dutch amyloid angiopathy (a disease with a remarkably similar molecular pathology to Alzheimer's disease) currently suggests that genes encoding proteins involved in amyloid processing are the most likely candidates (reviewed in reference 10). However, this lead is uncertain and it may be that amyloid deposition is a distant and late consequence of the primary pathogenic event.

Studying the molecular pathology of Alzheimer's disease will, therefore, lead to the identification of a plethora of candidate genes: the task of deciding which of these is the most likely to be causal would be extremely difficult in the absence of genetic information. However, since molecular genetics has allowed the localization of the causative gene relatively precisely, this simplifies the problem. Thus, molecular genetics and molecular pathology offer complementary routes to the pathogenesis of the disease: the former specifying a small chromosomal region, the latter a restricted range of protein functions. While there is no doubt that we are some way from understanding the disorder, the rate of progress in the study of both the molecular genetics and the molecular pathology of Alzheimer's disease gives some ground for optimism.

REFERENCES

1. Rommens JM, Iannuzzi MC, Kerem B, Drumm ML, Melmer G, Dean M, Rozmahel R, Cole JL, Kennedy D, Hidaka N, Zsiga M, Buchwald M, Riordan JR, Tsui LC, Collins FS. Identification of the cystic fibrosis gene: chromosome walking and jumping. Science 1989; 245: 1059-65.
2. Owen MJ, Mullan MJ. Molecular genetic studies of manic depression and schizophrenia. Trends Neurosci 1990; 13: 29-31.
3. St George-Hyslop PH, Tanzi RE, Polinsky R, Haines JL, Nee L, Watkins PC, Myers PC, Feldman RG, Pollen D, Drachman D, Growdon J, Bruni A, Foncin JF, Salmon D, Hobbs WJ, Conneally PM, Gusella JF. The genetic defect causing familiar Alzheimer's disease maps on chromosome 21. Science 1987; 235: 885-90.
4. St George-Hyslop PH, Myers RH, Haines JL, Farrer LA, Tanzi RE, Abe K, James MF, Conneally PM, Polinsky RJ, Gusella JF. Familial Alzheimer's disease: progress and problems. Neurobiol 1989; 10: 417-25.
5. Beaudet A, Bowcock A, Buchwald M, Cavalli-Sforza L, Farrall M, King MC, Klinger K, Lalouel JM, Lathrop G, Naylor S, Ott J, Tsui LC, Wainwright B, Watkins P, White R, Williamson R. Linkage of cystic fibrosis to two tightly linked markers: joint report from a collaborative study. Am J Hum Genet 1986; 39: 681-93.
6. Ott J. Cutting a Gordian knot in the linkage analysis of complex traits. Am J Hum Genet 1990; 46: 219-22.
7. Sing CF, Moll PP. Strategies for unravelling the bases of coronary artery disease. In Berg K, Rettersol N, Refsum S (eds). From phenotype to gene in common disorders. Copenhagen: Munksgard, 1990: 17-38.
8. Schellenberg GD, Bird TD, Wijsman EM, Moore DK, Boehnke M, Bryant EM, Lampe TH, Nochlin D, Sumi S, Deeb SS, Beyreuther K, Martin GM. Absence of linkage of chromosome 21q21 markers to familial Alzheimer's disease. Science 1988; 241: 1507-10.
9. St George-Hyslop PH, Haines JL, Farrer LA, Polinsky R, Van Broeckhoven C, Goate AM, Crapper McClachlan DR, Orr H, Bruni AC, Sorbi S, Rainero I, Foncin JF, Pollen D, Cantu JM, Tupler R, Vatanjan M, Mayeux R, Nee L, Backhovens H, Martin JJ, Rossor MN, Owen MJ, Mullan MJ, Percy ME, Karlinsky H, Rich S, Growdon J, Montesi MP, Heston L, Gusella JF, Hardy JA. Genetic linkage studies suggest that Alzheimer's disease is not a single homogeneous disorder. Nature 1990 (in press).
10. Selkoe DJ. Deciphering Alzheimer's disease: the amyloid precursor yields new clues. Science 1990; 248: 1058-60.

Address for correspondence:

John Hardy,
Dementia Research Group,
St Mary's Hospital Medical School,
Imperial College,
London W2 1PG, UK

54 Risk of Dementia in First-Degree Relatives of Patients with Alzheimer's Disease

C. M. VAN DUIJN, L. A. FARRER,
L. A. CUPPLES AND A. HOFMAN

There is much evidence for a genetic component in Alzheimer's disease. In a considerable number of families the disease is inherited as an autosomal dominant disorder. Still, 50% of the patients with Alzheimer's disease are sporadic, i.e. they have no first-degree relatives known with the disease (1-4). Since Alzheimer's disease does not express itself until middle age, it has been argued that those apparently sporadic patients may be due to reduced age-specific penetrance of a dominant disease (5). Survival analysis methods can be used to adjust for the age of relatives at the time of the study. Results of studies that have assessed the risk in relatives of Alzheimer patients using these methods have been controversial (6-8). One of the major problems in the interpretation of the former studies is that selection bias may have occurred in patient series derived from specialized clinical centers. We have assessed dementia in first-degree relatives of patients with Alzheimer's disease in a study with a complete ascertainment of early-onset patients within the period 1982-87 (4). The aim of our study was to estimate the genetic risk of dementia in relatives. If the disease can be explained solely by autosomal dominant inheritance, the lifetime risk of dementia among first-degree relatives of patients with Alzheimer's disease will approach 50%.

PATIENTS AND METHODS

The probands for this study comprised 198 patients with early-onset Alzheimer's disease (range age of onset 38-64 years). The patients were derived from a Dutch study of risk factors for the Alzheimer-type dementia (4). There were two study areas and in both study regions all patients with dementia diagnosed before the age of 70 years were ascertained with the help of geriatric services, neurology clinics, and nursing homes. The study may be considered as population based with a complete ascertainment of early-onset patients in the period 1980-87. For this study the diagnosis of Alzheimer's disease in the probands was verified independently by one of the investigators (9). All patients had a score on the clinical dementia rating

Alzheimer's Disease: Basic Mechanisms, Diagnosis and Therapeutic Strategies
Edited by K. Iqbal, D. R. C. McLachlan, B. Winblad and H. M. Wisniewski
©1991 John Wiley & Sons Ltd

scale of more than 0.5 (10), a score on the short portable mental status questionnaire below 20 (out of 30) (11) and a score on the Hachinski scale of 7 or less (12). For all patients there was an EEG or CT scan available.

Detailed data on family history were collected by interviewing a sibling or one of the parents of the patient. These data were always verified by either a second first-degree relative of the patient and/or by medical records. The age of onset of dementia in the relatives was determined as the age at which memory loss or change in behavior was first noted. If patients had been hospitalized, medical records were collected to verify the diagnosis of dementia. For nondemented relatives, the censoring age was assessed, i.e. the age at time of the study or the age at death. The study population comprised 1308 relatives, of whom 128 were known with dementia. For the 1180 nondemented relatives the average age at censoring was 62 years (SD = 19). The censoring age was unknown for 17 relatives.

Risks of dementia and the age of onset distribution among first-degree relatives were estimated using a maximum likelihood method (13). This method considers not only affected persons with known onset ages and unaffected persons with known censoring ages (i.e. those individuals typically included in the Kaplan–Meier life table analyses), but also persons for whom onset age or censoring age data are missing (13). For these latter relatives, a censoring age distribution was estimated based on the censoring distribution of the unaffected relatives with known data. The maximum likelihood estimates of risk of dementia and age of onset distribution allow for the possibility that (a) a proportion of relatives asymptomatic at the time of study may be susceptible and express the disease later in life, and (b) some deceased relatives may have succumbed to causes unrelated to Alzheimer's disease although they may have developed symptoms had they survived.

RESULTS AND DISCUSSION

The proportion of first-degree relatives with dementia is given in Figure 1. The risk of dementia in first-degree relatives of the Alzheimer probands increases rapidly after age 55 years. By the age of 102 years the risk of dementia was 0.38 (SE = 0.05). The estimated mean onset age among relatives (78 years; SE = 1.6) was 11 years greater than the observed mean age of onset of dementia in relatives, which was 67 years (SE = 1.2).

There was no significant difference in risk between male and female relatives. At age 83 years, the risk of dementia was 0.20 (SE = 0.04) for men and 0.28 (SE = 0.04) for women. After stratification for age at onset of the proband — early onset ≤ 58 years and late onset > 58 years (13) — we found that the risk of 0.49 (SE = 0.10) in relatives of patients with early onset of disease was higher than in relatives of late onset probands ($P < 0.10$) (Figure 2). There may be two explanations for this finding. First, since relatives with Alzheimer's disease tend to have similar onset ages, a higher proportion of susceptible relatives from early-onset than late-onset cases may have expressed the disease already at the time of censoring. Alternatively, in early-onset patients the disease may be more likely to be transmitted as an autosomal dominant trait.

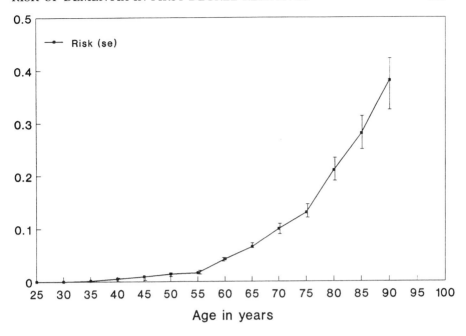

Figure 1. Risk of dementia in first-degree relatives of patients with Alzheimer's disease up to age 102 years

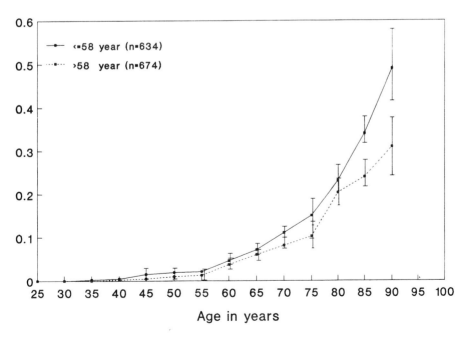

Figure 2. Risk of dementia in first-degree relatives of patients with Alzheimer's disease by onset age of probands

In agreement with earlier studies (7,8), our findings suggest that the risk of dementia in relatives is lower than expected for an autosomal dominant inherited disorder. Since we have studied dementia in first-degree relatives, and not Alzheimer's disease specifically, our data have probably overestimated the true risk of developing Alzheimer's disease. Only in relatives of patients with a disease onset before the age of 58 years, did the risk of dementia approach the value expected on the basis of autosomal dominant inheritance. If we assume that the penetrance of the disease is one by age 102, it is unlikely that all patients with Alzheimer's disease can be explained by autosomal dominant inheritance. Environmental factors or other genetic mechanisms may account for a considerable number of patients.

Acknowledgments

This work was funded by the Netherlands Organisation for Scientific Research and kindly supported by a Junior Travel Fellowship of the Alzheimer's Association (USA).

We thank H. de Bruyn, M. de Haes, J. Kamman, M. van Meurs and C. Valkenburg for their help in data collection and genealogy studies.

REFERENCES

1. Heyman A, Wilkinson WE, Stafford JA et al. Ann Neurol 1984; 15: 335-41.
2. Fitch N, Becker R, Heller A. Ann Neurol 1988; 23: 14-19.
3. Amaducci LA, Fratiglioni L, Rocca WA et al. Neurology 1986; 36: 922-31.
4. Hofman A, Schulte W, Tanja TA et al. Neurology 1989; 39: 1589-92.
5. Editorial. Science 1989; 232: 448-50.
6. Breitner JCS, Silverman JM, Mohs RC, Davis KL. Neurology 1988; 38: 207-12.
7. Farrer LA, O'Sullivan DM, Cupples LA et al. Ann Neurol 1989; 25: 485-8.
8. Sadovnick AD, Irwin ME, Baird PA, Beattle BL. Genet Epidemiol 1989; 6: 633-43.
9. McKhann G, Drachman D, Folstein M et al. Neurology 1984; 34: 939-44.
10. Hughes CP, Berg L, Danziger WL, Coben LA, Martin RL. Br J Psychiat 1982; 140: 566-72.
11. Pfeiffer E. JAGS 1975; 23: 433-41.
12. Hachinski VC, Lassen NA, Marshall J. Lancet, 1974; ii: 207-9.
13. Farrer LA, Myers RH, Cupples LA et al. Neurology 1990; 40: 395-403.

Address for correspondence:

Dr C. M. van Duijn,
Department of Epidemiology and Biostatistics,
Erasmus University Medical School,
PO Box 1738, 3000 DR Rotterdam, The Netherlands

55 Gene Expression in Embryonic, Normal and Alzheimer's Disease Brain

R. M. BAYNEY, A. S. LEE, S. K. PEKAR, M. E. KAMARCK
AND E. J. MUFSON

In the quest for the 'altered gene(s)', which possibly underlies the etiopathology or consequence of Alzheimer's disease (AD), numerous studies have documented alterations in gene expression, particularly changes in the relationship between amyloid deposition and the precursor holoprotein(s) (APP) in brain samples obtained at autopsy. Since it has been shown that the cellular distribution of mRNAs encoding APPs is not restricted to those cells which exhibit selective neuronal degeneration in AD, it is important to determine whether there is a consistent relationship between regions of the brain known to exhibit extensive neuronal degeneration and the expression of aberrant APP mRNAs in AD. Indeed, it is possible that in normal brain, there is a regionally specific, physiologically homeostatic relationship between the synthesis and degradation of APPs. The disruption of this equilibrium by pathologic events (e.g. trauma, neurotoxins, trophic depletion and neurotransmitter dysfunction) may lead to differential APP gene transcription resulting in amyloid deposition. Recently, several workers, using a variety of methodologies, have reported either increased (1-3), decreased (4-6) or unaltered (7-9) expression of the APP gene at the level of transcription in several brain subregions including cerebral cortex, hippocampus and basal forebrain in AD. The present investigation focuses on a comparison of levels of APP, microtubule-associated protein tau, and superoxide dismutase (SOD) transcripts by polymerase chain reaction amplification of reverse transcribed mRNA (PCR-RT) extracted from basal forebrain (nucleus basalis), frontal cortex (superior frontal gyrus), hippocampus, and lateral pole of the cerebellum from embryonic (3 months), neurologically normal young (28 years old) and aged (mean age 77 years, range 66-98 years), and clinically and histopathologically confirmed AD (mean age 80 years, range 69-89 years). These regions were chosen because they exhibit significant variation in amyloid deposition, neurotransmitter dysfunction, and neuronal degeneration in AD.

Alzheimer's Disease: Basic Mechanisms, Diagnosis and Therapeutic Strategies
Edited by K. Iqbal, D. R. C. McLachlan, B. Winblad and H. M. Wisniewski
© 1991 John Wiley & Sons Ltd

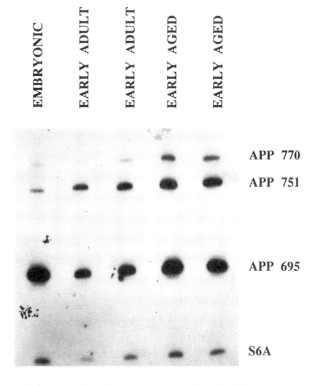

Figure 1. Developmental expression of APP gene

The utility and efficacy of PCR-RT is demonstrated by examining the ontogenic expression of the APP gene (Figure 1). Oligonucleotide primers flanking the point of alternative splicing of the APP gene (10) facilitate detection of the three major alternatively spliced gene transcripts termed APP_{695}, APP_{751} and APP_{770} from reverse transcribed mRNA isolated from tissue. This analysis demonstrates that in embryonic brain, APP_{695} is the predominantly expressed transcript accounting for 95% of total APP mRNAs (Figure 1, Table 1). In adulthood (cases a and b, Table 1),

Table 1. Developmental expression of APP gene transcripts

Stage	Total APPs[1]	% Total APPs			Ratio
		695	751	770	695 : 751 : 770
Fetal	18.7	95.7	3.4	0.9	90.0 : 3.6 : 1
Early[a]	23.9	69.1	28.3	2.6	26.9 : 11.0 : 1
Adult[b]	17.2	70.2	26.5	3.2	21.7 : 8.2 : 1
Early[a]	22.3	68.8	25.8	5.4	12.7 : 4.8 : 1
Aged[b]	22.8	65.5	28.4	6.1	10.7 : 4.6 : 1

[1]Total APP mRNAs expressed per unit of ribosomal protein S6A.
[a]Frontal cortex, [b]occipital cortex.

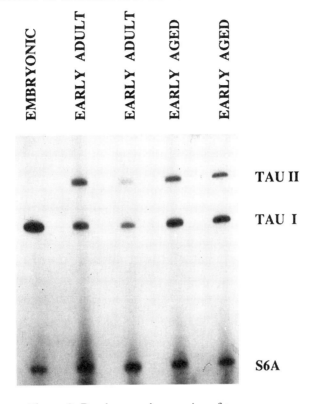

Figure 2. Developmental expression of tau gene

both APP_{751} and APP_{770} mRNA levels are increased while there is a significant reduction in APP_{695} mRNA.

Parenthetically, the ratio of APP 695 : 751 : 770 also shows a dramatic developmental decrease. These data corroborate to some extent the developmental work of Konig et al (11) using an S1 nuclease assay. Interestingly, these investigators did not observe any effect of aging on APP_{751} mRNA. A similar analysis of the developmental expression of the tau gene reveals that tau I is the exclusively spliced gene transcript in the embryonic brain (Figure 2) supporting the RNAse protection and in-situ data of

Table 2. Developmental expression of tau gene transcripts

Stage	Total taus[1]	% Total taus		Ratio Tau I : Tau II
		Tau I	Tau II	
Fetal	5.1	100	ND	
Early[a]	1.4	56.2	43.8	1.3 : 1
Adult[b]	0.6	75.2	24.8	3.0 : 1
Early[a]	2.2	67.9	32.1	2.1 : 1
Aged[b]	2.5	66.6	33.4	2.0 : 1

[1]Total tau mRNAs expressed per unit of ribosomal protein S6A.
[a]Frontal cortex, [b]occipital cortex; ND, not determined.

Table 3. APP gene expression in nucleus basalis

Case number	Total APPs	% Total APPs 695	751	770	Ratio 695 : 751
a C-M-76	5.5	57.6	38.3	4.1	1.5
b C-F-73	8.0	78.8	19.9	1.3	4.0
c C-M-71	7.3	67.5	30.0	2.5	2.3
d C-M-81	2.6	69.1	28.6	2.3	2.4
e C-F-98	2.5	63.3	29.4	7.3	2.2
f C-F-85	2.7	51.0	44.1	4.8	1.2
g AD-F-85	1.7	65.8	30.4	3.9	2.2
h AD-M-82	0.4	85.0	15.0	ND	5.7
i AD-M-69	2.0	67.8	29.7	2.6	2.3
j AD-M-89	11.7	69.0	29.4	1.6	2.3
k AD-F-78	1.3	51.9	42.6	5.5	1.2
l AD-M-76	14.8	60.1	36.1	3.8	1.7
m AD-M-80	1.9	80.9	19.1	ND	4.2

C, control; AD, Alzheimer's disease; M/F, sex; number after sex, age at death; ND, not determined.

Goedert et al (12). With age, the expression of tau II mRNA increases with a concomitant reduction in tau I mRNAs; the ratio of these transcripts ranges from 1.3–3.0 (Table 2).

Evaluation of the various forms of APP mRNA revealed their differential expression within the basal forebrain of both aged and AD patients. For example, PCR-RT demonstrated abundant (Table 3; C-F-73, AD-M-89, AD-M-76) and relatively reduced (C-F-85, AD-M-82, AD-F-78) levels of APP$_{695}$ mRNA (Figure 3). Similarly, we found variations in levels of APP$_{751}$ mRNA between normal aged and AD patients. Abundant expression was seen in cases C-F-85 and AD-F-78 whereas this mRNA was underrepresented in patients C-F-73, AD-M-82 and AD-M-80 (Table 3). Both relatively high and low levels of APP$_{770}$ mRNA are observed in both patient groups. While total APP mRNA content (expressed per unit of ribosomal

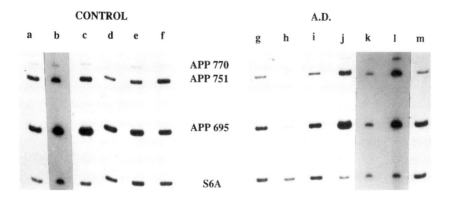

Figure 3. PCR-RT analysis of APP mRNAs in nucleus basalis of normal and AD patients

protein S6A) (13) varies over a 3.2-fold range in normal patients, this variation is significantly greater in the AD group (37-fold) (Table 3) and may be a reflection of such factors as neuronal loss, astrogliosis, and aberrant APP gene expression. In contrast to the in-situ data of Palmert et al (14) and Cohen and co-workers (15), substantial evidence was not found to correlate AD with increased expression of APP_{695} mRNA or total APP mRNAs. In frontal cortex, hippocampus and cerebellum, we observed considerable patient variability indicating both aberrant and unaltered expression independent of pathology, in the proportion of total APP mRNAs represented by APP_{695}, APP_{751} and APP_{770} mRNAs. In all but one case (data not presented) the general trend of abundance of APP mRNA transcripts was found to be APP 695 > 751 > 770. In these areas, APP_{695} accounted for between 47% and 93% of total APP mRNAs; this value was highest in cerebellum. In contrast, both APP_{751} and APP_{770} mRNAs varied over a wider range (up to 9-fold and 5-fold respectively). The PCR-RT data did not reveal a correlation between amyloid expression and an elevated APP 751 : 695 ratio as suggested by the northern and in-situ data of Johnson et al (6,16). Although in the adult brain non-neuronal cells located within the white matter (i.e. glial cells) produce appreciable APP mRNAs and changes in the levels of APP in this area may contribute to altered APP gene expression in AD (8), the present samples were composed predominantly of grey matter.

The present results indicate a heterogeneity of APP gene expression in both normal aged and AD brain. The question arose as to whether this heterogeneity was a unique feature of the APP gene. To determine this, we analysed alternative gene transcription of tau, a microtubule-associated protein, which may be aberrantly post-translationally modified and contribute to neurofibrillary tangle formation in AD. Recent findings indicate both altered (17) and unchanged (18) tau gene expression in AD. In cerebellum (Figure 4), for roughly equivalent cell copy numbers, considerable variation in total tau mRNA content was observed in both patient groups. Our data

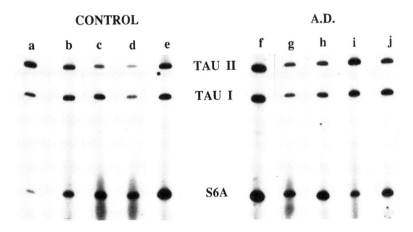

Figure 4. PCR-RT analysis of tau mRNAs in cerebellum of normal and AD patients

demonstrate that tau I mRNA is predominantly but not exclusively expressed in greater abundance than tau II mRNA. To illustrate this, tau II mRNA accounts for approximately 71% of the total tau mRNA content in patient C-M-68(a) with a calculated tau I : tau II ratio of 0.4. In other brain areas examined, with the exception of frontal cortex, cases are observed where, independent of pathology, the tau I : II mRNA ratio is < 1.0. No evidence was found to correlate AD with elevated levels of tau I mRNA.

In addition, we investigated the gene encoding Cu/Zn superoxide dismutase (SOD) which is located within the region (band q22) considered obligatory for Down's syndrome. SOD may be overexpressed (19,20) and act as a free radical scavenging enzyme in AD. Evaluation of the present PCR-RT data revealed approximately a 50% increase in SOD mRNA in the basal forebrain in AD. A similar overexpression is not observed in the other brain regions examined in this disease.

Both APP and tau genes are alternatively spliced and developmentally regulated in brain. In embryonic brain, APP_{695} and tau I mRNAs account for between 90% and 100% of their total complement of mRNAs. With age, reciprocal expression occurs between both APP and tau gene transcripts. The overall patterns of mRNA abundance are APP $695 > 751 > 770$ and tau I > tau II; these remain unaffected by AD. Evidence is found within the brain for regional variations in the absolute and relative levels of these gene transcripts. Despite significant variations in APP and tau mRNA levels in neurologically normal and AD patients, some interesting trends in the expression of these genes are observed. In frontal cortex, total APP mRNA content is reduced (mean 41%) in AD without affecting the relative levels of these transcripts. Reductions in APP_{695} mRNA in AD are correlated with an increase in APP_{770} transcript levels. Total tau mRNA content is reduced by 50% in frontal cortex in AD while the relative level of tau I : tau II is greatly reduced (mean 40%) in nucleus basalis. Like APP and tau, the abundance of SOD mRNA is regionally determined in the normal state, with an estimated increase of 50% in the nucleus basalis of AD patients. We suggest that the lack of a clear correlation between aberrant gene expression and AD may reflect, at least in part, the heterogeneous nature of gene expression in both normal and AD brain.

Acknowledgment

Support in part by the American Health Assistance Foundation (E.J.M.) is gratefully acknowledged.

REFERENCES

1. Tanaka S, Nakamura S, Ueda K, Kameyama M, Shiojiri S, Takahashi Y, Kitaguchi N, Ito H. Biochem Biphys Res Comm 1988; 157: 472-9.
2. Higgins GA, Lewis DA, Bahmanyar S, Goldgaber D, Gajdusek DC, Young WG, Morrison JH, Wilson MC. Proc Natl Acad Sci USA 1988; 85: 1297-301.
3. Tanaka S, Shiojiri S, Takahashi Y, Kitaguchi N, Ito H, Kameyama M, Kimura J, Nakamura S, Ueda K. Biochem Biophys Res Comm 1989; 165: 1406-14.
4. Goedert M. EMBO J 1987; 6: 3627-32.

5. Neve RL, Finch EA, Dawes LR. Neuron 1988; 1: 669-77.
6. Johnson SA, Rogers J, Finch CE. Neurobiol Aging 1989; 10: 267-72.
7. Zain SB, Salim M, Chou W-G, Sajdel-Sulkowska EM, Majocha RE, Marotta CA. Proc Natl Acad Sci USA 1988; 85: 929-33.
8. Golde TE, Estus S, Usiak M, Younkin LH, Younkin SG. Neuron 1990; 4: 253-67.
9. Koo EH, Sisodia SS, Cork LC, Unterbeck A, Bayney RM, Price DL. Neuron 1990; 2: 97-104.
10. Kitaguchi N, Takahashi Y, Tokushima Y, Shiojiri S, Ito H. Nature 1988; 331: 530-2.
11. Konig G, Beyreuther K, Masters CL, Schmitt HP, Salbaum JM. Prog Clin Biol Res 1989; 317: 1027-36.
12. Goedert M, Spillantini MG, Potier MC, Ulrich J, Crowther RA. EMBO J 1989; 8: 393-9.
13. Lott JB, Mackie GA. Gene 1988; 65: 31-9.
14. Palmert MR, Golde TE, Cohen ML, Kovacs DM, Tanzi RE, Gusella JF, Usiak MF, Younkin LH, Younkin SG. Science 1988; 241: 1080-4.
15. Cohen ML, Golde TE, Usiak MF, Younkin LH, Younkin SG. Proc Natl Acad Sci USA 1988; 85: 1227-31.
16. Johnson SA, McNeill T, Cordell B, Finch CE. Science 1990; 248: 854-7.
17. Kosik KS, Orecchio LD, Bakalis S, Neve RL. Neuron 1989; 2: 1389-97.
18. Goedert M, Spillantini MG, Jakes R, Rutherford D, Crowther RA. Neuron 1989; 3: 519-26.
19. Marklund SL, Adolfsson R, Gottfries CG, Winblad B. J Neurol Sci 1985; 67: 319-25.
20. Zemlan FP, Thienhaus OJ, Bosmann HB. Brain Res 1989; 476: 160-2.

Address for correspondence:

Dr R. M. Bayney,
Molecular Therapeutics Inc.,
400 Morgan Lane,
West Haven,
Connecticut 06516, USA

56 Down's Syndrome and Alzheimer Dementia: Clinical Evaluation and Genetic Association

J. J. A. HOLDEN, M. CHALIFOUX, C. CLAIRMAN, F. DALZIEL,
K. DITULLIO, D. GREER, M. KOROSSY, R. SMITH, M. WING,
L. CANBY, J. M. BERG, J. BURLEY, J. FOTHERINGHAM,
R. MACLACHLAN, D. ROBERTSON, D. STANISTREET,
I. SWIFT, B. N. WHITE AND B. D. McCREARY

Down's syndrome (DS) is the most common chromosomal disorder associated with developmental handicap, with an incidence of about 1/800 live births. Although the observation that adults with DS might develop dementia was first made more than a hundred years ago, it was not until the last few decades that the significance of the virtually universal presence of Alzheimer neuropathology found in those dying beyond age 40 years was widely appreciated (1). The importance of the association rests in part on current life expectancy findings for persons with DS: Canadian data, for example, indicate that at least 50% now survive into their 50s and 13.5% will still be alive at age 68 years (2). In addition, some investigators (3,4) have reported an excess of DS cases among relatives of individuals with Alzheimer's disease (AD). What are the clinical and health care implications of this remarkable association between the two conditions? What might systematic study reveal about the etiology and pathogenesis of each of them?

We report here our progress in a clinical and genetic research program concerned with characterizing the association between DS and AD, that was established at Queen's University in 1988 (5). A summary of our clinical assessment findings in the cohort being followed prospectively on an annual basis (including descriptions of two cases for whom both clinical and neuropathological observations are available) and the results to date of our genetic studies on families with a DS member are presented.

CLINICAL STUDIES

Until recently (6,7), relatively little published clinical and postmortem observations were available on DS subjects on whom prospective studies were initiated during life. Pooled cross-sectional information is of limited value in establishing the early

Alzheimer's Disease: Basic Mechanisms, Diagnosis and Therapeutic Strategies
Edited by K. Iqbal, D. R. C. McLachlan, B. Winblad and H. M. Wisniewski
©1991 John Wiley & Sons Ltd

features of dementia in DS and in forecasting its natural history and the services required by individual patients. In a 1986 review (8), only 45 case studies were available in which both clinical (usually retrospective) *and* pathological data were reported, and it was stressed that there was a need for prospective longitudinal studies followed by eventual postmortem examination.

Among the challenges faced by those who undertake such studies are:

(a) Establishing a clinical evaluation protocol that is useful in routine practice given that (i) available instruments (e.g. mini-mental state examination) are unsuitable for those with significant pre-existing intellectual impairment, (ii) neuro-psychological test batteries (however informative for research studies of cognitive decline) are too elaborate for routine practice, and (iii) the practical potential of various neurophysiologic and neuroradiologic procedures has yet to be established.

(b) Evaluating the additional impact on older persons with DS of (i) depression (which can mimic and coexist with dementia), (ii) mental effects of hypothyroidism (which is very prevalent in the DS population), and (iii) other chronic health problems, such as hearing and visual impairments.

(c) Maintaining the cooperation of subjects, their families and their professional advisors in completing the necessary studies, including the delicate matter of soliciting consent for postmortem examination.

Ongwanada — Queen's University program for Down's syndrome studies

A clinical-genetic program was established in 1988 (5), concerned with aging in persons with DS. The primary focus of the clinical component is to enrol and follow DS adults on an annual basis utilizing a standard protocol aimed at identifying early symptoms of AD. There are four main components for the clinical studies:

(a) *Annual neuropsychiatric review*: an informant (parent, caregiver) describes changes in personality, skills, memory, appetite, sleep and other behaviours, and a psychiatrist administers a modified mental state examination and examines gait, muscle tone and reflexes.

(b) *Laboratory assessments*: these are done in cooperation with the primary care physician and include a hemogram and thyroid function tests.

(c) *Genetic investigaiton of family*: this includes chromosome, DNA and dermatoglyphic studies on all available consenting individuals.

(d) *Neuropathological studies*: this involved postmortem brain examination when appropriate consent is provided.

Summary of clients

Of the 170 individuals with DS enrolled in our study to date, 137 (mean age 36.4 years; age range 18–60 years) showed no signs of deterioration during the previous three years, 23 (mean age 42.7 years; age range 33–62 years) had some deterioration during the past year and were classified as having possible AD, and 10 (mean age

53.2 years; age range 42–62 years) were considered to have probable AD since they had a history of deterioration during the past three years. The seizure rates for the three groups were 6%, 17% and 50%, respectively. Five clients, all with probable AD, died during the first 18 months of the study and autopsies have been completed on two cases and are in progress on two others.

In attempting to identify very early signs or changes which might be indicative of the onset of dementia in our subjects, we have examined several primitive reflexes, including the palmomental. Notably, about 50% of the subjects under 35 years old had a positive palmomental reflex compared to about 70% of those over 35 years old. We are interested in ascertaining whether individuals who test negative on first assessment change to a positive status prior to the onset of dementia. Nine individuals in our series had a negative palmomental test when first assessed and a positive one at follow-up; these persons ranged in age from 29–58 years, with a mean of 39.1 years. Clearly it is important to evaluate simple clinical tests which may serve as indicators of incipient dementia in persons with DS.

Case studies

Clinical and postmortem observations on two individuals who died after enrolment in the program are summarized below. In neither case did depression or thyroid hypofunction appear to play a significant role. In case 1 (C. H.), sensory impairments limited the scope for conducting a mental status examination. Case 2 (P. G.) obviously had advanced disease at the time of enrolment. Both had positive palmomental tests when first studied.

Case 1—C. H. (male, deceased at 60 years of age)

C. H., severely disabled for many years, remained at home until his mother could no longer care for him. At age 35 years, he began to wander and was confined to his room. He became lethargic and inactive. On institutionalization at age 45, he was obese, apathetic, had a shuffling gait, poor hearing and bilateral keratoconus and did not speak, but was able to feed and toilet himself. His Vineland social age was 1.2 years. There were no apparent changes until one week prior to death, when he refused to get out of bed, was incontinent of urine and had a stroke. He developed pneumonitis and died eight days later. His brain showed typical AD pathology and there was a large right hemisphere infarct. His case demonstrates the difficulties in recognizing AD in profoundly retarded persons and the need, already noted, for prospective longitudinal studies in order to delineate accurately the early manifestations and natural history of the disorder.

Case 2—P. G. (female, deceased at 59 years of age)

P. G.'s history reveals less severe mental retardation and a better 'quality of life'. As her maternal grandmother was schizophrenic, P. G. was admitted to an institution at 7 years. She was independent in self-help skills and worked in sheltered employment. At age 50 years, she began to have episodes of perplexity with rug hooking. At 54, she was apathetic, socially withdrawn and developed grand mal seizures. At 56, she was getting lost in familiar places. She lost toileting skills at 58, was mostly apathetic, but would also occasionally strike out at others. When enrolled in the study, she was 59 and had general increased muscle tone and positive grasp and palmomental reflexes. She died three months later. Postmortem findings showed severe Alzheimer neuropathology, with death due to aspiration pneumonia with severe tracheobronchitis. In P. G., the early development of apathy and social withdrawal, the onset of seizures, the duration of the dementia (five years, with the last two to three years in a state of confusion and dependence) and death secondary to aspiration pneumonia are quite typical of other cases reported in the literature (6,7).

GENETIC STUDIES

The observations (a) that there is an apparent excess of DS in some families with AD, and (b) that DS adults are at high risk for developing AD have led to many concerns among relatives of DS adults and health care workers as to future care and facilities for this growing group of handicapped individuals. Further, specific questions are frequently raised by family members regarding recurrence risks for DS and/or AD when one or both conditions have occurred in the family. Our study thus includes a genetic component and involves eliciting a detailed family history and undertaking chromosome, DNA and dermatoglyphic examinations on all consenting available family members.

Hypothesis

We hypothesize that some families in which both DS and AD occur have an unusual chromosome 21, involving a rearrangement (such as an inversion) which leads to less recombination on chromosome 21. This rearrangement could harbour a mutation causing AD or could result in an overproduction of some factor leading to the clinical signs of AD by position effect or some other intra/interchromosomal mechanism. Nondisjunction for chromosome 21 may be relatively common because of reduced pairing, due to the presence of an inversion. This could result in an increased probability of both AD and DS in a family. The presence of this abnormal chromosome in DS individuals could lead to symptoms of dementia at an earlier age than would occur in persons with DS without the abnormal 21-chromosome.

Predictions from the hypothesis are:

(a) Some persons with DS will have a parent or grandparent with AD, and nondisjunction will be in that parent's lineage.
(b) Reduced recombination should be evident on the nondisjoined 21s.
(c) Nondisjunction should be in meiosis I.
(d) Maternal age would not necessarily be advanced in these families.

To test the hypothesis, we are performing several genetic studies on families containing persons with DS alone or with both DS and AD. We have enrolled 42 such families to date, although only 20 have one or both parents available for study. Of the latter, 6 families have a parent or grandparent with suspected or probable AD.

Cytogenetics and DNA studies

The chromosome studies are aimed at identifying the parental origin of the extra 21-chromosome and tracing 21-chromosomes in the extended families. In addition, we are interested in identifying chromosome rearrangements, double nucleolus organizer regions (NORs), and variants which might be present and contribute to the etiology of DS. To this end, we perform G-banding, Q-banding and silver staining for NORs (9) on all available individuals. A minimum of 75 cells are examined for the presence of mosaicism and satellite association. One intellectually normal sibling has so far been found to have an unusual karyotype: 47,XX + mar, in which the marker appears to be an isochromosome-9p.

Chromosomal variants have been informative for most of the families studied. We have found the majority of nondisjunction to be maternal (14 in meiosis I; 2 in meiosis II), with only two cases of paternal meiosis II nondisjunction. We could not determine parental origin in three families.

DNA studies were performed on all individuals to confirm and extend the cytogenetic findings. DNA was extracted using an Applied Biosystems 340A Nucleic Acid Extractor. All manipulations were carried out as described elsewhere (10). Probes used for this study identified the following loci: D21S11, D21S13, D21S16, D21S24, D21S25, D21S26, D21S42, D21S82, D21S111, which span the length of chromosome 21.

Families with both DS and AD

Cytogenetic and DNA studies have proved useful in determining the origin of the extra chromosome in three of six families with both DS and AD studied to date. In all three, maternal age was advanced at the time of birth of the child with DS, so that the expectation was that the nondisjoined 21-chromosomes would be maternal. This was the case. In family DWN-040, for example, the father was diagnosed as having probable AD. The cytogenetics and a combination of D21S11, D21S82, D21S25 and D21S42 excluded a paternal origin of the extra chromosome 21, while D21S24 results excluded maternal MII. There was no evidence for recombination in the intervals examined in any of these three families.

Our results are not surprising since all three DS probands were born to mothers over the age of 35 years. Additional families are required to determine whether individuals with AD and DS probands born to mothers with lower maternal ages share the same 21 chromosome.

Dermatoglyphics

It has long been recognized that certain combinations of dermatoglyphic patterns are commoner in individuals with DS than in controls. It has been suggested that there may be unusual findings in persons with AD also (11). We therefore examined hand and footprints from all available family members to determine if there are any such unusual findings in some of the families.

Hand and footprints were studied in 131 individuals from 29 of our families. Both the Ford-Walker index (12) and the Indiana index (13) were used to analyze the prints. With the Ford-Walker index, a value of +3 characteristically occurs in DS, and with the Indiana index values of ≥ 103 are typical of the syndrome. The means for individuals with DS and those for their parents and siblings were as expected using both indices. There were no unusual findings in the three families described above with both DS and AD. However, in six other families of DS probands, parents and siblings had relatively high scores using both indices. Cytogenetic and DNA studies on these families are not yet completed, and so it is still uncertain whether higher indices are associated with a particular 21 chromosome or not.

CONCLUSIONS

Five of our clients with DS died during the first 18 months of this study. Their mean age was 55 years, similar to that found by other investigators (6,7). It appears that apathy, loss of skills and the development of seizures are typical early features of dementia in DS adults. The usual course is progressive, with death due to aspiration pneumonia 5-6 years later.

Of 20 families enrolled in the genetic study, 6 have a history of a family member with probable AD. In 3 cases, a parent of the DS proband is affected. Chromosome and DNA studies in 3 of the 6 families showed maternal origin of the extra chromosome 21, consistent with a maternal age-related etiology for the DS. Additional families in which maternal age apparently does not play a role are needed to test our hypothesis of the AD-associated 21 having a chromosome rearrangement which predisposes to nondisjunction.

The dermatoglyphic studies are interesting, in that 6 of 29 families studied showed apparent inheritance of hand and footprint characteristics which are commonly found in DS. The results of the cytogenetics and DNA studies should help to determine whether a particular chromosome 21 is associated with these unusual dermatoglyphic findings in these 6 families.

Acknowledgments

This program is sponsored in part from funds from the Ontario Ministry of Community and Social Services (to B. D. M. and J. J. A. H.) and from a research grant (MCSS Research Grants Program) administered by the Research and Program Evaluation Unit of that Ministry in cooperation with the Ontario Mental Health Foundation.

REFERENCES

1. Oliver C, Holland A. Psychol Med 1986; 16: 307-22.
2. Baird P, Sadovnick A. Hum Genet 1989; 82: 291-2.
3. Heston L. Science 1977; 196: 322-3.

4. Heyman A, Wilkinson WE et al. Ann Neurol 1983; 14: 507-15.
5. Holden JJA. In Denholm CJ (ed.) Preparing for the year 2000 national conference. Victoria: University of Victoria, 1990; 113-19.
6. Lai F, Williams R. Arch Neurol 1989; 46: 849-53.
7. Evenhuis H. Arch Neurol 1990; 47: 263-7.
8. Dalton A, Crapper-McLachlan D. Psychiatr Clin North Am 1986; 9: 659-70.
9. Holden JJA, Reimer DL, Higgins MJ, Roder JC, White BN. Cancer Genet Cytogenet 1985; 14: 131-46.
10. Sood R, White BN, Holden JJA. Am J Hum Genet 1990 (in press).
11. Weinreb HJ. Arch Neurol 1985; 42: 50-4.
12. Walker NF. Pediatr Clin N Am 1958; 5: 531-43.
13. Reed TE, Borgaonkar DS et al. J Pediatr 1970; 77: 1024-38.

Address for correspondence:

Dr J. J. A. Holden,
Cytogenetics and DNA Research Laboratory,
Ongwanada, 191 Portsmouth Avenue,
Kingston, Ontario, K7M 8A6, Canada.
Tel. 613-548-4417, ext 192
Fax. 613-548-8135

57 Characterization of Two Blocks of Cis-Acting Regulatory Elements Modulating the Expression of the Gene Encoding the Alzheimer's Amyloid Precursor Proteins

DEBOMOY K. LAHIRI AND NIKOLAOS K. ROBAKIS

The promoter region of the Alzheimer's amyloid precursor proteins (APP) contains several regulatory elements including five copies of the GGGCGC sequence located between positions -107 and -188, consensus sequences recognized by the transcription factors SP-1 and AP-1, a rich GC region characteristic of housekeeping genes and a heat shock element (9,10). It has been suggested that an increase in the transcriptional activity of this gene might result in the formation of the β-amyloid protein which aggregates to form the amyloid depositions observed in Alzheimer's disease and Down's syndrome. To determine the promoter sequence requirements for the expression of the gene encoding the APP, chimeric plasmids containing different parts of the promoter region of the APP gene linked to the bacterial chloramphenicol acetyl transferase (CAT) gene were constructed. Sequences derived from the 5'-flanking region were then tested for their effects on β-amyloid promoter activity by transfection and transient CAT expression in PC-12 and HeLa cells. In PC-12 cells there is a significant increase in basal promoter activity after deletion of certain sequences from the 5'-flanking region. The maximum increase was observed when the promoter sequences were reduced to 0.7 kb from 1.2 kb. Similar increase, though less pronounced, is observed in HeLa cells. However, further deletion of 150 base pairs (bps) resulted a sharp decrease in promoter activity in both cell lines indicating that this region contains cis-acting elements which stimulate the expression of APP gene. Interestingly, in both cell lines there was a gradual and significant increase in promoter activity upon further deletion, with a construct containing only 250 bps of flanking sequence displaying the strongest promoter activity. This construct contains three of the five GC boxes present in the amyloid promoter. Further deletion of 125 bps abolished all activity. These results indicate that there are two blocks of sequence which modulate the expression of APP gene promoter. One block extending from -600 to -460 bps acts as a positive regulator because its deletion results in a dramatic decrease in promoter activity. A second block of

Alzheimer's Disease: Basic Mechanisms, Diagnosis and Therapeutic Strategies
Edited by K. Iqbal, D. R. C. McLachlan, B. Winblad and H. M. Wisniewski
© 1991 John Wiley & Sons Ltd

sequences extending from −450 to −150 bps acts like a negative regulator as its removal results in increase in promoter activity. Our observations suggest that by imposing conformational constraints, these sequences might control the binding of *trans*-acting factor(s) on the APP gene promoter and thus modulate its expression.

INTRODUCTION

Alzheimer's disease (AD) is characterized by neuronal loss, the development of neurofibrillary tangles and amyloid depositions in the form of extracellular plaques and cerebrovascular amyloid. Amyloid depositions consist of a self-aggregating protein of 42 or 43 residues termed β-protein or A4 peptide (1,2). This peptide exists as a component of at least three distinct precursor proteins, referred to as APP_{695}, APP_{751}, and APP_{770}, encoded by a chromosome 21 gene (3-7). The human APP gene promoter has been cloned and shown to contain a high GC region with five GGGCGC boxes (8,9). The region upstream of the start site lacks any of the consensus sequence usually found in class II type eukaryotic promoters, such as CAAT and TATA boxes. Thus the APP gene promoter displays the characteristics of a 'housekeeping' gene. Other regulatory elements present in the APP gene promoter include a heat shock element and consensus sequences for the binding of the transcription factors AP-1 and SP-1 (9,10). Although the APP gene is expressed in the brain as well as in peripheral tissues, total APP mRNA levels seem to be highest in brain and kidney, intermediate in spleen, adrenal gland and lung, and lowest in liver, indicating that tissue-specific factors may regulate the expression of this gene. In the brain APP is expressed in both neuronal and non-neuronal cells (11). Interestingly, in-situ hybridization studies have indicated that various neuronal subpopulations contain different levels of APP mRNA (12,13) and in-vitro studies of primary rat neuroglia cultures have shown that APP is expressed only by astrocytes type I (14). In Down's syndrome there seems to be a dysregulation of the expression of this gene since the difference in the levels of total APP mRNAs between these patients and normal persons is much higher than the difference expected from the gene dosage ratio of 3:2 (15). In addition, it has been reported that in AD certain brain regions display a substantial increase in the level of the APP mRNA compared to normal persons (13,16). It is, therefore, important to characterize factors which regulate the expression of the APP gene. To this end we recently constructed plasmid pAmylCAT which contains 1.1 kb of 5'-flanking sequence of the APP gene and displayed promoter activity in several cell lines including HeLa and PC-12 cells. In the present study we present evidence showing that the promoter region of the APP gene contains at least two different regulatory elements which modulate its transcriptional activity.

EXPERIMENTAL PROCEDURES

Cell culture, transfection and CAT assay

HeLa cells were grown in Dulbecco's modified Eagle's medium (DMEM) with 10% horse serum and 5% fetal calf serum. Rat PC-12 cells were grown in RPMI media

(GIBCO). Twenty-four hours before transfection, the cells were seeded on polylysine coated dishes at a density of 10^5 cells per dish. Transfection was carried out by the calcium phosphate precipitate procedure using 25 μg of the CAT plasmids as described by Gorman et al (17). Cell extracts were prepared 48 hours after transfection. To assay for CAT activity (in total 100 μl), 25 μl of 1 M Tris Cl pH 7.2, 5 μl of 45 mM acetylCoA and 0.5 μl of [^{14}C] chloramphenicol were added to cell extracts, containing 25–40 μg of total protein. Transfection efficiency was adjusted by co-transfection with pRSV-βgal plasmid. After 2 hours of incubation at 37 °C, the chloramphenicol and acetylated derivatives were separated by ascending silica gel thin-layer chromatography (TLC) in chloroform:methanol (95:5) at room temperature. The TLC sheets were then air dried and autoradiographed. Radioactive spots were quantitated by liquid scintillation counter. Duplicate samples were used in each experiment.

Construction of deletion plasmids

The coding region of the enzyme chloramphenicol acetyl transferase (CAT) was used as a reporter for the activity of the AAPP promoter (17). Plasmid pAmylCAT was constructed by inserting a 1.2-kb PstI-BamHI fragment of the amyloid promoter into the polylinker region of pBLCAT3 in front of the CAT gene (18). This fragment contains 1100 bp upstream from the main transcription start site, and the first 105 bp of the transcribed sequence plasmid pAmylCAT is active in both PC-12 and HeLa cells (9). Deletion plasmids (pAmy1D^x) containing different lengths of upstream promoter sequences were constructed by linearizing pAmylCAT with restriction enzyme PstI followed by Bal31 nuclease digestion. The resultant plasmids were recircularized using Klenow and ligase enzyme. Eight deleted plasmids, pAmylD1 to pAmylD8, were obtained (Figure 1). The plasmids were isolated and purified by CsCl centrifugation and the exact deletion point was determined by Sanger's dideoxy sequencing method (19) using synthetic primers and the Sequenase kit (United States Biochemical Corporation). The 5'-end of the subcloned fragments is shown in Figure 1. The level of expression of these plasmids was measured by CAT assay following transfection.

Checking pAmylCAT in reverse orientation

To check the promoter activity of the 1.2-kb fragment in both orientations, the fragment was inserted in its natural orientation, in the polylinker region of plasmid pGCAT-A by forced cloning. Plasmid pGCAT-C was used to insert the promoter in the reverse orientation. These plasmids were kindly supplied to us by Dr T. Frebourg (Laboratory of Molecular Oncology, Cedex, France) and differ only by the orientation of their polylinkers (20).

RESULTS

Analysis of the sequence requirements for transcriptional activity of the APP promoter

A fragment containing 1100 bp of the APP gene promoter plus the first 100 bp of transcribed sequence (−1100 to +100) displayed high promoter activity when placed

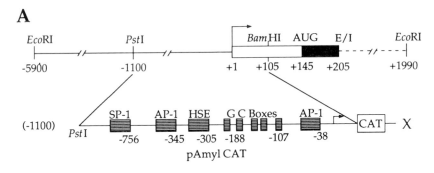

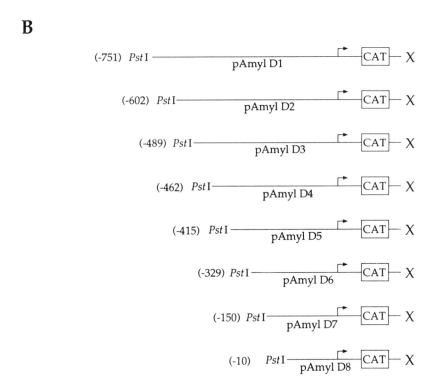

Figure 1. Schematic diagram of the APP gene promoter and construction of plasmids pAmylD1–D8. (A) An illustration of the transcriptional elements of the APP promoter region. Arrow indicates the direction of transcription. HSE is heat shock element and AP-1 and SP-1 are potential binding sites for transcriptional factors. Each GC box represents one copy of the sequence GGGCGC. The CAT box represents the coding sequence of the CAT enzyme. Solid line represents untranscribed region, open box and closed boxes denote 5'-untranslated and translated regions respectively. Broken line represents intron sequences and E/I is the site for exon–intron junction. (B) Construction of deletion plasmids pAmylD1–D8. Plasmids pAmylD1 through pAmylD8 were constructed by inserting different parts of the promoter into pBLCAT3 as shown above. Numbers at left represent the 5'-end of each deletion. X represents the remaining sequence of plasmid pAmylCAT

in front of the CAT gene in plasmid pAmylCAT (9). However, this fragment displayed no promoter activity when placed in front of the CAT gene in reverse orientation (see 'experimental procedures' section). To determine the sequences required for transcription of the APP gene, a series of progressive deletions from position -1100 bp to -10 bp, relative to the transcription start site of the APP promoter, was generated from plasmid pAmylCAT as described earlier (Figure 1). The resultant plasmids were then transfected into HeLa or PC-12 cells and the activity of the APP gene promoter was followed by measuring the CAT activity. To control for transfection efficiency, cells were co-transfected with pβgal-TK, a plasmid containing the bacterial β-galactosidase gene fused to the thymidine kinase (TK) promoter. To minimize anomalies specific to particular plasmid preparations, the experiment was repeated with two independent plasmid preparations. To quantitate the CAT activity, the radioactive TLC spots containing the acetylated derivatives of chloramphenicol were counted and the percentage conversion was calculated for each plasmid. For comparative purposes, the maximum conversion by plasmid D3 (for HeLa cells) and D2 (for PC-12 cells) was arbitrarily given a value of 100 and then the extent of conversion by other plasmids was expressed to this value.

In HeLa cells

As shown in Table 1, in HeLa cells there is a small decrease in the APP promoter activity after the first deletion, which is followed by an increase in promoter activity upon further deletions of up to 500 bp. The highest promoter activity in this cell line is observed with plasmid pAmylD3 (Table 1). Deletion of an additional 28 bp resulted in plasmid pAmylD4 which displayed a dramatic decrease in promoter

Table 1. Assay of the promoter activity of the deletion plasmids in HeLa and PC-12 cells. HeLa or PC-12 were transfected with deletion plasmids pAmylD1 to pAmylD8 shown in Figure 1 and CAT activity was measured in the cell extracts as described in the 'Experimental procedures' section. The spots of the autoradiogram of the TLC were counted and the promoter activity was quantitated as percentage conversion of [^{3}H] chloramphenicol to acetylated derivatives. In HeLa cells promoter activity was expressed relative to the activity of plasmid pAmylD3 (maximum activity) and in PC-12 cells relative to plasmid pAmylD2 (maximum activity)

Plasmids	HeLa cells	PC-12 cells
pAmylCAT	92	28
pAmylD1	51	80
pAmylD2	79	100
pAmylD3	100	31
pAmylD4	15	8
pAmylD5	30	20
pAmylD6	40	19
pAmylD7	58	28
pAmylD8	12	7
pBLCAT3	9	5

activity, suggesting the presence of a strong enhancer-like element within this DNA fragment. Interestingly, construction of further deletion plasmids resulted in a gradual although incomplete recovery of the promoter activity up to plasmid pAmylD7 which contains 150 bp of upstream sequences (Table 1). Similar results were obtained in PC-12 cells (see below), indicating the presence of a transcription attenuator. Further deletion of 140 bp results in total loss of promoter activity, indicating that essential functions of the APP promoter reside in this 150-bp fragment immediately upstream from the transcription start site.

In PC-12 cells

In PC-12 cells the first promoter deletion (plasmid pAmylD1) results in a substantial increase in promoter activity. This is in contrast to the effect of this deletion (pAmylD1) in HeLa cells where an almost 40% decrease in promoter activity was observed. This differential effect suggests that this promoter domain may respond to cell-specific *trans*-acting factors. Deletion of an additional 150 bp yields plasmid pAmylD2 which shows the highest activity in this system (Table 1). Elimination of the next 114 bp results in a threefold decrease in promoter activity in PC-12 cells. Since in HeLa cells deletion of the same region had little effect on the activity of the APP promoter (Table 1), this result suggests that the effect of this 114-bp portion on the activity of the amyloid promoter may be specific to PC-12 cells. Deletion of the next 28 bp resulted in a significant decrease in promoter activity. Since a similar response was observed in HeLa cells, this result indicates that this DNA region may act as a universal transcription stimulator for the APP gene. In agreement with the results obtained in HeLa cells, further deletions resulted in partial recovery of the promoter activity in PC-12 cells with maximum activity displayed by construct pAmylD7. In addition, and similar to the results obtained in HeLa cells, construct pAmylD8 displayed the promoter activity to the level of control plasmid in the PC-12 cell line.

DISCUSSION

Although APP is found in almost every tissue examined, its expression levels vary considerably (11–15). In the brain, the expression of this gene seems to depend both on the particular region examined as well as on the neuronal population. In addition different glial subpopulations may express different levels of APP (14).

These studies suggest that the expression of this gene is regulated by tissue or cell-specific factors which may modulate the synthesis of APP mRNA by interacting with specific regulatory sequences of the APP gene. The experiments described here constitute the first attempt to identify specific *cis*-acting regulatory regions of the APP gene promoter. The reporter CAT gene was used to measure the effect of sequence deletion on the APP promoter activity. Since previous experiments indicated that the expression of the APP gene is modulated by cell-specific factors, we used two different cell lines in our experiments: neuron-like pheochromocytoma cell line (PC-12) and HeLa cells. Our results indicate that the effect of certain regions of the amyloid promoter on its activity depends on the particular cell line used. Deletion of the first 500 bp seems to have very little effect on the activity of the APP promoter in HeLa cells, while in PC-12 cells deletion of the same region induced a threefold increase in the promoter activity. These results suggest that in PC-12 cells the region −1100 to −602 may act as a negative element and that this activity may be mediated by factors specific to PC-12 cells. Deletion of a 28-bp fragment from −489 to −462 resulted in a large decrease of the promoter activity in both cell lines, suggesting that this region may be part of an enhancer element. This conclusion was further supported by the stimulation of the activity of the heterologous TK promoter by a 38-mer synthetic oligonucleotide encompassing the region −489 to −452. Placement of one copy of this oligonucleotide in front of the TK promoter increased its activity threefold, while placement of three copies in tandem increased the TK promoter activity ninefold (data not shown). Further deletions of promoter sequences resulted in partial recovery of the promoter activity in both cell lines, suggesting that the region extending from −450 to −150 may act as a general negative regulator. Similarly acting sequences have been detected in the promoter of the collagen gene (21). Deletion of the next 140 bp resulted in a complete loss of the promoter activity in both cell lines, indicating that this region contains all the essential promoter elements of the APP gene. Interestingly this region includes three of the five GC boxes of the APP promoter, two of which are arranged in tandem between −146 and −134, the AP-1 site at position −41 and a region between −26 and −2 which displays a high degree of dyad symmetry with five other regions proximal to the transcriptional start site (9).

In summary, our results indicate that the activity of the APP gene promoter is mediated by at least two *cis*-acting elements: an enhancer-like element within the region from −600 to −450 bp and a negative element extending from position −450 to −150. In addition, the essential promoter elements of the APP gene seem to be present in a region extending about 150 bp upstream of the transcription start site. Further analysis of this region of the APP gene will determine the exact sequence requirements for its expression as well as any *trans*-acting factors which may interact with the APP promoter and modulate its activity.

Acknowledgments

This work was supported by grants AG08200 and AG05138. We thank Dr T. Frebourg (France) for providing us with the plasmids pGCAT-A and pGCAT-C. We are also grateful to Drs G. LaFauci and S. R. Salton for their help and comments.

REFERENCES

1. Glenner GG, Wong CW. Biochem Biophys Res Comm 1984; 122: 1131-5.
2. Masters CL, Simms G, Weinman NA, Multhaup G, McDonald BL, Beyreuther K. Proc Natl Acad Sci USA 1985; 82: 4245-9.
3. Kang J, Lemaire HG, Unterbeck A, Salbaum JM, Masters CL, Grezeschik K-H, Multhaup G, Beyreuther K, Muller-Hill B. Nature 1987; 325: 733-6.
4. Robakis NK, Ramakrishna N, Wolfe G, Wisniewski HM. Proc Natl Acad Sci USA 1987; 94: 4190-4.

5. Ponte P, Gonzalez-DeWhitt P, Schilling J, Miller J, Hsu D, Greenberg B, Davis K, Wallace B, Lieberburg I, Fuller F, Cordell B. Nature 1988; 331: 525-7.
6. Tanzi RE, McClatchey AI, Lomberti ED, Villa-Komaroff L, Gusella JF, Neve RL. Nature 1988; 331: 527-30.
7. Kitaguchi N, Takahashi Y, Tokushima Y, Shiojiri S, Ito H. Nature 1988; 331: 530-2.
8. Lahiri DK, LaFauci G, Salton S, Robakis NK. J Cell Biol 1988; 107: 293.
9. LaFauci G, Lahiri DK, Salton S, Robakis NK. Biochem Biophys Res Comm 1989; 159: 297-304.
10. Salbaum JM, Weidemann A, Lemaire HG, Masters CL, Beyreuther K. EMBO J 1988; 7: 2807-813.
11. Robakis NK, Lahiri DK, Brown HR, Rubenstein R, Mehta P, Wisniewski H, Goller N. In Swann JW (ed.) Disorders of the developing nervous system: changing views on their origins, diagnoses and treatments. New York: Alan R. Liss, 1988: 183-93.
12. Bahmanyar J, Higgins GA, Goldgaber D, Lewis DA, Morrison JH, Wilson ML, Shankar SK, Gajdusek DC. Science 1987; 237: 77-80.
13. Higgins GA, Lewis DA, Bahmanyar S, Goldgaber D, Gajdusek DC, Young WG, Morrison JH, Wilson MC. Proc Natl Acad Sci USA 1988; 85: 1297-301.
14. Berkenbosch F, Refolo LM, Friedrich VL, Casper D, Blum M, Robakis N. Neurosci Res 1990; 25: 431-40.
15. Neve RL, Finch EA, Dawes LR. Neuron 1988; 1: 669-77.
16. Palmert MR, Golde TE, Cohen ML, Kovacs DM, Tanzi RE, Gusalla JF, Usaiak MF, Younkin LH, Younkin SG. Science 1988; 241: 1080-4.
17. Gorman CM, Moffat LF, Howard BH. Mol Cell Biol 1982; 2: 1044-53.
18. Luckow B, Schutz G. Nucl Acids Res 1987; 15: 5490.
19. Sanger F, Nicklen S, Coulson AR. Proc Natl Acad Sci USA 1977; 74: 5463-67.
20. Frebourg T, Brison O. Gene 1988; 65: 315-18.
21. Mudryj M, Crombrugghe BD. Nucl Acids Res 1988; 16: 7513-26.

Address for correspondence:

Dr Nikolaos K. Robakis,
Department of Psychiatry and
Fishberg Research Center for Neurobiology,
Mount Sinai School of Medicine,
City University of New York,
New York, NY 10029, USA

58 The Common Origin of Familial Alzheimer's Disease in Calabria

A. C. BRUNI, M. P. MONTESI, G. GEI, I. RAINERO,
C. ERMIO AND J. F. FONCIN

The many problems encountered in familial Alzheimer's disease (FAD) linkage studies by molecular geneticists, and the discordant results obtained by different study groups, could be explained through genetic heterogeneity (1,2). The problems are aggravated when the families used are not large enough to generate reliable quantitative data, and occur mostly when dealing with late-onset FAD. To overcome these obstacles, linkage studies should ideally be done on single, very large kindreds with a sufficient number of informative matings. Three large plurigenerational families affected by dominant Alzheimer's disease — N (3,4), To (5) and RB — have been recently discovered; they originate from the same region of southern Italy and show a strong phenotypic similarity. Since family N has been instrumental in the mapping of the FAD gene (6), the addition of two other large genealogically related kindreds might be enough to reach significance within one kindred and thence to bypass difficulties arising from possible heterogeneity.

METHODS

All families were investigated through the same ascertainment method, that is the genealogical 'blanket method' (7,8). The following statistical methods were applied to quantitative and qualitative aspects in order to verify homogeneity. We used one-way analysis of variance (ANOVA) and the Kruskal-Wallis test to compare the age at death on the three families. We compared with the Student's t-test the age at onset and duration of disease in families N and To; in RB family, age at onset is known in too few instances to be informative. Chi-squared test was used to compare clinical symptoms of patients whose history was fully known.

RESULTS

Family N now numbers 6250 subjects in 13 generations. The earliest obligate carrier, born 1715 in the village of S. (province Catanzaro), is the common ancestor of 13 obligate carriers and 61 patients in successive generations (Figure 1); 9 were histopathologically confirmed. Family To groups more than 1500 subjects

Alzheimer's Disease: Basic Mechanisms, Diagnosis and Therapeutic Strategies
Edited by K. Iqbal, D. R. C. McLachlan, B. Winblad and H. M. Wisniewski
© 1991 John Wiley & Sons Ltd

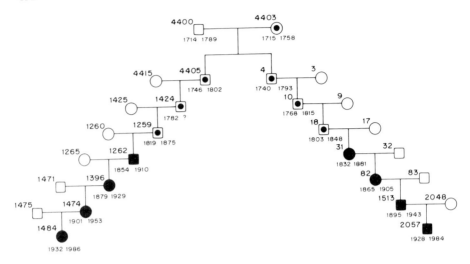

Figure 1. Common ancestors of different branches of family N. □ , male; ○, female; ■ ●, affected; ▣ ◉, obligate carriers; identifying number of subject in left upper corner; date of birth and death below symbols

in 8 generations with 22 affected. The apparent origin (in 1769) of family To is the city of C., near the village of S. in which N family originated. RB family has been studied only recently; it groups up to now 200 members in 7 generations starting at the beginning of the nineteenth century. Seven patients are identified. They originate from the village of R.B., 16 miles from C. and 22 miles from S. (Figure 2). Formal genetic data and quantitative phenotypic features of these families are given in Table 1. The frequency of typical clinical symptoms is shown in Table 2. Quantitative and qualitative traits are not significantly different in all three families. Transmission is autosomic dominant with sex ratio not significantly different from 1:1.

CLINICAL PICTURE

Early onset with anxiety, depression, loss of interest, personality change and progressive forgetfulness is followed by cognitive syndrome. Amnesia for recent events, disorientation, aphasia, agnosia and apraxia evolve smoothly but slowly, together with neurological signs: exaggerated deep tendon reflexes, rigidity, slow and stiff gait. Akinesia and amimia produce in the patient the aspect of a wax statue. Delusions and hallucinations often lead to a diagnosis of psychosis; combined with restlessness, they perturb the patient's family more than the dementia does and may lead to psychiatric institutionalization. With further evolution of dementia, the patients rapidly become totally bedridden; myoclonic jerks and epileptic seizures are the hallmarks of the terminal stage. Death from pneumonia or kidney infections comes, in most cases, after a total course of about eight years.

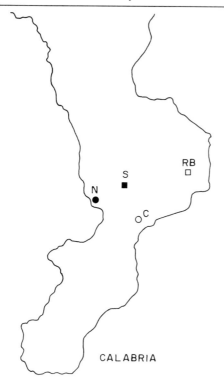

■ Origin of family 'N' (17th century)
● Present concentration of family 'N' (19th-20th century)
○ Present concentration of family 'TO' (18th-20th century)
□ Present concentration of family 'RB'

Figure 2. Calabria region (southern Italy) with the origin and the present concentration of FAD families.

Table 1.

	Family N	Family To	Family RB
Age of onset (years)			
mean	42.85	42.67	NC
SD	6.45	3.68	
Duration (years)			
mean	6.91	6.27	NC
SD	3.80	3.74	
Age at death (years)			
mean	49.76	49.44	49.50
SD	5.73	4.95	5.68
Segregation ratio	0.58	0.56	0.56
Sex ratio	1:1	1:0.47	1:2.5

Table 2.

Symptom	Family N	Family To	Family RB
PPS	30/36 (83%)	11/13 (85%)	4/4 (100%)
Myoclonus	23/36 (64%)	9/13 (69%)	2/4 (50%)
EPS	13/36 (36%)	1/13 (8%)	1/4 (25%)
Seizures	12/36 (33%)	4/13 (31%)	2/4 (50%)

PPS, Pseudopsychotic stage; EPS, extrapyramidal signs.

CONCLUSION

The strong symptomatologic similarity found in these three families could be explained by allelic identity by descent, as suggested by their close geographic origin. Many other (apparently) small clusters with early-onset FAD are found in our region. As a consequence it is fundamental to apply the methods of genetic epidemiology to verify this hypothesis. We think that a 'founder' effect could by postulated, due to the relative isolation and stability of the Calabrian population until the early twentieth century. These conditions are similar to those described by Bird (9) for the Volga Germans. We hope to be able to prove this hypothesis in the future through the identification of a common (carrier) ancestor, as we did in the past for apparently distinct branches of family N (10).

Acknowledgments

Work by the authors reported in this chapter was supported by SMID-Center; CNR grant 89.00326.75; Bilateral Project CNR–INSERM 1989-90.
    I. R. is recipient of an award from the French Foundation for Alzheimer Research.

REFERENCES

1. Bird TD, Shellemberg GD, Wijsman EM, Martin GM. Neurobiol Aging 1989; 10: 332-434.
2. Farrer LA, Myers RH, Cupples LA, St George-Hyslop PH, Bird TD, Rossor MN, Mullan MJ, Polinsky R, Nee L, Heston L, Van Broeckoven C, Martin J-J, Crapper-McLachlan D, Growdon JH. Neurology 1990; 40: 395-403.
3. Foncin JF, Supino-Viterbo V. Excerpta Medica International Congress Series 296 1973; 63-4.
4. Foncin JF, Salmon D, Supino-Viterbo, Feldman RG, Macchi G, Mariotti P, Scoppetta C, Caruso G, Bruni AC. Rev Neurol (Paris) 1985; 141: 194-202.
5. Bergamini L, Bruni AC, Gei G, Montesi MP, Ermio C, Pinessi L, Foncin JF. Alz Dis Assoc Disord 1989; 3 (suppl. 1): 4.
6. St George-Hyslop PH, Tanzi RE, Polinsky RJ, Haines JL, Nee L, Watkins PC, Myers R, Feldman R, Pollen D, Drachman D, Growdon J, Bruni AC, Salmon D, Frommelt P, Amaducci L, Sorbi S, Piacentini S, Stewart GD, Hobbs WJ, Conneally PM, Gusella JF. Science 1987; 235: 885-890.
7. Foncin JF, Salmon D, Bruni AC. In: Miner GD, Richter RW, Blass JP, Valentine JL, Winters-Miner LA (eds) Familial Alzheimer's disease. Molecular genetics and clinical perspectives. New York, Basel: Marcel Dekker, 1989; 45-53.

8. Foncin JF, Salmon D, Bruni AC. In Sinet PM, Lamour Y, Christen Y (eds) Genetics and Alzheimer's disease. Berlin: Springer, 1988; 13-30.
9. Bird TD, Lampe TH, Nemens EJ, Miner JW, Sumi SM, Schellenberg GD. Ann Neurol 1988; 23: 25-31.
10. Gei G, Foncin JF, Bruni AC. Fidia Biomed Inf 1988; 8: 8-11.

Address for correspondence:

Dr A. C. Bruni,
Centro Smid-Sud,
Via dei Campioni,
88046 Lamezia Terme (CZ), Italy

59 Construction of a Physical Map of Chromosome 21q in Relation to Alzheimer's Disease

WIM VAN HUL, GUY VAN CAMP, HUBERT BACKHOVENS,
PIET STINISSEN, ANITA WEHNERT,
JULIE KORENBERG AND CHRISTINE VAN BROECKHOVEN

A gene predisposing to Alzheimer's disease (AD) has been located on the proximal long arm of chromosome 21 close to the marker loci D21S13/D21S16 and D21S1/D21S11. However, a more precise localization of the AD gene has been hampered by lack of information on the relative positions and of the exact physical distances between the chromosome 21 markers located in this region. We aimed at constructing a complete physical map of the region between the centromere and D21S1/D21S11 using pulse field gel electrophoresis. At present our pulse field map consists of three major parts located around the marker loci D21S13/D21S16, D21S52 and D21S1/D21S11 and spanning in total 5700 kb of the proximal chromosome 21q arm.

INTRODUCTION

Conclusive linkage results were obtained in four families segregating autosomal dominant Alzheimer's dementia (AD) with early onset of the disease symptoms (< 60 years) and two marker loci, D21S16 and D21S1/D21S11 (1). The linked markers are located on the proximal long arm of chromosome 21 in the 21q11.2–21q22.2 region. However, at the time of the initial linkage report the relative positions of D21S16 and D21S1/D21S11 were unknown. Further linkage analysis studies suggested that D21S16 is tightly linked to the marker D21S13 (2), previously located centromeric of D21S1/D21S11 (3). Physical mapping using pulse field gel electrophoresis proved the close proximity of D21S13 and D21S16 (2). Additional linkage analysis studies with both D21S13 and D21S16 in early-onset AD families indicated that the AD gene is located centromeric of D21S1/D21S11, close to D21S13/D21S16 and therefore closer to the centromere (4,5). The physical map positions of the marker loci D21S13, D21S16 and D21S1/D21S11 have recently been confirmed and updated using an extended somatic cell hybrid panel and pulse field gel electrophoresis (6-8).

Alzheimer's Disease: Basic Mechanisms, Diagnosis and Therapeutic Strategies
Edited by K. Iqbal, D. R. C. McLachlan, B. Winblad and H. M. Wisniewski
© 1991 John Wiley & Sons Ltd

Significantly higher recombination rates have been suggested for the region centromeric of D21S1/D21S11 (3) preventing an accurate estimate of the physical distance between D21S16 and D21S1/D21S11. Further, the physical distance between D21S16 and the centromere is not yet known. Therefore, we aimed at constructing a complete physical map of the region between the centromere and D21S1/D21S11 by pulse field gel electrophoresis.

MATERIAL AND METHODS

Probes

The plasmid DNA probes pPW228C (D21S1), pPW233F (D21S4), pPW236B (D21S11) and pPW511–1H (D21S52) were kindly provided by P. Watkins (9); pGSE9 (D21S16), pGSM21 (D21S13), pGS4U (D21S110) and pJG90 (D21S95) by G. Stewart (10,11) and 26C (D21S26) by A. Millington-Ward (12). In the case of probe 26C we used a subclone pVH-ZT, containing a 1.2-kb EcoRI single copy DNA fragment in pUC18. The probes SF85 (D21S46) and SF105 (D21S48) were obtained from J. Korenberg (13).

Pulse field gel electrophoresis

Fresh human lymphocytes or chromosome 21 hybrid WA17 cells (14) were captured in agarose plugs (15) and the DNA was digested overnight with the rare-cutting restriction enzymes under conditions recommended by the supplier. The rare-cutting restriction enzymes BssHII, EagI, NotI, NarI, SfiI, SacII were obtained from New England Biolabs, MluI and NaeI from Boehringer. Electrophoresis was carried out in 1% agarose gels in 0.5× Tris borate buffer at 15 °C using the LKB 2015 Pulsaphor with a hexagonal electrode array. Separation of 50 kb to 1000 kb DNA molecules was achieved at 180 V for 40 hours using pulse times of 65 seconds. Fragments up to 2000 kb were resolved at 100 V during a 5-day run with pulse times starting at 100 seconds and linearly augmenting to 500 seconds. Chromosomes from *Saccharomyces cerevisiae* YP148 and *Candida albicans* were loaded on the gel as size markers.

Southern blot hybridization

The plasmid DNA probes were digested with the appropriate restriction enyzme, recovered from low melting point agarose gels and labelled with (α-^{32}P) dCTP using a random primer labelling kit (BRL).

After electrophoresis the genomic DNA was transferred in 10× SSC to Hybond N+ (Amersham) nylon membranes. The nylon filters were hybridized at 68 °C in buffer containing 7% SDS, 0.5 M Na$_2$HPO$_4$/NaH$_2$PO$_4$ pH 7.2, 1 mM EDTA (16) with the radiolabelled probes and washed in SSC containing 0.1% SDS. The SSC concentration in the wash solutions depended on the stringencies required.

RESULTS

We used eleven chromosome 21 DNA markers and pulse field gel electrophoresis to construct a physical map of the proximal long arm of chromosome 21 including the marker loci D21S13/D21S16, D21S52 and D21S1/D21S11. All three marker loci have been linked to familial AD (4,17). The order and subregional chromosomal localization of the chromosome 21 markers have recently been reanalyzed using an extended somatic cell hybrid panel (6). The marker D21S16 is the closest marker to the centromere, located in 21q11.1, D21S13 is in 21q11.2, D21S52 in 21q21.1 and D21S1/D21S11 in 21q21.2. The physical map order of the markers is consistent with their genetic map order (3): centromere—D21S13/D21S16—D21S52—D21S1/D21S11—telomere.

The region around D21S13/D21S16

We previously constructed a physical map of 1700 kb around the marker D21S13 comprising the marker D21S16 and using five rare-cutting restriction enzymes (8). The marker D21S13 contains an HTF island with sites for three of the five rare-cutting restriction enzymes and therefore acts as a linking probe, bringing together the two regions located on both sides of D21S13. In this study we were able to refine and extend the physical map to 2200 kb using higher resolution pulse field gels and fresh lymphocyte DNA digested with combinations of eight rare-cutting restriction enzymes. Further, we mapped three additional chromosome 21 markers D21S26, D21S46 and D21S48 to the 2200-kb region. A detailed map is presented in Figure 1. The marker D21S13 contains restriction sites for six of the eight rare-cutting restriction enzymes used, confirming the presence of the HTF island in this marker. The position of the marker D21S16 was slightly changed due to alterations in the positions of some of the rare-cutting restriction sites. The marker D21S16 is localized centromeric of D21S13 at a distance of 420 to 620 kb, results that are in agreement with those of Owen et al (7). Further, the clones D21S46 and D21S48 mapped on opposite sites of D21S13. Both these markers have previously been mapped in the 21pter-21q21.2 region but polymorphisms have not been reported (13). The marker D21S48 detected the same fragments as D21S16 and therefore mapped centromeric of D21S13 within the same distance as D21S16. The exact physical order of the probes D21S16 and D21S48 remains to be solved. The marker D21S46 is located 180 to 300 kb telomeric of D21S13. Similar mapping results for D21S46 and D21S48 have been reported by Owen et al (7). Further, physical and genetical mapping studies indicated that the marker D21S26 is located in 21q11.2-q21.1 and tightly linked to both D21S13 and D21S16 (18). On the pulse field map D21S26 is located telomeric of D21S13, separated by only one restriction site. The minimal distance between D21S26 and D21S13 is 10 kb; the maximal distance is 170 kb. Since D21S16 is the closest marker to the centromere the physical map order of this region is: centromere—D21S16/D21S48—D21S13—D21S26—D21S46—telomere.

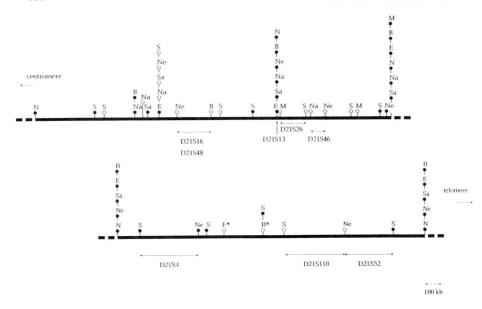

Figure 1. Physical map of the chromosome 21q arm. The map was constructed using DNA of fresh human lymphocytes or the chromosome 21 cell hybrid WA17 digested with the rare-cutting restriction enzymes: BssHII (B), EagI (E), MluI (M), NotI (N), NaeI (Ne), NarI (Na), SfiI (S) and SacII (Sa), separated by pulse field gel electrophoresis and hybridized with radiolabelled probes representing the chromosome 21 loci indicated by arrows below the map. Symbols: open and filled circles are restriction sites, respectively partially or completely cut by the restriction enzyme indicated. The restriction sites marked with an asterisk were detected only in DNA of the hybrid cell lines

The region around D21S52

In addition to the marker D21S52 we used two other markers, D21S4 and D21S110. The marker D21S4 is located physically closer to the centromere near the locus D21S13, while the marker D21S110 is in the same region as D21S52 (6). Our mapping results using DNA digested with six rare-cutting restriction enzymes, either single or in paired combinations, indicated that D21S52 shared one fragment of 1900 kb with both the markers D21S4 and D21S110 for four out of the six enzymes. These results are suggestive of the localization of the three markers between two HTF islands. The pulse field map between the two HTF islands is shown in Figure 1. Absence of sufficient restriction sites in DNA of fresh lymphocytes made it at first impossible to gain information on the exact order of the three markers between the HTF islands. Indeed, the ordering of markers using pulse field gel electrophoresis depends largely on the observation of overlapping fragments. It is, however, known that DNA in cultured cell lines is less methylated and therefore more frequently cut by the methylation-sensitive rare-cutting restriction enzymes. We used DNA of the chromosome 21 hybrid cell line WA17 and found two additional restriction sites, one BssHII and one EagI site, which were extremely helpful in determining the relative order of the markers D21S4, D21S110 and D21S52. Taking into account the centromeric position of the marker D21S4 the physical order of the markers in this region is: centromere−D21S4−D21S110−D21S52−telomere.

The region around D21S1/D21S11

The marker locus D21S1/D21S11 consists of two markers which proved to be genetically inseparable (1). The pulse field mapping results obtained on fresh lymphocyte DNA digested with several rare-cutting restriction enzymes indicated that the two markers D21S1 and D21S11 are physically close at a maximum distance of 150 kb. Further the markers D21S1 and D21S11 shared a BssHII fragment of around 1600 kb. A similar sized BssHII fragment is also recognized by the marker D21S95 previously mapped in the same chromosomal area as D21S1 and D21S11 (6). However, detailed mapping is needed to confirm the co-localization of the markers D21S95 and D21S1/D21S11 and to define the exact order and orientation of the markers towards the centromere.

DISCUSSION

Using pulse field gel electrophoresis we were able to construct a partial pulse field map covering 5700 kb of the 21q arm and consisting of three major parts located around the marker loci D21S13/D21S16, D21S52 and D21S1/D21S11, loci that have previously been linked to familial AD. No major discrepancies were found between our pulse field mapping results and those of Gardiner et al (6) and Owen et al (7). However, in contrast with the latter investigators, we obtained more detailed information in regard to the distances and physical map order of markers located in the candidate AD region.

The mapping results in Figure 1 illustrate that the map around D21S13/D21S16 ends with a cluster of rare-cutting restriction sites, while the map around D21S52 begins with one. The clustering of rare-cutting restriction sites is a first indication for the presence of an HTF island (19). Preliminary mapping results of Owen et al (7) indicated that D21S46 and D21S4 hybridized to one SalI fragment of 1500 kb obtained after partial DNA digestion, implicating that the two HTF islands are separated by a maximal distance of 1000 kb. It can, however, not be excluded that both HTF islands are in fact identical, connecting the two parts of the physical map together. Further, HTF islands are frequently present within the promoter sequence of housekeeping genes (20). Therefore clusters of rare-cutting restriction sites in a pulse field map may be considered as markpoints for genes. It has already been shown that the HTF island in D21S13 is associated with an expressed sequence (8,21). Each sequence isolated from the AD candidate region containing an HTF island may, if expressed, be considered part of a candidate gene for familial AD.

In order to obtain an accurate idea of the distance of D21S16 to the centromere and of the correlation between the genetical and physical map distances between the markers linked to familial AD, it is essential to bridge the three remaining gaps in our current physical map. To do so, additional chromosome 21 markers will be used together with high-resolution physical mapping techniques.

Acknowledgments

This work was in part funded by the National Fund for Scientific Research, the National Incentive Programme on Fundamental Research in Life Sciences, the Flemisch Biotechnology Programme and Innogenetics, Inc., Belgium.

G.V.C. is a research assistant and C.V.B. a research associate of the National Fund for Scientific Research, Belgium.

REFERENCES

1. St George-Hyslop PH, Tanzi RE, Polinsky RJ, Haines JL, Nee L, Watkins PC, Myers RH, Feldman RG, Pollen D, Drachman D, Growdon J, Bruin A, Foncin J-F, Salmon D, Frommelt P, Amaducci L, Sorbi S, Piacentini S, Stewart GD, Hobbs WJ, Conneally PM, Gusella JF. Science 1987; 235: 885-90.
2. Van Broeckhoven C, Van Hul W, Backhovens H, Raeymaekers P, Van Camp G, Stinissen P, Wehnert A, De Winter G, Gheuns J, Vandenberghe A. In Sinet PM, Lamour Y, Christen Y (eds) Genetics and Alzheimer's disease. Berlin: Springer, 1988: 124-9.
3. Tanzi RE, Haines JL, Watkins PC, Stewart GD, Wallace MR, Hallewell R, Wong C, Wexler NS, Conneally PM, Gusella JF. Genomics 1988; 3: 129-36.
4. Goate AM, Haynes AR, Owen MJ, Farral M, James LA, Lai LYC, Mullan MJ, Roques P, Rossor MN, Williamson R, Hardy JA. Lancet 1989; i: 352-5.
5. Van Broeckhoven C et al. In Bunney WE, Hippius H, Laakmann G, Schmauss (eds) Neuropsychopharmacology. Berlin, Heidelberg: Springer-Verlag, 1990: 86-91.
6. Gardiner K, Horisberger M, Kraus J, Tantravahi U, Korenberg J, Rao V, Reddy S, Patterson D. EMBO J 1990; 9: 25-34.
7. Owen MJ, James LA, Hardy JA, Williamson R, Goate AM. Am J Hum Genet 1990; 46: 316-22.
8. Stinissen P, Van Hul W, Van Camp G, Backhovens H, Wehnert A, Vandenberghe A, Van Broeckhoven C. Genomics 1990; 7: 119-22.
9. Watkins PC, Tanzi RE, Gibbons KT, Tricoli JV, Landes G, Eddy R, Shows TB, Gusella JF. Nucl Acids Res 1985; 13: 6075-88.
10. Stewart GD, Harris P, Galt J, Ferguson-Smith MA. Nucl Acids Res 1985; 13: 4125-32.
11. Galt J, Boyd E, Connor JM, Ferguson-Smith MA. Hum Genet 1989; 81: 113-19.
12. Millington-Ward A, Wassenaar ALM, Pearson PL. Cytogen Cell Genet 1985; 40: 699.
13. Korenberg JR, Croyle ML, Cox DR. Am J Hum Genet 1987; 41: 963-78.
14. Raziuddin A, Sarkar FH, Dutkowski R, Shulman L, Ruddle FH, Gupta SL. Proc Natl Acad Sci USA 1984; 81: 5504-8.
15. Van Ommen GJB, Verkerk JMH. In Davies KE (ed.) Analysis of human genetic disease. Oxford: IRL Press, 1986: 113-33.
16. Church GM, Gilbert W. Proc Natl Acad Sci USA 1984; 81: 1991-5.
17. St George-Hyslop PH et al. Nature 1990; 347: 194-7.
18. Van Hul et al (submitted for publication).
19. Brown WR, Bird AP. Nature 1986; 322: 477-81.
20. Lindsay S, Bird AP. Nature 1987; 327: 336-8.
21. Neve RL, Stewart GD, Newcombe P, Van Keuren ML, Patterson D, Drabkin HA, Kurnit DM. Gene 1986; 49: 361-9.

Address for correspondence:

Dr C. Van Broeckhoven,
Neurogenetics, Department of Biochemistry,
Born-Bunge Foundation, University of Antwerp,
Universiteitsplein 1, B-2610 Antwerp, Belgium

Part IX

ANIMAL MODELS

60 Model Systems Relevant to Alzheimer's Disease

DONALD L. PRICE, VASSILIS E. KOLIATSOS, LEE J. MARTIN,
LARY C. WALKER, RICHARD E. CLATTERBUCK,
EDWARD H. KOO, SANGRAM S. SISODIA,
WILLIAM C. MOBLEY AND LINDA C. CORK

The principal neuropathological abnormalities of Alzheimer's disease (AD) include degeneration of neurons in specific cell populations; neurofibrillary tangles; senile plaques (abnormal neurites around deposits of amyloid); and congophilic angiopathy (1,2). This review focuses on several models that provide significant new insights into processes relevant to several of these abnormalities, i.e. the mechanisms of amyloidogenesis and alterations in the viability of basal forebrain cholinergic neurons. First, we describe recent findings concerning the in-vitro processing, in-vivo localization, and axonal transport of the amyloid precursor protein (APP) (3–5). Second, we outline recent studies of the formation of plaques (with an emphasis on the evolution of neuritic abnormalities and the deposition of amyloid) in aged macaques (5–10). These animals develop age-related brain abnormalities, including swollen neurites, some of which accumulate APP; neurites in proximity to deposits of $\beta/A4$; the presence of $\beta/A4$ and α_1-antichymotrypsin (ACT) in plaques and around blood vessels; and neuronal atrophy and abnormal cytoskeletal immunoreactivities in perikarya of some nerve cells. Finally, we discuss investigations of animals with experimental lesions of the fimbria-fornix (11), which cause degenerative changes in basal forebrain cholinergic neurons, and the use of nerve growth factor (NGF) to prevent degeneration of these cells (12).

THE BIOLOGY OF APP IN VITRO AND IN VIVO

The APP gene, localized to human chromosome 21 (13), gives rise to alternatively spliced messenger ribonucleic acids (mRNAs) that encode APP_{695} (13); APP_{751}, which is identical to protease nexin-II (14,15); and APP_{770} (16–18). The two longer forms of APP mRNA contain sequences with homologies to the Kunitz family of protease inhibitors as does a fourth alternatively spliced transcript that encodes a 563 amino acid polypeptide lacking the $\beta/A4$ region and transmembrane and cytoplasmic domains of the other forms of APP (19). An integral membrane glycoprotein, APP, is secreted in cultured cells as a COOH-terminal truncated

Alzheimer's Disease: Basic Mechanisms, Diagnosis and Therapeutic Strategies
Edited by K. Iqbal, D. R. C. McLachlan, B. Winblad and H. M. Wisniewski
©1991 John Wiley & Sons Ltd

molecule. APP isoforms are present in brain, and, in AD, APP appears to be abnormally cleaved to form β/A4, the principal component of amyloid found in senile plaques and in the walls of blood vessels (20). Beta/A4 is a 4-kilodalton β-pleated molecule that includes between 12 and 14 amino acids of the transmembrane domain and between 24–28 amino acids of the adjacent extracellular domain of APP (21–23).

Processing in transfected cells

Following transfection of normal or mutated APP complementary DNAs into cultured mammalian cells, transmembrane APPs are cleaved, and the amino terminal domain is secreted (4,24). Sisodia and colleagues (4) have recently documented, for the first time, that the cleavage event is membrane associated and requires transmembrane sequences and the proximal 11 amino acids of the adjacent extracellular region. This finding implies that normal processing results in truncation of APP within the β/A4 domain, a conclusion confirmed by a recent study that obtained C-terminal amino acid sequence data of the secreted form of APP (25). It is not currently known if APP is identically processed in neurons as in transfected cells, but, if APP is processed in this way, it would not be possible for nerve cells to form β/A4 under normal circumstances. It is probable that the normal processing of APP is significantly compromised in affected cells in the brains of individuals showing amyloid deposits, i.e. aged nonhuman primates and older humans with Down's syndrome or AD. In these settings, we suggest that, in some degenerating neurons, APP is abnormally cleaved, leaving β/A4 intact and capable of self-assembling into amyloid fibrils.

Axonal transport

Koo and colleagues (3) recently demonstrated that, within neurons of the dorsal root ganglia of rats, APP is carried in axons by the fast anterograde transport system. In these studies, two classic ligation paradigms were used to study the transport of APP in sciatic nerve. In these peripheral nerves, APP accumulated progressively in segments adjacent to the proximal ligature. Rates of accumulation were consistent with APP being carried by rapid transport; the kinetics of APP accumulation resembled those of acetylcholinesterase (rapidly transported) but not β-tubulin (slowly transported) (26). When lumbar dorsal root ganglia were first microinjected with labeled methionine in the same experimental paradigm, immunoprecipitation demonstrated an accumulation of labeled APP proximal to the first ligature, indicating that the accumulation of APP in nerves originated from labeled neuronal perikarya. Finally, immunocytochemistry localized APP immunoreactivity within swollen axons of segments of nerve adjacent to the proximal ligature. Thus, APP is synthesized in neurons, is carried by fast axonal transport, and accumulates proximally in ligated axons. The fate of the molecule at the nerve terminal, however, is unclear.

Immunoreactivity in primate cortex

In monkey brain, APP mRNAs are expressed in cortical neurons (9,27), and APP immunoreactivity is readily detected in cell bodies and proximal dendrites of pyramidal neurons in layers III and V (5). APP immunoreactivity is also present in axon hillocks, in initial segments, and in axons; throughout the cortical neuropil, APP immunoreactivity is also seen in fine punctate deposits that have the light-microscopic appearance of synaptic terminals (5). Consistent with this interpretation is the presence of synaptophysin immunoreactivity in similar patterns of distribution.

AMYLOIDOGENESIS IN AGED MONKEYS

To date, the best animal model to study cerebral amyloidogenesis is the aged nonhuman primate. Macaques more than 25 years of age, which commonly exhibit impairments on a variety of tasks (28,29), develop senile plaques similar to those occurring in aged humans and in subjects with AD (6,7). Cork and colleagues have studied the temporal development of plaques in the brains of monkeys ranging in age from 15-35 years. Abnormal fibers and neurites appear in cortex at the end of the second decade (6,10,30), and these neurites are derived from a number of populations of cholinergic, catecholaminergic, and peptidergic neurons (30-35). Fiber and neuritic abnormalities increase with age and may precede the majority of β/A4 deposits (10), which, in turn, may precede the appearance of ACT, a serine protease inhibitor associated with amyloid (8,10). Although mature senile plaques and congophilic angiopathy appear somewhat later than neurites, both types of lesions are found in the majority of rhesus monkeys more than 25-28 years of age (6,10).

More recent investigations have focused on processes that underlie amyloidogenesis (5-7,9,10). Major age-related alterations in relative levels of APP expression in brain have not been detected in aged monkeys (9), and it seems unlikely that simple changes in levels of expression are the key event in amyloidogenesis in nonhuman primates. It appears more likely that aberrant translational processing in neurons may be important in the genesis of parenchymal amyloid deposits in these monkeys. Consistent with this idea is the observation that many APP-immunoreactive neurites are often decorated by or capped by β/A4 deposits. On the basis of our recent studies (4,5,10), we have hypothesized that some abnormal neurites accumulate transported APP, and, at these sites, APP may be abnormally processed (possibly by actions of proteases or their inhibitors); the result is the liberation of β/A4, which assembles into amyloid fibrils.

EFFECTS OF NGF ON EXPERIMENTAL DEGENERATION OF SEPTAL NEURONS

Basal forebrain cholinergic neurons, located in the medial septum, diagonal band, and substantia innominata (36-40), provide the principal cholinergic innervation of the amygdala, hippocampus, and neocortex of primates (41,42). NGF receptors are expressed on basal forebrain neurons of primates (43,44). In AD, some basal forebrain neurons become atrophic, and it is likely that some nerve cells may show reduced levels of ChAT activity (45,46). Eventually, these cells degenerate (47,48), leading to reductions in cholinergic markers in targets (49–51). Some of these features can be recapitulated in transection of axons of the fimbria-fornix (11). In this experimental paradigm, there is evidence of cell atrophy in these cholinergic neurons, reduced levels of ChAT immunoreactivity, and alterations in elements of the neuronal cytoskeleton. Moreover, there is progressive reduction in the number of ChAT-immunoreactive cell bodies (11,52–58). Following the lesion (3–4 weeks), there is evidence of cell loss (11,56,58–61). Because axotomized basal forebrain cholinergic neurons show some features in common with abnormal cholinergic nerve cells present in the basal forebrain in cases of AD, they provide a model to ask whether experimental degeneration of these cells can be prevented by intraventricular administration of NGF (62,63).

In rat, NGF prevents degenerative changes in basal forebrain cholinergic neurons axotomized by transection of the fimbria-fornix (57,64–68). Because the amino acid sequences of NGF and its receptor are highly conserved across species (69–73), we hypothesized that intraventricular administration of mouse NGF would also prevent degeneration of axotomized basal forebrain cholinergic neurons in nonhuman primates (74). Following transection of the fornix, animals were allowed to survive for two weeks, during which time half of the subjects were treated with NGF. In animals receiving vehicle alone, the number of ChAT-immunoreactive medial septal neurons was reduced by approximately 50% ipsilateral to the lesion. Remaining ChAT-immunoreactive neurons appeared smaller than those in control, unoperated animals. Treatment with NGF prevented reductions in the number and size of cholinergic neurons in the medial septal nucleus. Adjacent sections stained with ChAT and NGF receptor immunocytochemistry revealed that these markers are co-localized in >95% of neurons of the medial septal nucleus in all groups of animals. Thus, mouse NGF profoundly influences the process of axotomy-induced retrograde degeneration in these cholinergic neurons in nonhuman primates. Recent studies indicated that recombinant human NGF (rhNGF) prevents axotomy-induced abnormalities in basal forebrain cholinergic neurons of rats (12). Finally, preliminary studies suggest that rhNGF also has protective effects on nonhuman primate medial septal neurons damaged in the same experimental paradigm (12). The in-vivo effectiveness of mouse NGF and rhNGF on primate basal forebrain cholinergic neurons suggests that this trophic factor may be useful in ameliorating the acetylcholine-dependent, age-associated memory impairments that occur in nonhuman primates (28,29,75).

CONCLUSIONS

This review has focused on several models relevant to issues raised by studies of the neuropathology of AD: the biology of APP in vitro and in vivo; amyloidogenesis in the brains of aged nonhuman primates; and degenerative changes in basal forebrain cholinergic neurons following fimbria-fornix lesions and the effects of treatment with NGF on phenotypic alterations in these cells. In different ways, these investigations provide illustrations of the extraordinary utility of animal models for studies of the mechanisms and treatment of neurological disorders.

Acknowledgments

This work was supported by grants from the US Public Health Service (NIH NS 07179, AG 05539, AG 05146, NS 20471) as well as the Metropolitan Life Foundation, the Robert L. & Clara G. Patterson Trust, and the American Health Assistance Foundation. Dr Price is the recipient of a Javits Neuroscience Investigator Award (NIH NS 10580). Drs Price and Koo are recipients of an award from the National Institute of Aging, Leadership and Excellence in Alzheimer's Disease (AG 07914).

REFERENCES

1. Price DL. Annu Rev Neurosci 1986; 9: 489-512.
2. Selkoe DJ. Annu Rev Neurosci 1989; 12: 463-90.
3. Koo EH, Sisodia SS, Archer DR, Martin LJ, Weidemann A, Beyreuther K, Fischer P, Masters CL, Price DL. Proc Natl Acad Sci USA 1990; 87: 1561-5.
4. Sisodia SS, Koo EH, Beyreuther K, Unterbeck A, Price DL. Science 1990; 248: 492-5.
5. Martin LJ, Sisodia SS, Koo EH, Cork LC, Dellovade TL, Weidemann A, Beyreuther K, Masters C, Price DL. Proc Natl Acad Sci USA (in press).
6. Struble RG, Price DL Jr, Cork LC, Price DL. Brain Res 1985; 361: 267-75.
7. Selkoe DJ, Bell DS, Podlisny MB, Price DL, Cork LC. Science 1987; 235: 873-7.
8. Abraham CR, Selkoe DJ, Potter H, Price DL, Cork LC. Neuroscience 1989; 32: 715-20.
9. Koo EH, Sisodia SS, Cork LC, Unterbeck A, Bayney RM, Price DL: Neuron 1990; 2: 97-104.
10. Cork LC, Masters C, Beyreuther K, Price DL. Am J Pathol (in press).
11. Koliatsos VE, Applegate MD, Kitt CA, Walker LC, DeLong MR, Price DL. Brain Res 1989; 482: 205-18.
12. Koliatsos VE, Applegate MD, Clatterbuck RE, Burton LE, Mobley WC, Hefti F, Price DL. Soc Neurosci Abstr 1990; 16: 296.
13. Kang J, Lemaire H-G, Unterbeck A, Salbaum JM, Masters CL, Grzeschik K-H, Multhaup G, Beyreuther K, Müller-Hill B. Nature 1987; 325: 733-6.
14. Oltersdorf T, Fritz LC, Schenk DB, Lieburg I, Johnson-Wood KL, Beattie EC, Ward PJ, Blacher RW, Dovey HF, Sinha S. Nature 1989; 341: 144-7.
15. Van Nostrand WE, Wagner SL, Suzuki M, Choi BH, Farrow JS, Geddes JW, Cotman CW, Cunningham DD. Nature 1989; 341: 546-9.
16. Kitaguchi N, Takahashi Y, Tokushima Y, Shiojiri S, Ito H. Nature 1988; 331: 530-2.
17. Ponte P, Gonzalez-DeWhitt P, Schilling J, Miller J, Hsu D, Greenberg B, Davis K, Wallace W, Lieburg I, Fuller F, Cordell B. Nature 1988; 331: 525-7.
18. Tanzi RE, McClatchey AI, Lampert ED, Villa-Komaroff L, Gusella JF, Neve RL. Nature 1988; 331: 528-30.
19. de Sauvage F, Octave J-N. Science 1989; 245: 651-3.
20. Müller-Hill B, Beyreuther K. Annu Rev Biochem 1989; 58: 287-307.
21. Glenner GG, Wong CW. Biochem Biophys Res Comm 1984; 120: 885-90.
22. Masters CL, Multhaup G, Simms G, Pottgiesser J, Martins RN, Beyreuther K. EMBO J 1985; 4: 2757-63.
23. Wong CW, Quaranta V, Glenner GG. Proc Natl Acad Sci USA 1985; 82: 8729-32.
24. Weidemann A, König G, Bunke D, Fischer P, Salbaum JM, Masters CL, Beyreuther K. Cell 1989; 57: 115-26.
25. Esch FS, Keim PS, Beattie EC, Blacher RW, Culwell AR, Olstersdorf T, McClure D, Ward PJ. Science 1990; 248: 1122-4.

26. Grafstein B, Forman DS. Physiol Rev 1980; 60: 1167-83.
27. Bahmanyar S, Higgins GA, Goldgaber D, Lewis DA, Morrison JH, Wilson MC, Shankar SK, Gajdusek DC. Science 1987; 237: 77-9.
28. Presty SK, Bachevalier J, Walker LC, Struble RG, Price DL, Mishkin M, Cork LC. Neurobiol Aging 1987; 8: 435-40.
29. Bachevalier J, Landis LS, Walker LC, Brickson M, Mishkin M, Price DL, Cork LC. Neurobiol Aging (in press).
30. Kitt CA, Struble RG, Cork LC, Mobley WC, Walker LC, Joh TH, Price DL. Neuroscience 1985; 16: 691-9.
31. Struble RG, Hedreen JC, Cork LC, Price DL. Neurobiol Aging 1984; 5: 191-8.
32. Struble RG, Kitt CA, Walker LC, Cork LC, Price DL. Brain Res 1984; 324: 394-396.
33. Kitt CA, Price DL, Struble RG, Cork LC, Wainer BH, Becher MW, Mobley WC. Science 1984; 226: 1443-5.
34. Walker LC, Kitt CA, Cork LC, Struble RG, Dellovade TL, Price DL. J Neuropathol Exp Neurol 1988; 47: 138-44.
35. Walker LC, Kitt CA, Struble RG, Schmechel DE, Oertel WH, Cork LC, Price DL. Neurosci Lett 1985; 59: 165-9.
36. McKinney M, Struble RG, Price DL, Coyle JT. J Neurosci 1982; 7: 2363-8.
37. Hedreen JC, Bacon SJ, Cork LC, Kitt CA, Crawford GD, Salvaterra PM, Price DL. Neurosci Lett 1983; 43: 173-7.
38. Mesulam M-M, Mufson EJ, Levey AI, Wainer BH. J Comp Neurol 1983; 214: 170-97.
39. Mesulam M-M, Mufson EJ, Levey AI, Wainer BH. Neuroscience 1984; 12: 669-86.
40. Koliatsos VE, Price DL. In Richardson RT (ed.) Functional aspects of the basal forebrain. Boston: Birkhauser (in press).
41. Lehmann J, Struble RG, Antuono PG, Coyle JT, Cork LC, Price DL. Brain Res 1984; 322: 361-4.
42. Struble RG, Lehmann J, Mitchell SJ, McKinney M, Price DL, Coyle JT, DeLong MR. Neurosci Lett 1986; 66: 215-20.
43. Hefti F, Hartikka J, Salvatierra A, Weiner WJ, Mash DC. Neurosci Lett 1986; 69: 37-41.
44. Schatteman GC, Gibbs L, Lanahan AA, Claude P, Bothwell M. J Neurosci 1988; 8: 860-73.
45. Perry RH, Candy JM, Perry EK, Irving D, Blessed G, Fairbairn AF, Tomlinson BE. Neurosci Lett 1982; 33: 311-15.
46. Pearson RCA, Sofroniew MV, Cuello AC, Powell TPS, Eckenstein F, Esiri MM, Wilcock GK. Brain Res 1983; 289: 375-9.
47. Whitehouse PJ, Price DL, Struble RG, Clark AW, Coyle JT, DeLong MR. Science 1982; 215: 1237-9.
48. Arendt T, Taubert G, Bigl V, Arendt A. Acta Neuropathol (Berl) 1988; 75: 226-32.
49. Bowen DM, Smith CB, White P, Davison AN. Brain 1976; 99: 459-96.
50. Davies P, Maloney AJF. Lancet 1976; ii: 1403.
51. Perry EK, Gibson PH, Blessed G, Perry RH, Tomlinson BE. J Neurol Sci 1977; 34: 247-65.
52. Daitz HM, Powell TPS. J Neurol Neurosurg Psychiat 1954; 17: 75-82.
53. McLardy T. J Comp Neurol 1955; 103: 305-24.
54. Sofroniew MV, Pearson RCA, Eckenstein F, Cuello AC, Powell TPS. Brain Res 1983; 289: 370-4.
55. Pearson RCA, Sofroniew MV, Powell TPS. Brain Res 1984; 311: 194-8.
56. Gage FH, Wictorin K, Fischer W, Williams LR, Varon S, Bjorklund A. Neuroscience 1986; 19: 241-55.
57. Hefti F. J Neurosci 1986; 6: 2155-62.
58. Armstrong DM, Terry RD, DeTeresa RM, Bruce G, Hersh LB, Gage FH. J Comp Neurol 1987; 264: 421-36.
59. Applegate MD, Koliatsos VE, Price DL. Soc Neurosci Abstr 1989; 15: 408.
60. O'Brien TS, Svendsen CN, Isacson O, Sofroniew MV. Brain Res 1990; 508: 249-56.

61. Tuszynski MH, Armstrong DM, Gage FH. Brain Res 1990; 508: 241-8.
62. Phelps CH, Gage FH, Growdon JH, Hefti F, Harbaugh R, Johnston MV, Khachaturian Z, Mobley W, Price D, Raskind M, Simpkins J, Thal L, Woodcock J (Ad Hoc Working Group on Nerve Growth Factor and Alzheimer's Disease). Science 1989; 243: 11.
63. Phelps CH, Gage FH, Growdon JH, Hefti F, Harbaugh R, Johnston MV, Khachaturian ZS, Mobley WC, Price DL, Raskind M, Simpkins J, Thal LJ, Woodcock J. Neurobiol Aging 1989; 10: 205-7.
64. Williams LR, Varon S, Peterson GM, Wictorin K, Fischer W, Bjorklund A, Gage FH. Proc Natl Acad Sci USA 1986; 83: 9231-5.
65. Kromer LF. Science 1987; 235: 214-16.
66. Gage FH, Armstrong DM, Williams DR, Varon S. J Comp Neurol 1988; 269: 147-55.
67. Rosenberg MB, Friedmann T, Robertson RC, Tuszynski M, Wolff JA, Breakefield XO, Gage FH. Science 1988; 242: 1575-81.
68. Whittemore SR, Holets VR, Levy DJ. Mol Neurobiol Neuropharmacol 1989; 9: 85.
69. Angeletti RH, Bradshaw RA. Proc Natl Acad Sci USA 1971; 68: 2417-20.
70. Ullrich A, Gray A, Berman C, Dull TJ. Nature 1983; 303: 821-5.
71. Dunbar JC, Tregear GW, Bradshaw RA. J Protein Chem 1984; 3: 349-56.
72. Johnson D, Lanahan A, Buck CR, Sehgal A, Morgan C, Mercer E, Bothwell M, Chao M. Cell 1986; 47: 545-54.
73. Meier R, Becker-André M, Götz R, Heumann R, Shaw A, Thoenen H. EMBO J 1986; 5: 1489-93.
74. Koliatsos VE, Nauta HJW, Clatterbuck RE, Holztman DM, Mobley WC, Price DL. J Neurosci (in press).
75. Bartus RT, Dean RL III, Beer B, Lippa AS. Science 1982; 217: 408-17.

Address for correspondence:

Dr Donald L. Price,
Neuropathology Laboratory,
509 Pathology Building, The Johns Hopkins University School of Medicine,
600 North Wolfe Street, Baltimore, Maryland 21205-2181, USA.
Tel. (301) 955-5632
Fax. (301) 955-9777

61 Transgenic Mice and Alzheimer's Disease

JUSTINUS BEER, J. MICHAEL SALBAUM,
EVELINE SCHLICHTMANN, PETER HOPPE, SCOTT EARLEY,
GEORGE A. CARLSON, COLIN L. MASTERS
AND KONRAD BEYREUTHER

Alzheimer's disease (AD) is characterized by neuronal loss and massive depositions of amyloid β/A4 protein in the brain (1,2). The deposits of β/A4 protein appear at distinct locations: intracellular in association with the appearance of neurofibrillary tangles, as extracellular amyloid infiltrations of the neuropil and as perivascular amyloid. Brains from patients with Down's syndrome (DS) show the same pathology that is otherwise characteristic for AD. The major proteinaceous component of the corresponding fibrils isolated from brains of patients with AD and DS is a protein of 42-43 amino acid residues. This self-aggregating protein has a molecular weight of about 4 kDa and a proposed secondary structure of β-pleated sheets (1-3). Accordingly, this protein is termed β/A4. The β/A4 protein is part of a larger precursor protein called APP (amyloid precursor protein). The corresponding APP gene maps to the long arm of chromosome 21 close to the obligate Down's syndrome region (4-7). It gives rise to several alternatively spliced products. cDNAs coding for APP proteins of 695, 714, 751, 770 and 563 amino acid residues have been reported (4,8-13). APP_{695}, APP_{751} and APP_{770} are glycosylated transmembrane proteins (14,15). Compared to APP_{695} the two longer forms contain an additional domain with homology to the Kunitz type II family of serine protease inhibitors (8,10,11). APP_{714} and APP_{770} have an additional sequence of 19 amino acid residues, which is homologous to MRC OX-2, a rat cell surface glycoprotein of the rat MHC-complex (16). The secreted form $APRP_{563}$ (amyloid precursor related protein) lacks the transmembrane, the cytoplasmic and the β/A4 domains and therefore does not contribute to Alzheimer's disease (12).

APP primary translation products containing the transmembrane structure are heavily modified post-translationally. One notable modification is a specific proteolytic cleavage, which leads to the secretion of the ectodomain of APP proteins (15). The site of cleavage is located close to the membrane and lies within the β/A4 sequence. Thus aberrant proteolytic processing rather than a normal cleavage is involved in generating the N-terminus of the β/A4 protein and, consecutively, amyloid pathology (17,18). The secreted forms may contribute additional biological

Alzheimer's Disease: Basic Mechanisms, Diagnosis and Therapeutic Strategies
Edited by K. Iqbal, D. R. C. McLachlan, B. Winblad and H. M. Wisniewski
©1991 John Wiley & Sons Ltd

function to APP. The ectodomain of APP_{695} has been reported to exhibit growth factor-like activity (19), whereas those of APP_{751} and APP_{770} are presumed to be identical to protease nexin II (20,21), an inhibitor of serum serine proteases. These findings imply a role for APP proteins within the central nervous system (CNS) in guidance of axons and growth cones, and establishment and maintenance of synapses (22).

Messenger RNA analysis revealed that the alternative splicing products of the APP gene are not only expressed in brain but also in peripheral tissues (4–11,23–25) and in permanent cell lines of neuronal and non-neuronal origin (8,10,15). Quantification experiments showed that APP_{695} is the predominantly expressed alternative splicing product in the brain and spinal cord of humans and rodents (9,23). APP_{751} and APP_{770} are expressed in all other organs, whereas APP_{695} is a minor species outside of the CNS (9,23). The APP gene is not evenly expressed in the mouse brain but shows regional differences with the highest expression in frontal cortex areas, the olfactory system, pyramidal layers in the hippocampus, the granular layer in the cerebellum and in the hypothalamus (24). Comparison of APP gene expression in brains of patients with AD versus controls so far has generally not been conclusive. Recent investigations demonstrated that the mRNA expression is not selectively altered in the cortex of AD patients and that differential expression of the gene is not correlated with depositions in the brain of aged nonhuman primates (26). In-situ hybridization showed a contrasting picture since APP_{695} seems to be expressed in elevated levels in the nucleus basalis and locus ceruleus, in those brain areas which are most seriously affected with AD pathology (27). In rat brain most if not all neurons express the APP gene. The highest levels were detected in the olfactory areas, cerebral cortex, hippocampus, dentate gyrus, amygdala and cerebellum. Almost no hybridization signal was seen in cells of the white matter (22). Patients with DS, who without exception show AD pathology after they have passed the age of 30 years (28,29), have increased levels of APP transcripts presumably due to a gene dosis effect caused by the presence of three copies of chromosome 21 (23). In contrast to the SOD gene, which shows the expected 1.5-fold increase in expression in DS, the expression of the APP gene is elevated 3–5 fold, more similar to what is observed for the interferon alpha receptor, another gene on chromosome 21. It has been speculated that this gene dosage effect and the subsequent overexpression of APP is somehow involved in the amyloid pathology observed in aged DS individuals.

We set out to test the hypothesis that overproduction of APP_{695} may lead to $\beta/A4$ depositions in the brain since:

(a) APP_{695} is the major alternative splicing product in the brain (9).
(b) Overexpression of APP at mRNA and protein level in DS is correlated with earlier onset of amyloid $\beta/A4$ protein deposition (29). In these patients this onset precedes that of normal individuals by about 50 years (29,30).
(c) Transplants of hippocampal tissue from fetal mice with trisomy 16 into forebrain locations of 6-week-old normal mice showed $\beta/A4$ immunoreactivity (31). In-situ hybridization of mouse embryos with trisomy of chromosome 16, the

equivalent of the human chromosome 21, showed increased amounts of murine APP mRNA. This increase and the factors induced by the transplantation are presumably responsible for the $\beta/A4$ immunoreactivity in the transplants since control mice did not develop this pathology (31).

Overexpression of APP_{695} in HeLa cells did not lead to $\beta/A4$-aggregates (15). Because an animal model of AD in laboratory rodents rather than in primates would greatly facilitate research into diagnostics and therapy of AD, we chose mice transgenic for human APP as an in-vivo approach to investigate whether overexpression of APP_{695} would result in $\beta/A4$ amyloid pathology. The APP gene in mouse and rat is highly conserved (23,32). But the pathological changes similar to AD have so far not been found to occur spontaneously in rodents. This may be due to the short lifespan of these animals and not due to the three amino acid exchanges found in the $\beta/A4$ sequence of murine and rat APP, since the synthetic rodent amyloid sequence has been shown to form fibrils and amyloid in vitro (22).

For the expression of the human APP_{695} transgene in mice we selected the promoter hMTII of the human metallothionein IIA-gene (33). The 0.8-kb HindIII/BamHI fragment of the promoter was fused with the 3-kb SmaI-fragment of the human APP_{695} cDNA, which comprises the full-length coding region and the 3' untranslated part up to the first polyadenylation site (4). We used pUC19 as a vector (34). The DNA used for injection experiments was purified over a CsCl-density gradient and linearized with SspI site in pUC19. The transgenic mouse line MTA4 contained 2-3 copies of the APP_{695} transgene and was used for all further experiments.

The offspring of the transgenic mice were tested by Southern blotting of mouse-tail DNA. Analysis of DNA from MTA4 mice by Southern hybridization revealed a 7.5-kb BamHI fragment corresponding to the murine APP gene, whereas the 7.0-kb fragment represented the transgene. Comparison of the intensity of these signals usually allowed us to distinguish between heterozygous and homozygous transgenic animals.

The expression of the transgene at the mRNA-level was determined by S1-nuclease protection. This method allows not only to distinguish between the transcripts of the transgene and the endogenous transcripts but also to quantify the amount. The 0.8-kb PstI fragment of APP_{695} cDNA was used in these experiments as the probe, which gives a protected DNA-fragment of 378 bases. The intensity of this band reflects the activity of the gene.

The human APP_{695} transgene was found to be constitutively expressed in a number of tissues, notably in the brain. A short-term induction of the hMTII promoter was achieved by treating animals with 10 mM $CdCl_2$ for 8 hours (35). We did not find any enhancement of transgene activity in the brain. This is presumably due to the blood–brain barrier and, consecutively, the inability of Cd^{2+} ions to reach in time the cells in the brain. The additional activity of the transgene is due to induction of the hMTII promoter of the transgene by endogenous brain glucocorticoid levels through hormone-responsive elements. In kidney we were able to detect a 5-fold increase in transgene activity. In heart and lung, the activity was slightly above endogenous transcription, whereas spleen, muscle, thymus and testis did not react on that treatment with stronger transcription activity. The amount of total APP transcripts in the brain of MTA4 mice is increased by only 10% when compared to normal mice. Homozygous animals showed a 2–3 fold higher transcription in the brain than the heterozygous animals. Analysis of brain protein extracts from MTA4 as well as normal mice by western blotting revealed that extracts from the transgenic mice contained at total 300–500% of APP protein in comparison to the 100% from normal mice. This may be due to the fact that during construction of the transgene, parts of the 5'-nontranslated region of the human APP_{695} message was replaced by sequences derived from the 5'-nontranslated region of the hMTII gene, which could result in an altered translational specificity or efficiency. Long-term induction studies were performed by supplying the animals with drinking water supplemented with $ZnCl_2$, which is far less toxic than the $CdCl_2$ used in the short-term experiments. Analysis of transgenic mice after a six-month period of exposure to $ZnCl_2$ revealed a 2–3 fold increased level of transgene activity in the brain. Zn^{2+} ions are believed to cross the blood–brain barrier by using the transferrin receptor and thus be available to activate the hMTII promoter in brain cells.

In order to examine the cells that specifically overexpress the transgene in the mouse brain, we used immunoperoxidase methods for the localization of the transgenic product. In these immunocytochemical studies we used monoclonal and polyclonal antibodies raised against different epitopes of APP_{695}. The monoclonal antibody Mab22C11 and the polyclonal antibody 42 were raised against a fusion protein, which was expressed in E. coli. The construct contained the sequence of APP_{695} and the VH-domain of a murine IgM heavy chain (13). The epitope of the monoclonal antibody is near the N-terminus of the cysteine-rich domain of APP. Another polyclonal antibody was generated in rabbits immunized with a synthetic peptide representing the C-terminal 43 amino acid residues of the endodomain. The antibodies detect the membrane-bound APP forms since the epitopes are present in all these proteins.

In the brain of a normal mouse the staining is strongest for pyramidal cells of the cortex and hippocampus as well as the Purkinje cells in cerebellum. Analysis of transgenic mice revealed that total APP in pyramidal and Purkinje cells is increased, and that this overexpression is enhanced by further induction of the transgene with zinc chloride. This suggested that neurons overexpress the transgene. A 3–5 fold higher amount in total APP was found in the brain of transgenic animals induced with zinc chloride compared to controls.

We used a polyclonal antibody raised against a synthetic peptide representing amino acid residues 2–43 of the human β/A4 sequence to analyse sections of brain tissue from heterozygous or homozygous MTA4 mice with or without zinc induction, for we have been unable to demonstrate any β/A4 amyloid reactivity in the brains of these animals, some of which have been exposed to zinc for 20 months. This may suggest that overexpression of the human APP_{695} in the neurons of the CNS of these transgenic mice alone does not lead to β/A4 protein formation and that mechanisms other than overexpression are involved in developing the amyloid pathology that is characteristic for the brain of patients with AD. Deposition of amyloid in the brain is a slow process that in humans takes decades to develop. It might well be that the lifespan of a laboratory mouse is still not long enough, and the APP overexpression in brains of MTA4 mice not sufficiently high to result in amyloid pathology. However, a more likely assumption is that overexpression alone is not sufficient for the induction of amyloid β/A4 protein formation. This in turn would suggest that additional genes on chromosome 21 account for the earlier onset of AD amyloid pathology in DS.

Acknowledgments

This project is supported by the Deutsche Forschungsgemeinschaft through Sonderforschungsbereich 317, the Bundesminister für Forschung und Technologie of Germany, the Fonds der Chemischen Industrie. Justinus Beer was supported by the Boehringer Ingelheim Fonds and Colin L. Masters by the Alzheimer's Disease and Related Disorders Association and the National Health and Medical Research Council of Austrialia.

REFERENCES

1. Glenner GG, Wong CW. Biochem Biophys Res Comm 1984; 120: 1131–5.
2. Masters CL, Simms G, Weinman NA, Multhaup G, McDonald BL, Beyreuther K. Proc Natl Acad Sci USA 1985; 82: 4245–9.
3. Masters CL, Multhaup G, Simms G, Pottgießer J, Martins RN, Beyreuther K. EMBO 1985; 11: 2757–63.
4. Kang J, Lemaire HG, Unterbeck A, Salbaum JM, Masters CL, Grzeschik KH, Multhaup G, Beyreuther K, Müller-Hill, B. Nature 1987; 308: 733–6.
5. Goldgaber D, Lerman MI, McBride OW, Saffiotti U, Gajdusek DC. Science 1987; 235: 877–80.
6. Tanzi RE, Gusella JF, Watkins PC, Bruns GAP, St George-Hyslop P, Van Keuren ML, Patterson D, Pagan S, Kurnit DM, Neve RL. Science 1987; 235: 880–4.
7. Robakis NK, Ramakrishna N, Wolfe G, Wisniewski HM. Proc Natl Acad Sci USA 1987; 84: 4190–4.
8. Kitaguchi N, Takahashi Y, Tokushima Y, Shirohiri S, Ito H. Nature 1988; 331: 385–96.
9. Kang J, Müller-Hill B. Biochem Biophys Res Comm 1990; 166: 1192–200.
10. Ponte P, Gonzales-DeWhitt P, Schilling J, Miller J, Hsu D, Greenberg B, Davis K, Wallace W, Lieberburg I, Fuller F, Cordell B. Nature 1988; 331: 525–7.
11. Tanzi RE, McClatchey AI, Lamperti ED, Villa-Komaroff L, Gusella JF, Neve RL. Nature 1988; 331: 528–30.
12. DeSauvage F, Octave JN. Science 1989; 245: 651–3.
13. Tanaka S, Nakamura S, Kunihiro U, Kameyama M, Shiojiri S, Takahashi Y, Kitaguchi N, Ito H. Biochem Biophys Res Comm 157: 472–9.
14. Dyrks T, Weidemann A, Multhaup G, Salbaum JM, Lemaire HG, Kang J, Müller-Hill B, Masters CL, Beyreuther K. EMBO 1988; 7: 949–57.
15. Weidemann A, König G, Bunke D, Fischer P, Salbaum JM, Masters CL, Beyreuther K. Cell 1989; 57: 115–26.
16. Clark MJ, Gagnon J, Williams AF, Barclay AN. EMBO 1985; 4: 113–118.
17. Sisodia SS, Koo EH, Beyreuther K, Unterbeck A, Price DL. Science 1990; 248: 492–5.
18. Esch FS, Keim PS, Beattie EC, Blacher RW, Culwell AR, Oltersdorf T, McClure D, Ward PJ. Science 1990; 248: 1122–4.
19. Saitoh T, Sandsmo M, Roch JM, Kimura N, Cole G, Schubert D, Oltersdorf T, Schenk DB. Cell 1989; 58: 615–22.

20. Van Norstrand WE, Wagner SL, Suzuki M, Choi BH, Farrow JS, Geddes JW, Cotman CW, Cunningham DD. Nature 1989; 341: 546-9.
21. Oltersdorf T, Fritz LC, Schenk DB, Lieberburg I, Johnson-Wood KL, Beattie EC, Ward PJ, Blucher RW, Dovey HF, Sinha S. Nature 1989; 341: 144-7.
22. Shivers B, Hilbich C, Multhaup G, Salbaum JM, Beyreuther K, Seeburg PH. EMBO J 1988; 7: 1365-70.
23. Neve RL, Finch EA, Dawes LR. Neuron 1988; 1: 669-77.
24. Bendotti C, Forloni GL, Morgan RA, O'Hara BF, Oster-Granite ML, Reeves RH, Gearhart JD, Coyle JT. PNAS 1988; 85: 3628-32.
25. Zimmermann K, Herget T, Salbaum JM, Lemaire HG, Kang J, Müller-Hill B, Masters CL, Beyreuther K. EMBO J 1988; 7: 367-72.
26. Koo EH, Sisodia SS, Cork LC, Unterbeck A, Bayney RM, Price DL. Neuron 1990; 4: 97-104.
27. Palmert MR, Golde TE, Cohen ML, Kovacs DM, Tanzi RE, Gusella JF, Usiak MF, Younkin LH, Younkin SG. Science 1988; 241: 1080-4.
28. Beyreuther K, Multhaup G, Simms G, Pottgießer J, Schröder W, Martins RN, Masters CL. In: Bignami A, Bolis L, Gajdusek DC (eds) Discussions in neuroscience. Geneva: Fondation pour l'Etude du Système Nerveux, 1986; 4: 68-79.
29. Rumble B, Retallack R, Hilbich C, Simms G, Multhaup G, Martins R, Hockey A, Montgomery P, Beyreuther K, Masters CL. New Engl J Med 1989; 320: 1446-52.
30. Davies L, Wolska B, Hilbich C, Multhaup G, Martins R, Simms G, Beyreuther K, Masters CL. Neurology 1988; 38: 1688-93.
31. Richards SJ, Waters JJ, Rogers DC, Martel FL, Sparkman DR, White CL, Beyreuther K, Masters CL, Dunnett SB. Prog Brain Res 1990; 82: 215-23.
32. Yamada T, Susuki H, Funiya H, Miyata T, Goto I, Sahaki Y. Biochem Biophys Res Comm 1987; 149: 665-71.
33. Karin M, Haslinger A, Holtgreve H, Richards RI, Krauter P, Westphal HM, Beato M. Nature 1984; 308: 513-19.
34. Yanish-Perron C, Vieira J, Messing J. Gene 1985; 33: 103-19.
35. Rüther U, Garber C, Komitowski D, Müller R, Wagner E. Nature 1987; 325: 412-16.

Address for correspondence:

Justinus Beer,
Center for Molecular Biology,
University of Heidelberg,
Im Neuenheimer Feld 282,
D-6900 Heidelberg 1, Germany

62 Trisomy 16 Mouse Model of Alzheimer's Disease

AUDRIUS V. PLIOPLYS

Aging individuals with Down's syndrome (DS) develop the neuropathologic hallmarks of Alzheimer's disease (AD) and a large proportion display evidence of decreasing cognitive abilities (1–3). In addition, other lines of research suggest an association between DS and AD: extra copies of 21st chromosome genetic material are found in nonfamilial AD (4); genetic polymorphisms in genes coded on the 21st chromosome have been found in families with familial AD (5); the gene for β-amyloid, one of the abnormally stored materials in AD, has been mapped to the 21st chromosome (6). Cerebral cortical dendritic abnormalities similar to those found in DS have been described in AD (7–9). These morphologic changes may be due to underlying abnormalities in neuronal microtubules (10). Furthermore, cytoskeletal abnormalities are common to both DS and AD. A microtubule-dependent event, lymphocyte capping in response to concanavalin A, has been shown to be defective in both DS and AD (11). Similar findings have been made in cultured DS and AD fibroblasts (12). These DS and AD cytoskeletal related findings may be due to abnormal phosphorylation, suggestive of a defect in post-translation modification (13). The highly phosphorylated 210-kDa neurofilament subunit is redistributed to aberrant locations in AD (13) and is precociously expressed in DS (14). Nonphosphorylated neurofilament proteins are markers for vulnerable cortical neurons in AD (15). The Alz-50 antigen which is specific for AD (16) has kinase activity and may be involved in abnormal cytoskeletal phosphorylation (17). In AD protein kinase C dependent phosphorylation is abnormal (18). Early stages of AD are typified by the loss of neurofilament-rich axonal systems (19).

The proposed cytoskeletal abnormalities in DS may be on the basis of the enzymes coded on the 21st chromosome and this may be related to the interferon α and β receptors which are coded by this chromosome (20). In DS, cellular responsiveness to interferon is exaggerated such that a given dose of interferon elicits not a 1.5-fold antiviral response but a 3- to 15-fold response (21). In the initiation of the antiviral state, interferon treatment decreases the rates of cell mitosis, locomotion, membrane ruffling and saltatory movements of intracellular granules (22,23). Fibroblasts treated with interferon contain three times the number of actin fibers when compared to untreated cells (23). Interferon treatment of normal cells produces defective

Alzheimer's Disease: Basic Mechanisms, Diagnosis and Therapeutic Strategies
Edited by K. Iqbal, D. R. C. McLachlan, B. Winblad and H. M. Wisniewski
© 1991 John Wiley & Sons Ltd

lymphocyte capping following concanavalin A administration (23)—results which are similar to lymphocyte capping abnormalities in DS and AD (11). Interferon is present in the cerebrospinal fluid (24). In monkeys the CNS can produce interferon-dependent RNA following intrathecal administration of interferon (25). Neurons in vivo and in culture are sensitive to interferon, suggesting the possibility of functional interferon receptors in the CNS (26). In DS neuronal cytoskeletal changes may be due to enhanced responsiveness to interferon.

Murine trisomy 16 is an excellent model for DS (20,27). The human 21st chromosome and the mouse 16th chromosome both code for the free radical scavenging enzyme superoxide dismutase-1 (SOD-1), the purine biosynthetic enzyme phosphoribosylglycinamide synthetase (PRGS), the proto-oncogene ETS-2, interferon α and β receptors, and amyloid precursor protein (28). Phenotypic features of human DS and murine trisomy 16 are also similar including flat facies, shortened neck, ear abnormalities, congenital heart disease (endocardial cushion defects and aortic arch abnormalities), fetal edema, thymic hypoplasia and decreased T-lymphocyte and antibody responsiveness. Both conditions have high rates of fetal wastage. The electrical membrane properties of cultured dorsal root ganglion neurons from DS and trisomy 16 are similar (29,30). Brain development is likewise similar with decreased brain size, reduced neuronal numbers and decreased brain levels of catecholaminergic, cholinergic and serotonergic markers (20,31–33).

ELECTRON MICROSCOPIC OBSERVATIONS

Cytoskeletal EM observations in trisomy 16 revealed microtubular profiles which were more curved and coiled than in normals (34). The apparent numerical density and spacing of microtubules did not differ between normal and trisomy 16 mice as has been reported in AD (10). Paired helical filaments, one of the pathologic hallmarks of AD, were not observed in the trisomy 16 material. The ultrastructural microtubular differences in trisomy 16 may be related to reported cytoskeletal abnormalities in AD.

The EM also revealed increased cellular membrane fragility in trisomy 16 CNS neurons (34). During the processes of fixation, embedding and sectioning, trisomic neuronal membranes became fragmented and lost cell-to-cell apposition. CNS lipid abnormalities have been reported in DS. In particular, phosphatidylethanolamine content is decreased and the cholesterol/phospholipid ratio is increased (35,36). Significantly, in AD CNS neuronal membrane abnormalities have likewise been noted, including abnormalities in gangliosides (37–40). Possibly similar membrane lipid abnormalities occur in trisomy 16 which may account for the observed ultrastructural membrane fragility. Alternatively, anomalous expression of amyloid precursor protein (APP) may account for these membrane findings. In normal rodents, APP is widely expressed throughout the CNS as a cell surface receptor (41). APP is coded on the mouse 16th chromosome and may be anomalously expressed in trisomy 16. APP may play an important role in cell membrane integrity and in maintaining cell-to-cell contact (41,42).

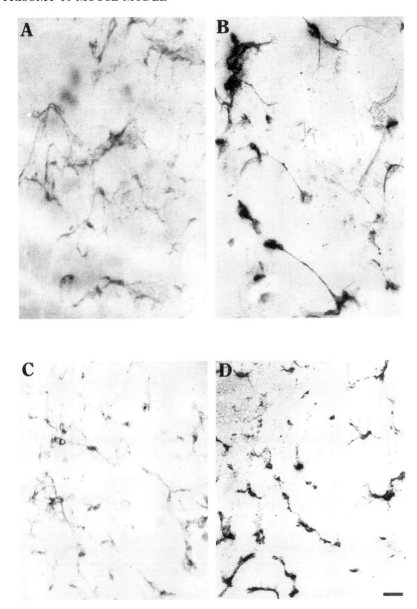

Figure 1. Photomicrographs of cultured CNS neurons taken from normal E17 mice (A and C) and trisomy 16 littermates (B and D), immunoperoxidase stained with a monoclonal antibody directed against the 210-kDa neurofilament subunit (mabN210, Dr Hawkes; A and B) and the 68-kDa neurofilament subunit (Boehringer Mannheim; C and D). There is greater 210-kDa subunit immunoreactivity in the trisomic culture (B) than in the normal culture (A), a result which confirms previously published results (32). There is likewise greater 68-kDa subunit immunoreactivity in trisomic cultures (D) as compared to controls (C). Scale bar 50 μm

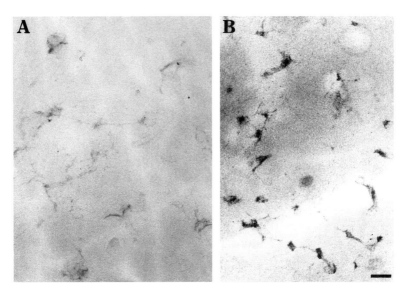

Figure 2. Photomicrographs of cultured CNS neurons taken from a normal E17 mouse (A) and a trisomy 16 littermate (B), immunoperoxidase stained with sera directed against microtubule-associated tau proteins (Sigma). There is greater immunoreactivity in the trisomic culture (B) than in the normal one (A). Scale bar 50 μm

Trisomy 16 neuronal nuclei are smaller and more irregular in size than normals (34). The trisomy 16 CNS nuclear observations may be a reflection of the additionally stored chromosomal material in each nucleus. Alternatively, abnormalities in chromatin and nuclear histones have been described in AD. For eukaryotic gene expression it is necessary for the genome to be accessible to RNA polymerase systems. The H1 histones can condense DNA and make it inaccessible for transcription (43). CNS chromatin in AD is in a much higher state of compaction (44), is less accessible to the enzyme micrococcal nuclease (45) and has increased H1 linker histones on dinucleosomes (46). Possibly, trisomy 16 nuclei have similar histone abnormalities and the observed nuclear morphologic differences are due to differences in these nuclear proteins.

The EM cytoskeletal, cellular membrane and nuclear contour observations strengthen the role of the trisomy 16 mouse as a model for AD.

CENTRAL NERVOUS SYSTEM NEURONAL CULTURES: EFFECTS OF INTERFERON

When a mixture of α and β mouse interferon was applied to normal cultured neurons, there was an increase in the immunohistochemical staining intensity of the 210-kDa neurofilament subunit in neuronal cell bodies (47). Significantly, there was a difference between untreated normal and trisomic CNS neurons: there was more 210-kDa neurofilament immunohistochemical expression in the trisomic cultures. When an inhibitor of the interferon mediated antiviral state, oxyphenbutazone,

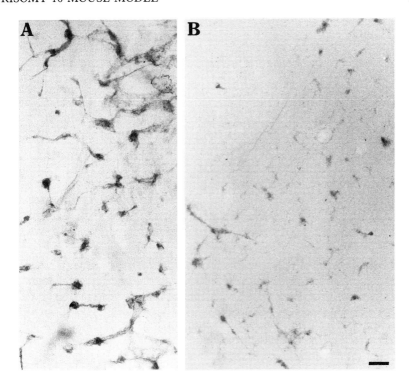

Figure 3. Photomicrographs of cultured CNS neurons taken from a normal E17 mouse (A) and a trisomy 16 littermate (B), immunoperoxidase stained with sera directed against tubulin (Sigma). There is greater immunoreactivity in the normal culture (A) than in the trisomic one (B). Scale bar 50 μm

without the presence of interferon, there was a significant reduction in the intensity of neurofilament immunohistochemical expression. It is postulated that the observed effects on trisomic neurons were due to the presence of interferon which is endogenously produced within the culture by concurrently growing fibroblasts.

These results have demonstrated that interferon has a regulatory effect on neuronal neurofilament expression. Also, a difference has been shown in neurofilament immunohistochemical expression between normal and trisomy 16 cultured CNS neurons. Finally, and possibly of greater importance, an interferon inhibitor has been shown to normalize trisomic CNS neurofilament expression.

These tissue culture investigations have been extended to other cytoskeletal components. As with the 210-kDa neurofilament subunit, the 68-kDa subunit has more intense immunohistochemical expression in trisomy 16 than in normals (Figure 1). A similar result was found with the immunohistochemical expression of the microtubule-associated tau proteins (Figure 2) (48). It should be noted that in AD tau proteins are abnormally distributed (49,50). Sera directed against the main constituent of microtubules, tubulin, produced the opposite effect with increased staining in normal as compared to trisomy 16 cultures (Figure 3). It has not yet been possible to delineate the effects of interferon on the immunohistochemical expression of these cytoskeletal components.

SUMMARY

All of these lines of investigation strengthen the T-16 mouse as a model for AD. Also, interferon-mediated neuronal hypersensitivity may be causally related to cytoskeletal misregulation in DS and set the stage for the eventual development of AD in DS. A similar process may be at play in AD.

Acknowledgments

The author would like to acknowledge the assistance rendered by Surrey Place Centre, Toronto, Ontario, the Alschuler and Crown Funds and by the Medical Research Institute Council of Michael Reese Hospital.

REFERENCES

1. Dalton AJ, Crapper-McLachlan DR. Psych Clin N Am 1986; 9: 659-70.
2. Malamud N. In Gatiz CM (ed.) Aging and the brain. New York: Plenum, 1972: 63.
3. Wisniewski KE et al. Neurology 1985; 35: 957-61.
4. Delabar JM et al. Science (Wash.) 1987; 235: 1390-92.
5. St George-Hyslop PH et al. Science (Wash.) 1987; 235: 885-90.
6. Goldgaber D et al. Science (Wash.) 1987; 235: 877-80.
7. Purpura DP et al. Dev Brain Res 1982; 5: 287-97.
8. Scheibel AB, Tomiyasu U. Exp Neurol 1978; 60: 1-8.
9. Tavares MA et al. Morfol Norm Patol 1981; 5: 81-6.
10. Paula-Barbosa M et al. Brain Res 1987; 416: 139-42.
11. Duijndam-Van den Burge M, Goekoop JG. J Neurol Neurosurg Psychiat 1986; 49: 595-8.
12. McSwigan JD. Neurosci Abstr 1986; 12: 1316.
13. Sternberger LA, Sternberger NH. Proc Natl Acad Sci USA 1983; 80: 6126-30.
14. Plioply AV. J Neurol Sci 1987; 79: 91-100.
15. Morrison JH et al. Brain Res 1987; 416: 331-6.
16. Wolozin BL et al. Science (Wash.) 1986; 232: 648-50.
17. Wolozin BL, Davies P. Neurosci Abstr 1986; 12: 944.
18. Ueda K et al. Arch Neurol 1989; 46: 1195-9.
19. De la Monte SM. Ann Neurol 1989; 25: 450-9.
20. Epstein CJ et al. Ann NY Acad Sci 1985; 450: 157-68.
21. Epstein CJ. In Epstein CJ (ed.) The neurobiology of Down syndrome. New York: Raven Press, 1986: 1-15.
22. Pfeffer LM et al. Exp Cell Res 1979; 121: 120.
23. Pfeffer LM et al. J Cell Biol 1980; 85: 9-17.
24. Gresser I, Naficy K. Proc Soc Exp Biol Med 1964; 117: 285-9.
25. Smith RA, Landel C. Neurology 1987; 37 (suppl. 1): 303.
26. Dafny N et al. J Neuroimm 1985; 9: 1-12.
27. Gropp A et al. Cytogenet Cell Genet 1975; 14: 42-62.
28. Reeves RH et al. Neurosci Abstr 1987; 13(2): 1121.
29. Orozco CV et al. Dev Br Res 1987; 32: 111-22.

30. Scott BS et al. Dev Br Res 1981; 2: 257-70.
31. Oster-Granite ML. Br Res Bull 1986; 16: 767-71.
32. Reeves RH et al. Br Res Bull 1986; 16: 803-14.
33. Wisniewski KE et al. N Engl J Med 1984; 311: 1187-8.
34. Plioplys AV, Bedford HM. Br Res Bull 1989; 22: 233-43.
35. Balazs R, Brookshank BWL. J Ment Defic Res 1985; 29: 1-14.
36. Balazs R, Brookshank BWL. In Epstein CJ (ed.) The neurobiology of Down syndrome. New York: Raven Press, 1986: 59-72.
37. Barany MY et al. Lancet 1985; i: 517.
38. Chia LS et al. Biochim Biophys Acta 1984; 775: 308-12.
39. Crino PB et al. Arch Neurol 1989; 46: 398-401.
40. Zubenko GS. Brain Res 1986; 385: 115-21.
41. Shivers B et al. Neurosci Abstr 1987; 13(2) 819.
42. Kang J et al. Nature (Lond) 1987; 325: 733-6.
43. Knezetic JA, Luse DS. Cell 1986; 45: 95-104.
44. Crapper DR et al. Brain 1979; 102: 483-95.
45. Lewis PN et al. J Neurochem 1981; 37: 1193-202.
46. Crapper-McLachlan DR et al. Ann Neurol 1984; 15: 329-34.
47. Plioplys AV. J Neurol Sci 1988; 85: 209-22.
48. Plioplys AV. Neurology 1989; 39 (suppl 1): 250.
49. Bancher C et al. Brain Res 1989; 477: 90-9.
50. Kowall NW, Kosik KS. Ann Neurol 1987; 22: 639-43.

Address for correspondence:

Dr Audrius V. Plioplys,
Department of Neurology (Main Reese 395),
Michael Reese Hospital,
2900 S. Ellis Ave.,
Chicago, Illinois 60616, USA

63 A New Model for Studying the Neuropathology of Alzheimer's Disease Derived from Transplantation of Trisomy 16 CNS Tissues

SARAH-JANE RICHARDS, JONATHAN J. WATERS,
CLAUDE WISCHIK, DENNIS R. SPARKMAN,
CHARLES L. WHITE III, KONRAD BEYREUTHER,
COLIN MASTERS, CARMELA R. ABRAHAM
AND STEPHEN B. DUNNETT

Alzheimer's disease (AD) is the commonest form of dementia, affecting 5% of the population over the age of 65 years (1). The age of onset may be as early as 35 years and the disease can occur either as a sporadic or familial form (2). Trisomy 21 individuals (Down's syndrome) are known to be at risk of developing AD in middle life (3,4). This has been attributed to the presence of gene(s) on chromosome 21 which in excess lead to the neuropathological changes observed in AD. The main neuropathological features of AD are amyloid plaques and neurofibrillary tangles, which occur at highest density in the neocortex and hippocampus (5-7). Immunocytochemical studies have shown that amyloid is deposited in the brains of trisomy 21 individuals approximately 50 years before that seen in the normal aging population (8).

The amyloid (A4) protein has been isolated from the neuropathological plaque core (9-11). It shares amino-acid sequence homology and is antigenically related to the amyloid protein isolated from AD cerebral vasculature (β-amyloid) (12,13). Although the gene encoding the A4 protein has been mapped on chromosome 21 (14,15) to the region 21q11-q22 (16), genetic familial linkage studies have shown a recombination event occurring between the amyloid A4 gene and the disease locus (17), thus suggesting amyloid A4 is not the causative gene of familial AD.

The major components of the neurofibrillary tangle are paired helical filaments (PHF) (5). The precise structural composition of these abnormally expressed filaments has still to be determined. However, several proteins may share epitopes with PHFs, including microtubule-associated protein 2 (18), microtubule-associated protein tau (19), ubiquitin (20) and amyloid A4 (13). In particular, microtubule-associated tau may be intrinsic to the structure of the PHF (21).

Alzheimer's Disease: Basic Mechanisms, Diagnosis and Therapeutic Strategies
Edited by K. Iqbal, D. R. C. McLachlan, B. Winblad and H. M. Wisniewski
©1991 John Wiley & Sons Ltd

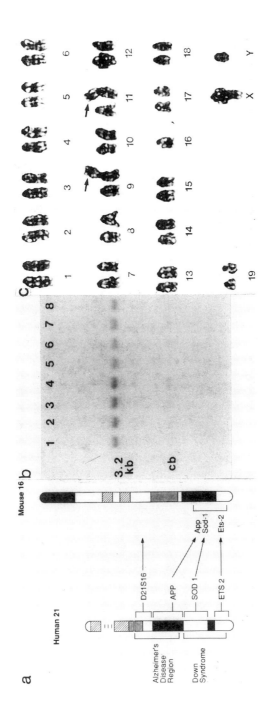

Figure 1. (a) Genes located on human chromosome 21 and mouse chromosome 16 (adapted from ref. 34). (b) Gene dosage for trisomic (lanes 1–4) and control (lanes 5–8) tissues confirmed by Southern blot analysis. Hybridization with a 1.1-kb fragment of the APP cDNA revealed dosage at a 3.2-kb band; cb, constant band. (c) Karyotyping of trisomic liver tissues confirmed Robertsonian translocations (arrows)

The serine protease inhibitor α_1-antichymotrypsin is predominantly located in association with amyloid deposits in the cores of neuritic plaques, in neurones and around blood vessels in the AD brain (22,23). While amyloid plaques may also be observed in Creutzfeldt–Jakob disease, the presence of α_1-antichymotrypsin immunoreactivity in association with β/A4 only in the AD pathology has made this protein a distinctive marker for distinguishing the two neurodegenerative disorders (22).

Trisomic strains of experimental mice can be derived using breeding regimens which select for specific Robertsonian translocations, and this has enabled gene dosage effects to be studied in vivo. Recent developments in cytogenetic techniques now permit mapping of human, single copy sequences onto animal chromosomes (24). In particular, human chromosome 21 sequences associated with the amyloid precursor protein (APP) and D21S16 (the closest marker associated with a familial Alzheimer's gene) have been mapped onto murine chromosome 16 (25) (Figure 1a). Consequently, it is of interest to ask whether overexpression of genes on chromosome 16 in the trisomy 16 mouse would produce similar neuropathological changes to those observed in the human disease and individuals with trisomy 21.

It has not previously been possible to address this issue since trisomy 16 mice rarely survive beyond day 20 of gestation, thus denying the opportunity for investigating the pathological changes associated with development or aging. However, techniques are well established for the transplantation of fetal neural tissues into adult recipient brain, where the grafted donor tissue is readily vascularized, survives and develops for the duration of the host lifespan. In this study we have transplanted neocortical and hippocampal tissues derived from trisomic and control fetuses into the brains of normal recipient mice, and monitored neuropathological changes over six months within the grafts.

MATERIALS AND METHODS

Litters containing trisomy 16 mice were generated by a breeding regimen in which male offspring from matings of homozygous Robertsonian translocations Rb(9:16)9Rma and Rb(11:16)2H were mated with females of the CFLP strain possessing acrocentric chromosomes only, to yield a Rb9Rma/Rb2H × CFLP cross. Normal littermates were used as a source of control tissue.

The trisomy 16 embryo may be visually selected from its normal littermates on the criteria of a shorter crown-to-rump measurement, severe oedema of the neck, flattened nasal bridge, shortened forelimbs and hindlimbs and prematurely opened eye. Confirmation of the assignment of tissues to either the trisomic or the normal control group was undertaken by Southern blot analysis (26) (Figure 1b) and karyotyping (27) (Figure 1c).

Transplantation procedures

Embryos for transplantation were staged by timed matings and their age confirmed by crown–rump length. Frontal cortex and hippocampal dissections were taken from

7 trisomic and 18 normal embryos assessed as E14–16. Young recipient CFLP mice were anaesthetized with 1 ml/100 g ketamine and transplantation cavities were surgically prepared by making fine burr holes through the skull and aspirating superficial cavities in the frontal (arrow) and retrosplenial (arrowheads) cortex. Each recipient received two grafts: neocortical donor tissue implanted into the frontal cavity, and hippocampal donor tissue into the retrosplenial cavity, by the delayed solid graft technique (28). The recipient mice were allowed to survive for up to 4–6 months before being sacrificed for histological analysis (Figure 2A).

Histology

Recipient brains were removed, immersed–fixed in formalin and paraffin wax embedded. A single E18 trisomy 16 embryo, a normal littermate, and postmortem Alzheimer cortical tissues were post fixed and embedded by the same procedure.

Tissue sections (8 μm) were de-waxed in xylene and rehydrated through graded alcohols to Tris-buffered saline at pH 7.2 (TBS). Cell bodies were visualized using a conventional cresyl violet stain and silver staining of nerve fibres and neurofibrils was undertaken using Palmgren's method (29). Thioflavine S was used as a conventional amyloid stain (29).

Immunohistochemistry

Sections for immunocytochemical analysis were de-waxed in xylene, dehydrated through graded alcohols and washed 2×15 min in TBS before being incubated with normal goat serum 1:30 (Dakopatts) for 1 hour at 22 °C. Polyclonal primary antisera APP—raised against the synthetic A4 protein (13), A128—raised against purified paired helical filaments (30), α_1-antichymotrypsin (22) β/A4—raised against a synthetic β-protein (13), and glial fibrillary acidic protein (GFAP—Dakopatts) were applied to sections at a dilution of 1:200 and incubated overnight at 4 °C. Sections were washed 2×15 min in TBS before being incubated with either (i) rabbit anti-goat IgG 1:50 (Sigma) for 1 hour at 4 °C followed by anti-rabbit PAP (Dakopatts) 1:30 for 1 hour at 4 °C with immunoreactivity being visualized with the chromogen 3,3'-diaminobenzidine (Sigma) 0.05 mg/ml in 0.1 M phosphate buffer pH 5.8, or anti-rabbit IgG conjugated FITC or rhodamine 1:50 (Dakopatts).

Monoclonal antibodies tau 6.423 (21) and ubiquitin (a generous gift of Dr B. H. Anderton, Institute of Psychiatry, London, UK) were applied to sections at a dilution of 1:50 following pre-incubation of the tissue with normal mouse serum. Immunoreactivity was either visualized by PAP/3,3'-diaminobenzidine chromogen or anti-mouse IgG conjugated FITC.

RESULTS

Routine histological assessment showed poor survival of neocortical grafts transplanted to the frontal cortex of host animals, irrespective of whether they were derived from trisomic or control donor embryos. In contrast, healthy hippocampal

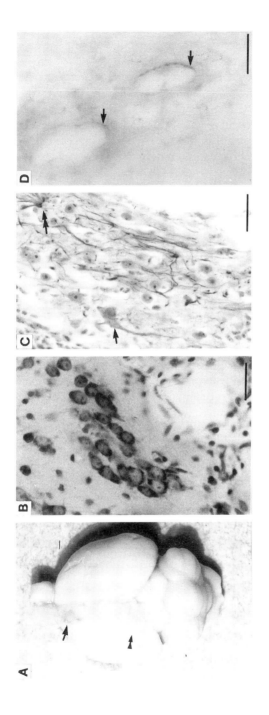

Figure 2. (A) Hippocampal grafts placed within frontal cortex (arrow) and retrosplenial cortex (arrowheads) at 4 months survival. (B) Cresyl violet staining of aggregated cells within a trisomic graft. (C) Palmgren silver staining demonstrating a pyramidal neuron with abnormal fibrils within the proximal dendrite (arrow), and developing extraneuronal tangle (double arrow) with a trisomic graft. (D) APP immunoreactive deposits around the cerebral vasculature with a trisomic graft (arrows). Scale bars B–D 40 μm

grafts were obtained from both groups of donors. Nissl body staining revealed no gross differences in either numbers or distribution of cells within the hippocampal grafts between the two groups. However, within the trisomic grafts, large cells judged to be neuronal by their morphology and GFAP negative, tended to form aggregates (Figure 2B). No differences were seen in the cellular composition of adjacent host parenchyma. Palmgren silver staining revealed occasional extraneuronal tangles of fibres (double arrows) and pyramidal neurons with abnormal fibrils within the proximal dendrite (arrow) (Figure 2C), although the abnormal staining was not as definitive as that observed in human Alzheimer tissue.

The trisomy 16 embryo appeared devoid of dense cellular immunoreactivity to APP, β/A4, α_1-antichymotrypsin, A128 or tau 6.423. However, the APP antibody produced high levels of background immunoreactivity which may be indicative of the presence of this protein at synapses. Postmortem Alzheimer cortical tissues were included in each batch of immunocytochemical staining to confirm the activity and appropriate patterns of immunoreactivity of the antibodies.

Immunocytochemical staining with the APP antibody demonstrated the presence of deposits of A4 immunoreactivity around the cerebral vasculature within the trisomic grafts (Figure 2D), and revealed numerous densely stained cells within the trisomic hippocampal tissues; however, no similar staining was observed within the control grafts, the host brain or within the trisomy 16 embryo. The localization of immunoreactive product appeared to be predominantly intracellular. However, in areas where positively stained cell bodies formed aggregates, there appeared to be some extracellular staining around the cell soma. This extracellular staining was also GFAP immunoreactive. Immunoreactivity produced high levels of background neuropil staining in all trisomic grafts but not in the control grafts. In one case of a trisomic graft, immunoreactive cell bodies appeared surrounded by extracellular matrix.

A similar pattern of immune reactivity was observed with α_1-antichymotrypsin within the trisomic grafts; while this protein was observed predominantly intracellularly, in areas where trisomic cells had aggregated and appeared to be degenerating, extracellular or a secreted form of α_1-antichymotrypsin was apparent.

Intracellular immunoreactivity of similar numbers of cells within trisomic grafts was observed with the A128, β/A4 and tau 6.423 antibodies. No immunoreactivity was observed in the control grafts, and background neuropil staining of both groups of grafts was low. GFAP-immunoreactive astrocytic cell bodies and processes were present in the host brain tissue, and a few processes were observed in the graft. Postmortem AD tissue revealed fibres and cell bodies immunoreactive for ubiquitin and this pattern of staining was also observed within the trisomic grafts. However, in host brain only immunoreactive fibres were observed. The number of ubiquitin-positive cells within the sections of trisomic graft tissue was lower than those immunoreactive for β/A4 and tau 6.423. While control grafts revealed ubiquitin-positive fibres they lacked any immunoreactive cell bodies.

Co-localization studies have demonstrated the intracellular co-existence of APP with A128 (Figure 3A,B), APP with α_1-antichymotrypsin (Figure 3C,D) and β/A4 with tau 6.423 (Figure 3E,F). In human AD tissue tau 6.423 was observed as

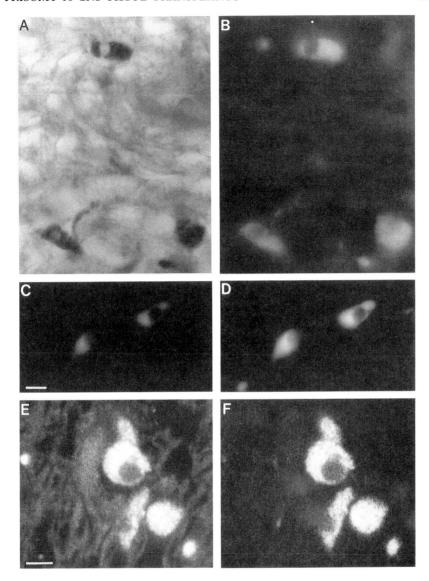

Figure 3. Immunocytochemical co-localization of AD neuropathological proteins in trisomic hippocampal grafts. (A) demonstrates cells immunoreactive for the pre-A4 protein and visualized with 3,3'-diaminobenzidine; (B) depicts the same section immunoreactive for A128 and visualized with a rhodamine conjugated secondary antibody (Dakopatts). (C) Cells in a different trisomic graft section immunoreactive for APP and visualized with a rhodamine-conjugated secondary antibody (Dakopatts). (D) Immunoractive co-localization of the same cells positive for the polyclonal α_1-antichymotrypsin antiserum and visualized with an FITC-conjugated secondary antibody (Dakopatts). (E) Cells containing small intracellular granular inclusions immunoreactive for β/A4 (FITC) are also immunoreactive for tau 6.423 (rhodamine) (F). Scale bars 10 μm; A–C are the same magnification

intracellular neurofibrillary tangles and granular inclusions. The tau 6.423-labelled granular inclusions have also been observed within the trisomic grafts and co-localize with small intracellular inclusions immunoreactive with β/A4 (31).

DISCUSSION

Alzheimer's disease is a progressive neurodegenerative disorder which is clinically diagnosed by the onset of dementia, and usually occurs in old age. Confirmation of the diagnosis of dementia as AD is usually only achieved after neuropathological examination postmortem. By this time loss of cortico-cortical connections is extensive and the advanced stages of cellular degeneration are observed in the form of amyloid plaques and neurofibrillary tangles. Due to the rarity of postmortem studies of newly diagnosed AD, it has not been possible to study the onset and progression of the neuropathology in a controlled and systematic way. Evaluation of postmortem studies on brain tissues from cases of trisomy 21 and the normal aging population suggests that amyloid deposition predates clinical diagnosis of AD by approximately 30 years (8). Furthermore, this amyloidogenic process in trisomy 21 occurs about 50 years earlier than in the normal aging population which in part may be attributed to the higher APP gene dosage in trisomy 21.

The observation of immunoreactivity for proteins associated with both aspects of Alzheimer's neuropathology within hippocampal grafts of trisomy 16 mice, together with the absence of staining in the trisomy 16 mouse at 18 days' gestation, indicates that extending the life of trisomic hippocampal tissues is necessary to reveal this pattern of immunoreactivity. Furthermore, it strongly suggests the presence of a gene (or genes) on mouse chromosome 16 whose overexpression can produce neuropathological features akin to human Alzheimer's disease (Table 1).

Co-localization of intracellular staining with β/A4 and tau 6.423 strongly suggests that either both proteins are being produced within the same cell, or that β/A4 amyloid and PHFs have shared epitopes. This possibility is supported by the demonstration of co-existence of immunoreactivity for β/A4 and neurofibrillary tangles in postmortem studies in Alzheimer's brain (31–34,36). In the event of both proteins

Table 1. Immunoreactivity in grafts and host brain

Antisera	Host brain	T-16 graft	Control graft
A4 precursor protein	—*	intra- and extracellular	—
β/A4 amyloid	—	intracellular	—
paired helical filaments	—	intracellular	—
tau 6.423	—	intracellular	—
α_1-antichymotrypsin	—	intra- and extracellular	—
glial fibrillary acidic protein	astrocytes	astrocytic processes	cell bodies and processes
ubiquitin	processes	processes and occasional cell bodies	processes

*—, no immunoreactivity

being produced within the same cell it would suggest that either the neurodegeneration observed within our trisomic grafts was in its early stages, or that the PHFs within the trisomic mouse do not become engulfed with the 'fuzzy' protein which comprises mainly tau protein (35). Immunohistochemical analysis favours the latter speculation. The few ubiquitin-immunoreactive cells may be accounted for by intracellular accumulations of tau 6.423 encapsulating the ubiquitin components of the PHFs and in consequence rendering them unavailable for antibody recognition. Often we see densely immunoreactive cells with immunoreactive product apparently spilling out into the extracellular space, along with an increase in extracellular matrix and GFAP immunoreactivity within the region of these aggregated degenerating cells. We have never observed neurofibrillary tangles within our grafts and in view of the short lifespan of a mouse (approximately 1 year) it is possible that the formation of these tangles does not have sufficient time to ocur within trisomic murine tissue. Instead, intracellular microtubule transportation becomes disrupted; accumulations of β/A4 amyloid and PHF proteins occur within the cell soma, leading to the rapid destruction of the outer cell membrane followed by cell death.

Immunocytochemical analysis of these trisomic grafts suggests the existence of an intracellular pathological pathway in which an antigenically distinct form of β/A4 (or its precursor protein) and tau protein both accumulate first in the cytoplasmic inclusions and then in intracellular tangles. Whether PHF formation represents a later stage of the trisomy 16 model is as yet unknown. Although many of the proteins that are abnormally expressed in AD such as tau, ubiquitin and α_1-antichymotrypsin and other proteases are not located on chromosome 21, the demonstration of AD-like pathology in murine trisomy 16 grafts strongly suggests that proteins central to the causation of AD are encoded on this chromosome.

Due to the rarity of postmortem studies of newly diagnosed AD, it has not been possible to study the onset and progression of the disease in a controlled and systematic way in humans, and there have been no adequate animal models. We propose that trisomy 16 murine grafts provide a powerful system in which to study the processes of neurodegeneration and to assess the viability of alternative therapeutic strategies to inhibit the development or reverse the pathological manifestations of Alzheimer's disease.

Acknowledgments

The authors are grateful to Dr Martin Bobrow and Mr John Crolla (Guy's Hospital, London) for making available the Robertsonian translocation mouse strains and for continued advice regarding breeding regimens. Sincere thanks are also extended to Dr Claude Wischik and Dr Gerd Multhaup for their helpful discussion and Dr David Mann for the provision of initial help on A4 immunohistochemistry. This work has been supported by the Medical Research Council and the Mental Health Foundation and is part of a study reported in EMBO J (1991).

REFERENCES

1. Terry RD. J Neuropath Exp Neurol 22: 629-42.
2. Heston LL, Mastri AR, Anderson VE, White J. Arch Gen Psychiat 1981; 38: 1085-90.

3. Burger PC, Vogel FS. Am J Pathol 1973; 73: 457–76.
4. Oliver C, Holland J. Psychol Med 1986; 16: 307–22.
5. Kidd M. Nature 1963; 197: 192–3.
6. Kidd M. Brain 1964; 87: 307–20.
7. Terry RD, Katzman R. Ann Neurol 1983; 114: 497–506.
8. Rumble B, Retallack R, Hilbich C, Simms G, Multhaup G, Martins R, Hockey A, Montgomery P, Beyreuther K, Masters CL. N Engl J Med 1989; 320: 1446–52.
9. Masters CL, Simms G, Weinman NA, Multhaup G, McDonald BL, Beyreuther, K. Proc Natl Acad Sci USA 1985; 82: 4245–9.
10. Roher A, Wolfe D, Palutke M, KuKuruga D. Proc Natl Acad Sci USA 1986; 83: 2662–6.
11. Selkoe DJ, Abraham CR, Podlisny MB, Duffy LK. J Neurochem 1986; 46: 1820–34.
12. Glenner GG, Wong CW. Biochem Biophys Res Comm 1984; 120: 885–90.
13. Masters CL, Multhaup G, Simms G, Pottgeisser J, Martins RN, Beyreuther K. EMBO J 1985; 4: 2757–63.
14. Goldgaber D, Lerman MI, McBride OW, Saffiotti U, Gajdusek DC. Science 1987; 235: 877–80.
15. Kang J, Lemaire H-G, Unterbeck A, Salbaum M, Masters CL, Grzeschik K-H, Multhaup G, Beyreuther K, Muller-Hill B. Nature 1987; 325: 733–6.
16. Robakis NK, Wisniewski HM, Jenkins EC, Devine-Gage EA et al. Lancet 1987; i: 384–5.
17. Van Broeckhoven C, Genthe AM, Vandenberghe A, Horstemke B, Backhovens H et al. Nature 1987; 329: 153–5.
18. Kosik KS, Joachim CL, Selkoe DJ. Proc Natl Acad Sci USA 1986; 83: 4044–8.
19. Brion JP, Couck AM, Passareiro E, Flament-Durand J. J Submicrosc Cytol 1985; 17: 89–96.
20. Mori H, Kando J, Ihara Y. Science 1987; 235: 1641–4.
21. Wischik CM, Novak M, Thorensen HC, Edwards PC, Runswick MJ, Jakes R, Walker JE, Milstein C, Roth M, Klug A. Proc Natl Acad Sci USA 1988; 85: 4506–10.
22. Abraham CR, Selkoe DJ, Potter H. Cell 1988; 52: 487–501.
23. Abraham CR, Shiramhama T, Potter H. Neurobiol Aging, 1990; 11: 123–9.
24. Lovett M, Goldgaber D, Ashley P, Cox DR, Gajdusek DC, Epstein CJ. Biochem Biophys Res Comm 1987; 144: 1069–75.
25. Reeves RH, Robakis NK, Oster-Granite ML, Wisniewski HM, Coyle JT, Gearhart JD. Mol Brain Res 1987; 2: 215–21.
26. Maniatis T, Fritsch EF, Sambrook J (eds). Molecular cloning: a laboratory manual. New York: Cold Spring Harbor, 1982; 382–9.
27. Waters JJ, Bartlett DJ. Clin Cytogen Bull 1988; 2: 30–1.
28. Stenevi U, Kromer LF, Gage FH, Björklund A. In Björklund A, Stenevi U (eds) Neural grafting in the mammalian CNS. Amsterdam: Elsevier, 1985: 41–51.
29. Ralis HM, Beesley RA, Ralis ZA. Techniques in neurohistology. Sevenoaks: Butterworth, 1973.
30. Sparkman DR, White CL III. In Milner GD, Richter RW Blass JP, Valentine JL, Winters-Miner LA (eds) Familial Alzheimer's disease. New York: Marcel Dekker, 1989: 269–86.
31. Richards S-J, Waters JJ, Wischik C, Beyreuther K, Masters C, Sparkman DR, White CL III, Abraham CR, Dunnett SB. EMBO J 1991 (in press).
32. Benowitz LE, Rodriquez W, Paskevich P, Mufson EJ, Schenk D, Neve RL. Exp Neurol 1989; 106: 237–50.
33. Grundke-Iqbal I, Iqbal K, George L, Tung Y-C, Kim KS, Wisniewski H. Proc Natl Acad Sci USA 1989; 86: 2853–7.
34. Hyman BT, Van Hoesen GW, Beyreuther K, Masters CL. Neurosci Lett 1989; 101: 352–5.
35. Wischik CM, Novak M, Edwards P, Klug A, Tichelaar W, Crowther RA. Proc Natl Acad Sci USA 1988; 85: 4884–8.

36. Harrington K, Edwards P, Hills R, Whitmore J, Richard S-J, Bondareff W, Crowther RA (submitted for publication).

Address for correspondence:

Dr Sarah-Jane Richards,
Department of Medicine,
Level 5, Addenbrooke's Hospital, Hills Road,
Cambridge, CB2 2QQ, UK

64 Effects of Combined Intracerebroventricular Infusion of Choline and Oral Administration of Cholinergic Drugs on Learning Impairment in Ventral Globus Pallidus-Lesioned Rats

AKINORI UEKI AND KOHO MIYOSHI

The nucleus basalis magnocellularis (NBM) of the rat, a group of cholinergic neurons in the ventral corner of the globus pallidus, is homologous to the human nucleus basalis of Meynert, i.e. the structure implicated in Alzheimer's disease.

To examine the neurochemical and histological consequence of loss of the cortical cholinergic system, the ventral globus pallidus of the rat was destroyed in the region of the NBM by kainic acid injection. Examination of coronal sections throughout the kainic acid lesion revealed that lesions in the NBM were located in the ventral globus pallidus. Examination of the injected regions in sections prepared by the immuno-histochemical method for choline acetyltransferase (CAT) revealed a marked loss of the large CAT-reactive neurons within the ventral globus pallidus (1). Examination of cerebral cortex in sections prepared by the histochemical method for acetylcholin-esterase (AChE) revealed a dramatic decrease in AChE staining in the injected side (2). The CAT activity in the cerebral cortex ipsilateral to the lesion was significantly lower than that on the contralateral side. No changes were seen in the glutamate decarboxylase (GAD) activity in the cerebral cortex (3). Thus, destruction of the NBM appeared to have selectively damaged the cholinergic neurons. A significant deficit was observed in the acquisition and retention of passive avoidance task following NBM destruction (4). Also, an ameliorating effect on the learning disturbance in ventral globus pallidus-lesioned rats was exhibited following oral administration of 1 or 3 mg/kg THA (9-amino-1,2,3,4-tetrahydroacridine hydrochloride) and NIK-247 (9-amino-2,3,5,6,7,8-hexahydro-1H-cyclopenta[b]quinoline monohydrate hydrochloride), which are cholinesterase inhibitors (5). The observation that choline administration can stimulate synthesis of acetylcholine in the brain has previously

Alzheimer's Disease: Basic Mechanisms, Diagnosis and Therapeutic Strategies
Edited by K. Iqbal, D. R. C. McLachlan, B. Winblad and H. M. Wisniewski
© 1991 John Wiley & Sons Ltd

provided a useful approach for modifying the functional activity of cholinergic neurons (6).

Our preliminary studies demonstrated that oral administration of choline could not increase cerebral acetylcholine level by a transient raising of the cerebral choline concentration. In the present study, we examined the effects of separate and combined oral administration of 0.5 mg/kg THA and NIK-247 and of intracerebroventricular infusion of choline, using an osmotic minipump, on the acquisition of memory task. If choline administration improves a hypocholinergic state, then it might be expected to partially reverse deficits that result from lesioning of the ventral globus pallidus.

METHODS

Subjects

The animals used for this study were 11 to 12-week-old Jcl:Wistar male rats weighing 260–290 g each. They were housed in pairs in cages in a temperature- and light-controlled room (22–25 °C, 12-h light–dark cycle starting at 7:00 a.m.). Food (Jcl, CE-2) and water were available ad libitum.

Surgical procedure

Rats were anesthetized with pentobarbital (40 mg/kg i.p.) and placed in a stereotaxic apparatus. Ibotenic acid (20 nmol in 1 μl of a 50 mM sodium phosphate buffer, pH 7.4) was infused into the bilateral ventral globus pallidus containing NBM following the stereotaxic atlas of Paxinos and Watson (7). Sham-operated rats underwent a similar surgical procedure including insertion of the injection needle but no drug was delivered.

Following a three-week recovery period, each ventral globus pallidus-lesioned rat was anesthetized with pentobarbital (40 mg/kg i.p.) and a permanent microcannula was stereotaxically implanted unilaterally into the left lateral ventricle. The cannula was then anchored firmly and permanently to the skull with dental resin. The tubing which was connected to an Alzet osmotic minipump was then passed subcutaneously between the shoulder blades. The size and location of ibotenic acid lesions and correct placement of the tip of the cannula were verified microscopically in brain sections made after the experiments were completed.

Infusion solutions

Pumps were filled with a phosphate buffer containing choline chloride in such concentrations that 1 μmol ($n = 15$) or 100 μmol ($n = 15$) were infused daily. The pump assures constant delivery of a test substance for a two-week period at a pumping rate of 0.46 μl/h.

Drugs administration

Ventral globus pallidus-lesioned rats with continuous intracerebroventricular infusion received 0.5 mg/kg THA ($n = 5$) and 0.5 mg/kg NIK-247 ($n = 5$). This did not enable a recovery from the learning disturbance or elevate the brain acetylcholine content. THA and NIK-247 were dissolved in physiological saline and given orally 20 min before the test trial.

Passive avoidance learning

Behavioral testing was begun one week after the implant surgery. The rats were submitted to seven habituation sessions (one per day). On days 1, 2 and 3, they were handled for five minutes. On days 4, 5, 6 and 7, they were allowed to explore the apparatus for five minutes.

A two-compartment step-through passive avoidance apparatus was used. The first compartment, an illuminated box, was separated by a guillotine door from the second compartment, a dark box. The passive avoidance procedure is used to measure an animal's ability to learn and remember to avoid a brief footshock by inhibiting a response which normally occurs with a high degree of probability. An electromechanical switching circuit was used to measure the animal's latency in entering the dark compartment of the shuttle box. In the acquisition trial, the animals gradually are to exhibit longer latencies as passive avoidance is acquired by repeated trials using the same procedure.

Shock sensitivity and locomotor activity measurements

After the passive avoidance learning, the rats were evaluated for differences in shock sensitivity using the same shock grid and source as had been used in the passive avoidance task. Vocalization (any audible response to shock) or a jump response (the lifting of at least two paws from grid) were recorded for each animal at each shock level.

Their locomotor activity was recorded using an electromagnetic activity meter at 10-minute intervals for a total period of 60 minutes immediately after the animal was placed in the activity cage.

Measurement of acetylcholine and choline in rat brain

On the seventh day after the implant surgery, ventral globus pallidus-lesioned rats that had been infused with either choline or phosphate buffer began to receive a drug solution (THA, 0.5 mg/kg; or NIK-247, 0.5 mg/kg) or saline once a day. Seven days later they were killed by microwave irradiation 20 minutes after the last oral administration. A piece of the cerebral cortex was then dissected from the brain of each animal. The concentrations of acetylcholine and choline were measured using high-performance liquid chromatography with an electrochemical detector (ECD-100, Eicom, Kyoto, Japan) as described elsewhere (5).

RESULTS

Acquisition of passive avoidance response

The mean acquisition trial latencies tended to lengthen in the ventral globus pallidus-lesioned rats at an intracerebroventricular infusion rate of 100 μmol/day choline. No significant difference in the mean acquisition trial latency was found between the intracerebroventricular choline infusion (100 and 1 μmol/day) group and the phosphate buffer group (Figure 1).

With the combination of intracerebroventricular choline infusion and oral THA administration (0.5 mg/kg) there was a much longer latency than with the combination of intracerebroventricular phosphate buffer infusion and oral saline administration. It became evident on the first and second day of the acquisition trial that the mean latency of the group that received a combination of intracerebroventricular choline infusion (100 μmol/day) and oral THA administration (0.5 mg/kg) was significantly different from that of the group that received a combination of intracerebroventricular phosphate buffer infusion and oral saline administration (Figure 2).

The results with NIK-247 were similar to those with THA, and there was no significant difference in the acquisition trial between the combination of intracerebroventricular choline infusion (1 μmol/day) and oral NIK-247 administration (0.5 mg/kg) and the combination of intracerebroventricular phosphate buffer infusion and oral saline administration.

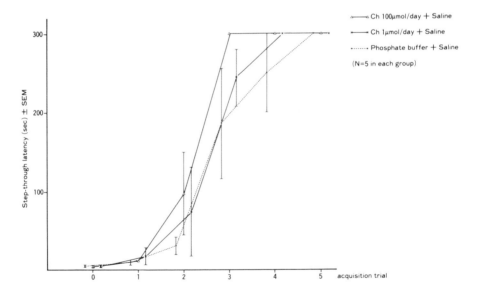

Figure 1. Effect of continuous intracerebroventricular infusion of choline (Ch) on acquisition of passive avoidance response in ventral globus pallidus-lesioned rats

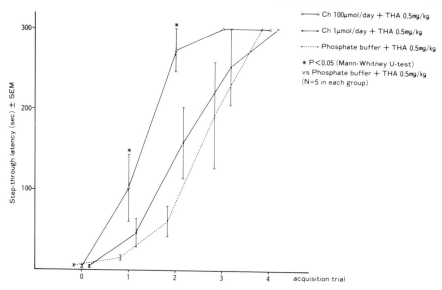

Figure 2. Effect of combined oral administration of tetrahydroaminoacridine (THA) and continuous intracerebroventricular infusion of choline (Ch) on acquisition of passive avoidance response in ventral globus pallidus-lesioned rats

Shock sensitivity and locomotor activity

Evaluations of sensitivity to shock did not reveal any sensory disturbances caused by the intracerebroventricular choline infusion or the combination of intracerebroventricular choline infusion and oral THA or NIK-247 administration (0.5 mg/kg).

There was no significant difference in terms of ventral globus pallidus-lesioned rat locomotor activity between the intracerebroventricular choline infusion and phosphate buffer infusion groups. There was a tendency toward increased locomotor activity with the combination of intracerebroventricular choline infusion (100 μmol/day) and oral THA administration (0.5 mg/kg) as compared to the combination intracerebroventricular phosphate buffer infusion and oral THA administration (0.5 mg/kg). No changes in locomotor acitivity were seen with the combination of intracerebroventricular choline infusion (100 μmol/day) and oral NIK-247 administration (0.5 mg/kg). Similar results were seen with the combination of intracerebroventricular phosphate buffer infusion and oral NIK-247 administration (0.5 mg/kg).

Measurement of acetylcholine and choline in rat brain

The concentrations of choline were significantly increased in the ventral globus pallidus-lesioned rats in the intracerebroventricular choline infusion group as compared to intracerebroventricular phosphate buffer infusion group. Similar results were obtained by combining oral THA or NIK-247 administration (0.5 mg/kg) with intracerebroventricular choline infusion. The concentration of acetylcholine (ACh) in the ventral globus pallidus-lesioned rats treated that underwent intracerebroventricular choline infusion was not significant. The concentration of ACh in the group that received the combination of intracerebroventricular choline infusion (100 μmol/day) and oral THA or NIK-247 administration (0.5 mg/kg) was significantly greater as compared to the group that received the combination intracerebroventricular phosphate buffer infusion and oral THA or NIK-247 administration (0.5 mg/kg).

DISCUSSION

In the present study, we examined the effect of choline administration on passive avoidance response and on the cerebral choline and acetylcholine concentrations in ventral globus pallidus-lesioned rats. Intracerebroventricular choline infusion had no effect on the cerebral acetylcholine concentration. The combination of intracerebroventricular choline infusion and oral THA or NIK-247 administration (0.5 mg/kg), in contrast, caused a significant increase in the acetylcholine concentration of the cerebral cortex. The findings of the present study on intracerebroventricular choline infusion in ventral globus pallidus-lesioned rats would seem to suggest that acetylcholine synthesis can be accelerated by a continuous rise in brain choline concentration. Intracerebroventricular choline infusion did not improve the impairment in passive avoidance learning caused by ventral globus pallidus lesions. However, the combination of intracerebroventricular choline infusion (100 μmol/day) and oral THA or NIK-247 administration (0.5 mg/kg) enabled recovery from learning impairment in ventral globus pallidus-lesioned rats. Separate administration of choline and THA or NIK-247, however, did not improve passive avoidance learning or the cerebral acetylcholine content in these rats. Since memory impairment of the ventral globus pallidus-lesioned rat may be attributed largely to reduction in cortical cholinergic activity, continuous intracerebroventricular infusion of choline may intensify the ameliorating effect of THA or NIK-247 without eliciting a marked change in general activity and sensitivity levels.

REFERENCES

1. Miyoshi K, Sato M, Nakaso S, Ueki A. Ann Rep Pharmacopsychiat Res Found 1987; 18: 20-30.
2. Miyoshi K, Takauchi S, Ueki A, Taira H, Furuhashi A, Sato M. Ann Rep Pharmacopsychiat Res Found 1989; 20: 10-20.
3. Ueki A, Miyoshi K. Jpn J Psychiat Neurol 1987; 41: 87-96.
4. Ueki A, Sato M, Nakaso S, Miyoshi K. Ann Rep Pharmacopsychiat Res Found 1988; 19: 6-15.
5. Ueki A, Miyoshi K. J Neurol Sci 1989; 90: 1-21.
6. Cohen EL, Wurtman RJ. Science 1976; 191: 561-62.
7. Paxinos G, Watson C. The rat brain in stereotaxic coordinates. London: Academic Press, 1989.

Address for correspondence:

Dr Akinori Ueki,
Department of Neuropsychiatry, Hyogo College of Medicine,
1-1, Mukogawa-cho, Nishinomiya, Hyogo 663, Japan

65 Protease Inhibitor, Leupeptin, Causes Irreversible Axonal Changes in Rats

SHIGERU TAKAUCHI AND KOHO MIYOSHI

Recently, it has been shown that amyloid β-protein precursor contains a peptide very similar to the Kunitz family of serine protease inhibitors (1–3), and another serine protease inhibitor α_1-antichymotrypsin has been detected in the brain amyloid deposits of Alzheimer's disease (4). These findings suggest that protease inhibitors participate in the mechanism of amyloid deposition by causing derangement of normal metabolism of precursor proteins, and this leads to cerebral amyloidosis which characterizes an important aspect of Alzheimer's disease.

Leupeptin is a potent cysteine protease inhibitor of microbial origin (5), which, experimentally, induces an accumulation of neurofilaments in axon terminals. This suggests a connection between protease inhibitor and neurofibrillar pathology (6,7). Continuous administration of leupeptin into the rat lateral ventricle resulted in a prominent accumulation of lipofuscin-like granules in neurons, indicating that protease inhibitor exaggerates the neuronal aging process (8). We also found an accumulation of lipofuscin-like dense bodies in the perikaryon, as well as a remarkable degeneration of neuronal processes following continuous administration of leupeptin into the rat lateral ventricle. The resemblance between aggregates of these degenerated neuronal processes induced by leupeptin and the degenerated neurites seen as an important constituent in senile plaque suggested that degenerated neurites are caused by amyloid protein acting as a protease inhibitor (9).

In this study, we investigated the long-term effect of leupeptin infusion in the rat brain and found that the intracytoplasmic accumulation of lipofuscin granules was reversible, but the degeneration of neuronal processes extended over the cerebral cortex, and a part of the cerebral neuron continued to shrink even after the leupeptin infusion was ended. These findings, in addition to the association of protease inhibitors with senile plaque formation, suggest that some derangement of protease activity in neurons plays a role in the pathological aging process of the CNS.

MATERIALS AND METHODS

Thirty Wistar albino rats, each weighing about 200 g, were used for the present study. Leupeptin, purchased from Peptide Institute Inc., was injected into the lateral ventricles of the rats using a constant infusion technique. Each rat was implanted

Alzheimer's Disease: Basic Mechanisms, Diagnosis and Therapeutic Strategies
Edited by K. Iqbal, D. R. C. McLachlan, B. Winblad and H. M. Wisniewski
©1991 John Wiley & Sons Ltd

with an osmotic minipump (Alzet model 2002) that was attached to a cannula stereotaxically guided into its right lateral ventricle. The leupeptin solution, which was prepared at 32.5 mg/ml with phosphate buffer solution, was continuously given for two weeks, with the daily dose and the total dose being 0.47 mg and 6.25 mg, respectively.

On the 15th day, 20 rats were sacrificed by perfusion with 2.5% glutaraldehyde solution from the left ventricle (group A). The other rats were allowed to survive for four additional weeks, following two weeks of leupeptin infusion, and were sacrificed by the same method on the 43rd day of the experiment (group B). Brains and spinal cords were dissected, and stored overnight in glutaraldehyde solution. Coronal slices of 3 mm and 1 mm thickness were made alternatively from the olfactory bulb to the lumbar cord. The former slices were rinsed with phosphate buffer, dehydrated through graded alcohol and embedded in paraffin. The latter slices were cut again into small pieces keeping the orientation of the anatomical structures. After rinsing with phosphate buffer, the tissue blocks were postfixed with 2% osmic acid for 2 hours, dehydrated through graded alcohol, and embedded in a mixture of Epon 812 and Epon 815. Paraffin section were stained with H-E stain, and 1 μm Epon sections were stained with toluidine blue for light microscopy. Ultrathin sections were made using a Porter-Blum MT-2 ultramicrotome with glass blades, and stained with uranyl acetate and lead acetate for examination under a JEOL 1200EX electron microscope.

RESULTS

Light microscopic findings

Light microscopic examination of H-E stained sections from group A rats showed numerous eosinophilic spherical structures of various sizes, resembling so-called spheroids in the hippocampus and corpus callosum. A smaller number of the same structures were found in other parts of the cerebral cortex as well as in the thalamus, caudate nucleus, and putamen. Cell bodies of cortical neurons were much more eosinophilic than they normally appear, although the nuclei were neither shrunken nor pyknotic. While the eosinophilic neurons were widely distributed from the rostral to caudal portions of the cerebral cortex, a marked predominance of these neurons was found in the hippocampus where almost all neurons had eosinophilic cell bodies. The architecture of the cerebral cortex was preserved and no neuronal loss was detectable. In the cerebellar cortex, however, a decreased population of Purkinje cells showed severe degeneration and were presumably responsible for the ataxia. Generally, glial cell proliferation was not remarkable, but in the hippocampus an increased number of glial cells was noticed. On semithin sections stained with toluidine blue (Figure 1A), dark spherical structures corresponding to spheroids were observed with the same distribution as the eosinophilic spherical structures seen with H-E stain. They were well demarcated, containing fine, dense granules, and sometimes enclosed by a thin layer of myelin sheath indicating the origin of an axon. Cortical neurons, especially neurons of the dentate gyrus, contained abundant, small,

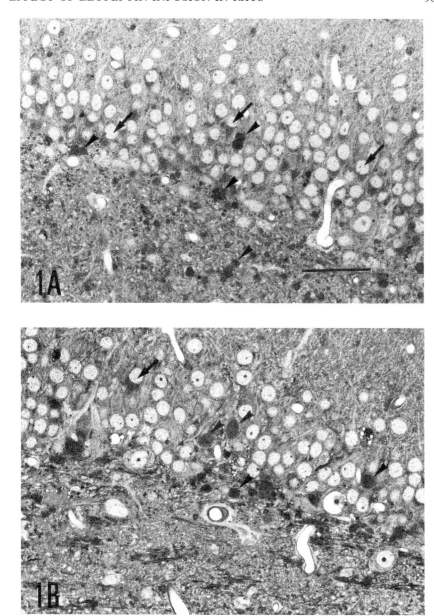

Figure 1. (A) The dentate gyrus of a rat treated with leupeptin. All neurons with dark-appearing perikaryon are filled with lipofuscin-like granules (arrows), and numerous degenerated neurites (arrowheads) are dispersed in the neuropil. Toluidine blue-stained 1-μm epoxy section. Scale bar 50 μm. (B) The region corresponding to (A) of a rat survived for four weeks following leupeptin infusion. An apparent decrease of neurons with intracytoplasmic granules is noted, but the degenerated neurites remain unchanged. Toluidine blue-stained 1-μm epoxy section

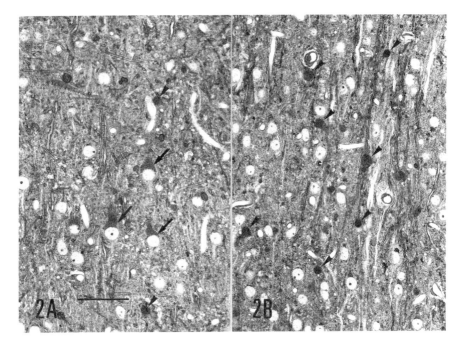

Figure 2. (A) The neurons of isocortex are also filled with lipofuscin-like granules (arrows), and there are a few swollen axons (arrowheads) in the neuropil of a rat sacrificed after two weeks of intraventricular leupeptin infusion. Toluidine blue-stained 1-μm epoxy section. Scale 50 μm. (B) Intracytoplasmic granules are decreased or absent, but degenerated axons are more noticeable (arrowheads). Isocortex of a rat allowed to survive for four weeks after intraventricular leupeptin infusion. Toluidine blue-stained 1-μm epoxy section

dark granules in the cytoplasm, which corresponded to the eosinophilic neurons seen by H-E stain (Figure 2A).

There were distinct differences between the neuroaxonal changes seen in group A rats and those of group B rats; that is, in group B rats, the granule-containing neurons were decreased in number, especially in the dentate gyrus (Figure 1B), and axonal swellings became more conspicuous in the isocortex (Figure 2B).

Electron microscopic findings

1. Changes of the perikaryon

In the group A rats, most neurons of the fascia dentata, subiculum, and a large part of the cerebral cortex contained numerous electron-dense granules resembling lipofuscin. The perikaryon was often occupied by aggregated granules, but the nucleus was situated normally and had no tendency to be pushed aside. In the group B rats, the neurons filled with the dense granules as described in group A rats were rarely encountered, but some cortical neurons contained clusters of dense granules.

The inner structure of the granules showed a range of variations: some granules were filled with a uniformly fine substance and had an appearance similar to lipofuscin granules. Most of the granules were revealed to be membranous dense bodies having a membranous whorl and an electron density higher than lipofuscin. A gradation of the granule density from dense body to vacuole through dense body with floccular inner material was assumed. Degenerating mitochondria showing a higher density and disrupted cristae were also observed, and a transition to dense bodies was strongly suggested. The dense granules also appeared in dendrites and were distributed not only in the vicinity of the perikaryon, but also in the distal portion of dendritic processes forming small clusters of granules.

2. Axonal changes

In both groups, in the regions where axonal swelling had been detected by light microscopic study, not only myelinated axons but also nonmyelinated axons, even the smallest ones, were variously enlarged and contained numerous mitochondria and membranous dense bodies. Especially in rats of group B, dystrophic axons containing disarranged neurofilaments, suggesting disturbed axonal transport, were sometimes observed (Figure 3). No microtubules were detected in the swollen axons,

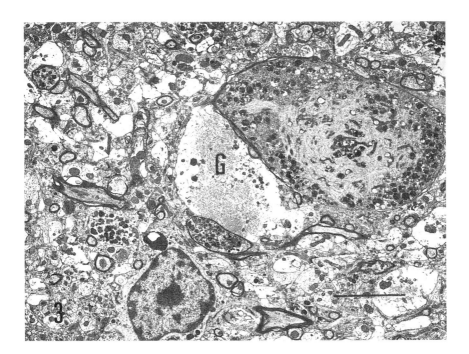

Figure 3. A dystrophic axon seen in the cerebral cortex of a rat surviving after leupeptin infusion. The disarranged bundle of neurofilaments suggests that some disturbance in axonal flow has taken place. A hypertrophic process of astroglia (G) is also visible. Scale Bar 5 μm

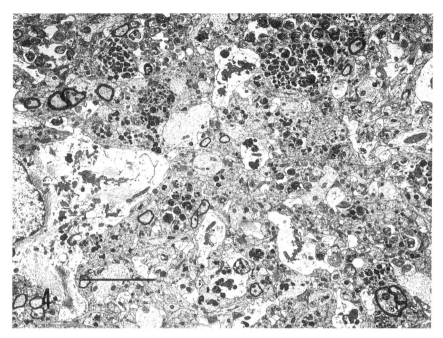

Figure 4. An aspect of the neuropil in the isocortex of a rat allowed to survive for four weeks following leupeptin infusion. Most of the neuronal processes are variously degenerated and mingled with swollen astroglial processes. Scale bar 5 μm

although, rarely, lamellated structures that are known to appear in dystrophic axons (10) were observed. Dense bodies were identical to those in the perikaryon showing various inner structures seemingly due to the degradation stage of abnormal products.

3. Neuropil

The general appearance of the neuropil of the cerebral cortex in rats of both groups, and especially in the hippocampus of leupeptin-treated rats, showed a distinct change from the normal appearance (Figure 4): namely, numerous degenerated neuronal processes consisting of small, swollen axons and dendrites containing dense granules, generally dispersed randomly, were mingled with glial cells and their processes with increased glial fibrils. Occasionally, small aggregates of degenerated neurites closely resembled the aggregation of degenerated neurites appearing in neuritic or senile plaque of Alzheimer's disease (Figure 5). Sometimes presynaptic terminals were enlarged and contained dense bodies or membranous whorls, suggesting synaptic degeneration. Neither amyloid fibrils nor degenerated neurites containing paired helical filaments, however, were found in the brains of leupeptin-treated rats.

DISCUSSION

Leupeptin is one of the protease inhibitors found in culture filtrates of various species of actinomycetes, and it has been shown to inhibit plasmin, trypsin, kallikrein, thrombokinase, papain, and cathepsin B (5). The ability of leupeptin to inhibit calcium-activated protease participated degradation of neurofilaments has been proved in vitro (11). Also, in goldfish, administration of leupeptin has induced accumulation of neurofilaments in synaptic terminals (6). Other morphological evidence concerning the effects of leupeptin has shown that intracellular protein degradation was retarded, autophagic vacuoles were increased, and autolysosomes persisted in hepatocytes of rats (12). Also, in neurons, accumulation of lipofuscin-like dense bodies has been observed in rats after intraventricular leupeptin infusion (8), and we have pointed out the changes of neuronal processes, another important finding in leupeptin-treated rats (9).

It is generally accepted that senile plaques are composed of masses of amyloid fibrils, degenerated neurites, glial cells, and their processes (13). In some cases, the amount of amyloid fibrils is so small that the major constituent within the plaque is thought to be neuronal processes (14). An interesting point found in the present study is that the aggregation of degenerated neuronal processes and synapses mingled with astroglial processes in the neuropil closely resembles the senile plaque of

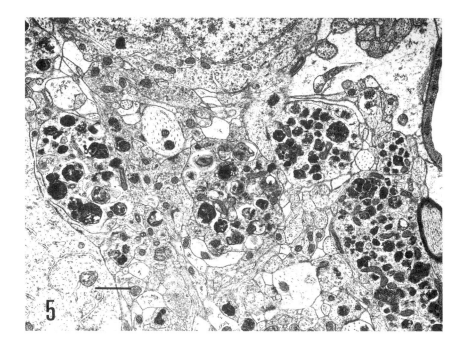

Figure 5. A small cluster of abnormal neurites resembles a primitive plaque in Alzheimer's disease. An electronmicrograph taken in the same section as Figure 4. Scale bar 1 μm

Alzheimer's disease. Although the intracytoplasmic accumulation of lipofuscin-like granules was ameliorated following the termination of leupeptin infusion, neuritic degeneration seemed to extend to a more widespread area of the isocortex. These findings suggest that the disturbance of protein catabolism caused by leupeptin has different effects on the neuronal cytoplasm than on the neurite: the former has the capacity to recover from the disturbance, but the latter does not. In addition, the disarrangement induced by leupeptin may stimulate secondary changes. A portion of the neurons is not able to recover, invoking an astroglial reaction, and the change as a whole becomes more similar to the aging brain.

Recently, a significant study concerning amyloid deposits of senile plaque has demonstrated that the serine protease inhibitor α_1-antichymotrypsin is one of the components of Alzheimer's disease amyloid deposits (4). Other leading studies have shown that amyloid precursor protein has a domain containing a protease inhibitor sequence (1-3), and the protease inhibitory activity has been detected in culture (3). The neurotoxicity of a peptide derived from the amyloid precursor has been demonstrated (15), although the amyloid β-protein itself appeared to have neurotrophic activity (16,17). So far, the role of protease inhibitor in the amyloid deposition and in the aging brain remains enigmatic.

Taking these facts into consideration, the irreversible changes of neuronal processes induced by leupeptin are suggestive of a means for understanding the mechanism not only of senile plaque formation, but also of the dystrophic axons and the neuronal cell loss which may be more important substrates than amyloid deposits for the dementia accompanying the pathological aging process. Although the role of protease inhibitor in senile plaque formation has not yet been clarified, it is possible that protease inhibitor not only takes part in the mechanism of amyloid deposition, but also causes changes in the axons and dendrites leading to degeneration in situ, by retarding degradation of sequestered materials and by deranging axoplasmic flow, or by some other unknown mechanism. Both the aggregated neurites in the hippocampus, which resemble the neuritic plaques, and the widespread neuritic dystrophy in the isocortex in the present study, suggest that leupeptin-induced changes in the CNS can be an animal model for the aging human brain.

REFERENCES

1. Ponte P, Gonzalez-DeWhitt P, Schilling J, Miller J, Hsu D, Greenberg B, Davis K, Wallace W, Lieberburg I, Fuller F, Cordell B. Nature 1988; 331: 525-7.
2. Tanzi RE, McClatchey AI, Lamperti ED, Villa-Komaroff L, Gusella JF, Neve RL. Nature 1988; 331: 528-30.
3. Kitaguchi N, Takahashi Y, Tokushima Y, Shiojiri S, Ito H. Nature 1988; 331: 530-2.
4. Abraham CR, Selkoe DJ, Potter H. Cell 1988; 52: 487-501.
5. Umezawa H, Aoyagi T. In Barrett AJ (ed.) Proteinases in mammalian cells and tissues. Amsterdam: Elsevier, 1977: 637-62.
6. Roots BI. Science 1983; 221: 971-2.
7. Ivy GO, Kitani K, Ihara Y. Brain Res 1989; 498: 360-5.
8. Ivy GO, Schottler F, Wenzel J, Baudry M, Lynch G. Science 1984; 226: 985-7.
9. Takauchi S, Miyoshi K. Acta Neuropathol 1989; 78: 380-7.
10. Lampert PW. J Neuropath Exp Neurol 1967; 26: 345-8.

11. Tashiro T, Ishizaki Y. FEBS Lett 1982; 141: 41-4.
12. Ishikawa T, Furuno K, Kato K. Exp Cell Res 1983; 144: 15-24.
13. Terry RD, Gonatas NK, Weiss M. Am J Path 1964; 44: 269-97.
14. Luse SA, Smith KR Jr. Am J Path 1964; 44: 553-63.
15. Yankner BA, Dawes LR, Fisher S, Villa-Komaroff L, Oster-Granite LM, Neve RL. Science 1989; 245: 417-20.
16. Whitson JS, Selkoe DJ, Cotman CW. Science 1989; 243: 1488-90.
17. Whitson JS, Glabe CG, Shintani E, Abcar A, Cotman CW. Neurosci Lett 1990; 110: 319-24.

Address for correspondence:

Dr Shigeru Takauchi,
Department of Neuropsychiatry,
Hyogo College of Medicine, 1-1, Mukogawa-cho,
Nishinomiya, Hyogo 663, Japan

Part X

BIOLOGICAL MARKERS/ SYSTEMIC MARKERS

66 Brain Nicotinic Receptor Deficits in Alzheimer Patients as Studied by Positron Emission Tomography Technique

A. NORDBERG, P. HARTVIG, A. LILJA, M. VIITANEN,
K. AMBERLA, H. LUNDQVIST, J. ULIN, Y. ANDERSSON,
B. LÅNGSTRÖM AND B. WINBLAD

Alzheimer's disease, senile dementia of Alzheimer type (AD/SDAT), is a progressive neurodegenerative disorder with global deterioration of cognitive function with preservation of many other brain functions. From studies in autopsy or biopsy human brain tissues the disease can neurochemically be characterized as changes of multiple transmitter systems (1). Among the afflicted neurotransmitters in AD/SDAT the cholinergic system shows the most consistent changes (2). It is also the system which best correlates with cognitive function (3,4). Since still no complete agreement exists between clinical diagnosis and final histopathological examination there is need for improved diagnostic resolution. Positron emission tomography (PET) is a technique suitable for in-vivo studies of central neuronal activity in brain. The method has already shown a great potential for psychopharmacological research (5). PET must therefore be considered as a putative diagnostic tool in neurodegenerative diseases such as AD/SDAT. Earlier PET studies performed in AD/SDAT patients have been limited to studies of cerebral blood flow and metabolism studied by oxygen and glucose utilization (6-9). A decrease in cerebral blood flow and oxygen consumption has been measured in vivo in AD/SDAT patients using $^{15}O_2$ and PET (6). A lower glucose utilization using the analogue $[2-^{18}F]$fluorodeoxyglucose has also been measured in cortical areas of AD/SDAT patients compared to age-matched controls (7,10). Recently, attempts have been made to visualize cholinergic markers in brain by PET technique. In this study $[^{11}C]$nicotine and PET were used in order to study in-vivo changes in nicotinic receptors in Alzheimer brains.

CHOLINERGIC TRACERS IN BRAIN VISUALIZED IN VIVO BY PET

Studies in postmortem brains indicate a cholinergic presynaptic defect in AD/SDAT. Attempts to measure the turnover of the cholinergic system in human brain by PET

Alzheimer's Disease: Basic Mechanisms, Diagnosis and Therapeutic Strategies
Edited by K. Iqbal, D. R. C. McLachlan, B. Winblad and H. M. Wisniewski
©1991 John Wiley & Sons Ltd

were initiated using [^{11}C]choline (11,12). A low penetration of intact [^{11}C]choline to the brain together with a rapid conversion of formed [^{11}C]acetylcholine to radiolabelled metabolites hampered this effort. An alternative to measuring precursor transport and transmitter turnover would be to visualize the cholinergic receptors. For the muscarinic receptors, PET studies using ligands for the muscarinic receptors (13,14) have not yet been extended to Alzheimer patients. In a limited study of one Alzheimer patient and one healthy volunteer, Holman et al (15) used single photon emission computerized tomography (SPECT) and [^{121}I]quinuclidinyl-4-iodobenzilate to visualize brain muscarinic receptors. Recently, attempts to visualize nicotinic receptors in vivo using [^{11}C]nicotine and PET have been made in monkeys (16,17) and humans (18,19). This strategy must be considered of high interest since a marked reduction in the number of nicotinic receptors has been measured by in-vitro receptor binding technique in autopsy AD/SDAT brain tissue (20).

NICOTINIC RECEPTORS IN HUMAN BRAIN

Multiple nicotinic receptors exist in human brain. The presence of the nicotinic receptors have been characterized in vitro in autopsy brain tissue using various radioactive ligands, mainly [^{3}H]nicotine. The nicotinic agonist binding sites in human brain can be rationalized in terms of superhigh, high and low affinity binding sites by competition studies between [^{3}H]nicotine and unlabelled nicotine (21-24). The regional distribution of high-affinity nicotinic receptors in human brain reveals a high content in areas such as the thalamus, caudate nucleus, putamen; intermediate in the cortical areas, hypothalamus, cerebellum; and low in the hippocampus, pons and globus pallidus (23-25). When [^{11}C]nicotine is intravenously injected in humans the ^{11}C radioactivity is rapidly taken up by the brain and distributed to various regions in a pattern which closely agrees with the distribution of nicotinic receptors measured by in-vitro receptor binding (18,19). Nicotine has recently been shown to stimulate the glucose utilization in areas of the rat brain that are rich in nicotinic receptors, which suggests that the nicotinic receptors might be coupled to energy metabolism (26).

UPTAKE AND BINDING OF [^{11}C]NICOTINE IN BRAIN OF ALZHEIMER PATIENTS

Neurochemical studies in postmortem brain tissue from AD/SDAT patients reveal a marked loss in the number of cortical nicotinic receptors (20,27). Furthermore, a change in the proportion of high to low affinity nicotinic receptors has been measured (22). In attempts to confirm these observations in vivo [^{11}C]nicotine was injected intravenously to Alzheimer patients and age-matched healthy volunteers. The study was performed by permission of the Ethical Committees at the Medical Faculty of Uppsala University and Karolinska Institute. The Alzheimer patients were assessed in the Geriatric Clinic, Huddinge Hospital, and the clinical diagnosis of Alzheimer's disease was determined according to DSMIII-R criteria. Clinical examination included blood and cerebrospinal fluid analysis, electroencephalography, computed tomography and magnetic resonance imaging. The healthy volunteers (mean age 68 ± 2 years, range 61–72 years) had no history of psychiatric or neurological disease. Both patients and controls underwent neuropsychological investigations such as Lurias's neuropsychological methods, trail making test, subtests from WAIS-R, WMS logical memory immediate recall and cued recall and recognition (28–31). The Alzheimer patients (mean age 68 ± 2 years, range 63–74 years) had a mean duration of the disease of 5 ± 1 years and the Hachinski score was less than 4. None of subjects were smokers. The (S)(−) and (R)(+) enantiomers of [^{11}C] nicotine were injected intravenously as tracer doses (less than 10% of the content of a cigarette) to both Alzheimer patients and controls. The uptake of (S)(−) and (R)(+)[^{11}C] nicotine to the brain was very similar in healthy volunteers, while in the Alzheimer patients a significantly markedly lower uptake of (R)(+)[^{11}C] nicotine was measured compared to (S)(−)[^{11}C] nicotine (19). The uptake of (S)(−)[^{11}C] nicotine was markedly lower in cortical areas, such as the temporal cortex, of the Alzheimer patients compared to age-matched controls (Figure 1). The uptake of (R)(+)[^{11}C] nicotine was also significantly lower in Alzheimer patients compared to control, which is illustrated for the frontal cortex in Figure 2. Thus a significantly lower uptake of both [^{11}C] nicotine enantiomers was observed in Alzheimer brains compared to controls.

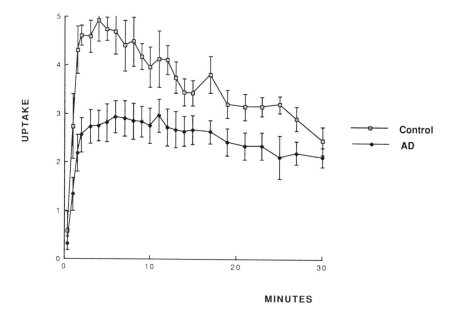

MINUTES

Figure 1. Uptake and time course of ^{11}C radioactivity in the temporal cortex of Alzheimer patients and age-matched healthy volunteers receiving an intravenous injection of (S)-(−)-N-[^{11}C] methyl nicotine. The uptake is expressed in nCi/cm³/dose·body weight^{-1}. Each curve represents the mean values $\pm$ SEM of six Alzheimer patients and four controls respectively

BIOLOGICAL/SYSTEMIC MARKERS

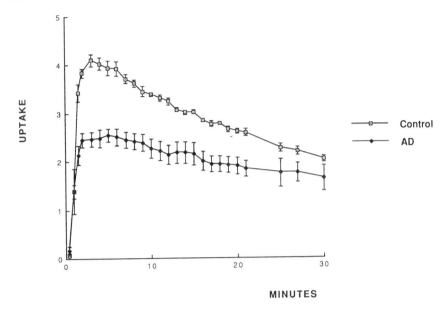

Figure 2. Uptake and time course of ¹¹C radioactivity in the frontal cortex of Alzheimer patients and age-matched healthy volunteers receiving an intravenous injection of (R)(+)-N-[¹¹C]methyl nicotine. The uptake is expressed in nCi/cm³/dose·body weight⁻¹. Each curve represents the mean value±SEM of five Alzheimer patients and five controls respectively

To exclude that the uptake of [¹¹C]nicotine and its concomitant distribution to the brain merely mimic the cerebral blood flow, studies using [¹¹C]butanol as a blood flow marker (32) were performed. The [¹¹C]butanol peaked in brain within 1–2 min after injection. While no significant difference in the regional distribution of [¹¹C]butanol was observed in the control subjects, a markedly lower uptake of [¹¹C]butanol was observed in the temporal and frontal cortex of the Alzheimer patients while the uptake to the thalamus was preserved (33). The elimination curve for [¹¹C]butanol in the brain was much more steep in comparison to both (S)(−) and (R)(+)[¹¹C]nicotine (Figures 3, 4). This might indicate that the (+) and (−) [¹¹C]nicotine enantiomers at least partly display specific binding profiles and that changes in uptake of [¹¹C]nicotine in Alzheimer patients might reflect changes in specific binding. Figure 3 illustrates the uptake of [¹¹C]butanol and (S)(−)[¹¹C]nicotine in the frontal cortex of two Alzheimer patients. The uptake of [¹¹C]butanol was markedly lower in the frontal cortex of both Alzheimer patients compared to healthy volunteers. The uptake of [¹¹C]nicotine was markedly lower in the frontal cortex of one of the Alzheimer patients compared to the other Alzheimer patient, although the uptake of [¹¹C]butanol (blood flow marker) was very similar in both patients (Figure 3). Interestingly, the uptake of (S)(−)[¹¹C]nicotine was similar in the temporal cortex of both Alzheimer patients (Figure 4). This observation illustrates that valuable information can be obtained by using tracers for neural activity in addition to solely blood flow markers.

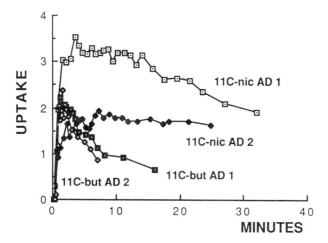

Figure 3. Uptake and time courses of ^{11}C radioactivity in the frontal cortex of two Alzheimer patients following intravenous injections of [^{11}C]butanol (11C-but) and (S)(−)-N-[^{11}C]methyl nicotine (11C-nic). The uptake is expressed in nCi/cm^3/dose·body weight^{-1}

CONCLUSION

PET studies of the brain following intravenous injections of (S)(−) and (R)(+)[^{11}C]nicotine have showed a marked reduction in the uptake of both enantiomers, especially the (R)(+), in Alzheimer patients compared to age-matched healthy volunteers. The larger difference in uptake of (S)(−) and (R)(+)[^{11}C]nicotine in Alzheimer patients compared to controls might be of diagnostic value. [^{11}C]Nicotine shows a time course in brain which is different from

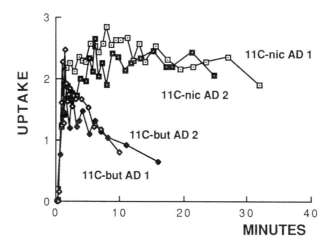

Figure 4. Uptake and time courses of ^{11}C radioactivity in the temporal cortex of two Alzheimer patients following intravenous injections of [^{11}C]butanol (11C-but) and (S)(−)-N-[^{11}C]methyl nicotine (11C-nic). The uptake is expressed in nCi/cm^3/dose·body weight^{-1}

that of solely blood markers such as [^{11}C]butanol. This observation might indicate a specific binding profile for both [^{11}C]nicotine enantiomers. Further studies are needed to evaluate how early in the course of Alzheimer's disease changes in uptake of [^{11}C]nicotine can be detected in brain. An early detection of the disease will favour new potential therapeutic strategies.

Acknowledgments

This study was supported by grants from the Swedish Medical Research Council, the Swedish Tobacco Company, Petrus and Augusta Hedlunds Foundation, Loo and Hans Osterman's Foundation, and Stohne's Foundation.

REFERENCES

1. Hardy JA, Adolfsson R, Alafuzoff I, Bucht G, Marcusson J, Nyberg P, Perdahl E, Wester P, Winblad B. Neurochem Int 1985; 7: 545-63.
2. Perry E. Br Med Bull 1986; 42: 63-9.
3. Drachman DA. Neurology 1977; 27: 783-90.
4. Drachman DA. In Katzman R, Terry RD, Bick KL (eds) Alzheimer's disease: senile dementia and related disorders. New York: Raven Press. 1978: 141-8.
5. Phelp ME, Maziotta JC, Huang SC. J Cerebr Blood Flow Metab 1982; 5: 138-46.
6. Frackowiak RSJ, Pozzilli C, Legg NJ, Boulay GH, Marshall J, Lenzi GL, Jones T. Brain 1981; 104: 753-78.
7. Ferris SH, de Leon MJ, Wolf AP, Farkas T, Christman DR, Reisberg B, Fowler JS, MacGregor R, Goldman A, George AE, Rampal S. Neurobiol Aging 1980; 1: 127-31.
8. Riege WH, Metter EJ. Neurobiol Aging 1988; 9: 69-86.
9. Burns A, Tune L, Steele C, Folstein M. Int J Geriatr Psychiatry 1989; 4: 67-72.
10. Foster NL, Chase TN, Mansi L, Brooks R, Fedio P, Patronas NJ, Di Chiro G. Ann Neurol 1984; 16: 649-54.
11. Eckernäs SÅ, Aquilonius SM, Bergström K, Hartvig P, Lindberg B, Lundqvist H, Långström B, Malmborg P, Någren K. IV World Congress of Biological Psychiatry, Philadelphia, Sept 1985. Amsterdam: Elsevier 1986.
12. Gauthier S, Diksic M, Yamamoto L, Tyler J, Feindel W. Can J Neurol 1985; 12: 214.
13. Dewey SL, Bendriem B, MacGregor R, King P, Fowler JS, Christman DR, Schlyer DJ, Wolf AP, Volkow N, Brodie JD. J Cerebr Blood Flow Metab 1989; 9: 1-S13.
14. Mazier M, Khalili-Varasteh M, Delforge J, Janier M, Leguludec P, Prenant C, Syrota A. Progr Brain Res 1990; 84: 347-59.
15. Holman BL, Gibson RE, Hill TC, Eckelman WC, Albert M, Rebz RC. JAMA 1985; 254: 3063-6.
16. Maziere M, Comar D, Marazano C, Berger G. Eur J Nucl Med 1976; 1: 255-8.
17. Nordberg A, Hartvig P, Lundqvist H, Antoni G, Ulin J, Långström B. J Neural Transm (P-D sect.) 1989; 1: 195-205.
18. Nybäck H, Nordberg A, Långström B, Halldin C, Hartvig P, Åhlin A, Swan CG, Sedvall G. Progr Brain Res 1989; 79: 313-19.
19. Nordberg A, Hartvig P, Lilja A, Viitanen M, Amberla K, Lundqvist H, Andersson Y, Ulin J, Windblad B, Långström B. J Neural Transm 1990; 2: 215-24.
20. Nordberg A, Windblad B. Neurosci Lett 1986; 72: 115-19.
21. Nordberg A, Adem A, Nilsson L, Winblad B. In Tomlinson B, Pepeu G, Wischik CM (eds) New trends in aging research. Padova: Liviana Press 1988: 27-36.
22. Nordberg A, Adem A, Hardy J, Winblad B. Neurosci Lett 1988; 317-21.

23. Nordberg A, Adem A, Nilsson L, Romanelli L, Zhang X. In Clementi F, Gotti C, Sher E (eds) Nicotinic acetylcholine receptors in the nervous system. Berlin: Springer 1988: 305-15.
24. Nordberg A, Nilsson-Håkansson L, Adem A, Hardy J, Alafuzoff I, Lai Z, Herrera-Marschitz M, Winblad B. Progr Brain Res 1989; 79: 353-62.
25. Adem A, Nordberg A, Singh Jossan S, Sara V, Gillberg PG. Neurosci Lett 1989; 101: 247-52.
26. London E. In The biology of nicotine dependence (Ciba Foundation Symposium 152) Chichester: John Wiley, 1990: 131-46.
27. Whitehouse P, Martino AM, Antuono PG, Lowenstein PR, Coyle JT, Price DL, Kellar KJ. Brain Res 1986; 371: 146-51.
28. Erkinjuntti T, Laaksonen R, Sulkawa R, Syrjäälinen R, Palo J. Acta Neurol Scand 1986; 74: 393-403.
29. Reitan RM. Percept Motor Skills 1958; 8: 271-6.
30. Wechsler DA. Wechsler adult inteligence scale — revised manual. New York: Psychological Corporation, 1981.
31. Weingartner H, Grafman J, Boutelle W, Kaye W, Martin PR. Science 1983; 122: 380-2.
32. Herscovitch P, Raichle ME, Kilbourn MR, Welch MJ. J Cerebr Blood Flow Metab 1987; 7: 527-42.
33. Nordberg A, Hartvig P, Lundqvist H, Lilja A, Viitanen M, Amberla K, Ulin J, Winblad B, Långström B. In Giacobini E, Becker RE (eds) Current research in Alzheimer therapy early diagnosis. New York: Taylor & Francis 1990: 329-38.

Address for correspondence:

Dr Agneta Nordberg,
Department of Pharmacology,
Box 591,
S-7511 24 Uppsala,
Sweden

67 Neurotransmitter Markers in the Cerebrospinal Fluid of Patients with Histologically Verified Alzheimer's Disease

K. J. REINIKAINEN, H. SOININEN, L. PALJÄRVI AND
P. J. RIEKKINEN Sr

Studies of neurotransmitter variables in the cerebrospinal fluid (CSF) of patients with Alzheimer's disease (AD) intended to find a specific diagnostic marker for the disease or to detect a reliable indicator for a certain abnormality of cerebral transmitter metabolism have given inconsistent findings (1,2). Since most studies have been performed in clinically diagnosed patients, inaccuracies in the diagnostics or coincidental presence of some other pathology may have confounded the findings. Therefore, to study this point further we have reanalyzed the neurotransmitter findings of autopsied dementia cases with the histological verification of AD.

PATIENTS AND METHODS

Patients

AD patients in this series were included in earlier reported studies (2-5). The patients had shown profound dementia during their lifetime. In each of the patients, symptoms of dementia had started insidiously and showed a steady progress. All patients had been evaluated for their dementia at the Department of Neurology, Kuopio University Central Hospital, according to a research scheme including history evaluation, clinical examination by a neurologist (H. S.), neuropsychological assessment, extensive laboratory examinations, CSF analysis, chest x-ray, electrocardiogram, electroencephalography and computed tomography of the head. Before lumbar punctures patients were kept on a tyrosine and tryptophan free diet; the lumbar punctures were performed in lateral decubitus position between 8.00 and 10.00 am after overnight bed rest and fasting. The CSF specimens were frozen ($-70\,^{\circ}$C) and stored until assayed.

All patients were diagnosed to have dementia according to DSMIII (6) and were found to fulfil the criteria of probable or possible AD of NINCDS-ADRDA (7). Those coming to autopsy and fulfilling the histopathological criteria of AD (8) were

Alzheimer's Disease: Basic Mechanisms, Diagnosis and Therapeutic Strategies
Edited by K. Iqbal, D. R. C. McLachlan, B. Winblad and H. M. Wisniewski
© 1991 John Wiley & Sons Ltd

included in this study. We were able to find 18 such cases who also had data of CSF neurotransmitter values analyzed by techniques used in the earlier reported clinical series. Variable time had elapsed since the lumbar punctures and autopsies; however, in the majority of cases CSF studies had been performed at a very advanced state of the disease, thus representing data of severe AD.

Control patients in the clinical series had been age-matched subjects without signs of dementia or any other abnormal neurological signs in the neurological evaluation (2-5). The values of the neurotransmitter findings of AD patients were compared with the findings of these corresponding control series.

Neuropathological methods

At autopsies after the brain had been weighed and divided, one half was immersed in 10% buffered formalin. After fixation, standard samples were taken from the frontal cortex (Brodmann area 9), temporal cortex (Brodmann area 21), hippocampus and parahippocampal cortex, thalamus, caudate nucleus, pallidum, putamen, substantia nigra and pons. Paraffin sections were stained with hematoxylin-eosin and Bielschowsky silver methods. The Bielschowsky preparations were used to detect senile plaques and neurofibrillary tangles. The number of senile plaques and neurofibrillary tangles in each case were checked to exceed the histopathological criteria for AD presented recently (8). The presence of possible parkinsonian disease (PD) pathology was examined in hematoxylin-eosin sections of the substantia nigra. The cell loss of the substantia nigra was based on 5-μm sections graded as being absent, mild (under 50% loss), moderate (50–70% loss) or severe (over 70% loss). Coexistent parkinsonian pathology was considered to be present if Lewy bodies and at least moderate cell loss were found in the substantia nigra (9).

Biochemical methods

In the CSF samples the activity of cholinesterase (ChE), as a marker of cholinergic neurons, was determined by the colorimetric method as described earlier (2,4). The concentrations of homovanillic acid (HVA), the main metabolite of dopamine, and of 5-hydroxyindoleacetic acid (5HIAA), the main metabolite of serotonin, were determined by the fluorometric method of Earley and Leonard (10) as described in the clinical paper (3). The activity of dopamine β-hydroxylase (DBH), as a marker of noradrenergic neurons, and somatostatin-like immunoreactivity (SLI) were determined by radioimmunoassay as described earlier (3,5).

Statistics

Comparisons between controls and AD patients were done by using Student's t-test for independent samples.

RESULTS

The activity of ChE was significantly lower (-27%) in AD patients as compared to the controls (Table 1). The level of HVA was reduced (-46%) significantly in the total group of AD patients. In the histopathological examination 5 out of these 18 AD cases showed coincident PD pathology in the substantia nigra, and HVA in the CSF of these patients was significantly lower compared both to AD cases without PD pathology (-64%, $P < 0.01$) and to the controls (-77%). The concentration of 5HIAA was also slightly lower (-22%) in AD patients when compared to the controls. The activity of DBH showed no significant difference between AD patients and controls. The CSF SLI was lower (-28%) in the AD group as compared to controls; this difference was statistically almost significant ($P = 0.052$).

The data of the transmitter markers between clinical series and those cases included in this study were closely comparable, as presented in Figures 1 and 2.

DISCUSSION

As the cholinergic deficiency is the most profound and consistently reported neurotransmitter abnormality in AD (2,11), several studies have been done in clinically diagnosed AD patients by assaying the activity of ChE or of more specific acetylcholinesterase in the CSF with the aim of finding a CSF marker for that cholinergic deficit of the brain, but with conflicting results. Some studies have found no difference between patients and controls (12-15), while others have reported

Table 1. Neurotransmitter markers in the CSF of 18 histologically verified AD patients. Values are means ± SD

Transmitter marker in CSF	AD patients	± % of control	P value	Controls
ChE (nmol/ml/min)	26.1 ± 6.7 ($n = 12$)	−27%	<0.01	35.6 ± 8 ($n = 29$)
HVA (ng/ml)				
all	42.0 ± 20.5 ($n = 18$)	−46%	<0.001	78.0 ± 25.2 ($n = 13$)
AD only	51.0 ± 14.0 ($n = 13$)	−35%	<0.01	78.0 ± 25.2 ($n = 13$)
AD + PD	18.6 ± 8.1 ($n = 5$)	−77%	<0.001	78.0 ± 25.2 ($n = 13$)
5HIAA (ng/ml)	32.9 ± 12.1 ($n = 18$)	−22%	<0.05	42.0 ± 10.8 ($n = 13$)
DBH (pmol/ml/min)	17.5 ± 9.1 ($n = 6$)	+6%	NS	16.9 ± 10.4 ($n = 20$)
SLI (pg/ml)	18.3 ± 3.1 ($n = 6$)	−28%	0.052	25.5 ± 7.6 ($n = 19$)

Abbreviations: ChE, cholinesterase; HVA, homovanillic acid; 5HIAA, 5-hydroxyindoleacetic acid; DBH, dopamine β-hydroxylase; SLI, somatostatin-like immunoreactivity. AD only means AD cases without additional histological features of parkinsonian changes in the histological examination of the substantia nigra, and correspondingly AD + PD means the presence of both changes.

a: CHE

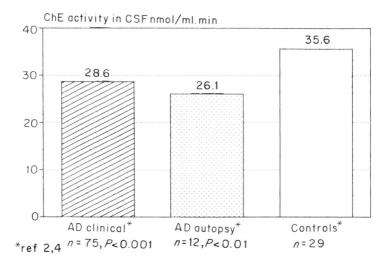

b: 5HIAA

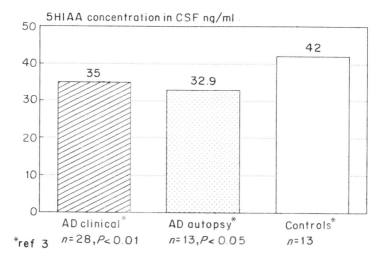

Figure 1. (a–d) Mean ChE activity, 5HIAA concentration, DBH activity and SLI in the CSF of clinically and histologically diagnosed AD patients. Data compared with the controls. Abbreviations as in Table 1. Statistical comparisons between AD patient groups and controls with Student's t-test

c: DBH

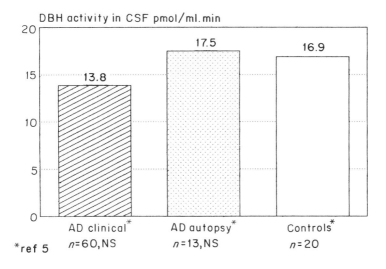

d: SLI

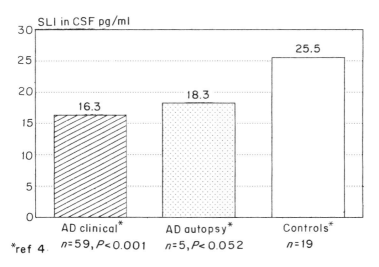

decreased ChE and acetylcholinesterase activities in the CSF in patients with AD diagnosed either by clinical methods (2,4,16–20) or confirmed by histology (2,21,22). However, when decreases have been found these have been only of moderate degree at greatest, and it seems that the reduced ChE activity in the CSF might be observed only in very severely demented patients in AD (2). In the present study the AD patients were at a very advanced state of the disease at the time of CSF sampling and the mean change was only modest (27%).

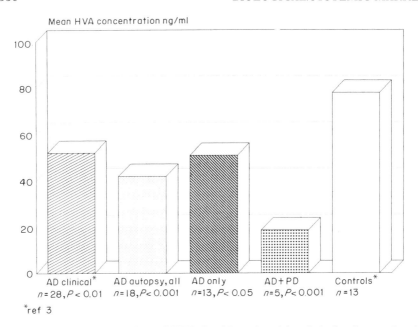

Figure 2. Mean concentration of HVA (in AD patients) in clinically diagnosed and in histologically diagnosed AD patients according to the presence of PD pathology in the substantia nigra. Data compared with the controls. Abbreviations as in Table 1. Statistical comparisons between AD patient groups and controls with Student's t-test

Also the methodological differences may contribute to the controversies in the findings. The method for ChE assay used in these patients measures both the activity of acetylcholinesterase and butyrylcholinesterase. In autopsy study the activity of butyrylcholinesterase was found to be increased in the postmortem brain tissue (23). On the other hand, acetylcholinesterase represents about 85–90% of the total ChE activity in the CSF (2), and thus our finding apparently indicates mainly the loss of the acetylcholinesterase activity as shown recently in our laboratory by Sirviö et al (20). In any case, present data further confirm the findings of earlier reports of clinically diagnosed AD patients that the cholinergic deficit of the brain is at least partly reflected in the CSF in patients with AD.

Unlike the cholinergic system, the dopaminergic neurons seem to be intact or only mildly affected in cortical areas of the brain in AD according to both postmortem (9,24,25) and antemortem studies (25), while many studies, though not all, have reported reduced levels of HVA in the CSF in AD (1). However, in some postmortem studies reduced concentrations of dopamine and HVA have been found in the subcortical brain areas, in the hippocampus and striatum (9,24,26). In the striatum this may reflect — at the structural level — pathology in the nigrostriatal tracts, coincidental cellular loss and presence of Lewy bodies in the substantia nigra as in Parkinson's disease (9), or in diffuse Lewy body disease or a Lewy body variant of AD (27). As shown recently, those AD patients having a PD pathology also had low striatal dopamine content and have had also considerably lower HVA levels in the CSF during their lifetime (9). In this study a few more cases were analyzed confirming our earlier findings, i.e. AD patients having noticeably reduced concentration of CSF HVA appeared to have pathology in the substantia nigra at the neuropathological examination.

However, also the AD patients without PD pathology were found to have significantly reduced CSF HVA. A similar finding was reported by others in a group of histologically verified AD cases (25). This might indicate reduced turnover of dopaminergic neurons associated with AD as proposed in one report (26), but not confirmed by others (9). Nevertheless, in these severely demented AD patients, the change was only moderate and thus not useful in early diagnosis of AD.

The serotonergic system has been shown to be involved by the disease process of AD, not only in late phase, as demonstrated by the postmortem studies (24,25,28), but also early in the course of the disease, as indicated by antemortem studies (25). However, as with the cholinergic system, this abnormality seems to be poorly expressed in the CSF as low 5HIAA concentrations (1). The 5HIAA in the lumbar CSF probably originates more from the spinal cord than from the brain and therefore the cerebral abnormality of serotonin metabolism needs to be very marked before it is detectable in the 5HIAA levels in the lumbar CSF (1). In the present study the reduction of 5HIAA level was only slight and represents an advanced state of the disease as found also in the clinical study (3).

As in our earlier clinical study (5) the activity of DBH was not significantly altered in the CSF in patients with AD. In a larger sample of 75 clinically diagnosed AD patients DBH activity was found to be marginally reduced only in a group of probable AD patients with most severe dementia — 21 out of 75 — by about 20% (1). Similarly, the level of main metabolite of noradrenaline is not clearly altered in the CSF in patients with AD (1).

The CSF SLI was reduced in this study as in the clinical series, but most probably due to the small number of cases available this was not statistically significant. However, the degree of the change was about the same as in several clinical series (1,4) thus supporting those findings. Although reduced CSF SLI may be detectable in mildly demented AD patients in larger series (1), the change is too subtle and too unspecific to be used as an adjunct to diagnostics.

In conclusion, present data of histologically verified AD patients confirms that, as in the brain, several neurotransmitter markers, including ChE, HVA, 5HIAA and SLI, are altered in the CSF in patients with AD. However, most of these changes are only subtle and detectable only in the very advanced state of AD and thus not useful in the diagnostics. Considerably lower HVA in CSF in AD patients may indicate the presence of concurrent pathology of the nigrostriatal system.

Acknowledgments

This study was supported partly by the research grant by the Medical Research Council of the Academy of Finland.

REFERENCES

1. Reinikainen KJ, Riekkinen PJ. In Fowler CJ, Carlson LA, Gottfries C-G, Windblad B (eds) Biological markers in dementia of Alzheimer type. London: Smith-Gordon, Nishimura 1990: 161-78.
2. Reinikainen KJ, Riekkinen PJ, Paljärvi L, Soininen H, Helkala E-L, Jolkkonen J, Laakso M. Neurochem Res 1988; 13: 135-46.
3. Soininen H, MacDonald E, Rekonen M, Riekkinen PJ. Acta Neurol Scand 1981; 64: 101-7.
4. Soininen HS, Jolkkonen JT, Reinikainen KJ, Haloen TO, Riekkinen PJ. J Neurol Sci 1984; 63: 167-72.
5. Soininen H, Pitkänen A, Halonen T, Riekkinen PJ. Acta Neurol Scand 1984; 69: 29-34.
6. Diagnostic and statistical manual of mental disorders, 3rd edn. Washington: APA, 1980.
7. McKhann G, Drachman D, Folstein M, Katzman R, Price D, Stadlan EM. Neurology; 1984: 939-44.
8. Khachaturian ZS. Arch Neurol 1985; 42: 1097-105.
9. Reinikainen KJ, Paljärvi L, Halonen T, Malminen O, Kosma V-M, Laakso M, Riekkinen PJ. Neurobiol Aging 1988; 9: 245-52.
10. Earley CJ, Leonard BE. J Pharmacol Methods 1978; 1: 67-79.
11. Perry EK. Br Med Bull 1986; 42: 63-9.
12. Johnsson S, Domino E. Clin Chim Acta 1971; 35: 421-8.
13. Deutsch SJ, Mohs RV, Levy MI, Rothpearl AB, Stockton D, Horvath T, Coco A, Davis KL. Biol Psychiat 1983; 18: 1363-73.
14. Lal S, Wood PL, Kiely ME, Etienne P, Gauthier S, Stanford J, Ford RM, Dastoor RM, Nair NPV. Neurobiol Aging 1984; 5: 269-74.
15. Ruberg M, Villageois A, Bonnet AM, Pillon B, Rieger F, Agid Y. J Neurol Neurosurg Psychiat 1987; 50: 538-43.
16. Tune L, Gucker S, Folstein M, Oshida L, Coyle TJ. Ann Neurol 1985; 17: 46-8.
17. Nakano S, Kato T, Nakamura S, Kameyama M. J Neurol Sci 1986; 75: 213-23.
18. Urakami K, Adachi Y, Awaki E, Takahashi K. Acta Neurol Scand 1989; 42: 232-7.
19. Atack JR, May C, Kaye JA, Kay AD, Rapoport. Ann Neurol 1988; 23: 161-7.
20. Sirviö J, Kutvonen R, Soininen H, Hartikainen P, Riekkinen PJ. J Neural Transm 1989; 75: 119-27.
21. Appleyard ME, Smith AD, Wilcock DK, Esiri MM. Lancet 1983; ii: 452.
22. Arendt T, Bigl V, Walther F, Sonntag M. Lancet 1984; i: 173.
23. Perry EK, Tomlinson BE, Blessed G, Bergman K, Gibson PH. Br Med J 1978; ii: 147-59.
24. Gottfries CG, Adolfsson R, Aquilonius SM, Carlsson A, Eckernäs SÅ, Nordberg A, Oreland L, Svennerholm L, Wiberg Å, Winblad B. Neurobiol Aging 1983; 4: 261-71.
25. Palmer AM, Bowen DM. In Fowler CJ, Carlson LA, Gottfries C-G, Winblad B (eds) Biological markers in dementia of Alzheimer type. London: Smith-Gordon, Nishimura 1990: 89-105.
26. Pearce BR, Palmer AM, Bowen DM, Wilcock GK, Esiri MM, Davison AN. Neurochem Pathol 1984; 2: 221-32.
27. Hansen L, Salmon D, Galsako D, Masliah E, Katzman R, DeTeresa R, Thal L, Pay MM, Hofstetter R, Klauber M, Rice V, Butters N, Alford M. Neurology 1990; 40: 1-8.
28. Reinikainen KJ, Paljärvi L, Huuskonen M, Soininen H, Laakso M, Reikkinen PJ. J Neurol Sci 1988; 84: 101-16.

Address for correspondence:

Dr Kari J. Reinikainen,
Department of Neurology, Kuopio University Central Hospital,
SF-70210 Kuopio, Finland. Tel. 358-71-173004

68 ELISA Quantitation of the Amyloid A4 Precursor Protein in Cerebrospinal Fluid

R. PRIOR, U. MÖNNING, A. WEIDEMANN, P. FISCHER,
K. BLENNOW, A. WALLIN, C. G. GOTTFRIES, C. L. MASTERS
AND K. BEYREUTHER

The amyloid β/A4 precursor protein (APP) is present in cerebrospinal fluid (CSF) in at least two C-terminal truncated forms of 91 kDa and 112 kDa molecular weight. Quantitative determination of APP content in CSF may be of value in understanding the mechanisms leading to amyloid deposition and plaque formation in Alzheimer's disease brains. Using a newly developed double sandwich ELISA we quantified total APP in 29 CSF samples from 14 patients with clinical Alzheimer's disease diagnosed according to the NINCDS-ADRDA criteria, 5 patients with multi-infarct dementia and 10 neurologically normal, aged control subjects. With an overall elevated degree of variability, the mean concentrations of APP were found to be slightly decreased in both Alzheimer's disease and multi-infarct dementia cases. APP CSF levels were not related to the CSF protein content or to the age in either dementia or control cases. CSF levels of APP may reflect mechanisms involved in both the pathogenesis and pathology of Alzheimer's disease such as altered intracerebral or choroid plexus APP expression, processing or secretion, neuronal death and reactive gliosis. Our CSF assay allows the quantitative analysis of APP in different stages of Alzheimer's disease and other neurological conditions and therefore represents a first step towards an understanding of the mechanisms underlying the CSF APP content variations and to evaluating the diagnostic utility of CSF APP measurements.

INTRODUCTION

As in many neurological diseases, the examination of cerebrospinal fluid (CSF) has been used in Alzheimer's disease (AD) in order to detect CSF changes associated with the course of AD, which still depends for its definite diagnosis on postmortem histopathological evaluation. Whereas the general CSF composition shows normal laboratory values, a large number of reports describe the CSF content of neurotransmitter markers and in particular of the cholinergic system enzyme acetylcholinesterase. Both unchanged and decreased values (1,2) are reported for this and for a variety of other neurotransmitter markers (3) that therefore partially

Alzheimer's Disease: Basic Mechanisms, Diagnosis and Therapeutic Strategies
Edited by K. Iqbal, D. R. C. McLachlan, B. Winblad and H. M. Wisniewski
© 1991 John Wiley & Sons Ltd

reflect neuronal dysfunction and cell death also observed in other neurodegenerative disorders. A more specific approach consists in the examination of CSF for the presence of proteins that are intimately associated to the intra- and extracellular neuropathology of AD, such as paired helical filament (4) and β/A4 amyloid related antigens (5). The presence of neurofibrillary tangles and amyloid deposits in many nondemented elderly people, however, is (in addition to the difficult solubilization of these antigens) the main reason that will preclude those tests from diagnostic routine use.

Of particular interest not only in this regard, but also from a pathogenetic viewpoint, is the presence of the β/A4 amyloid precursor protein (APP) in CSF. The CSF from both AD and normal controls shows on western blots at least two molecular-weight forms of APP (91 kDa and 112 kDa) that correspond to the APP_{695} and to the Kunitz-type II protease inhibitor containing APP_{751} and APP_{770} isoforms (6,7) (Figure 1). According to the alternative splicing pattern of APP mRNA in brain (8,9), APP_{695} is the major derivative in CSF respect to a small fraction of APP_{751} and APP_{770}. Intracerebral amyloid β/A4 protein deposition, though present also in non-AD cases, is greatly enhanced in AD. Increased APP expression in brain is suggested at least in Down's syndrome (10) as a relevant pathogenetic factor and may be reflected by increased APP levels in CSF. Since APP in CSF is present in a secreted, C-terminal truncated form (7,8), quantitative changes of the CSF content might also reflect a modification of its cellular secretion that could

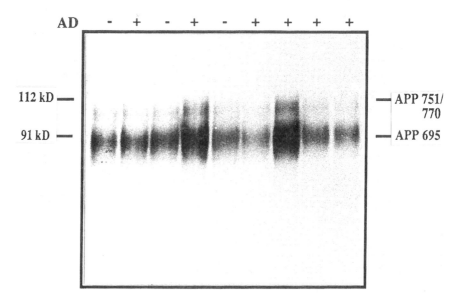

Figure 1. Secreted APP detected in CSF by western blot analysis. After immunoprecipitation with anti-FD-APP, proteins were separated by 8% polyacrylamide gel electrophoresis, electroblotted on nitrocellulose filter and immunostained with Mab22C11. The major reaction product corresponds to APP_{695}, whereas APP_{751} and APP_{770} are minor species. An identical pattern is detected in CSF samples from both AD patients and normal, aged control cases

favour the formation of amyloidogenic β/A4 fragments. The quantitative assessment of APP is therefore of critical value for an understanding of the mechanisms that lead to amyloid deposition. As a first step for the quantitative determination of APP concentrations we developed a double sandwich enzyme-linked immunosorbent assay (ELISA) that measures the total CSF APP content. The assay was used for the study of CSF samples from patients with AD, multi-infarct dementia (MID) and normal, aged control subjects.

MATERIALS AND METHODS

Patients and samples

CSF samples were obtained from three groups of patients:

I   Fourteen patients with early onset 'probable Alzheimer's disease' according to the diagnostic criteria of the NINCDS-ADRDA work group (11). The mean age in the AD group was 62 years (range 55–70 years).

II Five patients were classified as multi-infarct dementia cases according to the DSMIII-R and on the basis of a clear time relation between the vascular events (TIA/stroke) and the evolution of dementia symptoms; the mean age in this group was 71 years (range 63–76 years).

III As a reference group we selected 10 normal aged patients admitted for minor urologic or orthopedic surgery in spinal anaesthesia with a mean age of 68 years (range 62–77 years). The cognitive status in the control group was examined with the mini-mental state examination (12) excluding individuals with a score below 28. In addition, the control patients had no history, symptoms or signs of psychiatric, neurologic or other malignant, systemic or infectious disease.

All samples were stored frozen at $-70\,^{\circ}C$ within one hour of lumbar puncture.

Immunoreagents and solutions

The polyclonal and monoclonal antibodies used in this study were raised against purified Fd-APP fusion protein containing the APP_{695} protein and the Fd fragment of the murine IgM immunoglobulin heavy chain. Fd-APP and antibodies were prepared as described previously (7). The monoclonal antibody 22C11 is directed to the N-terminal region of all APP isoforms. For ELISA, ascitic fluid was purified by protein A affinity chromatography. The second anti-APP (anti-Fd-APP) antibody was raised as polyclonal antiserum in rabbit. To increase specificity of anti-Fd-APP in ELISA, we first prepared an IgG-fraction of this antiserum by protein A affinity chromatography. The IgG-fraction was subsequently preabsorbed with agarose-coupled mouse IgG (Sigma). For detection of bound anti-FD-APP we used a commercial alkaline phosphatase-coupled goat antiserum against rabbit IgG (Promega). The following buffers were used: phosphate-buffered saline (PBS) pH 7.6 as coating buffer; PBS + 3% bovine serum albumin (PBSA) as blocking buffer and for all antibody dilutions; 10 mM Tris HCl, 150 mM NaCl, 0.05% Tween

20 (TBST) was used as washing buffer. The chromogenic substrate p-nitrophenyl phosphate (PNPP) (0.04% mass/vol.) was dissolved in 10 mM diethanolamine (pH 9.5) containing 0.5 mM $MgCl_2$.

Standard ELISA procedure

Microtiter plates with 96 wells were coated with 100 μl of the monoclonal antibody 22C11 diluted in PBS to a final concentration of 5 μg/ml. The plates were incubated overnight at 4 °C and washed twice with PBS. Remaining binding sites were blocked by incubation with PBSA for 3 h at 37 °C (200 μl per well). After washing with TBST the CSF samples were applied after dilution in PBSA in the presence of 0.1% sodium dodecylsulfate and 0.2% Nonidet P40. CSF was diluted 1 : 10; in addition, a standard curve was prepared using serial dilutions from 10 nM to 0.3 nM of purified Fd-APP fusion protein obtained by electroelution after preparative polyacrylamide gel electrophoresis. The plates were incubated for 3 h at 37 °C and washed three times with TBST. In the next step, 50 μl of preabsorbed rabbit anti-Fd-APP IgG fraction were added to each well in a dilution of 1 : 5000 in PBSA for 2 h at 37 °C. After three times washing bound rabbit antibodies were detected with alkaline phosphatase conjugated goat anti-rabbit IgG (50 μl of a 1 : 7500 dilution added to each well and incubated for 2 h at 37 °C). The plates were then washed three times and 100 μl of 0.04% PNPP solution were added. The color development was stopped after 1 h at room temperature by addition of 100 μl of 5 mM EDTA. Absorbance values were measured at 405 nM with a Titertek Multiscan (Flow Laboratories) against blank wells where the addition of CSF samples was omitted. All samples were assayed in double and in two independent experiments. The specificity of the color reaction was confirmed by omitting single steps of the assay procedure. Total protein concentrations in CSF and in the APP standard samples were determined as described by Bradford (13) and expressed as OD at 595 nm.

RESULTS

The standard curve obtained with purified Fd-APP is shown in Figure 2. A relationship with good linearity between absorbance and concentration of Fd-APP was present for dilutions of the standard sample from 10 to 0.3 nM. When the CSF samples were applied in a 1 : 10 dilution, all obtained absorbance values were located within this linear range of the standard curve. As shown in Figure 3, in all groups there was considerable variability of the obtained absorbance for APP. The mean absorbance value (OD) was highest in the group of control patients ($OD_{405} = 937$, range 609–1087, standard deviation SD = 154) and slightly decreased in both the AD ($OD_{405} = 805$, range 216–1078, SD = 230) and the MID ($OD_{405} = 845$, range 538–1118, SD = 206) groups. The observed differences, however, were statistically not significant by evaluation with Student's t-test ($P > 0.05$). Similar and not significant ($P > 0.05$) results of decreased APP levels in AD and MID patients were obtained when the absorbance values for APP were compared to the total protein content of the CSF samples and expressed as ratio (r) between APP-OD and protein

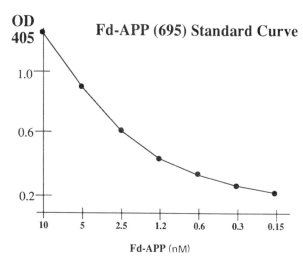

Figure 2. Standard curve obtained with purified APP_{695} fusion protein (Fd-APP). A linear relation between OD-values at 405 nm and Fd-APP concentrations is obtained for FD-APP concentrations ranging from 10 nM to 0.3 nM

concentration (control group: $r=3.1$, SD = 1.1; AD group: $r=2.6$, SD = 1.2; MID group: $r=2.3$, SD = 1.4). As indicated in Figure 4, no correlation could be observed between APP absorbance values and the age in either the AD or the control group $(P>0.2)$. A correlation between APP-OD and CSF protein concentration was also not found $(P>0.3)$.

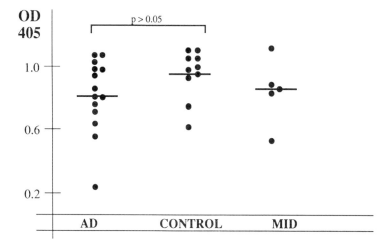

Figure 3. APP content of CSF samples from AD patients $(n=14)$, MID patients $(n=5)$ and normal, aged controls $(n=10)$. The APP content is expressed as OD at 405 nm. A broad range of values is obtained in all groups, with slightly decreased mean values for AD and MID. The differences are not significant when evaluated with Student's t-test $(P>0.05)$

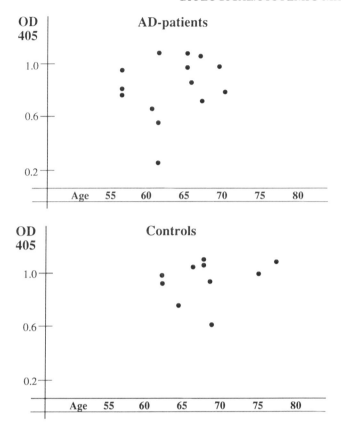

Figure 4. APP content in CSF related to age. APP content is expressed as OD at 405 nm. No correlation is seen in either the AD or the control group with linear regression analysis (regression line tested for statistical significance from zero: $P > 0.2$)

DISCUSSION

Our newly developed double sandwich ELISA uses antibodies that recognize all three isoforms of APP and allows a precise and sensitive quantitative determination of the total APP content in CSF. As readily appears, substantial differences of the total APP concentration in CSF between AD, MID and normal, aged control cases are not found. In both groups we observed a relatively broad range of absorbance values with minimum values in the AD patients. The mean absorbance indicates a slight reduction of the APP concentration in the AD and in the MID group. The APP levels in CSF are, in addition, not influenced by the total protein content, which was not correlated to the APP concentration, with nearly identical mean values for controls and AD patients and a similar result of slightly decreased APP/total protein ratios in AD and MID. These preliminary findings and, in particular, the tendency to reduced APP levels in AD and MID have to be corroborated by investigation of a larger number of patients.

The APP derivatives detected on CSF immunoblots show APP_{695} to be the most abundant form compared with APP_{751} and APP_{770} (7,8). A similar ratio has been found only in brain tissues or in cell lines of neuronal origin (7,10,14). A neuronal origin of the CSF APP therefore seems likely, although the CSF APP concentration might be influenced by choroid plexus secretion of APP or by increased APP production of reactive astrocytes as suggested from experimentally induced neuronal damage (15). Substantially unchanged CSF APP concentrations in AD are in line with recent evidence that the development of $\beta/A4$ amyloidosis in brain is related to aberrant processing of APP rather than to increased APP expression or secretion. APP cleavage in cell lines has been shown to occur within the $\beta/A4$ sequence (16) producing C-terminal membrane-associated and N-terminal secreted APP derivatives that both contain only part of the amyloidogenic region and cannot give rise to amyloid (17). The localization of the APP cleavage site in vivo will determine if CSF APP is derived from normal APP processing or if APP levels may reflect at least partially an alternative, amyloidogenic degradation pathway.

Several investigators describe AD-related changes in the APP mRNA splicing pattern. These results, however, are still controversial, since a selective increase of the respective mRNA in AD-affected brain regions is equally reported for APP_{695} (18), APP_{751} (19) and APP_{770} (20). One preliminary protein study based on the trypsin binding capacity of APP_{751} and APP_{770} describes an increase of these isoforms in the CSF of AD patients (21). Such an increase may be masked in our present assay by the abundance of APP_{695} in CSF and should be confirmed by ELISA quantitation that makes use of APP isoform specific antibodies. A similar assay is currently developed in our laboratory and will be essential to determine whether AD related changes in cerebral mRNA splicing are reflected by an altered CSF APP composition that, for diagnostic purposes, might be more useful than the quantitation of total APP. The determination of the latter will, however, be of interest for CSF samples of Down's syndrome, where increased levels of APP have already been described for serum and brain tissue (10). Longitudinal determinations of the CSF APP concentrations in sporadic and familial AD and in Down's syndrome will be needed to assess which physiological and pathological factors may influence the secretion of APP into the CSF and which role an altered APP content may have for the pathogenesis of AD.

Acknowledgments

The work was supported by the Deutsche Forschungsgemeinschaft through SFB 317 and a fellowship to R. P., the BMFT of Germany, the Boehringer Ingelheim Fonds, and the National Health and Medical Research Council of Australia.

REFERENCES

1. Elble R, Giacobini E, Scarsella GF. Arch Neurol 1987; 44: 403–7.
2. Appleyard ME, Smith AD, Wilcock GK, Esiri MM. Brain 1987; 110: 1309–22.

3. Atack JR. In Boller F, Katzman R, Rascol A, Signoret J-L, Christen Y (eds) Biological markers of Alzheimer's disease. Berlin: Springer 1984: 1-16.
4. Mehta PD, Thal L, Wiesniewski HM, Grundke-Iqbal I, Iqbal K. Lancet 1985; ii: 35.
5. Wisniewski HM, Mehta PD, Kim KS, Merz GS. In Boller F, Katzman R, Rascol A, Signoret J-L, Christen Y (eds) Biological markers of Alzheimer's disease. Berlin: Springer 1984: 23-29.
6. Weidemann A, König G, Bunke D, Fischer P, Salbaum JM, Masters CL, Beyreuther K. Cell 1989; 57: 115-26.
7. Palmert MR, Podlisny MB, Witker DS, Oltersdorf T, Younkin LH, Selkoe DJ, Younkin SG. Proc Natl Acad Sci USA 1989; 86: 6338-42.
8. Neve RL, Finch EA, Dawes LR. Neuron 1988; 1: 669-77.
9. Golde TE, Estus S, Usiak M, Younkin LH, Younkin SG. Neuron 1990; 4: 253-67.
10. Rumble B, Retallack R, Hilbich C, Simms G, Multhaup G, Martins R, Hockey A, Montgomery P, Beyreuther K, Masters CL. N Engl J Med 1989; 320: 1446-52.
11. McKhann G, Drachman D, Folstein M, Katzman R, Price D, Stadlan EM. Neurology 1984; 34: 939-44.
12. Folstein M, Folstein S, McHugh PR. J Psychiatry Res 1975; 12: 189-98.
13. Bradford MM. Anal Biochem 1976; 72: 248-54.
14. Kang J, Müller-Hill B. Biochem Biophys Res Comm 1990; 166: 1192-200.
15. Siman R, Card PJ, Nelson RB, Davis LG. Neuron 1989; 3: 275-85.
16. Sisodia SS, Koo EH, Beyreuther K, Unterbeck A, Price DL. Science 1990; 248: 492-5.
17. Esch FS, Keim PS, Beattie EC, Blacher RW, Culwell AR, Oltersdorf T, McClure D, Ward PJ. Science 1990; 248: 1122-24.
18. Palmert MR, Golde TE, Cohen ML, Kovacs DM, Tanzi RE, Gusella JF, Usiak MF, Younkin LH, Younkin SG. Science 1988; 241: 1080-84.
19. Johnson SA, McNeill T, Cordell B, Finch CE. Science 1990; 248: 854-7.
20. Tanaka S, Nakamura S, Ueda K, Kmeyama M, Shiojiri S, Takahashi Y, Kitaguchi N, Ito H. Biochem Biophys Res Comm 1988; 157: 472-9.
21. Kitaguchi N, Tokushima Y, Oishi K, Takahashi Y, Shiojiri S, Nakamura S, Tanaka S, Kodaira R, Ito H. Biochem Biophys Res Comm 1990; 166: 1453-9.

Address for correspondence:

Dr R. Prior,
Center for Molecular Biology,
University of Heidelberg,
Im Neuenheimer Feld 282,
D-6900 Heidelberg 1,
Germany

69 Alpha-1-Antichymotrypsin and Antitrypsin in CSF of Patients with Alzheimer-Type Dementia

YUKITO SHINOHARA, MASAHIRO YAMAMOTO,
HITOSHI OHSUGA, SACHIKO OHSUGA, KATSUNORI AKIYAMA,
FUMIHITO YOSHII, MICHIO TSUDA, HIROSHI KAMIGUCHI
AND MASAICHI YAMAMURA

Certain neuropathological lesions characterize the brains of Alzheimer's disease patients, including senile plaque, neurofibrillary tangles and so on. Recently, two approaches—molecular cloning and immunochemical analysis—have identified one of the components of Alzheimer's disease amyloid deposits in senile plaque as the serine protease inhibitor, α_1-antichymotrypsin (ACT) (1). It has been suggested that there is a special association between the β-protein and ACT in senile plaque, and perhaps an essential interaction between the two proteins in the formation of Alzheimer-type amyloid (2,3). In addition, the evidence of expression of mRNA of ACT in astrocytes in Alzheimer patients (2,3) and our observation (4) that the ACT inhibits DNA synthesis of cultured human carcinoma cell might support the hypothesis that ACT contributes to the pathological processes of Alzheimer's disease.

An increase in serum concentration of ACT (5) or antitrypsin (AT) (6), which is also one of the acute-phase reactant proteins, has already been reported in Alzheimer's disease patients. However, the concentrations of ACT or AT which normally exist in serum are very high and readily increase in patients with inflammation, malignancy and so on. In view of the known pathogenesis of Alzheimer's disease, the level of such proteins should be investigated in CSF, because CSF should far more sensitively reflect the changes in the central nervous system.

The purpose of this study was to measure the levels of ACT and AT in both CSF and serum of patients with senile dementia of Alzheimer type (DAT) and to evaluate the clinical significance of these measurements. A further aim of this study was to compare the results with those in nondemented controls and in patients with clinically diagnosed multi-infarct dementia (MID).

SUBJECTS AND METHODS

The subjects comprised 724 nondemented controls (mean age 47 ± 8 years) (CSF was obtained from 11 subjects), 12 patients with DAT (71 ± 6 years)

Alzheimer's Disease: Basic Mechanisms, Diagnosis and Therapeutic Strategies
Edited by K. Iqbal, D. R. C. McLachlan, B. Winblad and H. M. Wisniewski
© 1991 John Wiley & Sons Ltd

and 13 patients with MID (68±12 years). The diagnoses of DAT and MID were made based on the DSM III-R and NINCDS-ADRDA criteria, medical history, physical and neurological examinations, and CT and MRI findings. Hachinski's ischemic score was also calculated. Patients with dementia in whom the cause is undifferentiated and those with severe white matter changes on CT or MRI were excluded from this study. The measurements of ACT and AT in CSF and in serum were performed by using an ELISA method and a single radial immunodiffusion method, respectively. Since both ACT and AT are acute-phase reactants of inflammation, subjects who had high serum CRP values (>0.5 mg/dl) and high cell counts and protein in CSF were also excluded from this study. CSF was obtained by lumbar puncture, centrifuged and stored at −80 °C until the measurement. Serum was sampled simultaneously and stored at −80 °C.

In order to evaluate the integrity of the blood–brain barrier in these subjects, measurements of albumin concentration in CSF, and calculations of the ratios of CSF ACT to CSF albumin and CSF ACT to serum ACT and so on were made so that the specific significance of CSF ACT could be better assessed.

RESULTS

Serum ACT and AT levels

The concentrations of serum ACT and serum AT in nondemented controls were 298.2±48.5 μg/ml (*n*=724) and 2494.8±575.5 μg/ml (*n*=724), respectively. The corresponding values in DAT patients were 354.2±101.7 μg/ml (*n*=12) and 2461.0±487.9 μg/ml (*n*=10), respectively. The serum ACT levels in Alzheimer's disease patients were a little higher than in the controls. However, ACT and AT levels in serum showed a very slight increase with increasing age, and if a plot of

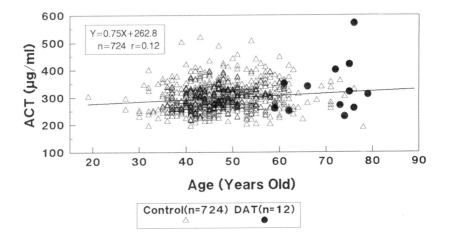

Figure 1. Serum ACT and age of subjects

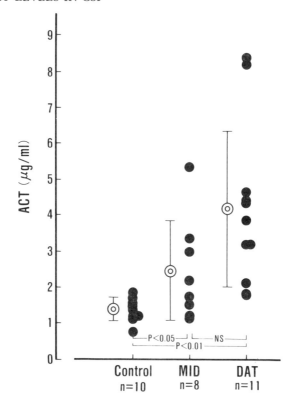

Figure 2. Comparison of CSF ACT values in controls, multi-infarct dementia (MID) and Alzheimer's disease (DAT)

serum ACT (Figure 1) and AT levels against age was made, the ACT and AT levels of the Alzheimer's disease patients were within the range of normal variation compared to the controls. The relationship between serum ACT and serum AT was also evaluated, but there was no apparent correlation between them.

ACT and AT levels in CSF

Figure 2 shows the concentrations of CSF ACT of the controls, MID and DAT patients. The CSF ACT level was much higher in patients with DAT in almost all cases (4.2 ± 2.2 μg/ml, $n = 11$) than that in controls (1.4 ± 0.3 μg/ml, $n = 10$), and this difference was statistically significant ($P < 0.01$). CSF ACT levels showed no correlation with age in the nondemented subjects.

CSF AT levels were also compared in nondemented subjects and in DAT patients. CSF AT level in DAT (15.4 ± 8.3 μg/ml, $n = 7$) was higher than that in controls (8.5 ± 3.6 μg/ml, $n = 9$), but the difference between them was not statistically significant. The relationships of CSF AT levels with age, and of CSF ACT levels with CSF AT levels were also investigated but there was no significant correlation, particularly in nondemented subjects.

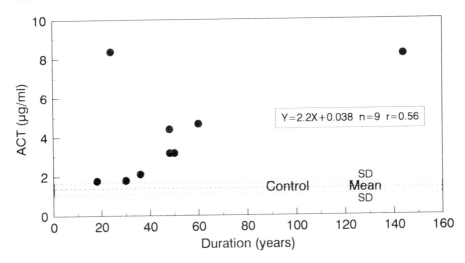

Figure 3. CSF ACT values and duration of illness

The degree of increase in CSF ACT in Alzheimer's disease was compared with duration of illness and severity of disease (FAST stage) (7). The results showed that CSF ACT seemed to increase with duration and progression of illness (Figure 3).

Integrity of blood–brain barrier

Since the serum ACT level is about 200 to 300 times higher than that in CSF, the possibility of breakdown of the blood-brain barrier was also investigated. However, there was essentially no difference in CSF albumin concentrations of controls and Alzheimer patients. On the other hand, the ratio of CSF ACT divided by serum ACT in DAT was statistically significantly higher than in the controls ($P < 0.001$). Both results suggested that there is no severe impairment of the blood-brain barrier in these subjects, although minimal breakdown of the barrier would not be detected by these evaluations.

CSF ACT in MID

The CSF ACT level in clinically diagnosed MID was 2.4 ± 1.3 µg/ml ($n = 8$). The mean value in MID was between those in nondemented subjects and in DAT, and the CSF ACT levels in MID patients could apparently be classified into a higher group and a lower group. The possibility that the group diagnosed here as MID may include patients with mixed-type dementia cannot be ruled out from this clinical study (8).

SUMMARY AND COMMENTS

The results obtained from this investigation can be summarized as follows:

1. There was no significant difference of serum ACT and AT levels between nondemented controls and DAT patients.
2. The CSF ACT level was increased highly significantly in patients with DAT, and this increase seems to be related to duration and progression of illness.
3. In patients who were diagnosed clinically as MID, CSF ACT measurement could be useful to suspect mixed-type dementia.

These results indicate that the measurement of CSF ACT level in DAT is useful and the increase may reflect the pathological processes of the illness. Further investigations should aim to (a) determine whether or not CSF ACT measurement is useful for early diagnosis of DAT, although present evidence is against this possibility, (b) identify the mechanisms of the pathological processes and progression of Alzheimer-type dementia and the increase in CSF ACT, and (c) evaluate a larger number of patients and obtain pathological confirmation, and so on.

REFERENCES

1. Abraham CR, Selkoe DJ, Potter H. Cell 1988; 52: 487-501.
2. Abraham CR, Potter H. Bio Technol 1889; 7: 147-53.
3. Abraham CR, Potter H. In Iqbal K, Wisniewski HM, Winblad B (eds) Alzheimer's disease and related disorders. New York: Alan R. Liss, 1989: 1037-48.
4. Tsuda M, Umezawa Y, Masuyama M, Yamaguchi K, Katsunuma T. Biochem Biophys Res Comm 1987; 144: 409-14.
5. Amari M, Matsubara E, Ishiguro K, Shoji M, Hirai S. Clin Neurol (Jap) 1989; 29: 1256-60.
6. Glimetto B, Argenitero V, Sanson F, Ongaro G, Tavolato B. Eur Neurol 1988; 28: 30-3.
7. Reiberg B. Geriatrics 1986; 41: 30-46.
8. Shinohara Y, Ohsuga H, Yamamoto M, Ohsuga S, Akiyama K, Yoshii F, Tsuda M, Kamiguchi H, Yamamura M. In Hartmann A et al (eds) Cerebral Ischemia and Dementia. Berlin: Springer (in press).

Address for correspondence:

Prof. Y. Shinohara,
Departments of Neurology and Biochemistry,
Tokai University School of Medicine,
Isehara, Kanagawa, 259-11, Japan

70 Circulating Forms of Amyloid Precursor Protein of Alzheimer's Disease

ASHLEY I. BUSH, KONRAD BEYREUTHER AND
COLIN L. MASTERS

Alzheimer's disease (AD) is characterized by cortical amyloid deposits associated with dementia in the elderly and adults with Down's syndrome. The deposits are principally composed of polymers of a 42–43 residue protein, A4 (1,2) or β-protein (3,4). Whether these deposits are the cause or a byproduct of neuronal dysfunction is still debated. The monomer, β/A4, appears to be produced by the abnormal proteolytic cleavage of a larger precursor protein (APP or PreA4), the predicted structure of which indicates that it is an integral transmembrane cell-surface receptor (5). The amyloidogenic β/A4 region spans part of the transmembrane region and part of the adjacent extracellular domain. Studies of the expression of APP have shown that it is almost ubiquitous. A greater knowledge of the location and topology of the potentially amyloidogenic APP and its physiology and metabolism will be essential in elucidating the pathogenesis of AD.

The APP gene, located on chromosome 21 within or near the boundary of 21q21 and 21q22.1 (5–11), produces at least five different mRNAs by alternate splicing. Some of these are expressed as a complex family of 90–130 kDa membrane-bound and soluble glycoproteins (12). The prototype is APP_{695} (5), and APP_{751} and APP_{770} are isoforms generated by the insertion of a serine protease inhibitory domain of the Kunitz type II family (13–15). APP_{714} and APP_{770} contain an OX-2 related domain (13,16). APP_{751} has been shown to be identical with protease nexin-II (PN-II) (17,18). The postulated splice product APP_{563} is homologous to APP_{751} but is carboxyl-terminally truncated and, therefore, could yield a nonamyloidogenic secreted form (19).

The tissue origin of the APP substrate for cerebral amyloidogenesis remains uncertain. Northern blot analysis has detected mRNA in brain, kidney, heart, spleen, pancreas, muscle, thymus, lung, adrenal gland, small intestine and liver (9), but so far no clear association has been observed between amyloidogenesis and mRNA species location or dosage in AD (reviewed by Müller-Hill and Beyreuther) (20). The mRNA for the inhibitory insert-lacking APP_{695} has been detected exclusively in the brain whereas mRNA coding for the inhibitory insert is found in both brain and periphery (21). APP is expressed in human brain and cerebrospinal fluid (12),

Alzheimer's Disease: Basic Mechanisms, Diagnosis and Therapeutic Strategies
Edited by K. Iqbal, D. R. C. McLachlan, B. Winblad and H. M. Wisniewski
©1991 John Wiley & Sons Ltd

rat brain (22) and many peripheral tissues. Of the tissues examined so far, APP_{695} is richest in the brain, but APP_{751} and APP_{770}, shown to possess protease inhibitory activity, were found predominantly in the kidney (23). Whereas it is easy to imagine how brain APP could be involved in aberrant amyloidogenic catabolism, for a distant precursor molecule to be involved in cerebral amyloidogenesis, it would need to be transported or contained within the blood. Although as yet unconfirmed, reports of β/A4 deposition in peripheral non-neural tissues in AD (24) are suggestive of a potentially hematogenous origin for the substrate of amyloidogenesis. Although the neuronal origin of β/A4 amyloid deposition still appears most consistent with currently known observations, a circulating form of APP and/or β/A4 should still be considered. The observation that APP undergoes vesicular release from platelets (25) immediately suggests one possible pathway. Moreover, the finding of APP in large quantities in platelets suggests that this blood element may provide a means for studying the normal catabolism and function of APP.

APP PROCESSING

Recent studies have demonstrated that the initial APP cleavage is a membrane-associated event occurring at a site located within the β/A4 region and yielding a secretable protein (26,27). Such carboxyl-terminal truncated molecules have been described in cell culture (12), human brain and cerebrospinal fluid (CSF) (12,28), platelet alpha granules (25,29,30) and plasma (25,29,31). Such cleavage near the membrane is consistent with the known processing of secreted growth factors such as epidermal growth factor (EGF) and transforming growth factor alpha (TGF-α). Sisodia et al transfected into mammalian cell cultures genes encoding authentic APP and hybrid APP lacking some or all of the extramembranous β/A4 domain (26). By observing which of the hybrids could still undergo cleavage and secretion of the ectodomain, they concluded that wild-type APP is normally cleaved within the β/A4 domain, making the formation of the amyloid impossible during normal processing. Esch et al purified the secreted amino-terminal and the membrane-associated carboxyl-terminal cleavage fragments from human embryonal 293 cells stably transfected with cDNA constructs encoding full-length forms of APP_{695} and APP_{751} (27). These workers sequenced the 9-kDa membrane-associated fragment and a carboxyl-terminal CNBr digestion fragment from the secreted portion. They found that the secreted forms of APP_{695} and APP_{751} terminate at Gln^{15} of β/A4, whereas the amino-terminus of the 9-kDa carboxyl-terminal APP fragment begins at Leu^{17}. Beta-A4 (Lys^{16}) is probably excised by a basic exopeptidase after the initial proteolytic cleavage of APP. If it can be shown that this exopeptidase selectively cuts at this site in vivo, then it may participate in the physiological secretion of carboxyl-truncated APP into CSF and plasma. Dysregulation of this pathway must be implicit in any pathophysiological model of AD.

Although carboxyl-terminal precursor fragments containing the β/A4 sequence tend to aggregate when not inserted into membranes (32), the cleavage and release of such fragments from membranes remains to be elucidated. In the Dutch familial congophilic angiopathies (hereditary cerebral hemorrhage with amyloidosis of Dutch type, HCHWA-D), an autosomal dominant condition where patients develop recurrent intracerebral hemorrhages associated with extensive cerebrovascular β/A4 deposition, a mutation causing the disease has been described (33) involving a glutamic acid to glutamine substitution at β/A4 position 22 (34). As the substitution is only six residues away from the putative constitutive cleavage site, it is possible that the responsible protease is unable to act at its binding site in a physiological manner and that the APP is subsequently catabolized by an alternative pathway producing an amyloidogenic cleavage product. The site of this proteolysis remains to be elucidated but platelet membranes are one possibility in this vasculopathic condition. A mutation has not yet been reported in the DNA for APP in sporadic AD, familial AD or Down's syndrome.

PLATELETS AND ALZHEIMER'S DISEASE

Studies of the platelet provide us with valuable data about the normal metabolism of APP and may also provide us with a potential clinical marker for AD, if not information about the pathogenesis of the disease itself. The presence of potentially amyloidogenic APP in the platelet (25) makes even more intriguing the known associations between AD and abnormal platelet membrane fluidity (35,36), and Down's syndrome (DS) and megakaryocytic leukaemia (37). Furthermore, the presence of significant amounts of APP released from the platelet α-granule (25,29,30,38) indicates that there will be an important, as yet undefined, physiological role for the molecule.

The human platelet, which carries out a number of biochemical processes that also occur in the brain, has been proposed as a peripheral model for neurons (39). The demonstration of abnormalities of function and morphology of platelets in Parkinson's disease (40), Huntington's disease (41) and depression (42) indicates that disease-specific abnormalities in the brain could be reflected in the platelet. Galtzin et al explored the possibility that the decrease in serotonin levels and density of serotonin uptake sites in AD brain neurons may be reflected in decreased [^{3}H]imipramine binding in platelet, but found no difference between AD and controls (43). In the search for a platelet marker of AD the findings of Zubenko and co-workers have yielded consistent differences between AD and controls. They have demonstrated variation in the fluorescence anisotropy of 1,6-diphenyl-1,3,5-hexatriene in labelled platelet membranes, an index of membrane fluidity, associated with an aggressive clinical subtype of AD (44). A single genetic platelet membrane fluidity locus has been postulated, which appears to explain 80% of the total variation of membrane fluidity within the families of patients with AD (45). Two studies so far have failed to detect differences between AD and controls on platelet protein immunoblots employing monoclonals against amino-terminal epitopes or a polyclonal against APP$_{695}$ fusion protein (25,29,30); the possibility of a platelet membrane abnormality in AD affecting APP release or cleavage warrants further investigation.

THE PLATELET AND APP

We purified and sequenced full-length APP from human platelets seen as 130 and 110-kDa bands on western blots employing either a monoclonal antibody recognizing

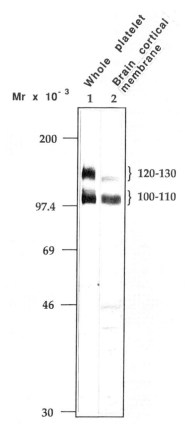

Figure 1. Detection of APP in platelets by western blot. SDS-PAGE immunoblot comparing homogenized whole platelets (lane 1) with human brain (cerebral cortex) membrane extract (lane 2). 100 μg protein was added to sample buffer and loaded into each lane. The blot was incubated with mAb 22C11 at 1 : 20 000 dilution. Molecular size markers on left. The major immunoreactive bands at 100–110 kDa and 120–130 kDa are indicated on the right

an amino-terminal epitope or a polyclonal antibody raised against an APP$_{695}$ fusion protein (Figure 1). The 110-kDa band may be a degradative product of the 130-kDa band because of the variability in the ratio of the two bands from preparation to preparation. These APP bands were found in platelet releasate as well as the soluble (cytosolic and granular content) and pellet (total membrane) fractions of ultra-centrifuged platelet homogenate, and there appeared to be approximately twice the amount of APP per unit protein in the soluble fraction of platelet homogenate compared to the total membrane fraction. The protein bands detected by amino-terminal antibody immunoblot were consistently broad, covering a molecular mass range of approximately 10 kDa from 120–130 kDa and 100–110 kDa. This finding was also observed by Smith et al, who detected a broad immunoreactive band from 100–120 kDa when employing a polyclonal antibody against an amino-terminal synthetic peptide (residues 45 to 62 of APP_{751}) on immunoblots of purified factor XIa inhibitor (XIaI) and platelet releasate (38). Both these reports also find that sharper immunoreactive bands within platelet releasate are achieved by use of antibodies against the Kunitz inhibitor region (~ 120 kDa), the β/A4 domain (~ 110 kDa) (38), or the carboxyl terminus (~ 120 kDa) (25). These findings could be explained by the existence of more than one species of APP being contained within the platelet, an amino-terminal antibody detecting several species at the same time.

Although the platelet is known to be capable of endocytosis, the finding of strong immunocytochemical labelling of megakaryocytes for APP (25,29) indicates that APP is probably synthesized in the bone marrow along with other platelet glycoproteins.

The release of APP from the platelet by degranulation stimuli such as thrombin, collagen or calcium ionophore (25,29,30,38) indicates that APP may have an

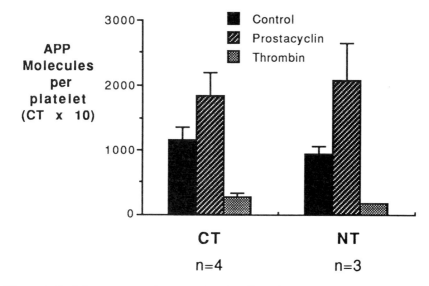

Figure 2. Radioimmunoassay demonstrating the effect of prostacyclin and thrombin upon APP in Triton-extracted platelets. Values are the means and standard errors of APP carboxyl-terminal (CT, pmol/ml × 10) and amino-terminal (NT, pmol/ml) radioimmunoassays on residual contents of Triton-X100-extracted whole platelets after exposure to prostacyclin (0.3 μg/ml) or thrombin (0.3 IU/ml), as compared to controls; n, number of individual experiments. The results indicate that prostacyclin treatment, which prevents degranulation of platelets, is associated with a greater retention of APP content. Thrombin treatment, promoting degranulation, causes a reduction in platelet APP content, as compared to controls. Method: washed platelets were suspended for 15 minutes at RT in 2 ml Tyrode's buffer lacking calcium and magnesium (136.9 mM NaCl, 2.68 mM KCl, 11.9 mM $NaHCO_3$, 0.42 mM NaH_2PO_4, pH 6.4) whereupon they were pelleted at $1500\,g$ for 15 minutes and the supernatant removed. The pellet was then extracted for 2 hours into 1 ml of the same buffer containing 2% Triton X-100 at 4 °C, whereupon unextracted debris was pelleted at 10 000 g for 15 minutes and the supernatant employed in a radioimmunoassay using synthetic peptides representing epitopes at either the amino-terminal (NT) or intracytoplasmic (CT) poles of the APP molecule, as previously described (25,53). The effects of the platelet degranulation inhibitor, prostacyclin (0.3 μg/ml), or the degranulation promoter, thrombin (0.3 IU/ml), when present in the suspension buffer was gauged by assaying the residual APP in the platelet pellet after extraction

important physiological role in events associated with coagulation (Figure 2). A breach of the vascular endothelium sets off a chain of events including the aggregation of circulating platelets and the degranulation of the glycoprotein contents of their α-granules. Alpha-granule contents include substrates for the coagulation cascade (such as thrombospondin and platelet factor 4) and growth factors (such as platelet-derived growth factor, fibroblast growth factor, EGF and TGF-β_2), the dual roles for which are the immediate repair of the vascular defect and the promotion of reparative tissue proliferation (46–48). It is possible that forms of APP released by the platelet may have a growth factor-related function. A 90-kDa form of APP has been shown to promote the growth of cultured fibroblasts (49) and neurons (50). Also, a secreted form of APP containing the Kunitz inhibitor region is identical to protease nexin-II (17,18). APP also binds epidermal growth factor binding protein (EGF BP), a fact that was used to detect its presence in the platelet α-granule, subsequently confirmed by immuno-blotting with a monoclonal antibody against an amino-terminal epitope and polyclonals against the full-length PN-II and against β/A4, and corroborated by the use of platelet subcellular markers (30). Van Nostrand et al have estimated the total PN-II in platelets as 160 ± 21 ng per 10^8 platelets (30). These data are comparable to our estimates of total platelet APP (measured by amino-terminal RIA, assuming a M_r of 130) as 45 ± 21 ng per 10^8 platelets (2076 molecules per platelet) and total platelet APP with intact carboxyl terminus (measured by carboxyl-terminal RIA, assuming a M_r of 130) as 4.0 ± 0.8 ng per 10^8 platelets (184 molecules per platelet) (25).

It is also likely that the released serine protease inhibitor-containing forms of platelet APP may participate in the coagulation cascade by providing negative feedback to activated coagulation pathway enzymes. Kitaguchi et al demonstrated that the protease inhibitor region of APP inhibits coagulation factor Xa at an equilibrium dissociation constant of 1.2×10^{-6} M (51), while Kido et al have shown that it inhibits plasmin with a K_i of 7.5×10^{-11} M (52). Similarly, the carboxyl-terminally truncated 120-kDa form of APP possessing the inhibitory insert released by HepG2 cells and activated platelets inhibits factor XIa at a dissociation constant of 4.5×10^{-10} M increasing to 2.5×10^{-11} M in the presence of 1 unit/ml heparin (38). In these three studies, the proteolytic activity of thrombin was not inhibited by APP.

Platelet studies have demonstrated that the forms of APP released by the platelet lack the carboxyl terminus (25,29,30,38). So far, only our study has found full-length APP with carboxyl terminus intact in association with the platelet (25). In that report, platelet releasate was found to possess a carboxyl terminus-containing form of 120-kDa APP that was sedimentable with ultracentrifugation, as well as soluble APP (120–130 kDa) that lacked the carboxyl terminus. We consider the vesicular release of platelet APP as a possible explanation. Platelet plasma membrane microparticles are known to be released following platelet activation and are found in normal plasma (reviewed in reference 53).

PLASMA APP AND ALZHEIMER'S DISEASE

Although it is likely that platelet APP is synthesized in the bone marrow megakaryocyte (25,29), the origin of plasma APP is still uncertain. The possibility that the kidney or other organ is a source of plasma APP cannot be excluded. The protein bands at 130 kDa and 110 kDa seen following anti-APP immunoblot of the heparin sepharose eluate of plasma are of the same molecular mass as those seen in platelet sub-fractions and in brain (25,29), but additional bands at 65 kDa and 42 kDa are apparent in plasma. Plasma APP purified by Affi-Gel Blue chromatography has been shown to contain the inhibitor insert and lack the carboxyl terminus (31). This latter study could detect neither the carboxyl terminal-containing APP nor the $\beta/A4$ epitope in the plasma.

Carboxyl-terminal immunoreactivity is found in human serum, where there is a 50% elevation by radioimmunoassay in Down's syndrome but no difference between AD and controls (54). Gel filtration of serum under reducing conditions indicated an apparent M_r of approximately 90 for this species.

FUTURE DIRECTIONS

Future studies of APP in the circulation will elaborate the origin and fate of the APP species containing the intact $\beta/A4$ domain, as these forms may be involved in AD-variant angiopathies if not in the pathogenesis of AD itself. The platelet now provides us with an easily accessible model for APP metabolism. The conditions for normal and abnormal proteolysis of APP and the elucidation of the proteases involved will yield information that will help elucidate the brain APP pathways. Understanding the physiological function of platelet and plasma APP may give insight into the nature of the pathophysiology of AD.

REFERENCES

1. Masters CL, Multhaup G, Simms G, Pottgiesser J, Martins RN, Beyreuther K. EMBO J 1985; 4: 2757-63.
2. Masters CL, Simms G, Weinman NA, Multhaup G, McDonald BL, Beyreuther K. Proc Natl Acad Sci USA 1985; 82: 4245-9.
3. Glenner GG, Wong CW. Biochem Biophys Res Comm 1984; 120: 885-90.
4. Glenner GG, Wong CW. Biochem Biophys Res Comm 1984; 122: 1131-5.
5. Kang J, Lemaire H-J, Unterbeck A, Salbaum MJ, Masters CL, Grzeschik K-H, Multhaup G, Beyreuther K, Müller-Hill B. Nature 1987; 325: 733-6.
6. Goldgaber D, Lerman MI, McBride OW, Saffiotti U, Gajdusek DC. Science 1987; 235: 877-80.
7. Robakis NK, Ramakrishna N, Wolfe G, Wisniewski HM. Proc Natl Acad Sci USA 1987; 84: 4190-4.
8. Robakis NK, Wisniewski HM, Jenkins EC, Devine-Gage GA, Hoock GE, Yao X-L, Ramakrishna N, Wolfe G, Silverman WP, Brown WT. Lancet 1987; i: 384-5.
9. Tanzi RE, Gusella JF, Watkins PC, Bruns GAP, St George-Hyslop P, van Keuren ML, Patterson D, Pagan S, Kurnit DM, Neve RL. Science 1987; 235: 880-4.
10. Van Broeckhoven C, Genthe AM, Vandenberghe A, Horsthemke B, Backhov H, Raeymaekers P, Van Hul W, Wehnert A, Gheuens J, Cras P, Bruyland Martin JJ, Salbaum M, Multhaup G, Masters CL, Beyreuther K, Gurl HMD, Mullan MJ, Holland A, Barton A, Irving N, Williamson R, Richa SJ, Hardy JA. Nature 1987; 329: 153-5.
11. Zabel BU, Salbaum JM, Multhaup G, Masters CL, Bohl J, Beyreuther K. Cytogenet Cell Genet 1987; 46: 725-6.

12. Weidemann A, König G, Bunke D, Fischer P, Salbaum JM, Masters CL, Beyreuther K. Cell 1989; 57: 115-26.
13. Kitaguchi N, Takahashi Y, Tokushima Y, Shiojiri S, Ito H. Nature 1988; 311: 530-2.
14. Ponte P, Gonzalez De-Whitt P, Schilling J, Miller J, Hsu D, Greenberg B, Davis K, Wallace W, Lieberburg I, Fuller F, Cordell B. Nature 1988; 331: 525-7.
15. Tanzi RE, McClatchey AI, Lamperti ED, Villa-Komaroff L, Gusella JF, Neve RL. Nature 1988; 331: 528-30.
16. Golde TE, Estus S, Usiak M, Younkin LH, Younkin SG. Neuron 1990; 4: 253-67.
17. Oltersdorf T, Fritz LC, Schenk DB, Lieberburg I, Johnson-Wood KL, Beattie EC, Ward PJ, Blacher RW, Dovey HF, Sinha S. Nature 1989; 341: 144-7.
18. Van Nostrand WE, Wagner SL, Suzuki M, Choi BH, Farrow JS, Geddes JW, Cotman CW, Cunningham DD. Nature 1989; 341: 546-9.
19. De Sauvage F, Octave J-N. Science 1989; 245: 651-3.
20. Müller-Hill B, Beyreuther K. Ann Rev Biochem 1989; 58: 287-307.
21. Spillantini MG, Hunt SP, Ulrich, J, Goedert M. Mol Brain Res 1989; 6: 143-50.
22. Card JP, Meade RP, Davis LG. Neuron 1988; 1: 835-46.
23. Tanaka S, Shiojiri S, Takahashi Y, Kitaguchi N, Ito H, Kameyama M, Kimura J, Nakamura S, Ueda K. Biochem Biophys Res Comm 1989; 165: 1406-14.
24. Joachim CL, Mori H, Selkoe DJ. Nature 1989; 341: 226-30.
25. Bush AI, Martins RN, Rumble B, Moir R, Fuller S, Milward E, Currie J, Ames D, Weidemann A, Fischer P, Multhaup G, Beyreuther K, Masters CL. J Biol Chem 1990; 265: 15977-83.
26. Sisodia SS, Koo EH, Beyreuther K, Unterbeck A, Price DL. Science 1990; 248: 492-5.
27. Esch FS, Keim PS, Beattie EC, Blacher RW, Culwell AR, Oltersdorf T, McClure D, Ward PJ. Science 1990; 248: 1122-4.
28. Palmert MR, Podlisny MB, Witker DS, Oltersdorf T, Younkin LH, Selkoe DJ, Younkin SG. Proc Natl Acad Sci USA. 1989; 86: 6338-42.
29. Bush AI, Martins RN, Rumble B, Moir R, Fuller S, Milward E, Currie J, Ames D, Weidemann A, Fischer P, Multhaup G, Beyreuther K, Masters CL. Neurobiol Aging 1990; 11: 333-4.
30. Van Nostrand WE, Schmaier AH, Farrow JS, Cunningham DD. Science 1990; 248: 745-8.
31. Podlisny MB, Mammen AL, Schlossmacher MG, Palmert MR, Younkin SG, Selkoe DJ. Biochem Biophys Res Comm 1990; 167: 1094-101.
32. Dyrks T, Weidemann A, Multhaup G, Salbaum JM, Lemaire H-G, Kang J, Müller-Hill B, Masters CL, Beyreuther K. EMBO J 1988; 7: 949-57.
33. Van Broekhoven C, Haan J, Bakker E, Hardy JA, Van Hul W, Whenert A, Vegter-Van der Vlis M, Roos RAC. Science 1990; 248: 1120-2.
34. Levy E, Carman MD, Fernandez-Madrid IJ, Power MD, Lieberburg I, van Duinen SG, Bots GTAM, Luyendijk W, Frangione B. Science 1990; 248: 1124-6.
35. Zubenko GS, Malinakova I, Chojnacki B. J Neuropath Exp Neurol 1987; 46: 407-18.
36. Zubenko GS, Cohen BM, Boller F, Malinakova I, Keefe N, Chojnacki B. Ann Neurol 1987; 22: 237-44.
37. Lewis DS, Thompson M, Hudson E, Liberman MM, Samson D. Acta Haemat 1983; 70: 236-42.
38. Smith RP, Higuchi, DA, Broze G. Science 1990; 248: 1126-8.
39. Da Prada M, Cesura AM, Launay JM, Richards JG. Experientia 1988; 44: 115-26.
40. Barbeau A, Campanella G, Butterworth RF, Yamada K. Neurology 1975; 25: 1-9.
41. Aminoff MJ, Trenchard A, Turner P, Wood WG. Lancet 1974; ii: 1115-16.
42. Garcia-Sevilla JA. Br J Psych 1989; 154 (suppl. 4): 67-72.
43. Galtzin A-M, Davous P, Roudier M, Lamour Y, Poirier M-F, Langer SZ. Psych Res 1989; 28: 289-94.
44. Zubenko GS, Huff FJ, Beyer J, Auerbach J, Teply I. Arch Gen Psych 1988; 45: 889-93.
45. Chakravarti A, Slaugenhaupt SS, Zubenko GS. Am J Hum Genet 1989; 44: 799-805.
46. Deuel TF, Huang JS. J Clin Invest 1984; 74: 669-76.

47. George JN, Nurden AT, Phillips DR. N Engl J Med 1984; 311: 1084-98.
48. Ross R. Ann Rev Med 1987; 38: 71-9.
49. Saitoh T, Sundsmo M, Roch JM, Kumura N, Cole G, Schubert D, Oltersdorf T, Schenk DB. Cell 1989; 58: 615-22.
50. Schubert D, Cole G, Saitoh T, Oltersdorf T. Biochem Biophys Res Comm 1989; 162: 83-8.
51. Kitaguchi N, Takahashi Y, Oishi K, Shiojiri S, Tokushima Y, Utsunomiya T, Ito H. Biochim Biophys Acta 1990; 1038: 105-13.
52. Kido H, Fukutomi A, Schilling J, Wang Y, Cordell B, Katunuma N. Biochem Biophys Res Comm 1990; 167: 716-21.
53. Sims PJ, Faioni EM, Wiedmer T, Shattil SJ. J. Biol Chem 1988; 263: 18205-12.
54. Rumble B, Retallack R, Hilbich C, Simms G, Multhaup G, Martins R, Hockey A, Montgomery P, Beyreuther K, Masters C. N Engl J Med 1989; 320: 1446-52.

Address for correspondence:

Professor Colin L. Masters,
Department of Pathology,
University of Melbourne,
Parkville, Victoria 3052,
Australia

71 Alzheimer Amyloid β/A4 Protein-Reactive Antibodies in Human Sera and CSF

U. MÖNNING, U. SCHREITER-GASSER, C. HILBICH,
D. BUNKE, R. PRIOR, C. L. MASTERS AND K. BEYREUTHER

The neuropathological hallmarks of Alzheimer's disease (AD) are intraneuronal and extraneuronal amyloid protein depositions associated with neurofibrillary tangles, amyloid plaques and vascular amyloid. They consist of the self-aggregating 42/43-residue amyloid β/A4 protein (1–3).

Molecular cloning based on the sequence of amyloid β/A4 protein has shown that the amyloid is synthesized as part of larger membrane proteins. They are encoded by the APP gene, which maps to chromosome 21. The APP gene is expressed in brain and peripheral tissues, such as muscle and epithelial cells (4).

The precursors of the β/A4 protein are integral, glycosylated membrane proteins which span the membrane bilayer once (5,6). Since the amyloidogenic β/A4 sequence includes the N-terminal half of the transmembrane domain of the precursor, it is suggested that membrane damage and proteolytic cleavage could be important events during amyloidogenesis.

It was recently proposed that AD may be a syndrome resulting from different etiologic subsets and that at least one is of immunological origin (7,8). Immunologic mechanisms play an important role in other neurological disorders such as myasthenia gravis and multiple sclerosis (9–11). Autoimmune responses to neuronal structures have been reported in these diseases. They are mediated by antibodies.

In contrast, Guilbert et al. (12) and Dighiero et al. (13) described natural antibodies which can bind to various antigens of healthy individuals. They can be detected, in broad occurrence, in normal preimmune serum of different species and are not pathogenic. A physiological role of these antibodies was proposed (14).

Here we describe a specific set of generally occurring antibodies that are reactive against the β/A4 protein of AD. They are present in the serum of all human individuals. The concentration of these antibodies is increased in the cerebrospinal fluid (CSF) of some AD patients. It is suggested that these naturally occurring antibodies may play a role in amyloid deposition in AD.

Alzheimer's Disease: Basic Mechanisms, Diagnosis and Therapeutic Strategies
Edited by K. Iqbal, D. R. C. McLachlan, B. Winblad and H. M. Wisniewski
©1991 John Wiley & Sons Ltd

RESULTS

Occurrence of β/A4-reactive antibodies in human sera

Sera from patients with AD and from control patients were tested for their ability to recognize a synthetic β/A4 protein. Since a major fraction of native β/A4 peptides starts with the second residue of the entire β/A4 sequence (3) binding studies were carried out with a synthetic peptide P2-43 corresponding to residues 598–639 of APP_{695} (15). In an enzyme-linked immunosorbent assay (ELISA) P2-43 was used as solid-phase ligand, coated to plastic microtiter plates. After incubation with human sera in different dilutions the binding of specific antibodies was detected by alkaline phosphatase-coupled anti-human IgG.

As shown in Figure 1, β/A4-reactive antibodies are present in sera of human individuals of different age. The content of P2-43-specific immunoglobulins is given as the ratio between P2-43-reactive Ig and total Ig content (determined by a direct ELISA). The antibody titers of P2-43-directed antibodies did not correlate with the clinical features of AD. Fab fragments obtained by papain digestions of IgG also bound to synthetic β/A4, thus proving that the reaction was not due to Fc-binding of IgG.

Immunoabsorption of β/A4-reactive antibodies

Immunoabsorptions were performed to confirm the specificity of binding observed in the direct ELISA. For this assay IgG of human sera was purified using a protein A affinity column. Pretreatment of purified IgG with P2-43 removed all amyloid

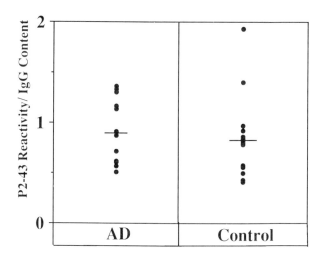

Figure 1. Content of antibodies specific to P2-43 in sera from AD patients (*n* = 12) and controls (*n* = 13). The content of P2-43-reactive IgG is given as ratio between P2-43 reactivity to absolute IgG content, both determined in an ELISA. A broad range of values is obtained in AD and control groups. The difference of the mean values is not significant

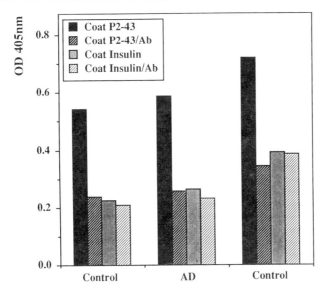

Figure 2. Reactivity of purified human serum IgG (*n* = 3) against P2-43 and bovine insulin before and after absorption with synthetic P2-43 (Ab) determined by a direct ELISA

specific antibodies from solution but had no effect on the binding to bovine insulin as a control peptide. The results are summarized in Figure 2. The difference between reactivities to P2-43 and to insulin accounts for the specific human IgG for peptide 2–43. Thus specific affinity corresponds to 60% of the total binding.

Specificity of isolated antibodies

We set out to determine whether the specific reactivity of human IgG to P2-43 was due to a specific set of antibodies. Immunoabsorption with sepharose-coupled P2-43 was performed to isolate the specific antibodies. Purified IgG of human sera were passed through a P2-43 immunoabsorbent and eluted with acid buffer. Immunoglobulin contents were determined from the absorption at 280 and 260 nm. Reactivities of eluate and void volume were tested by using P2-43 as antigen in direct immunoassay. The results obtained with antibody concentrations ranging from 0.6 μg/ml to 25 μg/ml are given in Figure 3. Fractions containing the eluted antibodies showed the expected high affinity to the antigen used for its isolation. The void volume of the immunoabsorbent was only weakly reactive.

The isolated P2-43-reactive antibodies showed a similar binding to native and synthetic β/A4 amyloid, indicating that these naturally occurring antibodies are indeed directed against a sequential epitope of β/A4 protein (Figure 4). Native amyloid plaques were isolated from postmortem tissue of a pathological confirmed case of AD.

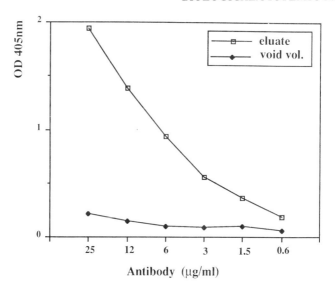

Figure 3. Affinity isolated P2-43-reactive antibodies. The antibodies in the eluate and void volume of a P2-43 affinity column were tested in concentrations of 0.6 μg/ml to 25 μg/ml on P2-43 in a direct ELISA. The reactivities are determined as OD at 405 nm

Detection of β/A4-reactive antibodies in human CSF

ELISA of CSF from AD patients and controls demonstrated that CSF also contained β/A4-reactive antibodies. The analysis was done as described for human sera. The reactivity is also given as the ratio of P2-43-reactive IgG to absolute Ig (Figure 5).

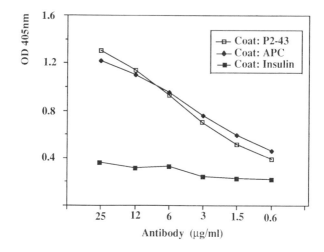

Figure 4. Reactivity of affinity isolated P2-43-reactive antibodies against native β/A4 amyloid (amyloid plaques, APC), synthetic β/A4 amyloid and bovine insulin. The reactivity is expressed as OD at 405 nm for antibody concentrations ranging from 0.6 μg to 25 μg/ml

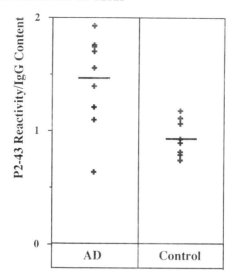

Figure 5. Content of P2-43-reactive IgG in CSF of AD patients ($n = 9$) and controls ($n = 8$). The content is given as the ratio between P2-43-reactivity and absolute IgG content

In contrast to human sera, the titer of CSF-specific β/A4-reactive antibodies was increased in two-thirds of the patients with a clinical diagnosis of AD included in our study. Elevated levels were not found in controls.

DISCUSSION

A set of naturally occurring antibodies reactive to amyloid β/A4 protein was detected in sera and cerebrospinal fluid of patients with a clinical diagnosis of AD and controls. The broad occurrence of these antibodies suggests that amyloid β/A4 protein-reactive antibodies represent a specific and perhaps obligatory component of the natural antibody repertoire.

Since these antibodies are present in sera of healthy human males and females, immunogenic stimulation by amyloid β/A4 for the origin of the antibodies seems to be highly improbable. The presence of amyloid β/A4-immunoreactivity in the periphery and in CSF of patients with AD has been suggested by Joachim et al. (16) and Pardridge et al. (17). The possibility that APP may be the antigenic target of those antibodies is intriguing, since secreted APP was detected in serum and CSF of human individuals (6,18). Secreted APP (APP$_{sec}$) can be generated from the transmembrane forms of APP (APP$_{mem}$) by proteolytic cleavage within the amyloidogenic β/A4 region (19,20). Since APP$_{mem}$ is ubiquitously expressed and present in brain and peripheral tissues as well as in body fluids, a physiological role of these naturally occurring antibodies (autoantibodies) in APP metabolism or catabolism may be possible.

The presence of autoantibodies has been described for various pathological conditions as well as for healthy individuals (9,11–13). A role of these normally occurring antibodies in 'self tolerance' by acting as blocking antibodies was suggested. (14). These autoantibodies may mask and protect self antigens against attack by the immune system. They could also be involved in the elimination of breakdown products.

Complement factors have been detected in amyloid protein depositions in the brain of patients with Alzheimer's disease (21,22). This indicates that immunological mechanisms might also be involved in APP degradation leading to plaque formation. Immunoglobulins have been detected within amyloid depositions by different investigators (23,24). However, a recent report showed that human immunoglobulins seem not to be associated with amyloid depositions in AD (22). Yet the elevated titer of the naturally occurring antibodies reactive against β/A4 protein in CSF may be possibly related to amyloid β/A4 depositions in the brain of Alzheimer patients. The difference in the titer of P2-43-reactive antibodies may correlate with the clinical features of Alzheimer's disease and thus might be of great diagnostic relevance.

Acknowledgments

The work was supported by the Deutsche Forschungsgemeinschaft through SFB 317, the BMFT of Germany, Cusanus Werk and the Fonds der chemischen Industrie. Colin L. Masters is supported by the National Health and Medical Research Council of Australia and by a grant from the Alzheimer's Disease and Related Disorders Association.

REFERENCES

1. Glenner GG, Wong CG. Biochem Biophys Res Comm 1984; 1120: 885-90.
2. Masters CL, Simms G, Weinman NA, Multhaup G, McDonald BL, Beyreuther K. Proc Natl Acad Sci USA 1985; 82: 4245-9.
3. Masters CL, Multhaup G, Simms G, Pottgieser J, Martins RN, Beyreuther K. EMBO J 1985; 4: 2757-63.
4. Müller-Hill B, Beyreuther K. Ann Rev Biochem 1989; 58: 287-307.
5. Dyrks T, Weidemann A, Multhaup G, Salbaum JM, Lemaire HG, Kang J, Müller-Hill B, Masters CL, Beyreuther K. EMBO J 1988; 7: 949-57.
6. Weidemann A, König G, Bunke D, Fischer P, Salbaum JM, Masters CL, Beyreuther K. Cell 1989; 57:115-26.
7. Fudenberg HH, Whitten HD, Arnaud P, Khansari N. Clin Immunol Immunopathol 1984; 32: 127-31.
8. Singh VK, Fudenberg HH, Brown FR. Mech Ageing Dev 1987; 37: 257-64.
9. Dawkins RL, Garlepp MJ. In Rose NR, MacKay IR (eds) The autoimmune diseases. New York: Academic Press 1985: 591-615.
10. Arnason BG. In Rose NR, MacKay IR (eds) The autoimmune diseases. New York: Academic Press 1985: 399-427.
11. Lindstrom J, Shelton D, Fugii Y. Adv Immun 1988; 42: 233-85.
12. Guilbert B, Dighiero G, Avrameas S. J Immun 1982; 128: 2779-87.
13. Dighiero G, Lymberi P, Mazié JC, Rouyre S, Butler-Browne GS, Whalen RG, Avrameas S. J Immun 1983; 131: 2267-72.
14. Grabar P. Immunol Today. 1983; 4: 337-9.
15. Kang J, Lemaire HG, Unterbeck A, Salbaum JM, Masters CL, Grzeschik KH, Multhaup G, Beyreuther K, Müller-Hill B. Nature 1987; 325: 733-6.

16. Joachim CL, Mori H, Selkoe DJ. Nature 1989; 341: 226-30.
17. Pardridge WM, Vinters HV, Miller BL, Tourtellotte WW, Eisenberg JB, Yang J. Biochem Biophys Res Comm 1987; 145: 241-8.
18. Palmert MR, Podlisny MB, Witker DS, Oltersdorf T, Younkin LH, Selkoe DJ, Younkin SG. PNAS 1989; 86: 6338-42.
19. Sisodia SS, Koo EH, Beyreuther K, Unterbeck A, Price DL. Science 1990; 248:492-5.
20. Esch FS, Keim PS, Beattie EC, Blacher RW, Culwell AR, Oltersdorf T, McClure D, Ward PJ. Science 1990; 248: 1122-4.
21. Eikelenboom P, Hack CE, Rozemuller JM, Stam FC. Virchows Arch B 1989; 56: 259-62.
22. Rozemuller JM, Eikelenboom P, Stam FC, Beyreuther K, Masters CL. J Neuropath Exp Neurol 1989; 48: 674-91.
23. Ishi T, Haga S. Neuropathol (Japan) 1983; 4: 31-6.
24. Ihara Y, Kurizaki H, Nukima N, Sugita H, Toyokura Y, Ebara C. Neurol Med (Japan) 1981; 15: 292-5.

Address for correspondence:

Dr U. Mönning,
Center for Molecular Biology,
University of Heidelberg,
Im Neuenheimer Feld 282,
D-6900 Heidelberg,
Germany

72 Normal Lactate Production and Altered Hexokinase Activity in Fibroblasts and Leukocytes from Familial Alzheimer's Disease Patients

M. MORTILLA, S. SORBI, S. LATORRACA, G. TESCO,
S. PIACENTINI, S. TONINI AND L. AMADUCCI

Alzheimer's disease is an age-related degenerative disorder of the nervous system that is characterized by the presence of neurofibrillary tangles, neuritic plaques and dystrophic neurites in susceptible areas of the brain. About 40% of people over 80 years old are affected (1).

Several earlier studies suggested that alterations in cerebral metabolic rate, cerebral oxygen consumption, cerebral blood flow and cerebral glucose utilization may occur among the earliest and best-documented abnormalities in dementias (2,3).

Besides these results a decreased activity of glycolytic enzymes has been documented in the brain of patients with AD, and more recently an increase of lactate production has been observed in cultured skin fibroblasts from AD patients. Some authors (4,5) have reported a decreased activity of the pyruvate dehydrogenase complex (PDHC) in affected areas of AD and Huntington's disease brain.

The activity of phosphofructokinase (PFK) in the cerebral cortex from cases of AD was reported to be less than 20% of that in control brains (6,7). The activity of hexokinase (HK) has also been found to be decreased in the nucleus basalis of Meynert in brains of patients affected with AD (8). Since PFK and HK are key enzymes in glycolysis and normally may be the rate-limiting enzymes of cerebral glucose utilization (9), any significant alterations in these enzymes in AD would have the potential to be significant for its pathophysiology. The abnormality in PFK and HK observed in postmortem brain seems to persist, in at least some patients, in cultured skin fibroblasts even after several passages (10,11).

Studies on cultured skin fibroblasts have also shown abnormalities in PDHC and PFK activities in patients with Down's syndrome (5,10), who are at very high risk of developing a dementia if they survive beyond 35 years of age.

Recently an increased lactate production and decreased CO_2 production in cultured skin fibroblasts from AD patients have been observed (12,13). Contrasting results, however, have been reported by a group (14) who failed to observe changes

Alzheimer's Disease: Basic Mechanisms, Diagnosis and Therapeutic Strategies
Edited by K. Iqbal, D. R. C. McLachlan, B. Winblad and H. M. Wisniewski
© 1991 John Wiley & Sons Ltd

in lactate production in similar cell cultures from AD patients. Moreover, that study indicated that in cultured skin fibroblasts an overall alteration of cell metabolism is present. They reported, in fact, changes in glucose oxidation, calcium content, protein and DNA synthesis in aged and AD fibroblasts.

The identification of changes in cultured cells consistent with known alterations in the brain in AD would provide an accessible and readily manipulable system for study and could be an important step toward defining the pathogenesis of AD. Thus we have studied lactate production, PFK, hexokinase (HK) and lactate dehydrogenase (LDH) activities in cultured skin fibroblasts and leukocytes from patients affected with familial Alzheimer's disease (FAD), their unaffected relatives, sporadic AD, apparently normal controls and pathological controls.

Skin fibroblasts have been studied from 3 FAD patients (2 brothers and a cousin from the same family), 3 non-blood relatives (spouses) of this family and 6 age-matched nonrelated apparently normal controls. Leukocytes were also used to study PFK and HK in 3 other FAD patients, 5 sporadic AD and 5 apparently normal age-matched controls.

Fibroblast cell cultures were obtained from forearm skin biopsy. Cells were grown in Dulbecco's modified Eagle's medium, supplemented with 20% FBS and harvested at confluence, 5 to 7 days after a 1 : 2 subculture, by mild trypsinization. Periodic testing revealed no contamination by PPLO. Protein content and cells numbers were similar in all lines studied as well as passage numbers. All cell lines were coded and studied in at least three different experiments, at least in triplicate in each experiment. Leukocytes were obtained by 30 ml of blood collected from overnight fasted patients using a plastic syringe containing eparine.

PFK activity was measured using the method of Racker (15) as modified by Sorbi and Blass (10). LDH activity was measured according to Clark and Nicklas (16). HK activity was measured according to Racker (15). Lactate production was measured according to Noll (17). Protein concentration was measured according to Lowry et al (18).

Lactate production was comparable in cultured skin fibroblasts from FAD affected members, their unaffected relatives and 3 controls (Table 1).

The activities of fibroblast PFK and LDH were comparable in all groups studied (Table 2).

Fibroblast HK activity was significantly decreased in FAD patients compared to the unaffected relatives. All affected members of this family had HK activity below the lowest of control values.

Table 1. Lactate production in Alzheimer's disease

	Lactase production nmol/mg protein·hour Mean ± SD
Controls (3)	676 ± 242
FAD (3)	858 ± 401
Unaffected relatives (5)	756 ± 126

Table 2. Fibroblast PFK, LDH and HK in Alzheimer's disease

	PFK	LDH	HK
Controls (6)	34.3±11	997±27	25.3±6
FAD (3)	39.6±11	621±12	19.3±2*
Unaffected relatives (3)	28.8±12	486±72	29.0±5

*P<0.05.
Enzyme activities are expressed as nmol/min. mg protein. All experiments were done in triplicate in at least three different experiments.

Leukocyte HK activity was also significantly decreased in patients with FAD, but not in sporadic AD, and PFK activity was normal in all AD patients (Table 3).

Cerebral metabolic rate for oxygen and glucose, and cerebral blood flow, were found to be significantly decreased in Alzheimer's brain, but there is now evidence that metabolic changes associated with AD are not confined to the brain.

In this study we have reported evidence of an alteration of the catalytic activity of the glycolytic rate-limiting enzyme HK in affected patients with the familial form of AD. Enzyme values were significantly decreased versus unaffected relatives and were also decreased versus apparently normal unrelated controls.

The decrease in HK activity was present either in cultured skin fibroblasts or in leukocytes from these patients. However, HK activity was normal in cells from patients with sporadic AD. In FAD patients lactate concentration was normal, contrasting with the earlier studies (11).

The significance of the finding of abnormalities in peripheral tissues in AD is not yet clear since the metabolic requirements of brain cells and fibroblasts are markedly different, particularly with respect to their dependence on oxidative metabolism and the primary substrate used in this process. It is difficult to assess the role of metabolic changes in peripheral cells on the pathogenesis of AD. The finding of any abnormality in cultured cells even after several cell passages should indicate that such alteration is independent from exogenous factors and linked to the cellular genome. Moreover, this kind of finding in peripheral cells may lead to a biological marker to be used as a test for the diagnosis.

Our results suggest a possible heterogeneity within AD patients, providing evidence that at least a subgroup with FAD have a modification in the activity of hexokinase.

Table 3. Leukocyte PFK and HK in Alzheimer's disease

	PFK	HK
Controls (5)	27.11± 9	55.9±12
FAD (3)	20.9 ± 9	36.1± 5*
AD (5)	40.5 ±19	56.3±24

* =P<0.05.
Enzyme activities are expressed as nmol/min. mg protein. All experiments were done in triplicate in at least three different experiments.

Further experiments are in progress to extend the study of these parameters to evaluate the frequency of this finding among FAD patients and to characterize this abnormality at a molecular level.

Acknowledgments

This work was supported by CNR (Consiglio Nazionale delle Ricerche), grants 88.00658.04 and 89.00223.70. We would like to thank the Alzheimer Society of Canada for the award (Junior Travel Fellowship).

REFERENCES

1. Rocca W, Bonaiuto S, Lippi A, Luciani P, Turtu' F, Cavarzeran F, Amaducci L. Neurology 1990; 40: 626-31.
2. Quastel JH. Lancet 1932; ii: 1417-25.
3. Sokoloff L. Res Publ Assoc Res Nerv Mental Dis 1966; 41: 237-41.
4. Perry EK, Perry RH, Tomlinson BE, Blessed G, Gibson PH. Neurosci Lett 1980; 18: 105-9.
5. Sorbi S, Bird ED, Blass JP. Ann Neurol 1983; 13: 72-3.
6. Bowen DM, White P, Spillane JA, Goodhart MJ, Curzon G, Iwangoff P, Mayer-Rouge W, Davison AN. Lancet 1979; i: 11-12.
7. Iwangoff P, Armbruster R, Enz A, Mayer-Rouge W. Mech Ageing Dev 1980; 14: 203-9.
8. Liguri G, Taddei N, Nassi P, Latorraca S, Neidani C, Sorbi S. Neurosci Lett 1990; 112: 338-42.
9. Lowrey OH, Passaneau J. J Biol Chem 1964; 139: 31-8.
10. Sorbi S, Blass JP. Banbury Rep 1983; 15: 297-307.
11. Sorbi S, Mortilla M, Piacentini S, Tonini S, Amaducci L. Neurosci Lett 1990; 117: 165-8.
12. Sims N, Finegan JM, Blass JP. N Engl J Med 1985; 313: 638-9.
13. Sims N, Finegan JM, Blass JP. Ann Neurol 1987; 21: 451-7.
14. Peterson C, Goldman JE. Proc Natl Acad Sci USA 1986; 83: 2758-62.
15. Racker R. J Biol Chem 1947; 167: 843-54.
16. Clark JB, Nicklas WJ. J Biol Chem 1970; 245: 4724-31.
17. Noll F. In Bergmeyer HU (ed.) Methods of enzymatic analysis, 2nd edn. NY, London: Academic Press 1974: 1475.
18. Lowry OH, Rosenbrough NJ, Farr AL, Randall RJ. J Biol Chem 1951; 193: 265-75.

Address for correspondence:

Dr M. Mortilla,
Department of Neurology and Psychiatry,
University of Florence,
Viale Morgagni 85,
50134 Florence, Italy

73 Alzheimer's Disease Associated Protein(s) in Human Brain Tissue: Detection, Measurement, Specificity and Distribution

HOSSEIN A. GHANBARI, BARNEY E. MILLER, JONATHAN K. CHONG, HENRY J. HAIGLER AND WILLIAM O. WHETSELL Jr

Alzheimer's disease (AD) is a neurodegenerative disease characterized by a chronically deteriorating course of impaired intellectual function and memory loss. The definitive diagnosis of AD is made by pathological examination of postmortem brain tissue in conjunction with a clinical history of dementia (1). This diagnosis is based on the presence in brain tissue of neuritic (senile) plaques (NPs) and neurofibrillary tangles (NFTs) which have been correlated with clinical dementia (2). NPs are thought to be composed of degenerating axons and nerve terminals as well as possible astrocytic elements (3) and often exhibit a central amyloid protein core (4). The NFT is an intraneuronal aggregate composed of normal and paired helical filaments and presumably consists of several different proteins (4).

Current diagnostic methods for AD are based on the neurohistopathological identification and counting of NPs and NFTs, a process that requires staining and microscopic examination of several brain sections (1). However, there are difficulties with using the NPs and NFTs as the basis for a diagnosis. For instance, the clinical and pathological progression of AD is marked by a continuing loss of neurons from the cerebral cortex, even though densities of NFTs and NPs within this region do not appear to correlate with the stage of the illness (5). Furthermore, NPs and NFTs also occur in nondemented elderly patients (1), histochemical staining is not very reproducible, NPs and NFTs are not uniformly distributed, and histopathological studies are time and labor intensive (6). Additionally, some studies have shown that NFTs and NPs are not necessarily correlated with the development of AD (5,7,8). Therefore, it would be useful to identify a readily measurable biochemical marker for Alzheimer's disease.

Alz-50 is a monoclonal antibody that reacts against brain tissue homogenates from patients with AD; it binds to a highly selective protein marker (A68) for this disorder (9–11). Immunocytochemical staining has established that Alz-50 recognizes an early cytological change that precedes the formation of NFTs and NPs. This early

Alzheimer's Disease: Basic Mechanisms, Diagnosis and Therapeutic Strategies
Edited by K. Iqbal, D. R. C. McLachlan, B. Winblad and H. M. Wisniewski
© 1991 John Wiley & Sons Ltd

cytological change is apparently specific for AD (7,12,13). However, Alz-50 crossreacts with normal components of the brain in direct immunoassay, western blot, and less frequently in immunocytochemical staining (11,14). In the present study, we used a sandwich enzyme immunoassay (developed at Abbott Laboratories) that minimizes Alz-50 crossreactivity and detects Alzheimer's disease associated proteins (ADAP) with high specificity (15,16). ADAP has three major Alz-50 reactive subunits including A-68 and is primarily associated with AD (17). In this study the measurement of ADAP has been described, specificity of the ADAP to AD has been determined, and the distribution of ADAP in 18 different regions of the human brain has been examined.

MATERIALS AND METHODS

Analysis

A rabbit polyclonal antibody (PR1) used in conjunction with the Alz-50 antibody is the basis of a rapid immunoassay (Alz-EIA) for brain tissue (15). The rabbit antibody (PR1) was developed using a highly purified ADAP fraction by differential centrifugation and detergent extraction (18). The assay employs 6-mm (¼ in) polystyrene beads coated with a purified (IgG) fraction of PR1. In the assay, the antigen in brain homogenate is first captured on the beads, and in the second step Alz-50 is allowed to specifically bind to the antigen immobilized on the bead. Alz- EIA activity is a measure of bound Alz-50 using an enzyme conjugated anti-mouse IgM. This configuration appears to minimize complications caused by the crossreactants from both AD and normal brain homogenates (15). The tissue (20–200 mg wet weight), was mixed with four volumes of homogenization buffer (0.05 M Tris HCl at pH 6.8, 1 mM EGTA and 150 mM NaCl) and then homogenized gently with a Kontes motorized pestle inside a 1.5-ml conical capped tube. The homogenate was centrifuged at $9500\,g$ for 5 minutes. A duplicate 50-μl aliquot of the supernatant (equivalent to 10 mg wet tissue) was used in the assay. The ADAP levels are expressed as absorbance units per 10 mg wet tissue or absorbance units per mg protein.

Specimens

Brain specimens used in the biochemical assay were fresh frozen. All the cases used in this study were clinically evaluated for dementia, and the specimens were examined histopathologically by neuropathologists.

RESULTS AND DISCUSSION

Detection and measurement of ADAP

The assay method for ADAP has been developed and optimized by Ghanbari et al (15). Sandwich enzyme-linked immunoassay configuration (Figure 1) appears to detect and measure ADAP only and seems to eliminate crossreactivity problems. There is strong evidence that ADAPs are present in aggregate form in the brain

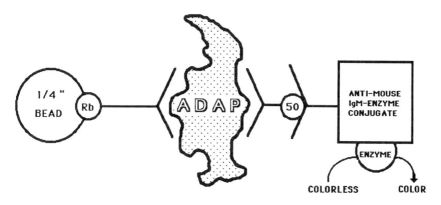

Figure 1. Assay configuration for Alz-EIA (Brain). Rb is rabbit anti-Alz IgG, ADAP is Alzheimer's disease associated proteins in the aggregate state, and '50' is Alz-50. Reproduced with permission from Ghanbari et al (15)

tissue and hence are multiepitopic. Even after solubilization ADAP has a molecular weight equivalent of 200 kDa and upon denaturation produces three Alz-50 immunoreactive major protein bands. In contrast the crossreactive proteins are in a soluble form in the brain and seem to have only one epitope. The multiepitopic ADAPs are favored in this sandwich assay. This method is referred to as Alz-EIA (Brain) and can reliably measure ADAP, providing a unique biochemical laboratory test for postmortem diagnosis of Alzheimer's disease. The method is very simple because it uses preformulated reagents and standard equipment and supplies. It is rapid: 120 data points (two trays) can readily be generated in less than four hours. This assay can become a powerful tool in the area of Alzheimer research and diagnostics and may help further research efforts to achieve a better understanding of the disease itself.

Specificity of ADAP

A multicenter clinical study was carried out to determine the specificity of ADAP (16). Figure 2 summarizes the results of this study for the following categories: normal control (NC), Alzheimer's disease (AD), and neurological disease control (NDC). The cases in the neurological disease control (NDC) category include Parkinson's disease ($n = 16$), multi-infarct dementia ($n = 5$), Huntington's disease ($n = 2$), amyotrophic lateral sclerosis ($n = 2$) Wernicke's encephalopathy ($n = 1$), and Korsakoff's syndrome ($n = 2$). There were 27 NC cases and 28 NDC cases, none of which contained any detectable level of ADAP; in the 46 cases in the AD category, however, 43 showed measurable levels of ADAP (Figure 2). Only frontal or temporal cortical tissues were analyzed for ADAP. In this study ADAP appears to be specific to AD cases; there were no false positives in the study. On further examination of the pathology reports, it was observed that one of the three false negatives had a brain tumor, one had a postmortem time of 96 hours, and a postmortem time was not reported for the third one. All three had questionable AD diagnosis and/or very long postmortem time.

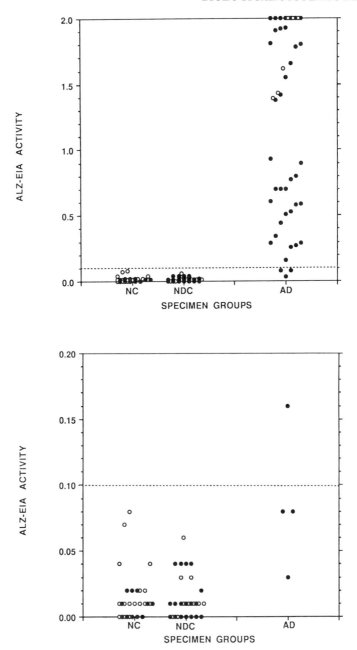

Figure 2. Scattergram of Alzheimer's disease associated protein (ADAP) concentrations for each diagnostic category. Top: a full-scale graph. Bottom: a *y*-axis scale 10-fold expansion. Closed circles indicate cases 65 years and older; open circles, cases under 65 years old. NC, normal control; NDC, neurologic disease control; AD, Alzheimer's disease. The circles on the 2.0 line (top) indicate values of 2.0 or higher (up to 16)

Based on this study, clinical dementia, NPs, and old age per se do not appear to be associated with the increased ADAP concentrations in the AD category. Dementia alone was not associated with an increase in ADAP concentrations, because there were 16 demented cases in the NDC category with no detectable level of ADAP. Furthermore, NPs were not always associated with the presence of ADAP; there were 5 NC cases and 16 NDC cases with NPs which had practically no detectable ADAP levels.

To examine the concentration of ADAP as a function of age, the data pertaining to ADAP concentrations for the cases aged 65 years or more were analyzed separately. Based on this analysis, the maximum value of ADAP in cases aged 65 years or more was actually lower in NC and NDC categories, and the median in AD category was decreased. Furthermore, in Figure 2, the ADAP concentrations for cases 65 years and older are presented in filled circles and for cases under 65 years old in open circles; there is no age-related pattern apparent in the figure. In fact, the highest 'values' of ADAP immunoreactivity in both NC and NDC categories correspond to cases under 65 years old (open circles, Figure 2). The Spearman correlation test showed a 15% (not significant) probability of ADAP concentration being negatively correlated with age. The oldest NDC case in this study was a 90-year-old female with multi-infarct dementia showing moderate NPs, and yet with ADAP concentration of only 0.01 absorbance unit/10 mg tissue, while the youngest AD case in the study was 46 years old and had an ADAP concentration of more than 2.0.

Distribution of ADAP in the brain

In order to determine the distribution of ADAP in brain, frozen hemispheres from five AD brains and five non-AD (NAD) brains were dissected into 18 discrete regions by an expert brain pathologist. Subsequently ADAP levels were assayed and expressed as absorbance units per mg protein. Table 1 is the summary of the patient information. The mean age for the AD group was 75 ± 7 years and for the NAD group was 57 ± 19 years. The average postmortem time was 6.0 ± 2.7 hours. Specimen 10 was clinically demented and diagnosed at autopsy as having vascular dementia.

Table 1. Specimen information. Pm/h refers to postmortem time in hours. Each specimen was quickly frozen at $-80\ °C$ after removal

Patient number	Diagnosis	Age, sex*	Pm/h
1	Alzheimer	68M	6.0
2	Alzheimer	77F	6.0
3	Alzheimer	70F	5.0
4	Alzheimer	76M	5.0
5	Alzheimer	85F	4.0
6	Normal	35F	5.0
7	Normal	43M	4.0
8	Normal	56M	12.0
9	Normal	75M	5.0
10	Vascular dementia	77F	8.0

*M, male; F, female

Table 2. ADAP level in 18 brain regions in Alzheimer's disease (AD) and non-Alzheimer's disease (NAD) brain

| | ADAP level (absorbance unit/mg protein) | | | | | | | | | |
| | AD | | | | | NAD | | | | |
Brain region	1*	2*	3*	4*	5*	6*	7*	8*	9*	10*
Frontal cortex	9.3	47.0	43.6	49.5	39.9	0.0	0.6	0.4	0.5	0.1
Temporal cortex	23.3	33.9	48.8	53.6	28.9	0.0	1.0	1.1	0.4	0.1
Parietal cortex	25.3	7.9	39.9	35.0	22.5	0.0	0.7	0.2	0.4	0.1
Occipital cortex	8.6	0.0	24.4	34.3	5.5	0.0	0.6	1.2	0.4	0.0
Hippocampus	31.5	21.2	40.2	37.2	27.1	0.0	0.8	1.0	0.5	0.0
Subiculum	21.1	26.9	55.4	41.1	30.7	0.1	0.8	1.9	0.4	0.1
Amygdala	ND†	39.4	95.2	38.8	14.8	0.0	0.8	1.5	0.4	0.6
Nucleus basalis	ND	13.0	6.5	11.5	4.1	0.0	0.0	0.8	0.9	0.2
Caudate nucleus	1.2	2.7	6.5	9.4	2.3	0.0	0.8	0.1	0.2	0.3
Putamen	1.4	1.7	3.8	3.9	2.4	0.0	0.7	0.6	0.5	0.5
Globus pallidus	ND	0.1	1.1	0.8	3.2	0.0	0.1	0.5	0.3	0.0
Thalamus	1.2	1.7	10.2	11.9	6.8	0.0	0.6	0.5	0.1	0.0
Hypothalamus	4.9	3.5	19.5	2.1	16.4	0.0	0.5	0.7	0.5	0.1
Subthalamus	1.2	1.5	1.9	10.8	ND	0.1	0.3	0.0	0.5	ND
Substantia nigra	ND	2.9	6.2	3.8	0.3	0.0	0.5	0.0	0.4	0.0
Locus ceruleus	ND	17.9	14.7	2.6	3.2	ND	ND	0.2	0.1	0.1
Medulla	0.5	0.2	0.8	8.3	0.0	0.0	0.9	0.0	0.3	0.3
Cerebellum	0.8	0.7	0.3	1.0	0.2	0.0	1.0	0.2	0.3	0.1

*For patient code numbers refer to Table 1.
†ND, not determined.

Table 2 shows the ADAP concentrations for each specimen in 18 brain regions expressed as Alz-EIA absorbance unit per mg protein. Essentially no ADAP (mean value for all 18 areas in the five brains was 0.36 ± 0.38 absorbance units/mg protein) was found in the NAD group or in the globus pallidus, medulla and cerebellum of the AD group means, respectively 1.3 ± 1.3, 1.96 ± 3.6 and 0.6 ± 0.34 absorbance units/mg protein. In the AD group there were significantly greater levels of ADAP (Student's t-test, $P < 0.05$) in all areas except globus pallidus, medulla, and cerebellum when compared to same areas in the NAD group. These three areas in the AD group were not different from the areas in the NAD group. As expected the areas globus pallidus, medulla and cerebellum in the AD group were not significantly different from each other (Student's t-test, $P > 0.1$).

Figure 3 shows a plot of the mean ± the standard deviation of five data points (ADAP levels for each region) for both the AD and NAD groups. Since the ADAP level in the cerebellum in all of the ten cases was significantly lower than the 15 other AD areas (and not different from reagent blank) it is proposed that this region could serve as an internal negative control for the distribution studies of ADAP.

The ADAP levels show a widespread distribution based on the analysis of 18 different brain regions of five AD brains. This study fully supports the findings that ADAP is highly associated with Alzheimer's disease (16). The fact that NAD and AD groups are not age matched may not be significant in this study because we

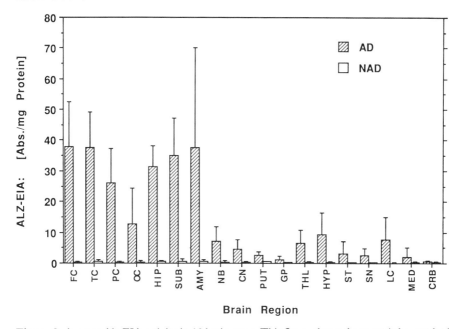

Figure 3. Average Alz-EIA activity in 18 brain areas. This figure shows the mean ± the standard deviation ($n = 5$) for both the non-Alzheimer's disease (NAD) and the Alzheimer's disease (AD) groups. The brain areas are in the same order as shown in Table 2 (the abbreviations in this figure correspond to the brain regions listed in Table 2)

have demonstrated that ADAP levels are not correlated with age (16). It is noteworthy, for example, that patient 10 (vascular dementia) was 77 years old (which is older than all but one of the AD patients), and like the other NAD specimens showed no significant ADAP concentrations in any of the 18 brain areas tested.

The highest concentrations of ADAP were found in the AD group's temporal cortex, hippocampus, subiculum and amygdala. Thus the ADAP is associated with those brain areas involved with AD (and cognitive function) based on previous reports using both similar (Alz-50 based) and different techniques (1,18,19). The wide variation in the ADAP levels for the amygdala, locus ceruleus, and nucleus basalis areas which are thought to be especially involved with Alzheimer's disease (1,19) is puzzling. However, the ADAP levels in these areas were significantly higher than that of the same areas in the NAD group. This finding may reflect the expected general cell loss (5,19,20) in these relatively small regions which are involved early in the disease. However, the similarities in the distribution of ADAP in areas thought to be involved with AD increase the probability that ADAP could mark the progression of the disease in brain.

Acknowledgments

We would like to especially thank Terry Kozuk, Sue Riesing and Allen Simon, without whose expert technical assistance this study would not have been possible.

REFERENCES

1. Khachaturian ZS. Arch Neurol 1985; 42: 1097-105.
2. Blessed G, Tomlinson BE, Roth, M. Br J Psychiatry 1968; 114: 797-811.
3. Birecree E, Whetsell W, Stoscheck C, King L, Nanney L. J Neuropath Exp Neurol 1988; 47: 549-60.
4. Davies, P. J Clin Psychiatry 1988; 49 (suppl.): 23-8.
5. Mann DMA, Marcyniuk B, Yates PO, Neary D, Snowden JS. Neuropath Appl Neurobiol 1988; 14: 177-95.
6. Wisniewski H, Rabe A, Zigman W, Silverman W. J Neuropath Exp Neurol 1989; 48: 606-8.
7. Katzman R, Terry R, DeTeresa R et al. Ann Neurol 1988; 23: 138-44.
8. Terry RD, Hansen LA, DeTeresa R, Davies P, Tobias H, Katzman R. J Neuropath Exp Neurol 1987; 46: 262-8.
9. Van Hoesen GW, Hyman BT, Wolozin B, Davies P, Damasio AR. Neurology 1987; 37 (suppl. 1): 332.
10. Wolozin B, Pruchnicki A, Dickson DW, Davies P. Science 1986; 232: 648-50.
11. Wolozin B, Davies P. Ann Neurol 1987; 22: 521-6.
12. Hyman BT, Van Hoesen GW, Wolozin B, Davies P, Damasio AR. Neurology 1987; 37: 225.
13. Hyman BT, Van Hoesen GW, Wolozin B, Davies P, Kromer L, Damasio A. Ann Neurol 1988; 23: 371-9.
14. Ksiezak-Reding H, Davies P, Yen S. J Biol Chem 1988; 263: 7943-7.
15. Ghanbari H, Kozuk T, Miller BE, Riesing S. J Clin Lab Anal 1990; 4: 189-92.
16. Ghanbari H, Miller B, Haigler H, Arato M, Bissette G, Davies P, Nemeroff C, Perry E, Perry R, Ravid R, Swaab D, Whetsell W, Zemlan F. JAMA 1990; 263: 2907-10.
17. Miller B, Simon A, Ghanbari H. Soc Neurosci Abstr 1989; 15: 1038.
18. Brun A, Englund E. Histopathol 1981; 5: 549-64.
19. Hardy JA, Mann DMA, Wester P, Winblad B. Neurobiol Aging 1986; 7: 489-502.
20. Neary D, Snowden JS, Mann DMA et al. J Neurol Neurosurg Psychiat 1986; 49: 229-37.

Address for correspondence:

Dr Hossein A. Ghanbari,
Abbott Laboratories,
Neuropsychiatric Markers,
D-9RR, AP20,
Abbott Park,
IL 60064, USA

74 Temporal-Frontal Differences in Alzheimer's Disease Associated Proteins—A Biochemical Study

R. RAVID, J. v. HEERIKHUIZE, D. F. SWAAB, W. KAMPHORST, H. J. HAIGLER, B. E. MILLER AND H. A. GHANBARI

Alzheimer's disease (AD) is a progressive neurodegenerative illness characterized by a persistent loss of memory and impairment in other cognitive functions. Antemortem diagnosis of this disease is primarily done by exclusion of other causes of dementia, while the postmortem diagnosis is based upon the presence of large numbers of neuritic plaques (NPs) and neurofibrillary tangles (NFTs) in conjunction with a clinical history of dementia (1,2). The classical hallmarks of AD have been extensively investigated and described in the scientific literature. Senile plaques in cerebral grey matter have been described already in 1892 by Block and Marinesco (3) and by Redlich in 1898 (4). Neurofibrillary changes were described by Alzheimer in 1907 (5) and dystrophic neurites have been described by Tomlinson et al in 1970 (6), as twisted processes which are probably identical with the neuropil threads visualized by Braak et al in 1986 (7). The use of NPs and NFTs as the basis for definitive diagnosis has some serious drawbacks: to start with, AD is characterized by neuronal loss in the cortex which is not always followed by concomitant change in densities of NPs and NFTs (8). In addition, these well-accepted markers of AD are also present in brains of aged controls and of patients with other neurological diseases (8–11). Moreover, NPs and NFTs are nonuniformly distributed over various brain regions, and the histopathological diagnosis of AD is mainly qualitative, is time-consuming and demands very experienced people. For the reasons listed above it is desirable to have an assay based on a specific marker of AD which combines reproducibility, rapidity and specificity for the disease.

A monoclonal antibody against AD brain homogenates has been developed (12,13). This antibody, called Alz-50, recognizes a neuronal antigen of 68 kDa (A68) which is expressed in AD and in some Down's syndrome brains (13–15). However, since some normally occurring brain proteins crossreact with Alz-50 in immunoassays and in western blots (16,17), a biochemical assay has recently been developed which is based upon a combination of the monoclonal Alz-50 and a polyclonal rabbit antibody (PR1) raised against a highly ADAP-enriched brain protein fraction. In

Alzheimer's Disease: Basic Mechanisms, Diagnosis and Therapeutic Strategies
Edited by K. Iqbal, D. R. C. McLachlan, B. Winblad and H. M. Wisniewski

this way the crossreactivity with normal brain components is minimized (18,19). The biochemical assay is thought to be an important contribution to the histopathological diagnosis of AD.

Diagnosis of AD

The patients have been clinically diagnosed as 'probable AD' according to the NINCDS-ADRDA criteria (20) and they all had a global determination scale (GDS) of 6–7 for severity of dementia (21). The neuropathological diagnosis of 'changes compatible with AD' or 'no pathology' for controls was performed by the same neuropathologists on formalin-fixed specimens (fixation duration, 1 month) and was based upon the distribution and amount of plaques and tangles in sections stained by the conventional histopathological staining procedures. The individuals carrying out the biochemical assay were blind to the clinical and neuropathological diagnoses.

Statistical analysis

Because the measured values of ADAP concentrations are truncated at 0 and 2, non-parametric statistics were chosen to analyze the data (22). The Mann–Whitney test was used to compare the non-AD group with the AD group. The Wilcoxon signed ranks test was used to compare frontal with temporal lobe in the three patient groups.

RESULTS

The concentration of Alzheimer's disease associated protein (ADAP) was measured in postmortem brain tissue samples of inferior temporal or superior frontal cortex from 30 human brains and results were expressed as absorbance units per mg protein. The normal group as well as the non-AD dementia group had essentially low levels of ADAP in both frontal and temporal lobe specimens: normal controls, 0.17 ± 0.06 and 0.33 ± 0.03 absorbance units/mg protein respectively; and non-AD dementia, 0.30 ± 0.06 and 0.58 ± 0.10 absorbance units/mg protein respectively. The AD group had substantial ADAP levels in frontal and temporal lobe specimens: 3.62 ± 0.90 and 7.43 ± 0.72 absorbance units/mg protein respectively.

CONCLUSIONS

1. The method described in this paper can reliably measure ADAP, providing a unique biochemical laboratory test for postmortem diagnosis of AD. This assay is rapid and simple to run, the supplies are standardized, the equipment is readily available and sample requirements are low (about 100 mg tissue for homogenization).

   The biochemical Alz-EIA offers a rapid, easily performed and quantitative diagnostic method which may serve as a valuable aid to the clinico-pathological diagnosis of AD.

2. It is apparent from these data that the enzyme-linked immunoassay (Alz-EIA) clearly distinguishes ADAP levels in AD brains from controls and other

neurological diseases. The ADAP levels in the AD group were significantly higher as compared with the non-Alzheimer dementia ($P < 0.002$) although the mean age of the NAD group (85.7 ± 2.1 years) was higher than the mean age of the AD patients (75.8 ± 2.0 years).

3. In addition, a regional variation was found between frontal and temporal lobe specimens which agrees with the classical neuropathological findings (23).

Acknowledgments

We would like to thank The Netherlands Brain Bank for supplying human brain tissue; Dr R. Verwer and E. J. van Zwieten for the statistical analysis of the data; Mrs S. de Waard and Mrs G. Beek for typing the manuscript.

REFERENCES

1. Khachaturian AS. Arch Neurol 1985; 42: 1097-105.
2. Blessed G, Tomlinson BE, Roth M. Br J Psychiatry 1968; 114: 797-811.
3. Blocq P, Marinesco G, Sem Med (Paris) 1892; 12: 445.
4. Redlich E. Jahrbücher Psych Neurolog Bel 1898; XVII: 208-12.
5. Alzheimer A. Allg Z Psychiat 1907; 64: 146-8.
6. Tomlinson BE, Blessed G, Roth M. J Neurol Sci 1970; 11: 205-42.
7. Braak H, Braak E, Grundke-Iqbal I, Iqbal K. Neurosci Lett 1986; 65: 351-5.
8. Mann DMA, Marcyniuk B, Yates PO, Neary D, Snowden JS. Neuropath Appl Neurobiol 1988; 14: 177-95.
9. Tomlinson BE, Blessed G, Roth M. J Neurol Sci 1968; 7: 331-56.
10. Katzmann R, Terry RD, DeTeresa R. Ann Neurol 1988; 23: 138-44.
11. Terry RD, Hansen LA, DeTeresa R, Davies P, Tobias H, Katzman R. J Neuropath Exp Neurol 1987; 46: 262-8.
12. Wolozin B, Pruchnicki A, Dickson DW, Davies P. Science 1986; 232: 648-50.
13. Wolozin B, Davies P. Ann Neurol 1987; 22: 521-6.
14. Hyman BT, Hoesen Van GW, Wolozin B, Davies P, Kromer L, Damasio A. Ann Neurol 1988; 23: 371-9.
15. Hyman BT, Kromer L, Hoesen Van GW. Brain Res 1988; 450: 392-7.
16. Davies P. J Clin Psychiatry (suppl.) 1988; 49: 23-8.
17. Ksiezak-Reding H, Davies P, Yen S. J Biol Chem 1988; 263: 7943-7.
18. Ghanbari H, Kozuk T, Miller BE, Reizing S. J Clin Lab Anal 1990; 4: 189-92.
19. Ghanbari HA, Miller BE, Haigler HJ, Arato M, Bissette G, Davies P, Nemeroff ChB, Perry EK, Perry R, Ravid R, Swaab DF, Whetsell WO, Zemlan FP. JAMA 1990; 263: 2907-10.
20. McKhann G, Drachman D, Folstein M, Katzman R, Price D, Stadlan EM. Neurology 1984; 34: 939-44.
21. Reisberg B, Ferris SH, de Leon MJ, Crook T. Am J Psych 1982; 139: 1136-9.
22. Conover WJ. Practical nonparametric statistics. Chichester: John Wiley, 1980: 280.
23. Brun A, Englund E. Histopathology 1981; 5: 549-64.

Address for correspondence:

Dr R. Ravid,
The Netherlands Institute for Brain Research,
Meibergdreef, 33, Amsterdam, The Netherlands

75 T-Cell Reactivity in Patients with Alzheimer's Disease

E. NIJHUIS, C. M. VAN DUIJN, C. WITTEMAN, A. HOFMAN, J. ROZING AND L. NAGELKERKEN

Compared to age-matched controls, life expectancy of patients with Alzheimer's disease (AD) is reduced, the primary cause of death being infection of the respiratory tract (1,2). Furthermore, in contrast to multi-infarct dementia, life expectancy in AD decreases with the severity of dementia (2). The increased mortality in AD due to infections is in agreement with several observations demonstrating a declining immune system in these patients (3–6).

The pathogenesis of the neurological symptoms as well as the impaired immune reactivity in AD is still largely unknown. Since the central nervous system (CNS) and the immune system interact quite intensively through neuroendocrine hormones and cytokines (7,8), it might be that defects in these two systems have a common etiology, related to homologous structures present on cells of these two systems (7). On the other hand, an impaired function of cells from the CNS or the immune system may also be related to altered plasma levels of cytokines or neuroendocrine hormones, active in both systems. Recently we demonstrated, however, that plasma levels of the cytokine interleukin-6, which are increased in various diseases with an inflammatory compound, were unchanged in AD (9).

For further studies on the immune system, we focused on three different pathways of T-cell activation, which may provide insight into the role of the different receptors involved.

Firstly, cells were activated via the T-cell receptor (TCR)/CD3 complex using phytohaemagglutin (PHA), a lectin that specifically binds to glycoproteins on T-cells, such as CD2 and CD3, and subsequently activates these cells in a monocyte-dependent manner (11).

Secondly, stimulation by an immobilized anti-CD3 monoclonal antibody (mAb) was performed. This system has been widely used to simulate antigen-specific proliferation and differentiation of T-cells in vitro, in a monocyte-independent way (12).

Thirdly, the alternative pathway of T-cell activation was investigated, using a combination of two anti-CD2 mAbs, recognizing different epitopes and an anti-CD28 mAb, which act synergistically with respect to T-cell proliferation (13). This mode

Alzheimer's Disease: Basic Mechanisms, Diagnosis and Therapeutic Strategies
Edited by K. Iqbal, D. R. C. McLachlan, B. Winblad and H. M. Wisniewski
©1991 John Wiley & Sons Ltd

of activation does not require TCR/CD3 complex triggering and therefore may provide us with a new point of view towards the role of the immune system in AD.

MATERIAL AND METHODS

Patients and cell preparations

Patients ($n = 29$) and age-matched controls ($n = 31$) were derived from an epidemiological study of early-onset AD patients (diagnosis ≤ 70 years) (9). The clinical diagnosis of AD was ascertained according to criteria described elsewhere (10). Peripheral blood mononuclear cells (PBMC) were obtained by Percoll density centrifugation ($\varrho = 1.078$) and subsequently cryopreserved. For experiments they were thawed according to standard procedures and viable cells were counted after trypan blue staining.

Proliferation assays

In flat-bottom wells, 4×10^4 PBMC were cultured in Iscove's modified Dulbecco's medium (IMDM), supplemented with penicillin (10^2 U/ml), streptomycin ($100 \, \mu g/ml$), glutamin (2 mM), β-mercaptoethanol ($50 \, \mu M$) and 10% fetal calf serum (FCS).

Anti-CD3 coated culture wells were prepared as described (11). Briefly, $100 \, \mu l$/well of a $1 : 10^3$ dilution of murine ascites CLB-T3/3 in phosphate-buffered saline (PBS) were incubated at $4 \, °C$ in 96-well plates. After overnight incubation the supernatant was removed and the wells were washed twice with PBS. Anti-CD2 (CLB-T11.1/1 and CLB-T11.1/2) and anti-CD28 (CLB-CD28/1) mAbs were all used in a $1 : 8 \times 10^3$ dilution of murine ascites. Phytohaemagglutinin was used at a concentration of $0.3 \, \mu g/ml$.

All cultures were performed with and without exogenous human recombinant IL-2 (hrIL-2; 50 U/ml; Cetus, Emeryville, CA). Cell proliferation was measured (expressed as counts per minute) on day 5 by [^{3}H]thymidine incorporation ($0.25 \, \mu Ci$) during the last 6 hours of culture.

Immunofluorescence

For membrane antigen analysis, 2×10^5 cells were incubated for 30 minutes with a saturating amount of a FITC-labeled mAb. Thereafter, cells were washed and 5000 cells were analyzed on a FACScan (Becton & Dickinson, Mountain View, California).

Statistics and calculations

Statistic analysis was performed using the two-tailed Mann–Whitney U test. Results are presented as percentages of the mean of matched controls. The displayed percentages were calculated as follows: the mean responses in counts per minute (c.p.m.) of age-matched controls were established from three different experiments and were set at 100%. The response of each individual (control and AD patient) was related to its corresponding mean value of 100%. In all cultures this represented about 20 000 c.p.m. Each experiment consisted of at least eight age-matched controls and AD patients.

RESULTS AND DISCUSSION

The ability of T-cells to proliferate was studied by stimulating PBMC from AD patients and age-matched controls with PHA. In anticipation of an eventually impaired IL-2 production, all cultures were also performed in the presence of an excess of hrIL-2 (50 U/ml). As can be seen in Figure 1, the T-cell response to PHA is significantly decreased ($P < 0.005$) in AD as compared to age-matched controls.

These differences in proliferation were, in any case, not solely due to an impaired IL-2 production since the proliferative response by T-cells from AD patients were still significantly lower ($P < 0.05$) after addition of excess hrIL-2.

The relative contribution of the TCR/CD3 complex to this defect was studied by activating the cells with immobilized anti-CD3 mAb, which is a monocyte-independent way of T-cell activation. As shown in Figure 2, the mean of the anti-CD3 response is slightly decreased. However, this decrease failed to prove to be statistically significant, irrespective of hrIL-2 addition to the cultures.

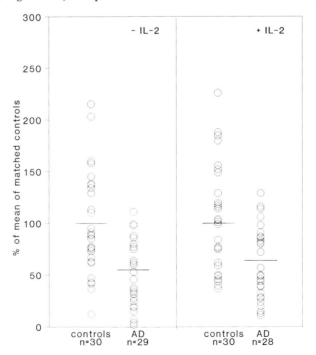

Figure 1. Decreased PHA response in AD patients; for the AD patients the mean response without addition of hrIL-2 was 53% and after addition of hrIL-2 61%

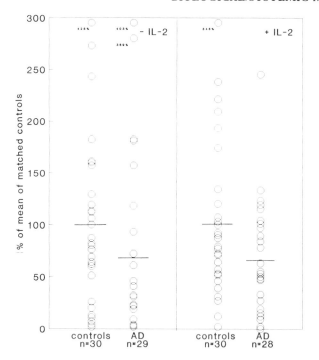

Figure 2. Anti-CD3 response is not significantly decreased in AD patients; for the AD patients the mean response without addition of hrIL-2 was 68% and after addition of hrIL-2 64%. Responses above 300% are shown with their actual values

These results imply that not the TCR/CD3 complex, but different structures may be the major cause of the declined T-cell reactivity. One of the possibilities is CD2, an adhesion molecule which is involved in the interaction between the T-cell and the monocyte during PHA activation, for instance (the natural ligand on the monocyte being leukocyte function-associated antigen-3; LFA-3). Therefore, we focused on the alternative pathway of T-cell activation using the combination of two different anti-CD2 mAbs and an anti-CD28 mAb. As can be seen in Figure 3, this way of T-cell activation again resulted in a significant decreased response in AD patients, not only in the absence ($P < 0.005$) but also in the presence of excess hrIL-2 ($P < 0.05$).

It appeared that AD patients with a low PHA response also responded poorly in the alternative pathway of T-cell activation.

Our results could not be explained by a diminished number of CD3$^+$ T-cells in our PBMC samples nor by major changes in the CD4/CD8 ratio in AD patients (data not shown). Therefore, it seems that these results may be related to an intrinsic defect. In this regard it will be worthwhile to study the role of CD2 and other cellular adhesion molecules involved in T-cell activation in patients with AD. For one of these, leucocyte function-associated antigen-1 (LFA-1), whose natural ligand on monocytes is the intercellular adhesion molecule-1 (ICAM-1), a role in T-cell activation has been established (14). It might be that the putative involvement of

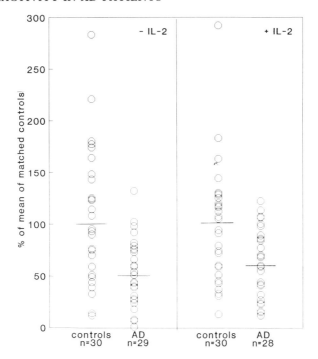

Figure 3. Decreased anti-CD2/anti-CD28 response in AD patients; for the AD patients the mean response without addition of hrIL-2 was 50% and 63% after addition of hrIL-2

cellular adhesion molecules in a declining immune system in patients with AD reflects a similar defect in the CNS of these patients. This is of particular interest in view of the homologies observed between several membrane structures in the CNS and the immune system, among which the homology between the cellular adhesion molecules ICAM-1 and NCAM-1 (neural cellular adhesion molecule) (15).

Acknowledgments

This work was funded by The Netherlands Foundation for Preventive Medicine grant 28-1802 and kindly supported by a Junior Travel Fellowship from the Alzheimer Society of Canada. We thank Dr R.A.W. van Lier for generously providing the CLB-T3/3, CLB-T11.1/1, CLB-T11.1/2 and CLB-CD28/1 monoclonal antibodies.

REFERENCES

1. Chandra V, Bharucha NE, Schoenberg BS. Neurology 1986; 36: 209–11.
2. Mölsa PK, Mattila RJ, Rinne UK. Acta Neurol Scand 1986; 74: 103–7.
3. Leonardi A, Arata L, Bino G, Caria M, Farinelli M, Parodi C, Scudeletti M, Canonica GW. J Neuroimmunol 1989; 22: 19–22.
4. Torack RM. Neurosci Lett 1986; 71: 365–9.
5. MacDonald SM, Goldstone AH, Morris JE, Morris JE, Exton-Smith AN, Callard RE. Clin Exp Immunol 1982; 49: 123–8.

6. Singh VK, Fudenberg HH, Brown III FR. Mech Ageing Dev 1987; 37: 257-64.
7. Fudenberg HH, Whitten HD, Arnaud P, Khansari N. Clin Immunol Immunopathol 1984; 32: 127-31.
8. Besedovsky HO, del Rey AE, Sorkin E. Immunol Today 1983; 4: 342-6.
9. van Duijn CM, Hofman A, Nagelkerken L. Neurosci Lett 1990; 180: 350-4.
10. McKhann G, Drachmann D, Folstein M, Katzman R, Price D, Stadlan EM. Neurology 1984; 34: 939-44.
11. Peacock JS, Colsky AS, Pinto VB. J Immunol Methods 1990; 126: 147-57.
12. van Lier RAW, Brouwer M, Rebel VI, van Noesel CJM, Aarden LA. Immunology 1989; 68: 45-50.
13. van Lier RAW, Brouwer M, Aarden LA. Eur J Immunol 1988; 18: 167-72.
14. van Noesel C, Miedema F, Brouwer M, de Rie MA, Aarden LA, van Lier RAW. Nature 1988; 333: 850-2.
15. Simmons D, Makgoba MW, Seed B. Nature 1988; 331: 624-7.

Address for correspondence:

Dr F. Nijhuis,
TNO Institute for Aging and Vascular Research,
PO Box 5815,
2280 HV Rijswijk, The Netherlands

76 Integrin Expression in Alzheimer Brain Tissue

P. L. McGEER, H. AKIYAMA AND T. KAWAMATA

The integrins are a superfamily of cell adhesion molecules which promote cell–cell and cell–matrix interactions. Each integrin has a unique α-subunit and one of three β-subunits (β-1, β-2, β-3). In brain, β-1 integrins are strongly expressed by capillary endothelial cells. The ligands for these are the capillary basement membrane proteins laminin and collagen type IV. The β-2 integrins, CD11a (LFA1), CD11b (MAC1, CR3) and CD11c (P150,95; CR4), as well as the common β-2 subunit, are constitutively expressed by all microglia. They are upregulated on reactive microglia in gray and white matter of Alzheimer's disease (AD) tissue. Ligands for the β-2 integrins are found in AD but not in normal brain parenchyma. The ligand for CD11a is ICAM-1, while those for CD11b and CD11c are complement proteins derived from C3 and C4. ICAM-1 is patchily distributed, but is associated with some plaques. Complement proteins are sharply localized to senile plaques, tangled neurons, dystrophic neurites and neuropil threads. An antibody to β-3 integrin stains only platelets. However, a polyclonal antibody against a vitronectin receptor, $\alpha_v\beta$-3, stains AD reactive microglia, while an antibody to its ligand, vitronectin, stains some senile plaques and tangled neurons.

INTRODUCTION

The integrins are a superfamily of adhesion molecules that promote interactions, principally between cells and extracellular matrix proteins, but also between different types of cells. They are highly involved in immune function, and thus play an important overall role in distinguishing self from non-self. They are α,β heterodimers, consisting of a carboxy terminal, intracellular domain, thought to be linked to the cytoskeletal apparatus, and an amino terminal, extracellular domain, often binding to an arginine-glycine-aspartate (RGD) prosthetic group on the target protein. The α chain of each integrin is unique; the β chain is common to groups of integrins which make up functional groups. So far, β-1, β-2 and β-3 subfamilies have been well described (1). However, other β units have been reported (2,3). A description of the best-known integrins and their ligands is given in Table 1.

Alzheimer's Disease: Basic Mechanisms, Diagnosis and Therapeutic Strategies
Edited by K. Iqbal, D. R. C. McLachlan, B. Winblad and H. M. Wisniewski
©1991 John Wiley & Sons Ltd

Table 1. General structure of integrins

β Subunit	α Subunit	Principal ligands
β-1	α-1 (VLA-1)	Collagen type IV
	α-2 (VLA-2)	Collagen type II
	α-3 (VLA-3)	Low affinity collagen, laminin, fibronectin
	α-4 (VLA-4)	Alternate fibronectin
	α-5 (VLA-5)	Fibronectin
	α-6 (VLA-6)	Laminin
β-2 (CD18)	α-1 (CD11a, LFA-1)	ICAM-1
	α-2 (CD11b, Mac-1)	Complement receptor CR3
	α-3 (CD11c)	Complement receptor CR4
β-3	11b (GpIIbIIIa)	Fibrinogen, von Willebrand factor
β-?	αVNR	Vitronectin

The β-1 integrins, also called very late antigens (VLAs), are made up of one of six known α units combined with the M_r 110 000 β-1 subunit (4). The β-1 integrins were originally identified on activated lymphocytes (4), but their primary role in brain appears to be in association with capillaries, where some members promote adhesion of endothelial cells to basement membrane basement proteins (5).

The β-2 family consists of three α subunits in association with the M_r 95 000 β-2 subunit. A congenital deficiency in production of the β-2 subunit exists in a disease known as leukocyte adhesion deficiency (6). Patients suffering from this disorder are vulnerable to repeated infections. This subclass of integrins seems to be exclusively associated with cells of the immune system. In brain, they occur on microglia.

The primary β-3 integrin is the protein GpIIbIIIa, where IIIa corresponds to the β-3 subunit. GpIIbIIIa is expressed on platelets (7) where it provides binding to fibrinogen, von Willebrand factor and vitronectin. It also occurs on malignant melanoma cells (8). The vitronectin receptor αVNR has been reported to be associated with β-3 (2), although it is also associated with other, as yet uncharacterized, β subunits (9–11).

In this paper, we report on the occurrence of β integrins and their principal ligands in Alzheimer and control brain tissue. The β integrins of greatest interest appear to be those associated with complement proteins. These include all β-2 integrins and the vitronectin receptor.

METHODS

Fifteen autopsied human brains obtained within 2–12 hours of death were employed in the study: 6 without neurological disorder and 9 with AD. Small blocks of brain tissue were fixed in 4% paraformaldehyde in 0.1 M phosphate buffer, pH 7.4, for 2 days and transferred to a maintenance solution of 15% sucrose in 0.1 M phosphate buffered saline (PBS), pH 7.4. Sections were cut on a freezing microtome at 30 μm thickness, collected in buffered 15% sucrose maintenance solution and stored until

Table 2. Antibodies used and structures they stain

Antigen	Antibody type	Source	Structures stained
VLA-1	Mab	M. Hemler	Capillaries
VLA-2	Mab	K. Pischel	Capillaries, trace
VLA-3	Mab	A. Albino	Negative
VLA-5	Rat Mab	C. Damsky	Negative
VLA-6	Mab	A. Sonnenberg	Negative
β-1	Rat Mab	C. Damsky	Capillaries
Collagen IV	Goat	South Biotech	Capillaries
Laminin	Rabbit	Gibco	Capillaries
CD11a (LFA-1)	Mab	Sanbio	Microglia
CD11b (Mac-1)	Mab	Sanbio	Microglia
CD11c (P150,95)	Mab	Bect-Dick	Microglia
CD18 (B-2)	Mab	Oncogene	Microglia
ICAM-1	Mab	Merck	Endothelial cells, some diffuse deposits
C3d	Mab	Quidel ⎫	⎧ Amyloid deposits, tangled
C4d	Mab	Quidel ⎭	⎩ neurons, dystrophic neurites
IIIa	Mab	Dakopatts	Platelets
αVNR	Rabbit	S. Dedhar	Microglia
C5b-9	Mab	Quidel	Dystrophic neurites, tangled neurons

Rabbit and goat are polyclonals; Mab, mouse monoclonal; Rat Mab, rat monoclonal.

used. Some unfixed brain blocks were immediately frozen on dry ice and sectioned in a cryostat. Unfixed cryostat sections were mounted on glass slides, air dried and fixed in acetone for 10 min.

The methods used for single and double immunostaining have previously been described in detail (14,15,19,20). A list of the antibodies used is given in Table 2.

RESULTS

The results of staining control and AD brain tissue for β-1 integrins is illustrated in Figure 1. In this figure, normal and AD brain cortex are shown stained for VLA-1 (α-1) and its receptor, which is collagen type IV, as well as VLA-6 (α-6) and its receptor, which is laminin. In each case, capillaries are strongly stained. Thus, endothelial cells express the β-1 integrins which then bind to basement membrane matrix proteins. No major alteration in the pattern of staining could be seen in the AD as compared to normal tissue. Other β-1 integrins that were tested, which included VLA-2, VLA-3 and VLA-5 (α-2, α-3 and α-5), showed negative or only trace staining of AD or control tissue (5).

Figure 2 illustrates staining of gray matter in control and AD angular gyrus for the β-2 integrins CD11a (LFA-1, Figures 2A and 2D), CD11b (MAC1, CR3, Figures 2B and 2E), and CD11c (P150,95, CR4, Figures 2C and 2F). In all cases, resting microglial cells were lightly to moderately stained. Microglia in AD tissue were

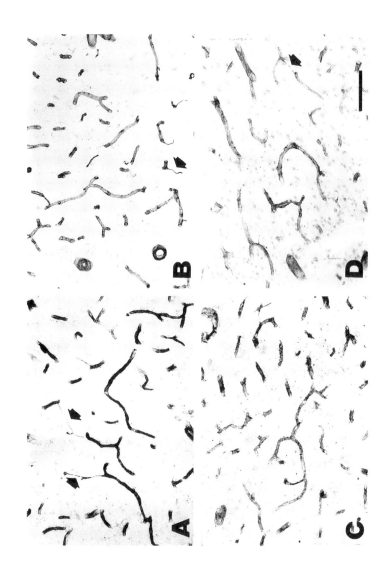

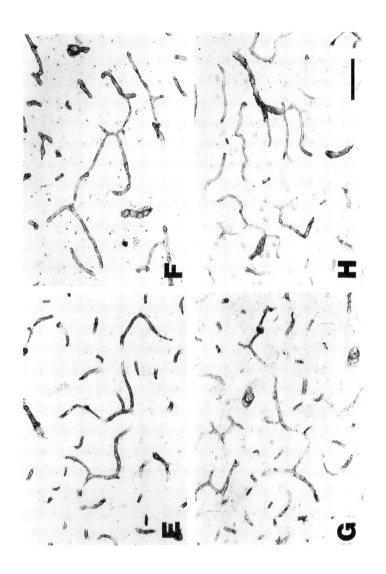

Figure 1. Staining of Alzheimer (A, B, C, D) and control (E, F, G, H) angular cortex for some β-1 integrins and their ligands. VLA-1 is shown in (A) and (E), and its ligand, collagen type IV, is shown in (B) and (F). VLA-6 is shown in (C) and (G), while its ligand, laminin, is shown in (D) and (H). In all cases, only capillaries are stained. In Alzheimer tissue, however, frequent 'strings' (arrows) are visible compared with control tissue. Scale bar 100 μm

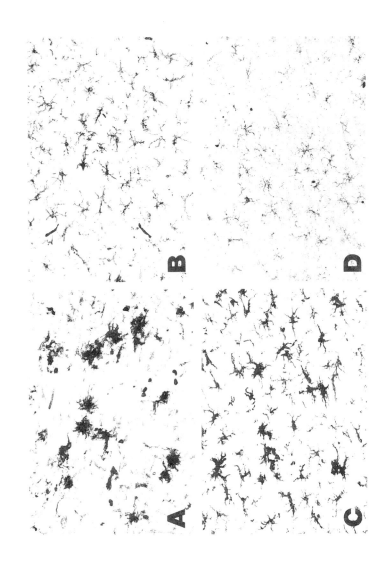

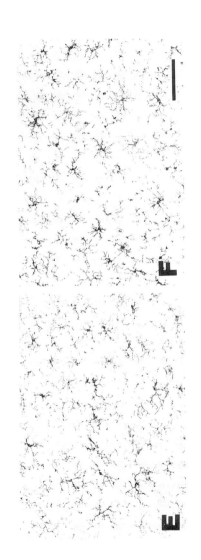

Figure 2. Staining of Alzheimer (A, B, C) and control (D, E, F) angular cortex for β-2 integrins. CD11a is shown in (A) and (D), CD11b in (B) and (E) and CD11c in (C) and (F). Microglial cells in AD and control tissue are universally stained, but notice the more intense staining for each of the β-2 integrins in Alzheimer's disease and the frequent association of microglial cells into agglomerates (same magnification as Figure 1). Scale bar 100 μm

594

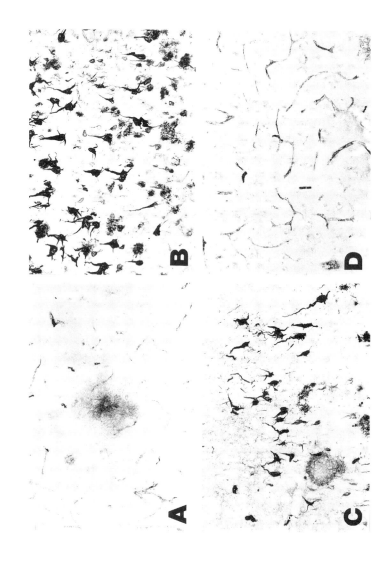

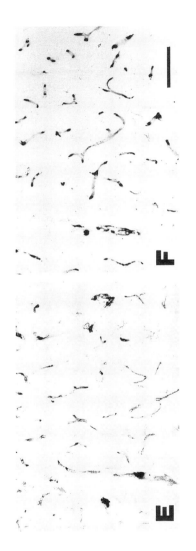

Figure 3. Staining of Alzheimer (A, B, C) and control (D, E, F) entorhinal cortex for presumed ligands of β-2 integrins or their degradation products. (A, D) staining for ICAM-1. Notice capillary staining in both AD and control tissue, but also diffuse staining of AD matrix. (B, E) staining for C3d. Plaques, tangles, neuropil threads and extracellular deposits are stained in AD tissue, while only capillaries are stained in control. (C, F) similar staining to C3d is obtained with antibodies to C4d. Scale bar 100 μm

stained much more intensely by each of the β-2 integrin antibodies than in control tissue. Moreover, a significant number of the positively staining microglial cells had altered morphology characteristic of reactive microglia (12,13). The staining was particularly intense in microglial aggregates which occur in the core of many senile plaques (14–17).

Figure 3 shows staining of AD and control brain with antibodies to proteins or fragments related to the presumed ligands for each of the β-2 integrins. These are: ICAM-1 for LFA-1; C3d, which is derived from the C3bi-like fraction of complement 3 protein which binds to CR3 (CD11b); and C4d, which is derived from a fraction of complement protein 4 which may bind to CR4 (18). Endothelial cells stain strongly for ICAM-1 in all cases (3A, 3D), but staining is also seen in patchy areas of the extracellular matrix in AD (3A). Antibodies to C3d and C4d stain senile plaques, diffuse amyloid deposits, tangled neurons, dystrophic neurites, and neuropil threads in AD tissue (3B, 3C) but only capillaries in controls (3E, 3F) (19,20). The identification of C3d and C4d in association with pathological elements in AD tissue is particularly significant since these complement proteins form chemical bonds with target tissue.

Staining of AD and control tissue with the antibody to the β-3 subunit (IIIa component of the protein GpIIbIIIa) is shown in Figure 4. It can be seen from the figure that only platelets stain positively.

A different type of staining was obtained with antibodies to the vitronectin receptor, αVNR. Staining for this protein, and its ligand, vitronectin, in AD and control tissue is shown in Figure 5. The antibody to the vitronectin receptor very weakly stains microglia in control tissue (Figure 5D), but strongly stains reactive microglia in AD

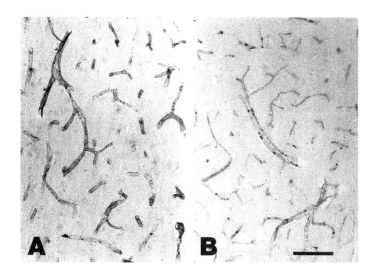

Figure 4. Staining of Alzheimer and control angular cortex for β-3 integrin (IIIa portion of GpIIbIIIa). Only scattered platelets within capillaries are visible in AD (A) and control (B) tissue. Scale bar 100 μm

tissue (Figure 5A). The antibody to vitronectin itself stains only residual plasma in the vessels of control tissue (Figure 5E), but in the cerebral cortex in AD, it associates with senile plaques and neurofibrillary tangles, as well as residual plasma (Figure 5B). This pattern of staining is highly similar to that seen with the membrane attack complex of complement (C5b-9). In control tissue, there is no staining for C5b-9 (Figure 5F), but in AD tissue, virtually the same elements are stained as with the antibodies to vitronectin (Figure 5C).

DISCUSSION

These results illustrate the very strong and universal presence of β-1 integrins on endothelial cells of brain capillaries and larger brain vessels. They provide binding between these cells and the basement membrane proteins collagen type IV and laminin. Collagen type IV and laminin constitute separate layers of the basement membrane (21). Thus, the β-1 integrins may be essential for building and maintaining the tight junctions which are characteristic of the blood–brain barrier. The other members of the β-1 family do not appear to play an important role in the maintenance of normal brain tissues.

The β-2 integrins appear to be acting as binding molecules on reactive microglia for the promotion of phagocytosis, while their ligands are acting as directional forces to guide them to the tissues targeted for destruction. ICAM-1 has a different distribution than C4d and C3d. Endothelial cells stain strongly for ICAM-1, and it may be that these cells serve as a source of this particular ligand. In AD tissue, there appear to be areas of diffusion from this source, so it may be that ICAM-1 is serving as a chemotactic agent to attract reactive microglia to the general area where phagocytosis is to take place. The complement proteins C3d and C4d, however, are tightly bound to targets marked for phagocytosis. Thus, they (or their precursors) act as opsonizing agents by promoting the direct binding of microglia to elements that are to be ingested.

Beta-3 integrin is associated with platelets and promotes their aggregation by providing binding to fibrinogen and von Willebrand factor. This does not seem to play a major role in the AD inflammatory process.

The vitronectin receptor, αVNR, is known to bind to the membrane attack complex (22). In some circumstances, it acts as an inhibitor by binding to soluble C5b-9, thus inhibiting insertion of the complex into the bilipid membrane layer. However, it has also been shown that, if the membrane attack complex does insert, vitronectin also binds to the complex (23). In this circumstance, it too may act as an opsonizing agent since, as we report here, the receptor for vitronectin is also found on reactive microglia.

These general findings in AD testify to the general inflammatory process which take splace in that disorder (14-20, 24,25). It would be anticipated that such inflammatory processes might exist simply as a requirement for the removal of damaged tissue caused by whatever primary process is responsible for AD. In addition, however, there may be autoimmune forces at work, since bystander lysis of neurons and their processes by the membrane attack complex seems to be occurring

598

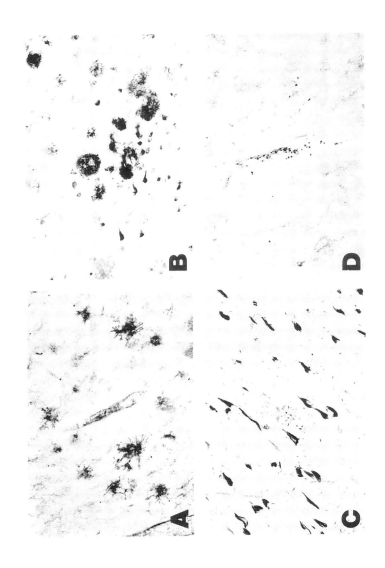

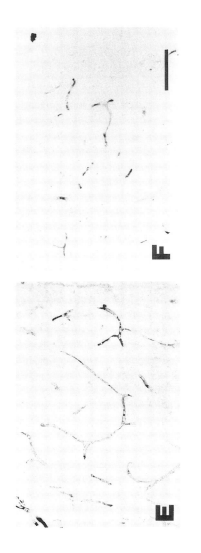

Figure 5. Staining of Alzheimer (A, B, C) and control (D, E, F) entorhinal cortex for the vitronectin receptor, αVNR (A, D), vitronectin (B, E) and the membrane attack complex, C5b-9 (C, F). Reactive microglia stained for αVNR can be seen in AD (A) but not control (D), although there is some very faint staining in white matter in the latter. Notice the strong staining of platelets in vessels. In AD tissue, plaques, tangles and neuropil threads are stained for vitronectin (B), while only residual plasma in capillaries is stained in controls (E). Extracellular amyloid staining is not obtained for the membrane attack complex, C5b-9, in AD tissue but some tangled neurons and dystrophic neurites are strongly stained (C); control tissue (F) shows positive staining only of residual plasma in capillaries. Same magnification as in Figure 1; scale bar 100 μm

(19,20). Indeed, the presence of the membrane attack complex suggests the possibility of unnecessary destruction of neurons. This, in turn, suggests that therapeutic approaches designed to block the inflammatory process might slow down the advance of AD.

To test this hypothesis, we sought statistics on the prevalence of AD amongst one class of patients who typically receive long-term anti-inflammatory therapy. These are patients suffering from rheumatoid arthritis. In keeping with the hypothesis that anti-inflammatory agents might be helpful in the treatment of AD, we found that the prevalence of AD amongst rheumatoid arthritics was several times lower than that reported for the general population (26). Several interpretations for this apparently low prevalence of AD amongst rheumatoid arthritics are possible. However, the hypothesis that this results from the treatment they have been receiving can be tested directly through clinical trials of anti-inflammatory agents in early Alzheimer's disease.

Acknowledgments

This research was supported by grants from the American Health Assistance Foundation, the Alzheimer Society of BC and the Canadian MRC, as well as donations from individual British Columbians. We thank Dr S. Dedhar, Dr Shi Gong Zhu, and Ms Joane Sunahara for discussion and technical assistance.

REFERENCES

1. Hynes RO. Cell 1987; 48: 549-54.
2. Ruoslahti E, Giancotti FG. Cancer Cells 1989; 1: 119-26.
3. Kajiji S, Tamura RN, Quaranta V. EMBO J 1989; 8: 673-80.
4. Hemler ME. Immunol Today 1988; 9: 109-11.
5. McGeer PL, Zhu SG, Dedhar S. J Neuroimmunol 1990; 26: 213-18.
6. Anderson DC, Springer TA. Ann Rev Med 1987; 38: 175-94.
7. Ginsberg MH, Loftus JC, Plow EF. Thromb Haemostasis 1988; 59: 1-6.
8. Boukerche H, Berthier-Vergnes O, Bailly M, Dore JF, Leung LLK, McGregor JL. Blood 1989; 74: 909-12.
9. Dedhar S, Gray V. J Cell Biol 1990; 110 (in press).
10. Cheresh DA, Smith JW, Cooper HM, Quaranta V. Cell 1989; 57: 59-69.
11. Freed EJ, Gailit P, van der Geer E, Ruoslahti E, Hunter T. EMBO J 19089; 8: 2955-65
12. del Rio Hortega T. Microglia. In Penfield's Cytology and cellular pathology of the nervous system, vol. 2 New York: Harper & Row 1932: 483-534.
13. Penfield W. Am J Pathol 1925; 1: 77-89.
14. Itagaki S, McGeer PL, Akiyama H, Zhu S, Selkoe D. J Neuroimmunol 1989; 24: 173-82.
15. McGeer PL, Itagaki S, Tago H, McGeer EG. Neurosci Lett 1987; 79: 195-200.
16. Rozemuller JM, Eikelenboom P, Pals ST, Stam FC. Neurosci Lett 1989; 101: 288-92.
17. Akiyama H, McGeer PL. J Neuroimmunol 1990, 30: 81-93.
18. Myones BL, Dalzell JG, Hogg N, Ross GD. J Clin Invest 1988; 82: 640-51.
19. McGeer PL, Akiyama H, Itagaki S, McGeer EG. Neurosci Lett 1989; 107: 341-6.
20. McGeer PL, Akiyama H, Itagaki S, McGeer EG. Can J Neurol Sci 1989; 16: 516-27.
21. Garbisa S, Negro A. Appl Pathol 1984; 2: 217-22.
22. Preisner KT. Blut 1989; 59: 419-31.
23. Parker CJ, Frane RN, Elstad MR. Blood 1988; 71: 86-93.

24. Luber-Narod J, Rogers J. Neurosci Lett 1988; 94: 17–22.
25. Rogers J, Luber-Narod J, Styren SD, Civin WH. Neurobiol Aging 1988; 9: 330–49.
26. McGeer PL, McGeer EG, Rogers J, Sibley J. Lancet 1990; 335: 1037.

Address for correspondence:

Dr Patrick L. McGeer,
2255 Wesbrook Mall,
University of British Columbia,
Vancouver, BC V6T 1W5,
Canada

Part XI

TREATMENT: CURRENT THERAPIES AND FUTURE DIRECTIONS/DRUG TRIALS

.

77 The Therapeutics of Alzheimer's Disease

KENNETH L. DAVIS AND VAHRAM HAROUTUNIAN

The therapeutics of Alzheimer's disease (AD) has made great advances in the last decade. Whereas ten years ago, drugs were developed with little regard to the fundamental changes in the Alzheimer's brain, a more rational scientific approach now drives the experimental therapeutics of AD. As a consequence, it can be anticipated that there will be a number of developments, both short-term and long-term, that will affect the therapy of AD in the future.

With the identification of specific cerebral neurotransmitter deficits in AD, therapeutic trials have been aimed at augmenting cerebral cholinergic neuro-transmission. Cholinesterase inhibitors may be considered the first generation of agents in the therapeutic armamentarium and include, among others, the amino acridines tetrahydroaminoacridine (THA) and its hydroxylated analog HRP-029. While these are the first available compounds, it should not be difficult to develop alternative cholinesterase inhibitors that possess very favorable brain penetrability, bioavailability, plasma stability, duration of action and few adverse events. Thus, it is a reasonable expectation that numerous safe and effective cholinesterase inhibitors can be anticipated.

However, cholinomimetic therapies for AD have met with only limited success (1). Table 1 summarizes the literature on cholinesterase treatments in AD. Not all patients respond to cholinesterase inhibitors, and even those who do, often have only a moderate response. The problem with using this purely cholinergic approach to the pharmacotherapeutics of AD is that there are numerous neurotransmitter deficits that exist in AD (14–17) that are unaffected by a cholinesterase inhibitor.

Animal models can be used to study the effects of neurotransmitter deficits. Neurotoxins such as ibotenic acid, quisqualate, NMDA, cysteamine, 6-hydroxy-dopamine and parachloroamphetamine can produce multiple neurotransmitter deficits in the rodent's brain. For example, ibotenic acid can produce lesions of the nucleus basalis of Meynert (nbM) (18–20), resulting in selective cholinergic depletions. Animals with nbM lesion show a deficit in passive avoidance learning which can be reversed with cholinomimetics. Figure 1 shows that the administration of a dose of 0.06 mg/kg of the cholinomimetic physostigmine normalizes this passive avoidance behavior (21). In order to mimic AD patients more closely, subsequent experiments have

Alzheimer's Disease: Basic Mechanisms, Diagnosis and Therapeutic Strategies
Edited by K. Iqbal, D. R. C. McLachlan, B. Winblad and H. M. Wisniewski
© 1991 John Wiley & Sons Ltd

Table 1. Clinical trials of cholinesterase inhibitors in patients with Alzheimer's disease. Reproduced with permission from Mohs and Davis (1)

Study	Patients	Drug and doses	Major findings
Beller et al (2)	4M, 4F 58-83 years	Oral physostigmine 0.5, 1.0, 2.0 mg q2h	Significant increase in word recall at 2.0-mg dose
Blackwood and Christie (3)	4M, 8F 54-68 years	Physostigmine i.v. 0.75 mg	Significant improvement in recognition memory
Caltagirone et al (4)	8 patients with onset before age 65	Oral physostigmine 1.0 mg qid	No improvement in memory or behavior
Christie et al (5)	11 patients with onset before age 65	Physostigmine i.v. 0.25, 0.375, 0.75 mg	Significant increase in picture recognition at 0.375-mg dose
Davis and Mohs (6)	8M, 2F 50-68 years	Physostigmine i.v. 0.125, 0.25, 0.5 mg	Significant increase in recognition memory at individual best dose
Kaye et al (7)	10 patients 51-71 years	Oral THA 30 mg plus 60 g lecithin	Significant increase in serial learning for least demented patients
Mohs et al (8)	8M, 4F 52-76 years	Oral physostigmine 0.5, 1.0, 1.5, 2.0 mg q2h	Cognitive improvement correlated with cortisol rise on best individual dose
Muramoto et al* (9)	3M, 3F 51-63 years	Physostigmine i.v. or s.c. 0.3 to 1.0 mg	3 of 6 showed improvement in praxis
Peters and Levin* (10)	4M, 1F 58-79 years	Physostigmine s.c. 0.005-0.015 mg/kg plus 3.6 g lecithin	4 of 5 showed significant improvement in verbal learning
Summers et al* (11)	3M, 9F 42-85 years	THA i.v. 0.25-1.5 mg/kg	Significant improvement in orientation for some patients at individual best dose
Thal et al (12)	5M, 3F 55-78 years	Oral physostigmine 0.5-2.5 mg q2h plus lecithin 10.8 g/day	Significant increase in verbal memory at individual best dose correlated with AChE inhibition of CSF
Wettstein (13)	5M, 3F 50-70 years	Oral physostigmine 1-2 mg q2h plus lecithin 18 g/day	No improvement in praxis, language orientation, or behavior

*Studies not conducted under double-blind conditions.

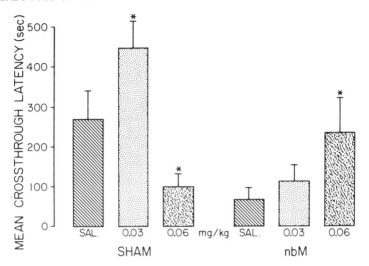

Figure 1. Effects of a 0.06 mg/kg dose of physostigmine on the 72-h retention of passive avoidance in sham-, nbM-, ANB- and nbM/ANB-lesioned rats

been designed where rats were administered a series of other neurotoxic agents that produced additional neurotransmitter deficiencies.

The first experiments focusing on other neurotransmitter deficits examined the role of somatostatin, since somatostatin depletion is relatively ubiquitous in AD patients (14,16). Cysteamine in a dose selective for somatostatin depletion was administered to nbM-lesioned rats (22–24). In these animals, physostigmine produced the same positive effect as it did in animals with only a cholinergic (nbM) lesion (21), implying that some other deficiency than somatostatin must account for the lack of effect of this cholinomimetic in AD.

The cholinergic and noradrenergic system interact dynamically. The depletion of CNS catecholamines by DSP-4 can block cholinomimetic effects such as oxotremorine-induced catalepsy (25). This raises the question of whether the loss of the intactness of the noradrenergic system would alter the memory-enhancing properties of cholinergic drugs. In one study, rats received ibotenic acid-induced lesions of the nbM and 6-hydroxydopamine-induced lesions in the ascending noradrenergic bundle (ANB) (21). Physostigmine was administered in increasing doses to controls and animals with the nucleus basalis/ANB lesion. The sham control responded to increasing doses of physostigmine with the usual inverted U-shaped curve, with maximal improvement at 0.03 mg/kg. In nucleus basalis-lesioned animals, 0.06 mg/kg would have been the ideal dose. In contrast, the animals with the double lesion showed no effect of the drug over a broad range. Therefore the efficacy of the cholinergic agent to improve performance on a passive avoidance test had been completely lost in the rats with the ANB and nucleus basalis lesions.

Since an intact noradrenergic system seems to be required for the integrity of some central cholinergic functions, the question was whether or not the positive effect of physostigmine could be restored by treating the animals with a noradrenergic

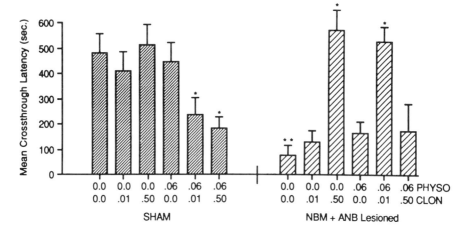

**VS SHAM P<.01
* VS 0.0 P<.03

Figure 2. Effects of post-acquisition administration of clonidine (CLON) (0, 0.01 and 0.5 mg/kg) and physostigmine (PHYSO) (0 and 0.06 mg/kg), either alone or in combination, on the 72-h retention of passive avoidance in nbM/ANB-lesioned rats. Reproduced with permission from Haroutunian et al (21)

agent such as clonidine. The results of experiments presented in Figure 2 show that cognitive deficits resulting from combined nbM/ANB lesions can be reversed by the simultaneous administration of physostigmine and the α_2-adrenergic receptor agonist, clonidine (9).

These results encourage combining cholinergic and noradrenergic agents in patients with AD. However, such studies are very complex. Cholinomimetic plus adrenergic agents could provide complex interactions on the cardiovascular system and therefore studies have proceeded with caution. Alpha-2 agonists combined with cholinesterase inhibitors are a rational first choice.

Palliative treatment, centered around the reversal of neurotransmitter deficits, will do little to alter the progression of AD. Longer-term approaches to the therapeutics of AD must therefore focus on developing drugs that may change the course of the illness. One approach would be to study the expression and processing of the precursor to amyloid, a protein that is found in large amounts in the brains of AD victims. The elucidation of the process from which β-amyloid is generated from the amyloid precursor protein may hold the promise of eventually offering a therapeutic intervention that could slow the progress of the disease.

The ultimate goal of the therapeutics of AD is to prevent this illness. Heredity seems to be a major risk factor for AD, thereby giving hope that this disease may be preventable. Fifty per cent of first-degree relatives of AD patients develop the symptoms of a progressive dementia by the late ninth decade of life. This finding is independent of the fact that only a subgroup of patients have been shown to have a locus on chromosome 21 linked to AD. Thus, there are likely to be multiple genetic foci for AD that share some common pathophysiology. Unraveling that pathophysiology and identifying a genetic loci for even a small subgroup of Alzheimer's patients offers the hope of developing a therapeutic strategy that can lead to the prevention of this most horrible human affliction.

REFERENCES

1. Mohs RC, Davis KL. In Meltzer HY (ed.) Psychopharmacology: the third generation of progress New York: Raven Press, 1987: 921-8.
2. Beller SA, Overall JE, Swann AC. Psychopharmacology 1985; 87: 147-51.
3. Blackwood DHR, Christie JE. Biol Psychiatry 1986; 21: 557-60.
4. Caltagirone C, Gainotti G, Masullo C. Int J Neurosci 1982; 16: 247-9.
5. Christie JE, Shering A, Ferguson J, Glen AIM. Br J Psychiatry 1981; 138: 46-50.
6. Davis KL, Mohs RC. Am J Psychiatry 1982; 139: 1421-4.
7. Kaye WH, Sitaram N, Weingartner H, Ebert MH, Smallberg S, Gillin JC. Biol Psychiatry 1982; 17: 275-80.
8. Mohs RC, Davis BM, Johns CA, Mathe AA, Greenwald BS, Horvath TB, Davis KL. Am J Psychiatry 1985; 142: 28-33.
9. Muramoto O, Sugishita M, Ando K. J Neurol Neurosurg Psychiatry 1984; 47: 485-91.
10. Peters BH, Levin HS. Ann Neurol 1979; 6: 219-21.
11. Summers WK, Viesselman JO, Marsh GM, Candelora K. Biol Psychiatry 1981; 16: 145-53.
12. Thal LJ, Fuld PA, Masur DM, Sharpless NS. Ann Neurol 1983; 13: 491-6.
13. Wettstein A. Ann Neurol 1983; 13: 210-12.
14. Beal MF, Mazureck MF, Tran VT, Chattha G, Bird ED, Martin JB. Science 1985; 229: 289-91.
15. Davies P, Terry RD. Neurobiol Aging 1981; 2: 9-14.
16. Davies P, Katzman R, Terry RD. Nature (Lond) 1980; 288: 279-80.
17. Perry EK. In Meltzer HY (ed.) Psychopharmacology: the third generation of progress New York: Raven Press, 1987: 887-95.
18. Haroutunian V, Kanof PD, Davis KL. Life Sci 1985; 37: 945-52.
19. Murray CL, Fibiger HC. Neuroscience 1985; 19: 1025-32.
20. Murray CL, Fibiger HC. Behav Neurosci 1986; 100: 23-32.
21. Haroutunian V, Kanof PD, Tsuboyama G, Davis KL. Brain Res 1990; 507: 261-6.
22. Brown MR, Fisher LA, Sawchenko PE et al. Regul Pept 1983; 5: 163-74.
23. Sagar SM, Landry D, Millard WJ et al. J Neurosci 1982; 2: 225-31.
24. Szabo S, Reichlin S. Endocrinology 1981; 109: 2255-7.
25. Mason ST, Fibiger HC. Nature 1979; 277: 396-7.

Address for correspondence:

Dr Kenneth L. Davis,
Department of Psychiatry,
The Mount Sinai School of Medicine,
1 Gustave Levy Place,
New York, NY 10029, USA

78 The Effect of THA on Cognitive Functions and Spectral Power EEG in Alzheimer's Disease: Preliminary Results of an Open Study

K. ALHAINEN, P. RIEKKINEN Sr, E.-L. HELKALA,
J. PARTANEN, V. LAULUMAA, K. REINIKAINEN,
H. SOININEN AND M. AIRAKSINEN

Tetrahydroaminoacridine (THA) is a reversible choline esterase (ChE) inhibitor. THA has a direct effect on muscarinic and probably on nicotinic receptors, too (1,2). Besides its ChE inhibitor effect, THA has been reported to decrease re-uptake of noradrenaline (NA) and serotonin (5-HT) in the cortex and dopamine (DA) in the striatum in rat. It also facilitates release of NA and 5-HT in cortical slices and DA in striatal slices (3). THA also blocks potassium channels in excitable cells causing elevation of intracellular K^+ concentration, which will in turn prolong duration of the action potential in hippocampal pyramidal neurons (4). This results in stimulation of neurotransmitter release.

As there is a well-documented cholinergic deficit in several brain areas of patients suffering from Alzheimer's disease (AD) (5-7), and also other neurotransmitter systems — such as noradrenergic (8,9) and serotoninergic (10) systems — are damaged during the disease process, it can be assumed that a compound like THA may have a therapeutic effect in this disorder. Because the cell damage in AD is predominantly presynaptic, the direct postsynaptic receptor binding of THA may be also favorable.

Recently, several clinical trials have been conducted using THA or physostigmine (11-19), another ChE inhibitor. Variation of treatment response in these trials may be due the proposed heterogeneity of AD patients (20). Some AD patients benefit from cholinergic treatment, but there is a problem how to discriminate responders and nonresponders for the treatment. A recent study by Soininen and co-workers (21) showed that only a proportion of AD patients had typical slowing of EEG during the disease process: in a one-year follow-up study electrical activity deteriorated in only half of the patients, while the severity of dementia progressed significantly in both groups. As recent data suggested that general disturbance and slowing of EEG in patients with AD may be related to cell loss and hypofunction of ascending cholinergic neurons from nucleus basalis of Meynert (NB) to cortex (22), it can be

Alzheimer's Disease: Basic Mechanisms, Diagnosis and Therapeutic Strategies
Edited by K. Iqbal, D. R. C. McLachlan, B. Winblad and H. M. Wisniewski
© 1991 John Wiley & Sons Ltd

assumed that spectral power analysis of EEG could be used in discrimination of responders to THA treatment.

The aim of this open treatment trial with THA was to find out effects of THA on cognitive functions and EEG of AD patients. Especially we were interested in whether the responders and the nonresponders would have a different pattern in a single-dose pharmaco-EEG and in a follow-up EEG during THA treatment.

PATIENTS AND METHODS

Patients

Eighteen patients fulfilling the NINCDS-ADRDA work group criteria (23) for probable AD were selected for the study. The study protocol was approved by the local ethics committee. The patients gave their informed consent for their participation in the study; if the patient was unable to give the consent, it was given by a near relative.

Before inclusion to the study the patients had a complete neuropsychological assessment including mini-mental state examination (MMS) (24), the cognitive subscale of Alzheimer's disease assessment scale (ADAS) (25), Buschke's selective reminding task (BSRT) (26), Heaton's visual reproductions (HVR) (27), verbal fluency test (VFT) (28), digit span (DS) (29) and trail-making test (TMT) (30). All the tests were repeated at the end of the trial.

EEG for spectral analysis was recorded on two consecutive days at the same time of the day (8–10 a.m.). A baseline EEG recording and another recording after a peroral single dose of THA 50 mg were performed. Fifteen of the AD patients did not have any medication with central nervous system (CNS) activity. Three AD patients had a low-dose neuroleptic medication, which was gradually ceased five days before the EEG recordings.

After the acute pharmaco-EEG the patients continued in an open THA treatment trial. They had a gradual 25-mg weekly increase of THA (Tacridon, Cedona) up to 100 mg/day. The maintenance dose was continued for four weeks and thereafter clinical response was evaluated and a further EEG was recorded. The main criterion for response was increase of MMS score three points or more as compared to baseline. During the trial the spouses of the patients were asked to assess questionnaires of instrumental activities of daily living (IADL) (31) and clinical global impression (CGI) (32).

EEG recording

Silver–silver chloride electrodes were applied according to the international 10/20 system. A bipolar montage was used and computerized spectral analysis was done on the following six derivations: T6-O2, T5-O1, C4-P4, C3-P3, F8-F4, F7-F3. An additional channel with an electrode placed at the outer canthus of the right eye and referred to an electrode below the right eye was used to monitor eye movements (EOG). A 16-channel Siemens Elema electroencephalograph was used with the amplifier bandwidth of 0.5–70 Hz (3 dB). In the beginning of each recording four 8.192-second, artefact-free epochs of EEG were digitized on-line at 125 samples per channel per second and stored on digital media by a Hewlett–Packard 310 (Motorola MC 68010) computer-based data acquisition system. Epochs containing eye movements or excessive muscle artefacts were identified by visual inspection of the EEG and EOG on the computer screen and were immediately eliminated. A standard paper recording was obtained in parallel at the same time. The subjects were instructed to relax and close their eyes. Verbal communication was used, if necessary, to maintain alertness of the subject. The recordings were thus made in a relaxed awake state.

Spectral analysis of EEG

For each epoch the fast Fourier transform (FFT) was computed on a series of half-overlapping sections of 4.1 seconds comprising 512 points (i.e. half of the epoch length). To reduce leakage and time truncation errors, the time-domain waveform of each section was multiplied by a cosine (Hanning) window before the FFT operation. The FFTs from a total of twelve sections were averaged to obtain the frequency spectrum of the whole EEG sample of 32.772 seconds for each site. The spectrum was further compressed into six frequency bands: delta (1.46–3.91 Hz), theta (4.15–7.32 Hz), alpha (7.57–13.92 Hz), beta (13.92–20.02 Hz), 20–30 Hz and 30–60 Hz. Two upper bands were calculated mainly for artifact estimation purposes. The absolute and relative amplitude and power in each band were calculated. The ratios of power in different bands, i.e. alpha/theta, alpha/delta, alpha/(theta + delta) and (beta + alpha)/(theta + delta) were also calculated. The relative values were computed as a percentage of the total EEG amplitude or power in the range of 1.46–20.02 Hz. Also the peak frequency as well as amplitude and power weighted mean frequencies in the ranges 4.15–13.92 Hz and 1.46–20.02 Hz were calculated.

Data analysis

The statistical analysis of the results was performed by SPSS/PC + V. 3.01 software. To find out differences between groups analysis of variance was used (ANOVA). The statistical significance of the treatment effect of THA was analysed using Student's t-test for paired samples (between baseline and the 4-week treatment). To change the EEG data into gaussian distributions the following transformations were used: for power parameters $\log(x/(1-x))$, where log is the natural logarithm and x is the absolute power in a frequency band, and for ratio parameters $\log(x)$, where x is the ratio of powers.

RESULTS

Mean age of the patients ($\pm$ SE) was 69.4 $\pm$ 1.9 years. Duration of disease was 4.3 $\pm$ 1.1 years. The AD patients had 5.2 $\pm$ 0.6 years of school education. At baseline the mean MMS score of the patients was 15.5 $\pm$ 1.4 (range 1.0–23.0).

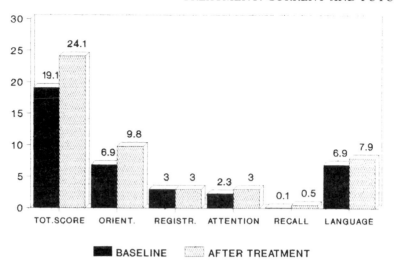

BASELINE   **AFTER TREATMENT**

Figure 1. Single items of mini-mental state examination of the responders at the baseline and after THA treatment. Significant increases are seen in total score, orientation, attention and language

After the 4-week treatment at the maintenance dose 8 patients (50%) were regarded as responders and the rest of the patients as nonresponders. Artefact-free EEG samples were obtained from 6 responders and 7 nonresponders for statistical analysis.

The mean MMS scores at the baseline and after the 4-week THA treatment were 19.1 ± 2.4 and 24.12 ± 2.4 ($P = 0.000$) for the responders, and 11.8 ± 2.0 and 12.1 ± 1.9 for the nonresponders, respectively. Single items of MMS of the responders are presented in Figure 1. A significant increase was observed in orientation ($P = 0.001$), attention ($P < 0.05$), and language ($P < 0.05$). The mean ADAS scores at the baseline and after the treatment were 16.6 ± 2.3 and 14.6 ± 2.0 ($P = 0.03$) for the responders and 44.1 ± 6.6 and 42.5 ± 6.3 for the nonresponders, respectively. Orientation improved also in ADAS significantly ($P < 0.05$). Some items of ADAS of the responders are presented in Figure 2. Total number of words recalled in BSRT increased in the responders from 13.1 ± 2.6 to 16.6 ± 3.1 ($P < 0.03$). Intrusions, words that were not a part of the wordlist, also increased in the responder group. Thus the number of correct words did not increase. Long-term retrieval of BSRT increased significantly from 3.22 ± 2.1 to 6.2 ± 2.7 ($P < 0.01$). Immediate recall of HVR increased also significantly for the responders from 1.5 ± 0.4 to 3.8 ± 0.8 ($P < 0.01$). The IADL scores of the responders improved significantly from 7.3 ± 1.3 to 9.7 ± 0.9 ($P < 0.01$). No improvement was seen in the nonresponders. During the treatment CGI improved in the responders when compared to that of nonresponders ($P < 0.01$, ANOVA). No significant changes were seen in VFT, DS and TMT.

EEG spectra of both groups at the baseline and after the treatment are presented in Figures 3 and 4 (T5-O1 derivation). In the responders there was a significant increase in the absolute alpha power ($P < 0.05$) and in the alpha-theta ratio ($P < 0.05$). Also the peak and the mean frequencies increased significantly ($P < 0.05$). No statistically

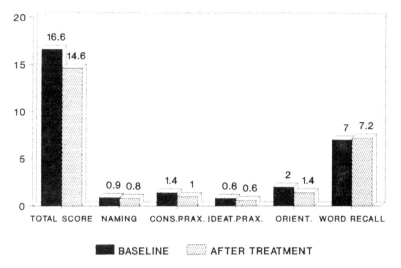

Figure 2. Some items of the cognitive subscale of Alzheimer's disease assessment scale (ADAS) at the baseline and after THA treatment (responders). Significant improvement of total score and orientation is observed (cons. prax., constructional praxis; ideat. prax., ideational praxis)

significant changes were observed in the nonresponders. In the acute single dose pharmaco-EEG there was seen a significant ($P < 0.01$) increase of the alpha-theta ratio in the responders as compared to the nonresponders, Figure 5. Relative change of the alpha-theta ratio from the baseline is presented in Figure 6.

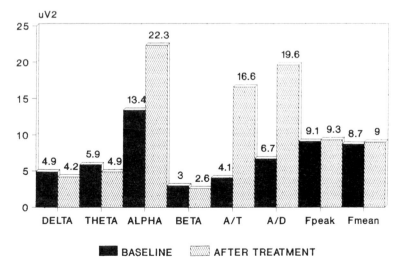

Figure 3. Spectral power EEG (derivation T5-O1) of the responders at the baseline and after THA treatment. Notice the increase of the absolute alpha power and the mean frequency. Significant changes are seen also in alpha-theta (A/T) and alpha-delta (A/D) ratios

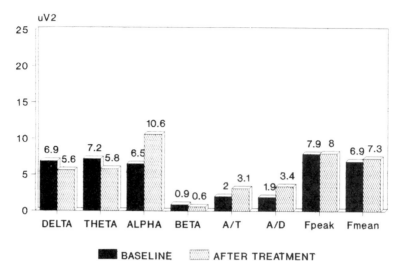

Figure 4. Spectral power EEG (T5-O1) of the nonresponders. No statistically significant changes are seen. The nonresponders had significantly less absolute alpha power at the baseline than the responders

DISCUSSION

The present study suggests that there is a subgroup of AD patients who respond to THA treatment. Our results demonstrate that orientation, attention and some cognitive functions other than memory will most likely respond to the treatment. Moreover, we observed that a single-dose pharmaco-EEG, which may reflect existing cholinergic dysfunction in AD, at least partially predicts treatment response.

It can be assumed that EEG abnormalities in AD are due to pathological function of the neocortex, at least partly caused by subcortical deafferentation, e.g. degeneration of direct cholinergic projections from the nucleus basalis and of indirect ones via the thalamus. This hypothesis is supported by the results of experimental studies showing that the cholinergic deafferentation of the cortex results in increased slow wave activity (33–35), which can at least partly be reversed by THA (Riekkinen P Jr, unpublished observations). If the subcortical deafferentation is severe enough, the possibilities for cholinergic treatment may be lost. Furthermore, in advanced cases of AD cortical damage may be too severe to allow any therapeutic effect of cholinomimetic agents. In addition, in AD isolation of the hippocampus disrupting information flow from the entorhinal cortex to the hippocampus leads to severe cognitive deficits, which may be resistant to cholinergic therapy (36). The role of monoaminergic effects of THA as regards EEG and cognition of AD patients is not determined yet.

The baseline MMS scores of the nonresponders were low and the ADAS scores high when compared to those of the responders. This might be caused by the more advanced disease process, e.g. the more profound subcortical deafferentation of the

Responders

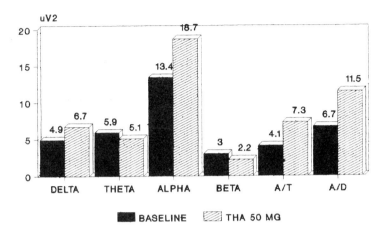

BASELINE   THA 50 MG

Nonresponders

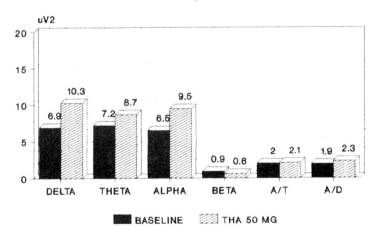

BASELINE   THA 50 MG

Figure 5. The effect of a single dose of 50 mg THA on spectral power EEG (T4-O1). The greatest change between the groups is seen in the alpha-theta (A/T) ratio, which increased significantly in the responders

nonresponders. At the baseline the nonresponders had significantly less occipito-temporal alpha power ($P < 0.05$) than the responders did. In other EEG measures the subgroups did not differ.

In the early stages of AD an increase of the theta power is seen in the EEG, while in more advanced cases there is a significant decrease of the alpha and increase of the delta power (21,37–39). The decrease in alpha-theta and alpha-delta ratios are also known to be sensitive to indicate the progress of the disease process. We observed a reverse phenomenon in AD patients responding to THA treatment both by the acute pharmaco-EEG and by follow-up EEG (after the treatment). The most sensitive

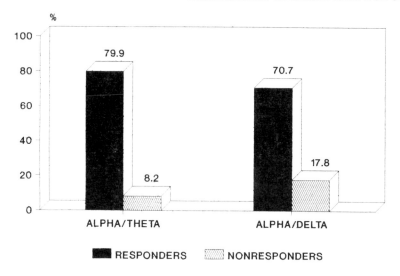

Figure 6. Relative change of alpha-theta and alpha-delta ratios from baseline in the single dose pharmaco-EEG (after 50 mg of peroral THA). There is a significant increase of the alpha-theta ratio in the responders

indicator of response was the increase of the alpha-theta ratio. The improvement of EEG in the acute pharmaco-EEG trial concomitantly with improvement of cognitive functions after the 4-week treatment in the responders suggests that this kind of approach may be useful in predicting responders to cholinergic treatment.

THA is by no means an optimal symptomatic treatment for AD. It has a nonspecific effect on arousal, which is reflected by better orientation and attention. Efficacy for memory disorder is minor. Better orientation and attention are also seen in the everyday life of the patients: the activities of daily living improve significantly in those who respond. Because THA has a potential liver toxicity (19) and only a proportion of AD patients benefit from it, it is desirable that further studies will be undertaken to develop methods for discrimination of AD patients responding to cholinergic treatment.

Acknowledgments

The present study was financially supported by the Academy of Finland, Neuroscience Center of Kuopio University, Yrjö Jahnsson Foundation, and the Research and Science Foundation of Farmos.

REFERENCES

1. Bradley D, Potter P, Potter LT. Neurosci Lett 1988; 88: 281–5.
2. Nilsson L, Adem A, Hardy J, Winblad B, Nordberg A. J Neural Transm 1987; 70: 357–68.
3. Drukarch B, Leysen JE, Stoof JC. Life Sci 1988; 42: 1011–17.
4. Stevens DR, Cotman CW. Neurosci Lett 1987; 79: 301–5.
5. Perry EK, Perry RH, Blessed G, Tomlinson BE. Lancet 1977; i: 289.

6. Perry EK, Tomlinson BE, Blessed G et al. Br Med J 1978; ii: 147-59.
7. Bartus RT, Dean RL, Beer B, Lippa AS. Science 1982; 217: 408-17.
8. Adolfsson R, Gottfries CG, Roos BE et al. Br J Psychiat 1979; 135: 216-23.
9. Reinikainen K, Paljärvi L, Huuskonen M, Soininen H, Laakso M, Riekkinen PJ. J Neurol Sci 1988; 84: 101-16.
10. Carlsson A, Adolfsson R, Aquilonius S-M et al. In Goldstein M, Calne DB, Lieberman A, Thoner MO (eds) Ergot compounds and brain function: neuroendocrine and neuropsychiatric aspects. New York: Raven Press, 1980: 295-304.
11. Summers WK, Majovski LV, Marsh GM, Tachiki K, Kling A. N Engl J Med 1986; 315: 1241-5.
12. Forsyth DR, Surmon DJ, Morgan RA, Wilcock GK. Age and Ageing 1989; 18: 223-9.
13. Gauthier S, Masson H, Gauthier L, et al. In Giacobini E, Becker R (eds) Current research in Alzheimer therapy. New York: Taylor & Francis, 1988: 237-45.
14. Fitten LJ, Perryman KM, Gross PL, Fine H, Cummins J, Marshall C. Am J Psychiat 1990; 147: 239-42.
15. Stern Y, Sano M, Mayeux R. Neurology 1988; 38: 1837-41.
16. Ashford JW, Sherman KA, Kumar V. Neurobiol Aging 1989; 10: 99-105.
17. Harrell LE, Jope RS, Falgout J et al. J Am Geriatr Soc 1990; 38: 113-22.
18. Gauthier S, Bouchard R, Lamontage A et al. N Engl J Med 1990; 322: 1272-6.
19. Chatellier G, Lacomblez L. Br Med J 1990; 300: 495-9.
20. Mayeux R, Stern Y, Spanton S. Neurology 1985; 35: 453-61.
21. Soininen H, Partanen J, Laulumaa V, Laakso M, Riekkinen PJ. Electroenceph Clin Neurophysiol 1989; 72: 290-7.
22. Riekkinen PJ, Riekkinen P Jr, Soininen H et al. In Mauer K, Riederer P, Beckman H (eds) Key topics in brain research. Alzheimer's disease: epidemiology, neuropathology, neurochemistry, clinics. New York: Springer-Verlag, 1990: 437-45.
23. McKhann G, Drachman D, Folstein M, Katzman R, Price D, Stadlan EM. Neurology 1984; 34: 939-44.
24. Folstein MF, Folstein SE, McHugh PR. J Psychiatr Res 1975; 12: 189-98.
25. Rosen WG, Mohs RC, Davis KL. Am J Psychiatry 1984; 141: 1356-64.
26. Buschke H, Fuld•PA. Neurology 1974; 24: 1019-25.
27. Wechsler D. Psychiatr Bull 1917; 2: 403-51.
28. Isaacs B, Kennie AT. Br J Psychiatry 1973; 123: 467-70.
29. Wechsler D. J Psychol 1945; 19: 87-95.
30. Reitan RM. Percept Mot Skills 1959; 8: 271.
31. Lawton MP, Brody EM. Gerontologist 1969; 9: 179-86.
32. Guy W. In ECDEW Assessment manual for psychopharmacology, Publication 76-338. Washington, DC: US Department of Health, Education and Welfare, 1976.
33. Buzsaki G, Bickford RG, Ponomareff G, Thal LJ, Mandel R, Gage FH. J Neurosci 1988; 8: 4007-26.
34. Vanderwolf CH. Int Rev Neurobiol 1988; 30: 225-340.
35. Riekkinen P Jr, Sirviö J, Riekkinen PJ. Neurosci Res 1990; 8: 12-20.
36. Hyman BT, Damasio AR, Van Hoesen GW et al. Science 1984; 225: 1168-70.
37. Coben LA, Danziger WL, Berg L. Electroenceph Clin Neurophysiol 1983; 55: 372-80.
38. Penttilä M, Partanen VJ, Soininen H, Riekkinen PJ. Electroenceph Clin Neurophysiol 1985; 60: 1-6.
39. Rae-Grant, Blume W, Lau C, Hachinski VC, Merskey H. Arch Neurol 1987; 44: 50-4.

Address for correspondence:

Professor Paavo Riekkinen,
Department of Neurology, University of Kuopio,
PO Box 6, SF-70211 Kuopio, Finland

79 THA in Alzheimer's Dementia: Clinical, Biochemical and Pharmacokinetic Findings

A. ÅHLIN, H. NYBÄCK, T. JUNTHE, G. ÖHMAN AND
I. NORDGREN

The intellectual decline of Alzheimer's disease has been shown to correlate with a reduction of markers for brain cholinergic neurotransmission. Accordingly treatment attempts have been performed using cholinomimetic drugs such as muscarinic and nicotinic receptor agonists and cholinesterase inhibitors. A clinical trial of tetrahydroaminoacridine (THA), a potent cholineesterase inhibitor, has attracted considerable interest due to the positive results obtained in Alzheimer patients (1). We recently finished a double-blind crossover study where therapeutic effects were correlated to the occurrence of side-effects and bioavailability of the drug in individual patients.

SUBJECTS AND METHODS

Fifteen patients fulfilling the DSMIII-R and NINCDS-ADRDA criteria for Alzheimer's disease were included in the study. Following a dose titration over 1–3 weeks the patients were given capsules of THA (75–150 mg/day) according to a double-blind crossover design. The treatment and placebo periods were four weeks with one week of wash-out in between. During the total of nine weeks of the study 7 of the patients were kept as inpatients, whereas 8 were seen daily as outpatients.

Treatment response was evaluated using a battery of neuropsychological tests (WAIS, WMS, Benton, Trails) and several clinical rating scales (Mini-Mental State, NOSIE-30, the Geriatric Rating Scale). Side-effects were monitored by weekly physical examinations and laboratory tests of blood and urine. The pharmacokinetics of THA were studied by comparing plasma levels of the drug following its administration by intravenous, peroral and rectal routes.

Fifteen patients entered the double-blind part of the study (Table 1). One patient was subsequently omitted from the treatment evaluation as his diagnosis was re-evaluated to pseudodementia.

Before breaking the code of the blind procedure we decided which period the patient did best as judged from tests, ward behavior and home situation. Our best guesses turned out to be no better than expected by chance (Table 2).

Alzheimer's Disease: Basic Mechanisms, Diagnosis and Therapeutic Strategies
Edited by K. Iqbal, D. R. C. McLachlan, B. Winblad and H. M. Wisniewski
© 1991 John Wiley & Sons Ltd

Table 1. Patient characteristics

No.	Sex (m/f)	Age (years)	MMS	GDS (scores)	THA dose (mg/day)
15	7/8	60 (49–72)	18 (6–30)	4 (2–5)	127 (75–150)

Figures in parentheses indicate range. MMS: Mini-Mental State; GDS: Global Deterioration Scale.

Table 2.

Patient no.	Sex	Psychol. tests	Clinical ratings	Side-effects	Best guess	Correct order
1	f	1	1	1	1	1
2	m	1	1	1	1	1
3	f	1	2	2	2	2
4	f	1	1	1	1	1
5	m	2	2	2	2	2
6	m	1	1	1	1	1
7	f	1	1	1	1	2
8	f	2	2	2	2	1
9	m	1	2	1	1	1
10	f	1	1	1	1	1
11	f	2	2	2	2	1
12	m	1	1	2	1	2
13	m	2	1	2	2	1
14	f	1	1	1	1	2
Correct		7/14	8/14	8/14	8/14	14/14

At the end of the dose titration period levels of acetylcholine (ACH), homovanillic acid (HVA) and 5-hydroxyindoleacetic acid (5-HIAA) were determined in the cerebrospinal fluid one hour following a morning dose of 50 mg of THA. The levels of these transmitters and metabolites were elevated (black columns) as compared to pretreatment levels (white columns) (Figure 1).

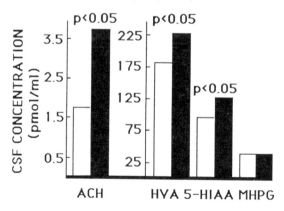

Figure 1. Levels of acetylcholine (ACH), homovanillic acid (HVA) and 5-hydroxyindoleacetic acid (5-HIAA) one hour following a morning dose of 50 mg THA (black columns) compared with pretreatment levels (white columns)

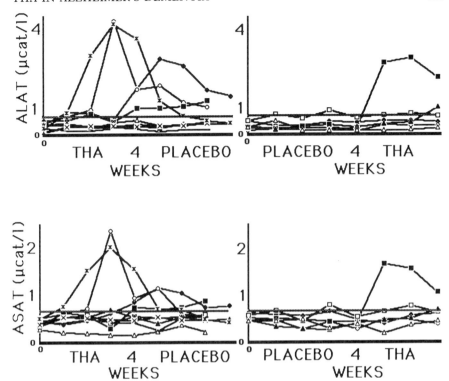

Figure 2. Liver transaminase levels during THA and placebo administration

RESULTS

The patients tolerated the drug without complaints of adverse effects and no patient had to be withdrawn from the study due to side-effects. Elevations of liver transaminases were seen on THA in about one third of the patients. These elevations returned towards normalization during the subsequent placebo period or after the end of the study. (Figure 2).

The overall clinical results were not overwhelming. However, indications of improvements of test scores were seen in patients with elevations of liver enzymes during THA treatment (Figure 3, black columns) as compared to their scores during placebo period (white columns). This tendency was not seen in the patients without elevations of liver enzymes (striped columns).

The evidence of improvement on THA was seen above all in subjects with elevated liver enzyme levels. Thus a significant correlation ($r = 0.57$, $P < 0.05$) was seen between plasma alanine aminotransferase (ALAT) and change of the clinical state according to NOSIE-30 (Figure 4).

By comparison of plasma levels of THA following intravenous and oral administrations the calculated bioavailability was found to be low and greatly varying between patients. In order to increase the bioavailability of the drug a preparation

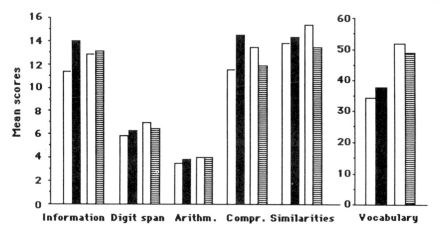

Figure 3. An improvement in Wechsler adult intelligence scale score was seen in patients with elevations of liver enzymes during THA treatment (black columns) compared to their scores during placebo periods (white columns). This tendency was not seen in patients without elevations of liver enzymes (striped columns)

of THA for rectal administration, which bypasses liver metabolism, was manufactured. The bioavailability of rectally administered THA was slightly increased as compared to the oral capsules (Table 3).

CONCLUSIONS

The clinical results of our study were less positive than expected from the study by Summers et al (1), but were more in accordance with other recently published studies with negative results, e.g. Chatellier et al (2).

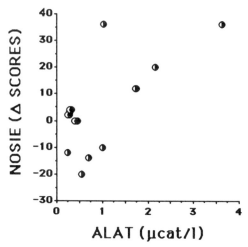

Figure 4. A significant correlation was seen between plasma alanine aminotransferase (ALAT) levels and NOSIE-30 score

Table 3

	Oral (50 mg) n = 7	Rectal (25 mg) n = 12
Half-life (hours)	2.5 (1.5–3.2)	2.7 (0.8–3.9)
Bioavailability (%)	19 (2.3–65)	34 (3–77)

The elevated levels of acetylcholine and monoamine metabolites in the CSF following THA indicates that the drug interacts with central neurotransmitter mechanisms.

Comparison of plasma levels following oral, rectal and intravenous administration revealed a great variance in the bioavailability of THA. Patients with a good bioavailability had increased liver enzyme levels and seemed to improve in measures of clinical effect.

When THA was administered per rectum the bioavailability became slightly higher compared to per os administration, probably due to a diminished first pass metabolism in the liver.

These results indicate that THA has a therapeutic potential although its liability to produce liver damage and its disadvantageous pharmacokinetic properties may constitute an obstacle for its introduction into clinical practice.

Acknowledgments

The present investigation was supported by the Swedish Medical Research Council (grants no. 21P-08891 and no. 21X-09120), the Salus Insurance Foundation and the Karolinska Institute.

REFERENCES

1. Summers WK, Majovski LV, Marsh GM, Tachiki K, Kling A. N Engl J Med 1986; 315: 1241-5.
2. Chatellier G, Lacomblez L. Br Med J 1990; 300: 495-9.

Address for correspondence:

A. Åhlin,
Department of Psychiatry and Psychology,
Karolinska Institute and Hospital,
S-10401 Stockholm, Sweden

80 New Cholinesterase Inhibitors for Treatment of Alzheimer's Disease

EZIO GIACOBINI AND ROBERT BECKER

The finding of a severely damaged and underactive cholinergic system in the brain of Alzheimer's disease (AD) patients has led to clinical trials of cholinomimetics including cholinesterase inhibitors (ChEI); for review see (1). Based on available experimental and clinical information (2), an ideal ChEI suitable for symptomatic treatment of memory and cognitive impairment should satisfy the following requirements: (a) produce a long-term acetylcholinesterase (AChE) inhibition in brain with a steady state of increased cortical acetylcholine (ACh); (b) not inhibit ACh synthesis or release in nerve endings; and (c) produce only mild side-effects at therapeutic doses. Such requirements have not been met by the ChEI used so far (1). We have studied a number of new ChEI in our laboratory (2). Based on our experimental results in animals we have proposed two new ChEI for experimental therapy of AD, heptyl-physostigmine (heptyl-Phy), a physostigmine (Phy) derivative, and metrifonate (MTF), a slow-release formulation (3-6) (Table 1).

METRIFONATE

Metrifonate is an organophosphorous ChEI with a duration of inhibition of brain cholinesterase (ChE) four times longer than Phy (3). In contrast to Phy it is not a directly acting inhibitor of ChE but requires nonenzymatic metabolism to form the active compound, dichlorvos (2,2-dichlorovinyl dimethyl phosphate) (7). Our results (3) and that of Nordgren et al. (7) show that the maximal concentration of the active drug which reaches the brain is only around 2%. This suggests a considerable blood–brain barrier for the compound or a rapid metabolism which does not allow a high concentration to build up in brain. This is a safety mechanism that, together with the slow reversibility of inhibition, explains the long-lasting effect and the minimal side-effect level. Differences in levels and metabolism in brain between MTF and Phy explain the difference in time of maximal inhibition and rate of enzyme activity recovery seen between the two drugs in the rat (3). When given acutely i.m., Phy and MTF show significant differences. First, ACh levels reach peak values in brain faster and are higher with Phy (500 μg/kg) than with MTF (80 mg/kg), even if ChE inhibition is four times longer with MTF (3,4). In humans, a dose of 10 mg/kg of oral MTF produces an 80% inhibition of plasma ChE, which

Alzheimer's Disease: Basic Mechanisms, Diagnosis and Therapeutic Strategies
Edited by K. Iqbal, D. R. C. McLachlan, B. Winblad and H. M. Wisniewski
©1991 John Wiley & Sons Ltd

Table 1. Cholinesterase inhibitors undergoing clinical trials for treatment of Alzheimer's disease

Drug	Study adminis- tration	Country	Side-effects	Number of patients	Memory effect	Cognitive effect
Physo- stigmine	oral i.v. i.c.v.	USA	nausea, antichol- inergic effects	Several hundreds	+ + +	(+) ? −
THA and THA analogues	oral oral oral oral oral oral	USA Japan Canada Sweden France Finland	hepatotoxicity, nausea, anti- cholinergic effects	300 − 52 (+lecith.) 20 67 (+lecith.) 14	? ? (+) + 0 +	? ? (+) + 0 +
Metrifonate	oral	USA	very mild	20	+	+ + +
Huperzine A	oral	China	−	Several hundreds	+	−
Heptyl- physo- stigmine	oral	Italy USA	−	10 20	− −	− −
E2020	oral	Japan	−	−	−	−

endures for 2–3 days without inducing significant side-effects (8). In AD patients, over 80% inhibition of plasma and red blood cell (RBC) ChE was achieved with only minor side-effects (7).

Becker et al. (9) performed a first study of a multiple dose trial of MTF conducted over a prolonged period of time in humans. They administered MTF to 20 patients who met NINCDS-ADRDA criteria for probable AD. Patients were given, under open conditions, single oral doses of MTF, 2.5, 5, 7.5 and 15 mg/kg per week. A statistically significant improvement in the Alzheimer disease assessment scale (ADAS) scores was observed with the 5 mg/kg weekly dose. Maximal improvement on the ADAS was associated with a mean 55.9% ($\pm$ 12.6% standard deviation) activity level of RBC AChE. Over 80% inhibition of plasma and RBC ChE was achieved with only minor side-effects (Table 1). Cholinesterase inhibition in the CSF of two patients was 37% and 47.5%, 24 hours after a second dose of 5 mg/kg per week of MTF separated by 7 days from the first dose.

ANALOGUES OF PHYSOSTIGMINE

Several authors (10–13) demonstrated the effect of a number of lipophilic derivatives of Phy characterized by reduced toxicity and reduced activity in the peripheral nervous system. The inhibitory effect (in vitro versus in vivo) of these drugs on AChE has been reported (5,14,15). One of these lipophilic derivatives, the heptyl-Phy (C8) derivative, produced an increase of ACh levels in brain and behavioral modifications suggesting a possible therapeutic use (5,12). The toxicity (LD_{50}) of

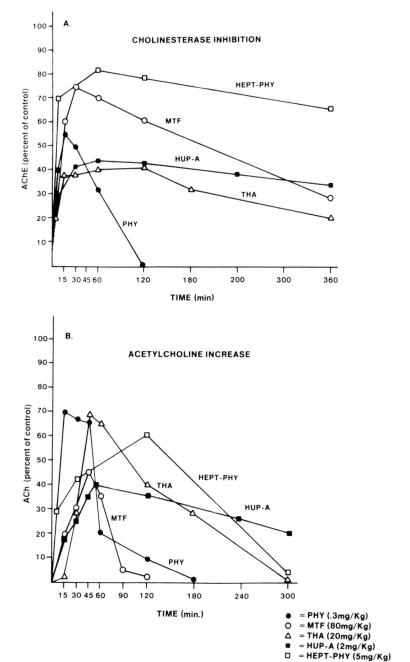

Figure 1. Comparison of the effect of five ChEI on percentage AChE inhibition (A) and ACh increase (B) in whole rat brain following a single dose of the drug administered i.m. PHY, physostigmine; MTF, metrifonate; THA, tetrahydroaminoacridine; HUP-A; Huperzine A: HEP-PHY, heptyl-physostigmine. Adapted from (18)

heptyl-Phy (35 mg/kg) is about 60 times lower than that of Phy (0.6 mg/kg) (16). At doses ranging between 0.1 mg/kg and 3.0 mg/kg, heptyl-Phy does not affect spontaneous activity in mice (16). At higher doses (3 mg/kg) its administration results in a depressant effect and in an inhibition of the activity-stimulating effect induced by scopolamine (1 mg/kg). Passive avoidance (step-through latencies) of mice injected post-trial with different doses of heptyl-Phy is significantly modified (10). Longer step-through latencies are present 24 h and 48 h following the post-trial injection of heptyl-Phy, indicating that the drug acts on consolidation mechanisms, by facilitating memory.

In human volunteers, 40 mg of a single oral dose of heptyl-Phy produced 40% plasma butyrylcholinesterase (BuChE) inhibition at 1 h and 17.7% at 6 h (Table 1). Red blood cell AChE was 46% and 30% inhibited at the same time points (17). No side-effects were recorded. The results suggest that heptyl-Phy produces different duration of effects on AChE and BuChE. This could explain the low level of peripheral side-effects mainly mediated by BuChE inhibition seen with this compound, as compared to Phy and tetrahydroaminoacridine (THA).

COMPARISON OF CHOLINESTERASE INHIBITOR EFFECTS AND GENERAL CONCLUSIONS

Table 1 is an overview of the clinical trials presently in progress with ChEIs in various countries.

Figure 1 compares the effect of five ChEI on AChE inhibition and ACh levels in rat brain following i.m. administration of one single dose of the drug. The dosage has been selected according to the criteria of assuring a maximal increase in ACh levels in brain with high ChE activity inhibition at a zero mortality level. Figure 1A shows that with MTF and heptyl-Phy it is possible to reach peak levels of 70–80% AChE inhibition within 30–60 min from the administration. Huperzine A and THA produce lower peak levels of inhibition (49%); however, this is maintained for almost 6 hours with HUP-A and 3 hours with THA. Physostigmine produces a rapid (15 min) peak of 55% inhibition but this effect is over within 2 hours.

The effect on brain ACh levels is also markedly different for the different drugs (Figure 1B). High ACh increases (70%) are obtained following both Phy and THA administration; however, particularly with Phy, this effect is short-lasting (1 h). Heptyl-physostigmine shows the most prolonged effect on brain ACh levels with a peak at 2 hours. The effect of MTF instead is rather short-lasting (1.5 h).

These results reveal major differences in biochemical effects on rat brain including extent and duration of ChE inhibition, inhibition of ACh release and increase in levels of ACh. Side-effects are also markedly different in time of appearance, duration and severity. These findings suggest significant differences in mechanisms of action of various ChE inhibitors with potential clinical implications for a future symptomatic therapy of AD patients.

REFERENCES

1. Becker R, Giacobini E. Drug Devel Res 1988; 12: 163-95.
2. Giacobini E, Becker R. In Miner GD, Richter RW, Blass JP, Valentine JL, Winters-Miner LA (eds) Familial Alzheimer's disease molecular genetics and clinical perspectives. New York: Marcel Dekker, 1989: 223-68.
3. Hallak M, Giacobini E. Neuropharmacology 1987; 26: 521-30.
4. Hallak M, Giacobini E. Neuropharmacology 1989; 28: 199-206.
5. DeSarno P, Pomponi M, Giacobini E, Tang XC, Williams E. Neurochem Res 1989; 14: 971-7.
6. Tang XC, DeSarno P, Sugaya K, Giacobini E. J Neurosci Res 1989; 24: 276-85.
7. Nordgren I, Bergstrom M, Holmstedt B, Sandoz M. Arch Toxicol 1978; 41: 31-41.
8. Nordgren I, Holmstedt B, Bengtsson E, Finkel Y. Am J Trop Med Hyg 1980; 29: 426-30.
9. Becker RE, Colliver J, Elble R, Feldman E, Giacobini E, Kumar V, Markwell S, Moriearty P, Parks R, Shillcutt SD, Unni L, Vicari S, Womack C, Zec RF. Drug Devel Res 1990; 19: 425-34.
10. Oliverio A, Castellano C, Iacopino C, Pavone F, Brufani M, Marta M, Pomponi M. In Biggio G, Spano PF, Toffano G, Gessa GL (eds) Modulation of central and peripheral transmitter function, Fidia Research Series, Symposia in neuroscience III. Padova: Liviana Press, 1986: 305-9.
11. Pavone F, Castellano C, Oliverio A, Brufani M, Marta M, Pomponi M. 2nd Congresso della Società Italiana di Neuroscienze, 1986: 424.
12. Brufani M, Castellani C, Marta M, Oliverio A, Pagella PG, Pavone F, Pomponi M. Pharmacol Biochem Behav 1987; 26: 625-9.
13. Castellano C, Oliverio A, Jacopino C, Pavone F, Brufani M, Marta M, Pomponi M. In Trends in the pharmacology of neurotransmission. Sofia: Bulgarian Academy of Sciences, 1987: 57-64.
14. Marta M, Pomponi M. Acta Med Rom 1987; 25: 433-7.
15. Marta M, Pomponi M. Biomed Biochem Acta 1988; 47: 285-8.
16. Marta M, Castellani C, Oliverio A, Pavone F, Pagella PG, Brufani M, Pomponi M. Life Sci 1988; 43: 1921-8.
17. Unni L, Becker RE, Hutt V, Bruno P. Intl Congr Pharmacol (Amsterdam) 1990; 183: 536.
18. Giacobini E, Becker R, McIlhany M, Kumar V. In Giacobini E, Becker R (eds) Current research in Alzheimer therapy. New York: Taylor & Francis, 1988: 113-22.

Address for correspondence:

Dr Ezio Giacobini,
Department of Pharmacology,
Southern Illinois University,
School of Medicine,
Springfield, IL 62794-9230, USA

81 Phosphatidylserine Restores Spatial Memory and Morphofunctional Cholinergic Markers in Basal Forebrain Nuclei of Aged Rats

A. MORANDI, D. GUIDOLIN, P. POLATO, A. ZANOTTI
AND M.G. NUNZI

Direct and indirect evidence indicates that the basal forebrain cholinergic nuclei, hippocampal formation and the connection between them are crucial structures in learning and memory functions (1,2). In fact, lesion-induced (3) or age-related (4) degeneration of these brain areas results in a severe impairment of cognitive function. In Alzheimer's disease (AD), degeneration of the central cholinergic system, and especially of basal forebrain neurons, is one of the most consistent pathologic features (5,6) and correlates with the degree of cognitive impairment (7–9). Thus, therapeutic intervention in AD and cognitive age-related disorders has been focused on either a correction of the cholinergic function or the prevention of further damage of the affected cell population.

Aged rodents with impairment in memory and learning show dysfunction of the basal forebrain cholinergic system (10,11). In particular, evidence has been provided that age-associated decline in spatial memory correlates with degenerative changes in forebrain cholinergic nuclei (12). We used this model to study the morpho-functional relationship between forebrain cholinergic cell groups and spatial memory and to evaluate the effects of chronic oral phosphatidylserine (BC-PS) administration on age-related changes. BC-PS, a pharmacologically active phospholipid (13), normalizes acetylcholine release from the cerebral cortex of aged rats (14) and increases their learning and memory functions (15). Moreover, BC-PS treatment is effective in improving cognitive functions of moderately impaired elderly humans (16) and Alzheimer's patients (17).

Young adult (4 months) and aged (22–24 months) male Sprague–Dawley rats were tested for spatial memory in the Morris water maze, as previously described (15). Aged rats, selected as memory-impaired in the screening test, were equitably allocated into control and treatment groups. All groups of animals were retested 7 and 12 weeks after the beginning of BC-PS treatment, which lasted till the end of behavioural testing (50 mg/kg daily, suspended in the drinking water). Animals were then

Alzheimer's Disease: Basic Mechanisms, Diagnosis and Therapeutic Strategies
Edited by K. Iqbal, D. R. C. McLachlan, B. Winblad and H. M. Wisniewski
©1991 John Wiley & Sons Ltd

perfused with a mixture of aldehydes and the brains processed for choline acetyltransferase (ChAT) and nerve growth factor receptor (NGFr) immunocyto-chemistry, according to the peroxidase–antiperoxidase method. Morphometric analysis was performed by means of a computerized image analysis system. ChAT optical density was measured in single neurons by photometric analysis.

SPATIAL MEMORY

In agreement with previous results (15), a subpopulation of aged rats showed impairment in the acquisition of the spatial task, relative to the young and aged nonimpaired groups, as indicated by mean escape latencies in the screening test (Figure 1). Whereas performance of aged impaired control rats did not change across behavioural testing, BC-PS-treated rats significantly improved their performance at both retesting weeks, compared to the screening test (Figure 1).

SEPTAL–HIPPOCAMPAL COMPLEX: IMAGE ANALYSIS

The septal complex (medial septum and Broca's diagonal band) provides the largest source of hippocampal cholinergic innervation (18). Recently, NGF has been shown to act as a neurotrophic factor for basal forebrain cholinergic neurons (19). Therefore, a dysfunction of the NGF–NGF receptor system would cause the retrograde degeneration of forebrain cholinergic nuclei. Thus, age-dependent decrement in NGF receptors may be crucial in deterioration of cholinergic neurons and determine the loss of cognitive ability. To evaluate the involvement of basal forebrain cholinergic

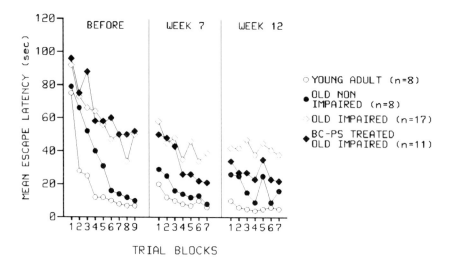

Figure 1. Effect of chronic BC-PS administration on the performance of old impaired rats in the Morris water maze ('before', screening test; 'week 7' 'week 12', after 7 and 12 weeks of BC-PS administration respectively)

neurons in age-related memory impairment and the therapeutic effects of BC-PS, we used a monoclonal antibody to ChAT and an immunoaffinity-purified antibody to NGFr.

ChAT

In the aged group, morphometric analysis of cholinergic neurons displayed a significant decrease in the area covered by the immunoreactive profiles (-31.7%; $P<0.05$) and soma size (-25%; $P<0.05$), compared to young controls. Moreover, preliminary results indicate a decrement in the optical density of the immunoreaction end product, suggesting a decline in ChAT neuronal content. However, aged memory-impaired rats were significantly different from the aged nonimpaired group, with respect to ChAT-positive cell number (-24%; $P<0.01$). No significant differences in any of the above-mentioned parameters were observed between young controls and BC-PS treated aged impaired rats.

NGFr

The cholinergic neuronal population of the septal complex of aged impaired animals showed a marked loss of NGFr reactivity ($P<0.01$), compared to young controls, while aged nonimpaired rats showed only a slight, not significant decrease. On the contrary, aged impaired rats chronically treated with BC-PS did not show any significant difference in NGFr immunoreactivity with respect to young controls (Figure 2).

DISCUSSION

This study provides evidence that degenerative changes of basal forebrain cholinergic neurons, as evidenced by loss of NGF and ChAT immunoreactivity, occur in aged rats with spatial memory impairment. NGF acts as a neurotrophic factor for forebrain cholinergic neurons (19). The decrease of NGFr density may thus be causal of atrophic changes in NGF responsive neurons and result in cognitive impairment associated with aging.

Moreover, the parallel decline of both ChAT and NGFr in aged memory-impaired animals further confirms the relation between trophic action of NGF and cholinergic function and the physiological role of NGF on forebrain cholinergic neurons (20).

Chronic treatment with BC-PS had a global effect: it restored morphological and functional parameters of cholinergic neurons, including NGF receptor density, while improving spatial memory. These data are consistent with previous results indicating that long-term BC-PS treatment prevents, in old rats, the decrement in hippocampal interneuronal connectivity (21) and restores ACh release and content in the cerebral cortex (14,22).

During aging, membrane lipid composition undergoes many changes, such as reduction in phospholipid synthesis (23) and increase in cholesterol/phospholipid ratio (24).

636

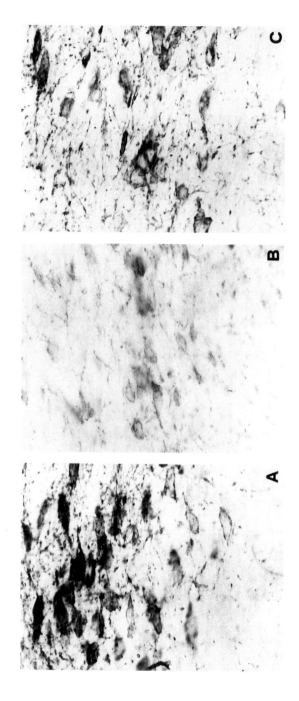

Figure 2. NGF receptor immunoreactivity of diagonal band. (A) young rat; (B) old impaired rat; (C) old impaired rat+BC-PS

These changes may play a key role in central nervous system (CNS) function, since alterations in cholesterol and phospholipids of CNS membranes dramatically affect a variety of receptor molecules (25). It has been previously demonstrated that BC-PS reduces the cholesterol/phospholipid ratio in aged CNS membranes (24). Moreover, lysophosphatidylserine, the active metabolite of PS, stimulates the incorporation of polyunsaturated fatty acids into membrane phospholipids (26). Furthermore, in aged rodents, chronic treatment with BC-PS has been reported to restore the density of M-cholinoreceptors (27) and to enhance membrane-bound enzymatic activities involved in membrane excitability (24) and signal transduction (28).

Restoration of NGFr immunoreactivity in the aging brain further highlights the beneficial effect of BC-PS on membrane structural properties and function and may explain BC-PS effects on trophic degree of cholinergic neurons and interneuronal connectivity. In particular, restoration of NGFr may ensure trophic support to cholinergic neurons in aged brain, by enhancing their responsiveness to NGF.

Altogether these data may represent the morphofunctional basis of the observed improvement in learning and memory function. This experimental evidence supports BC-PS as pharmacological treatment on cognitive dysfunction in old people.

REFERENCES

1. Hepler DJ, Olton DS, Wenk GL, Coyle JT. J Neurosci 1985; 5: 866-73.
2. Salomone JD. Trends Neurosci 1986; 9: 256-8.
3. Olton DS, Walker JA, Gage FH. Brain Res 1978; 139: 295-308.
4. Ingram DK, London ED, Goodrick CL. Neurobiol Aging 1981; 2: 41-7.
5. Whitehouse PJ, Price DL, Struble RG, Clark AW, Coyle JT, De Long MR. 1982; 215: 1237-9.
6. Pearson RCA, Sofroniew MV, Cuello AC, Powell TPS, Eckenstein R, Eiszi M, Wilcock GK. Brain Res 1983; 289: 375-9.
7. Jacobs RW, Butcher LL. In Scheibel AB, Wechsler AF (eds) The biological substrates of Alzheimer's disease. New York: Academic Press, 1986: 86-100.
8. Perry EK, Tomlinson BE, Blessed G, Bergman K, Gibson PH, Perry PH. Br Med J 1978; 2: 1457-9.
9. Perry EK, Blessed G, Tomlinson BE. Neurobiol Aging 1981; 2: 251-6.
10. Hornberger JC, Buell SJ, Flood DG, McNeill TH, Coleman PD. Neurobiol Aging 1985; 6: 269-75.
11. Biegon A, Greenberger V, Segal M. Neurobiol Aging 1986; 7: 215-17.
12. Fischer W, Gage FH, Bjorklund A. Eur J Neurosci 1989; 1: 34-45.
13. Toffano G, Bruni A. Pharmacol Res Comm 1980; 12: 829-45.
14. Pedata F, Giovannelli L, Spignoli G, Giovannini MG, Pepeu G. Neurobiol Aging 1985; 6: 337-9.
15. Zanotti A, Valzelli L, Toffano G. Psychopharm 1989; 99: 316-21.
16. Villardita C, Grioli S, Salmeri G, Nicoletti F, Pennisi G. Clin Tri J 1987; 24: 84-93.
17. Palmieri G, Palmieri R, Inzoli MR, Lombardi G, Sottini C, Tavolato B, Giometto B. Clin Tri J 1987; 24: 73-83.
18. Wenk H, Bigl V, Meyer V. Brain Res Rev 1980; 2: 295-316.
19. Hefti F. J Neurosci 1986; 6: 2155-62.
20. Vantini G, Schiavo N, Di Martino A, Polato P, Triban C, Callegaro L, Toffano G, Leon A. Neuron 1989; 3: 267-73.

21. Nunzi MG, Milan F, Guidolin D, Toffano G. Neurobiol Aging 1987; 8: 501-10.
22. Vannucchi MG, Pepeu G. Neurobiol Aging 1987; 8: 403-7.
23. Porcellati G, Gaiti A, Brunetti M. In Giacomini E, Filogamo G, Giacobini G, Vernadakis A (eds) The aging brain: cellular and molecular mechanisms of aging in the nervous system. New York: Raven Press, 1982: 77-86.
24. Calderini G, Aporti F, Bellini F, Bonetti AC, Rubini R, Teolato S, Xu C, Zanotti A, Toffano G. In Horrocks LA, Kanfer JN (eds) Phospholipids in the nervous system. New York: Raven Press 1987: 11-19.
25. Schroeder F. Neurobiol Aging 1984; 5: 323-33.
26. Sbashing-Agler M, Pullarkat RK. Neurochem Int 1985; 7: 295-300.
27. Amaducci L, SMID Group. Psychopharm Bull 1988; 24: 130-4.
28. Muller WE, Gelbmann MC, Pilch H. In Krieglstein J (ed.) Pharmacology of cerebral ischemia. Stuttgart: WVG 1989: 353-8.

Address for correspondence:

Dr A. Morandi,
Fidia Research Laboratories,
Via Ponte della Fabbrica 3/A,
35031 Abano Terme (PD),
Italy

82 Basic Fibroblast Growth Factor Protects Septal–Hippocampal Cholinergic Neurons Against Lesions Induced by AF64A

PAMELA E. POTTER AND RICHARD S. MORRISON

Nerve growth factor (NGF) prevents both the loss of septal–hippocampal cholinergic neurons induced by transection of the fimbria–fornix pathway (1,2), and the reduction in cortical choline acetyltransferase (ChAT) activity caused by injection of the excitatory neurotoxin ibotenic acid into the nucleus basalis (3). This has led to the hypothesis that NGF might be useful in treating Alzheimer's disease (4). Basic fibroblast growth factor (bFGF), originally identified in brain and pituitary extracts, was recently shown to have neuronotrophic activity for CNS neurons (5,6). Administration of bFGF also prevents degeneration of cholinergic neurons after fimbria–fornix lesions, and is even effective when administered subsequent to the lesion (7,8). Recently, two other growth factors, epidermal growth factor (EGF) and transforming growth factor α (TGF-α) have been shown to promote neuronal survival in vitro (9). Our preliminary studies suggest that EGF, like NGF and bFGF, protects neurons after fimbria–fornix lesion (Potter and Morrison, unpublished data). With the identification of these different trophic factors, it would appear that neurons may require multiple trophic factors for survival.

In addition to establishing the range of neuronal subtypes supported by specific trophic factors, it is of interest to determine whether these factors are active during growth and development and/or following various types of lesions to the nervous system. It is possible that not all growth factors will be protective against all types of lesions. For example, Johnson et al (10) found that a single application of NGF did not prevent loss of hippocampal ChAT activity following treatment with the cholinergic neurotoxin ethylcholine mustard aziridinium (AF64A). NGF also did not protect neurons in culture from the effects of AF64A (11), suggesting either that the neurons affected by AF64A did not have NGF receptors, or that NGF was incapable of protecting against the type of injury produced by AF64A. In this study, we have compared the effects of chronic infusion of NGF, bFGF, EGF, and TGF-α on loss of hippocampal ChAT activity induced by AF64A, in order to determine whether multiple trophic factors are capable of protecting cholinergic neurons against this type of lesion.

Alzheimer's Disease: Basic Mechanisms, Diagnosis and Therapeutic Strategies
Edited by K. Iqbal, D. R. C. McLachlan, B. Winblad and H. M. Wisniewski
©1991 John Wiley & Sons Ltd

METHODS

Preparation and administration of AF64A and growth factors

A 1 mM AF64A solution was prepared from acetylethylcholine mustard HCl (purchased from RBI, Natick, MA) as described by Fisher et al (12). Male Sprague-Dawley rats weighing approximately 200 grams were anesthetized with sodium pentobarbital, 50 mg/kg i.p., and placed into a stereotaxic holder. Two nmol of AF64A in 2 μl, or 2 μl of vehicle for sham operated animals, were infused at a rate of 0.5 μl/min through 26-gauge cannulae into each lateral ventricle at coordinates (from Bregma): AP-0.6; L$\pm$1.3; V-3.7. The cannulae were removed 5 min after AF64A infusion, then a 26-gauge Teflon cannula was inserted into the right lateral ventricle at the same coordinates, fixed into place with dental cement, and attached to an Alzet mini-pump containing 200 μl of either a growth factor (500 ng/ml) or vehicle (phosphate buffered saline, pH 7.4, with 1% heterologous rat serum). The pumps were pre-incubated at 37 °C for 4 hours in saline, so that they immediately began to deliver a flow of 0.5 μl/h. The mini-pumps were placed into a small pouch of skin at the back of the neck.

Measurement of ChAT activity

ChAT activity was determined by the radioenzymatic assay of Fonnum (13), in which the transfer of the [^{3}H]acetyl group from acetyl CoA to choline is measured. Data are expressed as pmol acetylcholine formed per minute per mg tissue, with the exception of septum, in which data are expressed as nmol per minute per mg protein. Protein was determined by the method of Lowry et al (14).

RESULTS

The results of these experiments are shown in Tables 1-3. The growth factors alone had no effect in any of the three nonlesioned tissues examined, suggesting that they do not by themselves cause any increase in ChAT activity. As shown previously (15), AF64A treatment decreased ChAT activity only in the hippocampus, where

Table 1. Effect of growth factors on hippocampal ChAT activity

	ChAT activity (pmol/min.mg tissue)		
	Sham	AF64A	% Control
Control	96.5 ± 3.9 (10)	45.9 ± 3.2 (12)	48
bFGF	87.2 ± 3.1 (10)	67.8 ± 5.9 (11)*	78
TGF-α	89.2 ± 4.9 (10)	57.1 ± 3.5 (15)	64
EGF	86.7 ± 5.5 (8)	51.8 ± 5.4 (6)	60
NGF	N.D.	61.9 ± 5.4 (6)	68

*$P < 0.05$ compared with untreated value, ANOVA.
Percentage of control for NGF was based on a combined control value from all samples.
ND, not determined.

Table 2. Effect of growth factors on septal ChAT activity

	ChAT activity (nmol/min.mg protein)		
	Sham	AF64A	% Control
Control	5.20±0.59 (10)	4.93±0.46 (7)	95
bFGF	5.24±1.16 (5)	4.42±0.60 (7)	84
TGF-α	4.37±0.55 (8)	4.25±0.29 (9)	97
EGF	4.33±0.52 (4)	6.23±0.46 (8)	143
NGF	N.D.	5.79±0.76 (6)	111

Table 3. Effect of growth factors on cortical ChAT activity

	ChAT activity (pmol/min.mg tissue)	
	Sham	AF64A
Control	56.1±1.2 (8)	50.6±2.8 (8)
bFGF	45.3±1.6 (8)	54.5±2.1 (8)
TGF-α	50.3±1.7 (8)	50.7±1.7 (8)
EGF	48.9±2.9 (8)	46.7±2.9 (8)

it was reduced to 48% of the control value. Basic FGF significantly ($P < 0.01$, ANOVA) attenuated this decrease in ChAT activity, to 78% of control. The other three factors, NGF, TGF-α and EGF, had no statistically significant effects, although NGF and TGF-α did bring ChAT activity back up to 64–68% of control.

DISCUSSION

The results described here indicate that the effects of the cholinergic neurotoxin AF64A can be partially reversed by a variety of growth factors. Basic FGF was the most effective of the growth factors tested, and caused a significant attenuation or reversal of the effects of AF64A treatment. Surprisingly, NGF also had some effect, in contrast to a previous report (10). In the present study, NGF was administered chronically, as opposed to a single injection, which may explain why an effect was seen. The other two factors, TGF-α and EGF, were slightly less effective than NGF, although there was no significant difference between the effects of all three of these factors. The observation that ChAT activity could not be fully restored by a single growth factor suggests that subpopulations of cholinergic neurons may vary in their requirements for trophic factors. Another possibility is that the location of growth factor receptors on the neurons may modify that neuron's response to trophic factors following injury. Both bFGF and NGF are extremely effective at protecting septal–hippocampal cholinergic neurons against the effects of fimbria-fornix transection, and EGF, which was the least effective growth factor in this study, also protected cells against this lesion (Potter and Morrison, unpublished observations). It seems likely that the receptors that would be effective in this paradigm would be located on the cell body in the septum, in order to promote regrowth of the neuron and maintenance of the cell body after axotomy. However, these receptors may not effectively protect against the actions of a toxin like AF64A, which, although its mechanism of action is still somewhat obscure, appears to affect cholinergic cells through an interaction with the high-affinity choline transport site located at the nerve terminal (16). Instead, a compound with receptors located near the nerve terminal might be more effective against this type of lesion. It remains to be seen whether the growth factors act synergistically, proving more effective in combination than singly. Treatment with selected combinations of growth factors may ultimately prove effective at restoring function in a variety of neurodegenerative diseases such as Alzheimer's disease.

REFERENCES

1. Hefti F. J Neurosci 1986; 6: 2155-62.
2. Montero CN, Hefti F. J Neurosci 1988; 8: 2986-99.
3. Haroutunian V, Kanof PD, Davis KL. Brain Res 1986; 386: 397-9.
4. Hefti F, Weiner WJ. Ann Neurol 1986; 20: 275-81.
5. Morrison RS, Sharma A, deVellis J, Bradshaw R. Proc Natl Acad Sci USA 1986; 83: 7537-41.
6. Walicke P, Cowan WM, Ueno N, Baird A, Guillemin R. Proc Natl Acad Sci USA 1986; 83: 3012-16.
7. Anderson KJ, Cam D, Lee S, Cotman CW. Nature 1988; 332: 360-1.
8. Otto D, Frothscher M, Unsicker K. J Neurosci Res 1989; 22: 83-91.
9. Morrison RS, Kornblum HI, Leslie FM, Bradshaw W. Science 1987; 238: 72-5.
10. Johnson GVW, Simonatao M, Jope RS. Neurochem Res 1988; 13: 685-92.
11. Atterwill CK, Collins P, Meakin J, Pillar AM, Prince AK. Biochem Pharmacol 1989; 38: 1631-8.
12. Fisher A, Mantione CR, Abraham DJ, Hanin I. J Pharmacol Exp Ther 1982; 222: 140-5.
13. Fonnum F. Biochem J 1969; 115: 465-72.
14. Lowry OH, Rosebrough NJ, Farr AL, Randall RJ. J Biol Chem 1951; 193: 265-75.
15. Potter PE, Hársing LG Jr, Kakuscka I, Gaál Gy, Vizi ES. Neurochem Int 1985; 7: 1047-53.
16. Potter PE, Tedford C, Kindel G, Hanin I. Brain Res 1989; 487: 238-44.

Address for correspondence:

Dr Pamela E. Potter,
Department of Anesthesiology,
Albert Einstein College of Medicine,
Montefiore Medical Centre,
111 East 210th Street,
Bronx, NY 10467, USA

83 Therapeutic Potential of Thyrotropin-Releasing Hormone and Lecithin Co-administration in Alzheimer's Disease

T. H. LAMPE, J. NORRIS, S.C. RISSE, E. OWEN-WILLIAMS
AND T. KEENAN

Thyrotropin-releasing hormone (TRH) is a small neuropeptide which is widely distributed throughout the mammalian central nervous system (CNS) and which is also available in synthetic drug form. Pharmacologic actions of TRH include potent facilitatory effects on CNS cholinergic transmission (1–4). A progressive deterioration of major CNS cholinergic pathways is considered to play an important role in the pathogenesis of Alzheimer's disease (AD), and TRH or TRH analogues have been suggested as potential therapeutic agents in this disorder (3–10). Recent studies have delineated apparent salutary cognitive effects of both TRH and a TRH analogue, respectively, in human (8) and animal (9) experimental models of AD. One recent report is the first to describe the apparent safety of a 'high-dose' TRH infusion in probable AD patients (10).

Lecithin (phosphatidylcholine) is a dietary precursor for neuronal synthesis of acetylcholine. The adjunctive co-administration of oral lecithin with TRH or TRH analogues for posited therapeutic purposes in AD is supported by several theoretical considerations: co-administration of lecithin may exert 'protective' effects and/or beneficial synergistic effects under such circumstances. TRH and lecithin co-administration as a potential therapeutic regimen in AD has been specifically suggested (5,6).

We conducted a pilot study to examine the effects of TRH and lecithin co-administration in probable AD patients. This pilot study was devised to accomplish two primary objectives: (a) to verify the anticipated safety and reasonableness of the investigative methods; and (b) to examine possible acute effects of TRH and lecithin co-administration on cognitive performance in AD patients. Because the effects of TRH and lecithin co-administration in humans or animals have not been described in any existing reports, deliberately cautious TRH and lecithin dosages were employed and safety issues were also emphasized in other aspects of the inpatient study protocol.

Alzheimer's Disease: Basic Mechanisms, Diagnosis and Therapeutic Strategies
Edited by K. Iqbal, D. R. C. McLachlan, B. Winblad and H. M. Wisniewski
©1991 John Wiley & Sons Ltd

METHODS AND SUBJECTS

This study was reviewed and approved by the Human Subjects Committee at American Lake VA Medical Center (Tacoma, Washington). The effects of sequential daily dosages of TRH (2 mg, 4 mg, 6 mg, 8 mg and 12 mg), administered intravenously in ascending order to AD study subjects over 5 consecutive days, were carefully assessed in the context of a 5-week inpatient study protocol (Table 1). As a prudent and theoretically salutary methodological adjunct, a daily oral dosage (6 g/day) of purified lecithin (90–95% soy phosphatidylcholine; American Lecithin Co.) was systematically administered to each participating subject, prior to and concurrent with the period of TRH administration (i.e. daily lecithin during weeks 2, 3 and 4 of the study). TRH (protirelin; Abbott Laboratories) and placebo (isotonic saline) infusions were administered under double-blind conditions to AD subjects during separate study weeks (weeks 3 and 4); the order of administration (TRH first or placebo first) was randomized.

Cognitive performance of AD subjects was assessed weekly (Fridays) during their participation in the 5-week protocol and twice-weekly (Wednesday and Friday) during study weeks 3 and 4 (infusion weeks); testing commenced 45 minutes post infusions (TRH, placebo). A cognitive battery of 11 test measures which assess areas of cognition known to be affected in Alzheimer's disease was administered at each testing session. Equivalent forms of the cognitive tests were systematically utilized to minimize the presentation of identical cognitive tasks in successive testing sessions and thereby reduce the risk of across-session bias.

Eight men aged 64.1 ± 6.6 years (mean $\pm$ SD) fulfilling NINCDS–ADRDA criteria for probable Alzheimer's disease were enrolled in this study. In all subjects, the initial onset of dementia symptoms occurred before age 68 years. All subjects were medication-free, normotensive, free of coexisting major medical problems and in generally sound physical health. None had prominent agitation or sleep disturbance. Baseline scores of the eight participating AD subjects on the mini-mental state examination (MMSE) ranged from 0 to 23; six of the eight AD subjects had moderate to severe baseline cognitive impairment (MMSE < 15).

RESULTS

All eight probable AD subjects enrolled in this study completed the 5-week inpatient study protocol as planned; in all, study procedures were consistently well tolerated.

Table 1. TRH and lecithin co-administration in 5-week study protocol

Week 1	Week 2	Week 3	Week 4	Week 5
Pre-drug baseline	Lecithin*	Lecithin* TRH** or placebo	Lecithin* TRH** or placebo	Post-drug baseline

* Lecithin dose 6 g daily.
**TRH doses (2 mg, 4 mg, 6 mg, 8 mg, 12 mg) administered i.v. in ascending order for 5 successive days.

Cardiovascular effects of study procedures

TRH administration causes prompt and transient increases in systolic and diastolic blood pressure (pressor responses) in humans (11), and consistent TRH-evoked pressor responses were evident in each AD subject in this pilot study. In all instances, pressor responses to TRH were brief, asymptomatic and self-limited. Prompt pressor responses during the 30-minute interval following TRH administration were of similar magnitude (about 30 mmHg systolic BP and about 16 mmHg diastolic BP) following each of the five i.v. TRH dosages. Daily assessments of subjects' vital signs during the 5-week protocol did not reveal any sustained changes or discernible pattern(s) of alteration associated with study participation. Serial electrocardiograms (ECGs) were monitored in each AD subject at regular intervals; no ECG changes associated with study participation were observed.

Other transient TRH side-effects with study procedures

Four of eight AD subjects exhibited transient shivering with an onset within the initial several minutes following infusions of the larger TRH dosages (8 mg, 12 mg) and with a duration of several minutes or less. This side-effect was reasonably well tolerated and apparently related to TRH dosage. Shivering is a recognized side-effect of high-dose TRH infusion in humans (12).

Most of the eight AD subjects experienced one or more of the typically minor side-effects associated with TRH administration in humans (e.g. abdominal sensations, urge to micturate, cutaneous warmth, 'funny' taste, nausea). In all instances, these miscellaneous visceral phenomena were reasonably well tolerated and disappeared within several minutes. Within subjects, the occurrence of these 'visceral' side-effects was not consistently apparent with successive TRH doses and did not appear to be dose-related; rather, these side-effects were typically isolated and nonrecurring phenomena.

Cognitive effects of study procedures

Two of the eight AD subjects who completed the study protocol were severely demented and proved to be too impaired to generate relevant responses to the tests comprising the cognitive battery. In the remaining six AD subjects, measures of cognitive performance during their study participation have been analyzed.

Differences between cognitive test scores obtained in AD subjects during study periods of TRH–lecithin and placebo–lecithin administrations have been examined. On 10 of 11 cognitive test measures, the mean scores of the six AD subjects were higher (better performance) during TRH–lecithin than placebo–lecithin; this distribution of test scores is unlikely to be due to chance ($P < 0.02$; binomial test). Differences (mean $\pm$ SD) between test scores associated with TRH and placebo infusions were further examined with t-tests for repeated measures. Mean TRH-associated increments in test scores on 4 of the 11 cognitive measures, while modest in magnitude, were sufficiently consistent in the six AD subjects to approach

Table 2. Comparison of mean differences in cognitive test scores between study weeks

Cognitive battery	Difference (TRH – placebo) $(x \pm SE)$	$P^\star$	Difference (TRH – week 1) $(x \pm SE)$	$P^\star$	Difference (baseline/ week 5 – baseline/ week 1) $(x \pm SE)$	$P^\star$
1. Word fluency — letters	1.4 ± 1.3		-1.5 ± 2.3		-2.3 ± 1.3	<0.06
2. Word fluency — animals	0.8 ± 1.5		0.0 ± 2.0		2.5 ± 2.2	
3. Trails	0.9 ± 0.9		3.7 ± 2.6		3.0 ± 2.3	
4. Naming	1.4 ± 0.7	<0.06	2.4 ± 1.5	<0.09	1.5 ± 1.6	
5. Benton visual — correct	0.5 ± 0.3	<0.06	-0.2 ± 0.3		-1.0 ± 0.6	<0.09
6. Benton visual — errors	0.4 ± 0.6		-0.3 ± 0.3		1.0 ± 0.9	
7. Buschke — total	1.4 ± 0.7	<0.06	2.3 ± 0.7	<0.02	2.5 ± 2.3	
8. Buschke — cued	0.7 ± 0.3	<0.04	0.8 ± 0.7		0.5 ± 0.4	
9. Buschke recall — total	0.2 ± 0.2		0.4 ± 0.3	<0.10	0.7 ± 0.5	
10. Buschke recall — cued	0.4 ± 0.3		0.9 ± 0.5	<0.08	0.5 ± 0.3	
11. Buschke recognition	1.1 ± 0.8		2.4 ± 1.1	<0.04	1.2 ± 0.3	<0.01

*Tests for significance (P values) are based on t-tests for repeated measures (one-tailed probabilities).

statistical significance (one-tailed probabilities): Boston naming ($P<0.06$); Benton visual correct ($P<0.06$); Buschke total ($P<0.06$); Buschke cued ($P<0.04$). These results are presented in Table 2.

Differences (mean $\pm$ SD) between test scores obtained from six AD subjects at drug-free baseline (study week 1) and during the period of TRH–lecithin administration were also examined with t-tests for repeated measures; the cognitive performance of AD subjects during the period of TRH–lecithin administration relative to initial baseline tended to be better on 5 of the 11 cognitive measures; see Table 2.

Differences (mean $\pm$ SD) between test scores obtained from the six AD subjects during drug-free intervals at the beginning of the study (initial baseline; study week 1) and at the conclusion of the study (post-study baseline; study week 5) were also examined with t-tests for repeated measures. The cognitive performance of AD subjects tended to be better at initial baseline (week 1) on 2 of the 11 cognitive measures; on 1 of the other cognitive measures, performance tended to be better at post-study baseline (week 5) than at initial baseline. These comparisons, which are presented in Table 2, do not suggest the occurrence of consistent longitudinal changes in AD subjects' cognitive performance as a consequence of their study participation (e.g. 'practice effects' from sequential testing; 'carry-over effects' from TRH and/or lecithin administrations).

INTERPRETATION OF STUDY RESULTS

1. In this 5-week pilot study, the effects of TRH and lecithin co-administration were examined in a small number of probable AD subjects, most of whom were moderately to severely demented. The 'high' TRH dosages and the lecithin dosage employed in this study were purposely cautious, relative to other recent applications of each agent for putative therapeutic purposes in humans.

2. Results from this pilot study suggest that 'high-dose' TRH and lecithin co-administration is likely to be reasonably safe in otherwise healthy patients with probable AD and are of value in this regard. The effects of TRH and lecithin co-administration in humans or animals have not been described previously. Study results provide initial evidence that systemic effects and side-effects of TRH and lecithin co-administration in humans are reasonably well tolerated and not appreciably different in quality or quantity from side-effects typically associated with parenteral administrations of TRH alone.

3. Analyses of the possible effects of study participation on the cognitive performance of AD subjects suggest the possibility that their cognitive performance may have been relatively improved during the period of TRH and lecithin co-administration in this pilot study. These findings, while of heuristic interest, are preliminary in nature and should be interpreted cautiously. The potential effects of TRH and lecithin co-administration on cognitive performance in probable AD patients appear to warrant further resolution.

4. In concert with other relevant findings (8,10,12), the findings of this pilot AD treatment study with TRH and lecithin co-administration suggest that the incorporation of somewhat larger TRH and lecithin dosages in AD treatment investigations may be reasonable and warranted at this time. Any such additional TRH/lecithin studies initially should be restricted to probable AD patients in otherwise good health, and side-effects should be carefully monitored and quantified.

CONCLUSIONS

1. Further studies will be necessary to clarify the potential therapeutic effects of TRH and/or TRH analogues on cognitive performance in AD patients and to clarify the possible value of adjunctive lecithin co-administration with TRH for such therapeutic purposes. Two important questions will need to be addressed:

(a) What specific method(s) of TRH and lecithin co-administration (i.e. dosages, routes, frequency, duration) are most effective in producing significant acute enhancement of cognitive function in patients with probable Alzheimer's disease?

(b) What are the cognitive and other effects of sustained TRH and lecithin co-administration in patients with Alzheimer's disease? Can any demonstrable acute beneficial effects be sustained over time?

2. Present findings provide support for the anticipated safety and potential merit of undertaking additional treatment studies with TRH and lecithin co-administration in Alzheimer's disease. Consideration also should be given to biologically active TRH analogues which may be appropriate for initial trials with adjunctive lecithin co-administration in patients with probable Alzheimer's disease.

Acknowledgments

This investigation was supported by a pilot research grant from the Alzheimer's Association (PRG-88-134) and by the Research Service and the Geriatric Research, Education and Clinical Center (GRECC) at the American Lake VA Medical Center in Tacoma, Washington. Diana Stevenson, Lindy Cubberley, Hal Kopeikin, and the staffs of the American Lake VAMC Alzheimer's Disease Research Unit, Pharmacy Service, and Dietetics Service provided important direct assistance with this study.

Discussions with A. Horita, M. Raskind, G. Yarbrough and T. Sunderland have been of considerable value. Helpful support was provided by J. Eichberg, P. Johnson, R. Stoll, S. Wheeler and B. J. Hoffman. TRH (protirelin) for use in this study was kindly provided by Abbott Laboratories, and purified lecithin was kindly provided by the American Lecithin Company.

REFERENCES

1. Kalivas PW, Horita A. J Pharm Exp Ther 1980; 212: 203-10.
2. Horita A, Carino MA, Lai H. Fed Proc 1986; 45: 795.
3. Yarbrough GG. Prog Neurobiol 1979; 12: 291-312.
4. Yabrough GG. Life Sci 1983; 33: 111-18.
5. Yarbrough GG, Pomara N. Prog Neuro-Psychopharmacol Biol Psychiat 1985; 9: 285-9.
6. Davies P. In Crook T, Gershon S (eds) Strategies for the development of an effective treatment for senile dementia. New Canaan: Mark Powley 1981: 19-34.
7. Metcalf G. Brain Res Rev 1982; 4: 389-408.
8. Molchan SE, Mellow AM, Lawlor BA, Weingartner HJ, Cohen RM, Cohen MR, Sunderland T. Psychopharmacology 1990; 100: 84-9.
9. Horita A, Carino MA, Zabawska J, Lai H. Peptides 1989; 10: 121-4.
10. Mellow AM, Sunderland T, Cohen RM, Lawlor BA, Hill JA, Newhouse PA, Cohen MR, Murphy DS. Psychopharmacology 1989; 98: 403-7.
11. Lampe TH, Veith R, Plymate SR, Risse SC, Kopeikin H, Cubberley L, Raskind MA. Psychoneuroendocrinology 1989; 14: 311-20.
12. Mitsumoto H, Salgado ED, Negroski D, Hanson MR et al. Neurology 1986; 36: 152-9.

Address for correspondence:

Dr Thomas H. Lampe,
GRECC 182(B), American Lake VA Medical Center,
Tacoma, WA 98493, USA

84 Therapy with a Combination of Coenzyme Q_{10}, Vitamin B_6 and Iron for Alzheimer's Disease and Senile Dementia of Alzheimer Type

MASAKI IMAGAWA

I have tried megavitamin—B_6, coenzyme Q_{10} (CoQ_{10})—therapy for Alzheimer's disease (AD) or senile dementia of Alzheimer type (SDAT) (1). In these diseases, cerebral blood flow is seen to be low from the appearance of [^{123}I] IMP. Therefore I inferred the metabolic disturbances in the brain tissue, especially the abnormal change of the component of respiratory chain in mitochondria. I have tried combination therapy with B_6, CoQ_{10} and iron; this therapy was more effective than vitamins alone (B_6, CoQ_{10}).

SUBJECTS AND METHOD

Twenty-three females (71.6 ± 7.2 years old, mean $\pm$ SD) and 4 males (73.2 ± 7.3 years old) were treated. AD had been diagnosed in 8 females and 1 male, and SDAT in 15 females and 3 males. Diagnosis and the grade of the patient's dementia was based on DSMIII-R. Therefore the mild grade was 4, the middle grade was 13 and the severe grade 10. The clinical course was followed by two methods: Hasegawa's dementia score (HDS) (2) and criteria for severity based on DSMIII-R, that is, normal 0, mild I, middle II, severe III. These numbers are changed according to the severity of the patient's symptoms and signs. Both HDS and clinical severity were marked on the time scale (each week). The dose of the drugs taken by the patients was CoQ_{10} 60–180 mg, B_6 180 mg, iron 150 mg daily.

RESULTS

Changes in both HDS and clinical severity are shown in Tables 1 and 2, and illustrated in Figures 1 and 2. HDS reached a plateau at 4 weeks. The first week showed the greatest response to therapy.

Alzheimer's Disease: Basic Mechanisms, Diagnosis and Therapeutic Strategies
Edited by K. Iqbal, D. R. C. McLachlan, B. Winblad and H. M. Wisniewski
© 1991 John Wiley & Sons Ltd

Table 1. Changes in Hasegawa's dementia score over the eight-week period

Patient	Pre-treatment value	Week				
		1st	2nd	4th	6th	8th
SDAT+AD (27)	15.1±5.2 $n=27$	20.6±7.7** $n=19$	19.7±8.7** $n=17$	23.4±7.3** $n=21$	23.6±6.8** $n=19$	23.1±7.1** $n=20$
SDAT (18)	14.7±4.7 $n=18$	20.4±8.2** $n=12$	18.2±8.6* $n=10$	23.5±6.9** $n=13$	23.6±7.0** $n=12$	23.0±7.5** $n=15$
AD (9)	16.0±6.3 $n=9$	20.9±7.2** $n=7$	22.0±8.9** $n=7$	23.1±8.4** $n=8$	23.4±6.9** $n=7$	23.1±6.7** $n=5$

*$P<0.05$, **$P<0.01$, Wilcoxon test.

Table 2. Changes in evaluation of activities of daily living (ADL) through the therapy (AD and SDAT patients)

ADL	Pre-treatment value	Week				
		1st	2nd	4th	6th	8th
III	11/27 40.7%	4/19* 21.1%	3/17* 17.6%	1/21* 4.8%	1/19* 5.3%	2/19* 10.5%
II	13/27 48.1%	8/19* 42.1%	7/17* 41.2%	9/21* 42.9%	6/19* 31.6%	5/19* 26.3%
I	3/27 11.1%	6/19* 31.5%	4/17* 23.5%	3/21* 14.3%	5/19* 26.3%	4/19* 21.1%
0	0/27 0.0%	1/19* 5.3%	3/17* 17.6%	8/21* 38.1%	7/19* 36.8%	8/19* 42.1%

$P<0.01$, Wilcoxon test.

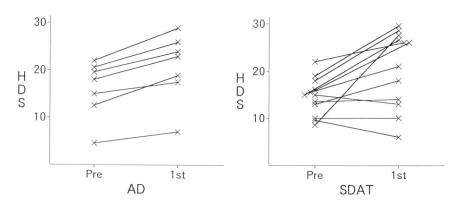

Figure 1. Changes in Hasegawa's dementia score (HDS) in Alzheimer's disease (AD) and senile dementia of Alzheimer type (SDAT) after one week of therapy

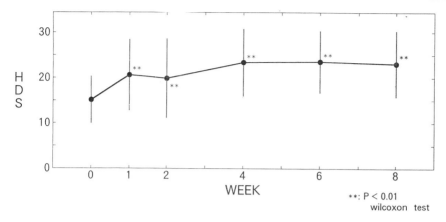

Figure 2. Changes in Hasegawa's dementia score (HDS) over 8 weeks of therapy (all patients)

DISCUSSION

The patients of AD, SDAT generally had lowered cerebral blood flow. This therapy is the point or focus for the integration of both information and energy systems on the patient's brain; that is, in the energy system, ATP will be increased in mitochondria (component of the respiratory chain). In poor cerebral blood flow, mitochondria will probably be damaged. Therefore, with CoQ_{10}, iron was administered to the patients. Here, ATP will be utilized for decarboxylation (B_6, B_6-enzyme). As a result, neurotransmitters will be produced on neuronal cells. The disappearance of symptoms and signs (for example, lower power of memory and learning, wandering, delirium, loss of dialogue, loss of habitual behavior) of AD and SDAT may be data to support this theory.

REFERENCES

1. Imagawa M. J Clin Exp Med 1989; 151: 345.
2. Masayuki M, Hiroshi S. J Card Ultrason 1988; 7: 315-20.

Address for correspondence:

Dr Masaki Imagawa,
Neuropsychiatric Clinic,
Hyogo Prefecture Amagasaki Hospital,
Hyogo, Japan

List of Contributors

Index

Index compiled by June Morrison